FIFTH EDITION

Drugs in Modern Society

Charles R. Carroll
Ball State University

With contributions by
Lynne H. Durrant
University of Utah

McGraw Hill

Boston Burr Ridge, IL Dubuque, IA Madison, WI New York San Francisco St. Louis
Bangkok Bogotá Caracas Lisbon London Madrid
Mexico City Milan New Delhi Seoul Singapore Sydney Taipei Toronto

McGraw-Hill Higher Education

A Division of The **McGraw-Hill** *Companies*

DRUGS IN MODERN SOCIETY: FIFTH EDITION

This book is printed on acid-free paper.

1 2 3 4 5 6 7 8 9 0 VNH/VNH 0 9 8 7 6 5 4 3 2 1 0

ISBN 0–697–29448–X

Vice president and editorial director: *Kevin T. Kane*
Publisher: *Edward E. Bartell*
Senior marketing manager: *Pamela S. Cooper*
Project manager: *Joyce M. Berendes*
Senior production supervisor: *Mary E. Haas*
Coordinator of freelance design: *Rick D. Noel*
Photo research coordinator: *John C. Leland*
Senior supplement coordinator: *David A. Welsh*
Compositor: *Shepherd, Inc.*
Typeface: *10/12 Minion*
Printer: *Von Hoffmann Press, Inc.*

Cover designer: *Kristyn A. Kalnes*
Photo research: *Connie Gardner Picture Research*

The credits section for this book begins on page 383 and is considered an extension of the copyright page.

Library of Congress Cataloging-in-Publication Data

Carroll, Charles R.
Drugs in modern society / Charles R. Carroll : with contributions by Lynne H. Durrant. — 5th ed.
p. cm.
Includes index.
ISBN 0–697–29448–X
1. Drug abuse. 2. Substance abuse. 3. Drugs—Physiological effect. 4. Neuropsychopharmacology. I. Durrant, Lynne H. II. Title.
RM316. C37 2000
616.86—dc21 99–16250
CIP

www.mhhe.com

contents

Chapter 3

part two

Chapter 4

Chapter 5

Chapter 6

Chapter 7

part three

Chapter 8

Chapter 9

boxes

preface

The continuing interest of Americans in the wellness and human potential movements, stress management, holistic health care, natural foods, and physical fitness suggests that people are increasingly concerned about their health and about preventing health problems. This emphasis on "self-care" and health enhancement and empowerment is, in part, a reaction to the recognized limits of medical care for those already sick or injured. More important, "self-care" and wellness-promoting activities are the result of a growing awareness that one's lifestyle and personal health habits play critical roles in the development of avoidable diseases and injuries.

According to supportive data for *Healthy People 2010: National Health Promotion and Disease Prevention Objectives*[1] and its Midcourse Review,[2] many of our most pressing health problems are related to the use of alcohol and other drugs, including tobacco.

After a recent ten-year decline in the-use of illegal drugs and tobacco use, surveys indicate increasing numbers of young Americans are again abusing marijuana, engaging in binge drinking, and starting to smoke cigarettes. Many others have become fascinated with heroin and the perceived thrill of "club drugs" and "herbal remedies," and cigar smoking has again become fashionable, after nearly three generations of decreasing use. The staggering toll that alcohol and other drug problems place on society, health status, and the economy is also growing once more.

Alcohol use is implicated in nearly half of all intentional injuries, such as homicides and suicides. In addition, alcohol-related traffic accidents are still one of the leading killers of young Americans.

Abuse of alcohol and other drugs significantly increases the risk of transmission of the human immunodeficiency virus (HIV). This can take place directly, through the sharing of contaminated needles, sexual contact with intravenous drug abusers and other drug injectors, or *in utero* infection, or indirectly through adverse effects on immune system functioning and the increased risk of unwanted or unsafe sexual practices.

Tobacco use is responsible for more than one of five deaths in the United States and is the most important preventable cause of death and disease in our society. The use of tobacco products is an acknowledged, major risk factor for diseases of the heart and blood vessels; chronic bronchitis and emphysema; cancers of the lung, larynx, oral cavity, esophagus, pancreas, and bladder; and other problems, such as respiratory infections and stomach ulcers.

Although the individual's role in promoting health and preventing disease is becoming more important, it is recognized that people usually make personal lifestyle choices within a society that glamorizes many hazardous behaviors through advertising and the mass media. Social influences involving peer pressure and the encouragement of risk-taking activities have a tremendous impact, especially on young people. In addition, society continues to support industries that produce unhealthful products, unevenly enacts and enforces laws against behaviors

1. *Healthy People 2010 Objectives: Draft for Public Comment*, U.S. Department of Health and Human Services. Office of Public Health and Science, September 15, 1998.
2. *Healthy People 2000: Midcourse Review and 1995 Revisions* (Hyattsville, Md.: U.S. Public Health Service, Centers for Disease Control and Prevention, National Center for Health Statistics, 1995).

such as driving while intoxicated, and offers somewhat ambiguous messages about those behaviors that are not advisable.[3]

In light of the widespread use and abuse of drugs and medications in America, this text is designed for use in drug education courses for students from a variety of disciplines. *Drugs in Modern Society* provides current, accurate, and documented information about drug substances presented in a scientific, logical, and objective manner. Mind-changing or psychoactive drugs are the major focus of this text, but consideration is also given to nonpsychoactives that are frequently misused and to the legal recreational or social drugs infrequently viewed as part of the real drug problem in America.

From a philosophical perspective this book seeks to enhance freedom of choice in terms of drug use or nonuse. Free choices can be made in consideration of how personal actions affect oneself. However, truly free choices also concern one's relations with other people, ". . . relations involving love, trust, integrity, responsibility, honor, and sacrifice."[4]

Changes in This Edition

- In this revised and updated fifth edition, the number of chapters has been increased to sixteen.
- A modified and **shortened introductory chapter** considers basic drug definitions, health-related consequences of drug-taking behavior, an overview of the current drug scene, a focus on the drug-crime relationship, and prospects for the future use and abuse of mind-changing drugs.
- The original chapter on alcohol and alcoholism has been divided into **two distinct and enhanced chapters.** The first deals with alcohol as America's drink-drug and focuses on cultural, historical, psychological, and physical aspects of alcohol and drinking. The second alcohol chapter pertains to alcohol abuse and alcoholism.
- Also added is **a new chapter on alcohol and other drugs in special populations.** New dimensions of drugging, drinking, and medicating are explored in relation to women; racial and ethnic minorities, in other words, African Americans, Hispanic Americans, Native Americans and Alaskan Natives, and Asians and Pacific Islanders; athletes; and the elderly.
- Throughout the text, **new or modified boxes and figures** have been included. Within each of the drug-specific chapters, the role of neurotransmitters in the production of drug effects has been featured.
- **New or expanded material** has been introduced on the following topics:
  - the recent increase in drug abuse among teenagers
  - the closing of the "gender gap" between female and male drug abuse
  - Rohypnol (the "date rape" drug)
  - club drugs
  - herbal remedies
  - proposals to limit alcohol and tobacco advertising and accessibility to youth
  - the role of neurotransmitters in the production of various drug effects
  - drinking and altered consciousness
  - alcohol consumption among college students
  - alcohol abuse in relation to work performance, law violations and violence, and alcohol-related accidents
  - drug therapy for alcoholics
  - secular alternatives to Alcoholics Anonymous
  - the new heroin epidemic
  - potentiating and synergistic drug interactions
  - the relationship between tobacco tars and the P53 gene in the development of lung cancer
  - voter approval of medical marijuana
  - major changes in marijuana and its use
  - increase in the number of prescription drugs being switched to OTC medications
  - introduction of a new analgesic, ketoprofen
  - a new use for oral contraceptives
  - chemically induced abortions
  - alcohol and other drug use and abuse among racial and ethnic minorities
  - gender-related drug hazards affecting women
  - major congressional legislation regarding alcohol and other drugs
  - alternatives to urine testing for detection of illegal drug use
  - elements of successful drug education prevention programs
  - and top-rated school-based drug prevention programs
- Finally, with regard to changes in this edition, we have added **important World Wide Web sites** at the end of each chapter. In addition, the following list of web sites on the Internet contain general alcohol, tobacco, and other drug information, statistics, and current research. These web sites will provide the reader with a wealth of information on specific drug-related topics to expand the information contained in the chapters.

ACDE (American Council for Drug Education):
http://www.acde.org

CADCA (Community Anti-Drug Coalitions of America):
http://www.cadca.org

CASA (Center on Addictions & Substance Abuse):
http://www.casacolumbia.org

Corporation for National Service Drug Alliance Office:
http://www.cns.gov

3. Julius B. Richmond, *Healthy people—The surgeon general's report on health promotion and disease prevention* (Washington, D.C.: GPO, 1979), 17.
4. Robert D. Russell, "*Holistic health.*" chap. 1 in *Education in the 80's: Health education,* ed. Robert D. Russell, (Washington, D.C.: National Education Association, 1981), 21.

CSAP (Center for Substance Abuse Prevention): http://www.samhsa.gov/csap/

CSAT (Center for Substance Abuse Treatment): http://www.samhsa.gov/csat/csat.htm

DEA (Drug Enforcement Agency): http://www.usdoj.gov/dea/

Drug Strategies: http://www.drugstrategies.org

Drug Watch International: http://www.drugwatch.org

Family Research Council: http://www.frc.org

Higher Education Center for Alcohol and Other Drug Prevention: http ://www.cdc.org/hec

Join Together: http://www.jointogether.org

National Clearinghouse for Alcohol & Drug Information: http://www.health.org

National Families in Action: http://www.emory.edu/NFIA

National Inhalant Prevention Coalition: http://www.inhalants.org

NIAAA (National Institute on Alcohol Abuse and Alcoholism): http://www.niaaa.nih.gov

NIDA (National Institute on Drug Abuse): http ://www.nida.nih.gov

NIH (National Institutes of Health): http://www.nih.gov

ONDCP (Office of National Drug Control Policy): http://www.whitehousedrugpolicy.gov

Partnership for a Drug-Free America: http://www.drugfreeamerica.org

PRIDE (Parents Resource Institute for Drug Education): http://prideusa.org

Reader's Digest and Parent Soup (cohosted): http://www.drugfreekids.com

Robert Wood Johnson Foundation: http://www.rwjf.org

SAMHSA (Substance Abuse and Mental Health Services Administration): http://www.samhsa.gov

Source: Pat Carpenter, Policy Analyst, Specific Drugs, Office of National Drug Control Policy (ONDCP)

Organization of the Text

Although each of the sixteen chapters is self-contained, this edition is organized into six major parts that provide a measure of sequential development and interrelatedness of subjects pertaining to psychoactive drugs and drug-taking behaviors.

Part 1 presents an overview of drugs, medicines, and drug problems in America; an understanding of the continuing popularity of mind-changing drugs despite legal, moral, and socials restrictions; and a simplified explanation of drug actions within the human body and of the frequently observed components of drug dependency.

Part 2 examines psychoactive drugs collectively referred to as the depressants; those substances that tend to slow the function of the central nervous system. Major consideration is given to alcohol, the nation's number one drug problem. Additional chapters discuss the narcotics and the sedative-hypnotics.

Part 3 looks at stimulants, the psychoactive drugs that tend to speed up central nervous system function. Primary emphasis is focused on tobacco products, because cigarette smoking is still considered the nation's leading preventable cause of death. A separate chapter considers the ongoing popularity of cocaine use, the amphetamines, and caffeine.

Part 4 is concerned with the mind-expanding euphoriants, namely the psychedelics, phencyclidine, and marijuana. The latter drug is a unique and controversial psychoactive, deserving its own distinct classification.

Part 5 addresses the less obvious aspects of America's drug problem: the frequent misuse and even abuse of over-the-counter and prescribed medications, many of which are not psychoactive in their effects.

Part 6 describes frequently overlooked dimensions of drugging, drinking, and medicating as seen in special populations—females, racial and ethnic minorities, athletes, and the elderly. The last two chapters offer a variety of insights into the prevention of alcohol, tobacco, and other drug (ATOD) abuse, and the variety of mechanisms employed to reduce the severity of drug-related problems in a drug-using society. The final chapter will be of primary interest to those developing ATOD prevention education programs in schools, churches, community-health agencies, and businesses and industries.

Learning Aids

Included in this text are various learning aids that should make your study of drugs and drug-taking behavior more effective and more meaningful. As the reader, you can choose those study aids that seem most valuable for enhancing your knowledge and the adoption of health-promoting and disease-preventing behavior in a drug-using society.

Key Terms

At the beginning of each chapter is a listing of some important terms related to various aspects of drugs, drug-taking behavior, or drug-abuse prevention. These words are defined or described in the chapter and are sometimes used frequently within that chapter and subsequent chapters of the text.

Chapter Objectives

Also at the beginning of each chapter are several statements that will indicate what the reader can expect to learn or be able to do after mastering the chapter contents. By reading the objectives before studying the chapter, you will identify important sections of the narrative. These can be used as guides in your study.

Chapter Introductions

The opening paragraphs of each chapter provide a brief preview of or commentary on the chapter's contents. After reading these comments, browse through the chapter, paying particular attention to topic headings, illustrations, charts, and boxed material so that you get a feeling for the kinds of ideas and major concepts included in the chapter.

At Issue: Point Versus Counterpoint Boxes

Appearing again in this edition are a series of controversial issues dealing with various drugs, drug use and abuse, and mechanisms for resolving or preventing alcohol and other drug problems. Each "At Issue" box presents a "point" and a "counterpoint" stance or philosophical position representing extreme viewpoints on a particular topic. As you read each "At Issue" box, decide how you would respond to the various points and counterpoints. You will encounter a range of beliefs that prove there is no universal agreement on many of the thorny problems and issues that abound in that area of drug use, abuse, and drug dependence. But developing a better understanding of the contrasting "points" and "counterpoints" may enable informed individuals to arrive at workable solutions to the numerous dilemmas associated with drug use and abuse.

Chapter Summaries

At the end of each chapter a summary reviews the significant ideas presented in the narrative. A few days after you have read the chapter, you may want to reread this short section. If you discover some terms or major concepts that seem unfamiliar, reread the related portions of the chapter narrative. You may also find it useful to again refer to the key terms and chapter objectives at the beginning of the chapter to determine your familiarity with the content of the chapter.

Review Questions and Activities

Appearing at the end of each chapter are several review questions that can be used to check your basic understanding of the major ideas presented in the narrative. The activities are intended to enhance the factual content of the chapter. If you can answer these questions or perform the tasks suggested, you have developed a significant comprehension of the chapter subject matter. If you cannot do this, reread certain sections of the narrative to increase your understanding of the ideas involved

Glossary

After the last chapter, a glossary compiles drug-related terms with definitions. You may wish to consult this extensive listing for a concise explanation of a particular word or phrase. Sometimes the glossary definition of an important term will provide a more inclusive meaning than the one found in the narrative of a chapter. The glossary can also be a useful guide to the correct spelling of a term or process.

Ancillary Materials

An outstanding ancillary package has been created to meet the needs of instructors.

- The *Instructor's Manual and Test Item File* contains lecture outlines for each chapter, teaching activities, discussion questions, research topics, essay questions, thought provokers tied to the At Issue boxes, suggested audiovisual aids, and supplemental readings. In addition, more than forty test questions are included for each chapter.
- A *Computerized Test Item File* is available to qualified adopters of the text. MicroTest is easy to use and allows the instructor to build custom tests and answer keys. MicroTest is available in Macintosh and Window versions.
- The *WCB McGraw-Hill Drug Transparencies* include more than forty images with an annotated guide. These transparencies will help the instructor present the most important concepts from the book in a visually appealing way. The transparencies are available to qualified adopters of the text.

Additional Resources

Photo/Illustration CD for Drugs provides the instructor with thirty-nine images that can be used in an electronic presentation.

The AIDS Booklet is updated every six months with the latest information on this devastating disease.

Annual Editions® is a collection of current, carefully selected articles from some of the most important magazines, newspapers, and journals published. Articles explore such challenging contemporary topics as the worldwide drug scourge, the global tobacco epidemic, the pitfalls of marijuana reform proposals, the resurgence of pot, deadly drug gangs, drugs and violence, and the "harm reduction" approach to solving America's drug woes.

Taking Sides® uses a pro/con approach to issues. It is designed to introduce the student to controversies in drugs and society. Seventeen issues are grouped into three parts: Drugs and Public Policy; Researching Tobacco, Caffeine, and Alcohol; and Drug Prevention and Treatment. The issues are self-contained and designed to be used independently.

acknowledgments

I wish to express my deepest thanks to the many people who have contributed to the evolution of *Drugs in Modern Society.* Without their support and assistance, this fifth edition would never have been accomplished.

In particular, I want to acknowledge the valuable contributions of the Center for Substance Abuse Prevention (formerly named the Office for Substance Abuse Prevention), the National Institute on Drug Abuse, the National Institute on Alcohol Abuse and Alcoholism, the U.S. Food and Drug Administration, the U.S. Department of Justice, and the Drug Enforcement Administration for their numerous publications and detailed responses to my unending inquiries. Such assistance in no way constitutes any official endorsement of this textbook.

I extend my very special thanks to the following individuals for their significant help in the preparation of specific portions of the manuscript: Margaret Henningson of CompCare Publications; Robert Kirk, formerly of the Distilled Spirits Council of the United States, Inc., and now with the American Council on Alcoholism; John Langer of the Drug Enforcement Administration, Department of Justice; Dr. Max M. Glatt; the National Council on Alcoholism and Drug Dependence; the Michigan Substance Abuse & Traffic Safety Information Center; Mr. Alex Fundock III of the *Journal of Studies on Alcohol;* and Alcoholics Anonymous World Services, Inc.

In addition, I gratefully acknowledge the expert research assistance provided by Mrs. Amy Wright and Health Resources Library of Greene Memorial Hospital, Xenia, Ohio; the Greene County Public Library, Xenia, Ohio; the Medical Library of Ball Memorial Hospital, Muncie, Indiana; and the Science-Health Science Library of Ball State University, Muncie, Indiana

I also want to recognize the valuable contributions of the following professional colleagues, who reviewed the prior edition and provided many detailed criticisms and ideas for improving this new edition as it was being developed:

Augustine Aryee, *Fitchburg State College*

Jack Benson, *Eastern Washington University*

Naydean Blair, *Houston Community College*

Sandra Bonneau, *Golden West College*

Ann R. Bristow, *Frostburg State University*

Linda A. Corrente, *Community College of Rhode Island*

Marvin D. Feit, *University of Akron*

John E. Gay, *Ohio University*

Richard Hurley, *Brigham Young University*

John J. Janowiak, *Appalachian State University*

Wayne D. Jones, *Southeastern Oklahoma State University*

Georgia Lynn Keeney, *University of Minnesota-Duluth*

Earl W. Patterson, *Nova Southeastern University*

Thomas Rowe, *University of Wisconsin-Stevens Point*

Jeffrey A. Schaler, *American University*

Martin S. Turnauer, *Radford University*

Marie Shaun Walter, *The College of St. Catherine*

Hugh T. Wilson, *California State University-Sacramento*

And, finally, thanks to Lynne H. Durrant of the University of Utah for her extraordinary talents in editing the revised manuscript. Her valuable contributions have enhanced the currency of the text, and added to the readability and integrity of each chapter. Such efforts reflect a significant commitment, that is deeply appreciated.

I want to thank my most effective teachers and consultants in the area of chemical dependence and drug-abuse prevention—those professionals who labor in prevention, therapeutic, and rehabilitation programs, and those precious souls who are in the long process of recovering from their illness.

The members of the editorial and production staffs of McGraw-Hill also deserve special recognition for their professional expertise and stimulating assistance.

Finally, I wish to express my heartfelt thanks to my family, who supported, encouraged, and sustained me during this labor of love. Emma and Margaret, you have meant so very much to me!

Charles R Carroll

Ball State University

Muncie, Indiana

Part One

Introduction

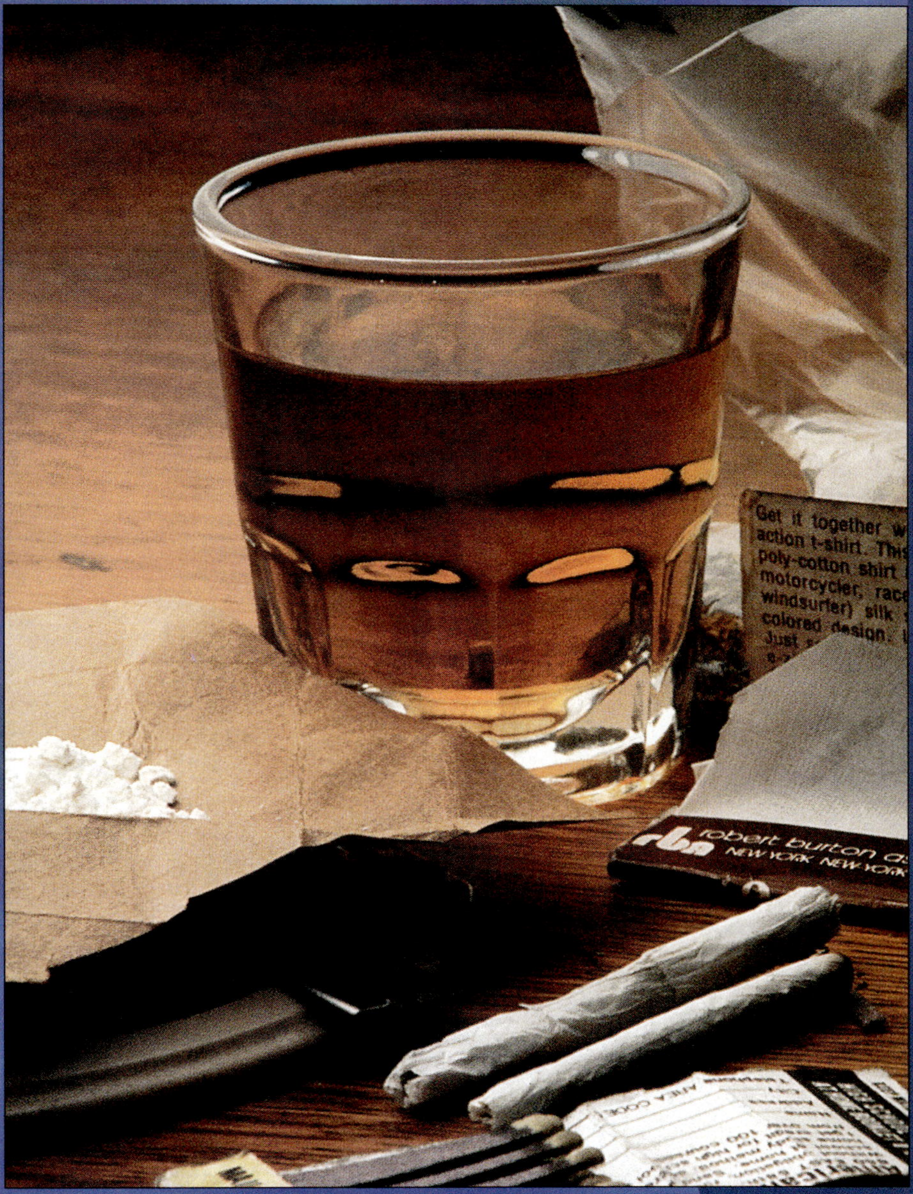

Questions of concern

1. Why do so many people continue to use and abuse psychoactive drugs now that the hazards of such behavior are so well-known and publicized?
2. What would our society be like if there were no mind-altering drugs to use or abuse?
3. Why are the consequences of using legal psychoactives so often tolerated or minimized, while the hazards of using illegal drugs are frequently exaggerated?

Chapter 1

Drugs, drinks, and medications

KEY TERMS

Acquired Immunodeficiency Syndrome (AIDS)
Adulteration
Controlled Substances Act
Depressant
Drug
Drug Abuse
Drug Abuse Warning Network
Drug Dependence
Drug Misuse
Flashback
HIV Infection
Inhalant
Marijuana
Medicine
Narcotics
National Drug Control Strategy
Over-the-Counter Drug
Panic
Prescription Drug
Psychedelics
Psychoactive Drug
Psychopathology
Stimulant
Therapeutics
Toxic Reaction

chapter objectives

After you have studied this chapter, you should be able to do the following:

1. Define the key terms.
2. Describe the nature of modern drug problems in terms of medical versus social use of drugs and the use of legally procured drugs versus illegal use of drugs.
3. Compare the successes and the failures of the "war on drugs" and the National Drug Control Strategy in terms of the use and abuse of alcohol, tobacco, and other drugs.
4. Explain how drug problems are frequently people problems.
5. Identify the costs to society resulting from the use and abuse of alcohol, tobacco, and other illegal drugs.
6. Identify five major types of illegal psychoactive drugs that are often abused.
7. Explain three different ways of classifying psychoactive drugs.
8. Identify several psychoactive drugs that can be purchased over-the-counter without a prescription.
9. Discuss the use of psychoactive drugs in relation to their potential for individual and social hazards.
10. Identify several major consequences that may accompany drug-taking behavior, other than the potential for adverse reactions.
11. Distinguish among the following adverse conditions associated with taking psychoactive drugs: toxic reaction, panic, flashback, psychopathology, and drug or chemical dependence.
12. Describe the current psychoactive drug scene in terms of the use, abuse, and nonuse of mind-changing drugs in the United States.
13. Explain the growing use and abuse of mind-changing drugs among young people.
14. List three predictive factors that will likely determine the American drug scene of the future.

Drug Problems in America

A recent national survey revealed that nearly 39 percent of American adults admitted that they had used illegal drugs. Although many people do not believe this drug use is their problem, these users represent a broad cross section of the American population. Fifty-one percent of our population currently drinks alcohol, 29 percent smoke cigarettes, and 6 percent use an illegal drug. Among our youth between the ages of 12 and 17, over 11 percent reported using illegal drugs in the previous 30 days, with marijuana being the most common drug of choice. Persons between the ages of 18 and 25 are most likely to use illegal drugs or alcohol, and drug use usually decreases as people get older. Caucasians, African Americans, and Mexican or Hispanic Americans do not differ greatly in their illicit drug use or heavy drinking. The majority of drug users are in the workforce. It is apparent that no American is immune and that all families are at risk.[1]

Although drugs are not only a problem for inner-city residents, the poor, or members of a minority group, the poor are disproportionately affected. Poorer neighborhoods have a higher incidence of drug-induced crimes and violence, and poorer people have less access to treatment facilities.

There is no doubt that widespread and persistent use of mind-changing drugs remains firmly entrenched in our society—part of the American way of life that affects users and nonusers. Indeed, the news media continue to feature "drug busts" in which law enforcement agents seize marijuana and raid secret, illegal "speed" labs in the suburbs as well as the inner city. School children are taught to say no to illegal drugs, while advertisers promote the sale of alcohol and cigarettes. As judges sentence drug abusers to long prison terms, many experts believe that treatment and rehabilitation of drug abusers would be more effective than law enforcement in reducing the number of drug addicts. Meanwhile, federal and state governments consider further restrictions on legal drugs—tobacco and alcohol.

In many ways our national concern with controlling and preventing the abuse of alcohol, tobacco, and other drugs continues a thirty-year effort. Proclaimed as a "war on drugs" by the federal government in the 1960s, it became the **National Drug Control Strategy** under President Clinton. The strategy aims at reducing drug use and availability by half over a ten-year period. This national antidrug policy views illegal drug use and its consequences as a major disease, similar to a virus that spreads from person to person and from community to community. These counter-drug efforts, like antivirus measures, will require endless prevention activities. On-going efforts include education, legal intervention, treatment, rehabilitation, compassion, and a willingness to commit prevention resources intelligently.

The federal expenditure of $10 billion to $16 billion annually since 1990 has produced mixed results in combating illegal drug use and drug abuse. Some observers believe that our antidrug crusade has been a monumental failure with no noticeable impact on illegal drug importation, manufacture, distribution, or consumption. Over fourteen million people, age twelve and over, currently use an illicit drug, and drug availability remains high.[2]

But others point to recent successes. Casual, illegal drug use among Americans has declined from its peak in 1979 of 14.9 percent to 6.1 percent in 1996. Use of cigarettes by adults has dropped by more than one-third since the 1960s, although smoking has increased again among teenagers. Hard liquor sales have fallen greatly, and deaths caused by alcohol-related motor vehicle crashes have been reduced significantly.

In spite of these accomplishments, the continuing costs of legal and illegal drug abuse represent an on-going threat to our society and are illustrated by the following consequences of drug-taking behavior:

Since 1990, America has experienced more than four million deaths related to alcohol, tobacco, and other drugs. Each year, just over 25,000 citizens die because of illegal drugs and drug-related AIDS, injury, homicide, tuberculosis, and hepatitis; 100,000 fall victim to alcohol-related illnesses, conditions, and accidents; and at least 400,000 are claimed by the disease effects of using tobacco products.

Currently, the estimated price tag for alcohol and drug abuse problems is about $276 billion annually, with most of the expenses related to productivity losses associated with illness and death; the annual cost of smoking is thought to be at least $72 billion, most is spent on losses due to premature deaths and medical treatment of tobacco-related diseases. However, many such costs cannot be easily determined, as noted in table 1.1

Drug-related hospital emergency room visits continue at record levels. At present, over one-half million such visitations are made each year, due largely to the consequences of illegal drug overdose and addiction (See fig. 1.1).

Legal and illegal drug use and abuse contribute to property and violent crime. In addition, more than one million people are arrested each year on drug-related charges.

Annually, Americans spend an estimated $49 billion getting illegal drugs, while federal, state, and local governments together spend nearly $30 billion to reduce illegal drug use and trafficking and to deal with their consequences.

Despite the high social and personal costs associated with mind-changing drugs, the United States remains a drug-oriented and, to some degree, a chemically dependent society. Although casual use of illegal drugs has fallen, as the federal government maintains, the variety of intoxicating substances has actually increased.[3] Not only are millions dependent on the legal "recreational" drugs, alcohol and tobacco, but countless others are addicted to physician-prescribed drugs and the illegal substances distributed everywhere, in America.[4]

In an attempt to ensure the safety of our airlines, railroads, highways, and merchant marine fleet, expensive drug detection programs have become standard procedures in the workplace as well as among college, professional, and even some high school athletic teams. Numerous officials, politicians, judges, entertainers, prominent sports figures, and business executives have been exposed, or voluntarily revealed, that they have used and abused cocaine, heroin, alcohol, tranquilizers, and marijuana. Even more common are the numbers of people who are multiple drug abusers.

In many ways, drug abuse and drug dependence have become as American as apple pie.

Drugs and Medicines

The mind- and behavior-changing substances mentioned involve legal, illegal, or potentially harmful chemicals known collectively as *drugs.* Drugs are substances that by their chemical nature can change the way the body functions and the way that people think, feel, and act. Drugs are often perceived as being "bad" for people: irresponsible people use them in illegal and harmful ways.

On the other hand, *medicines,* which are drugs also, are more frequently perceived as being "good" for people: sick people take medicines to get well. Perhaps we could better determine the goodness or badness of any drug, or better yet, the harmfulness, by considering how and why the drug is used and the consequences of using the drug.

While the news media tend to spotlight celebrities, such as Jonathan

table 1.1 Unspecified Costs to Society of Illegal Substance Use

Categories of Costs			
Criminal Justice Expenditures on Drug-Related Crime	**Health Care Costs**	**Lost Productivity Costs**	**Other Costs to Society**
• Investigating robberies, burglaries, and thefts for drug money and adjudicating and punishing the offenders • Investigating assaults and homicides in the drug business (or by a drug user who has lost control) and adjudicating and punishing the offenders	• Injuries resulting from drug-related child abuse/neglect • Injuries from drug-related accidents • Injuries from drug-related crime • Other medical care for illegal drug users, including volunteer services and outpatient services, such as emergency room visits • Resources used in nonhospital settings	• Lost productivity of drug-related accident victims • Lost productivity of drug-related crime victims • Time away from work and homemaking to care for drug users and their dependents • Drug-related educational problems and school dropouts • Offenders incarcerated for drug-related or drug-defined crimes	• Loss of property values due to drug-related neighborhood crime • Property damaged or destroyed in fires and in workplace and vehicular accidents • Agricultural resources devoted to illegal drug cultivation/production • Toxins introduced into public air and water supplies by drug production • Workplace prevention programs such as drug testing and employee assistance programs • Averting behavior by potential victims of drug-related crime • Pain and suffering costs to illegal drug users and their families and friends

Melvoin, Chris Farley, Robert Downey Jr., and Courtney Love, who become involved with illegal drugs, a major part of our widespread drug problem is just as often the result of people's using pills and capsules that are legally manufactured for use as medicines.

Aided by unprincipled physicians and compounded by our personal efforts of self-medication in a search for mental and physical pain relief, we often attempt to function with numerous combinations of tranquilizers, cough medicines, and headache remedies in our systems.

Critics of this supermedicated, tranquilized way of life contend that we are often sedated before birth if our mothers are prescribed antidepressant medication, during birth if they are given painkillers, and at school if our teachers think we have an attention-deficit disorder we are then placed on Ritalin. Once in the world of work, we are prescribed antianxiety drugs to combat tension and painkillers to ease discomfort. If we survive to old age, we may once again be given antidepressants or even major tranquilizers to make us more subdued, manageable patients.

Drug problems related to such legally prescribed medication were seldom thought about by most people, until physician-prescribed drug dependency adversely affected some famous Americans. Elvis Presley, Elizabeth Taylor, and Michael Jackson have been victims—to varying degrees—of drug abuse and chemical dependency related to prescription drugs.

Our national drug problems have another dimension—the use of legally approved "social" or "recreational" drugs. Until recently, smoking tobacco products and drinking alcoholic beverages were infrequently regarded as drug-taking behaviors. Tobacco cigarettes, chewing tobacco, cigars, and alcoholic beverages, have been widely advertised, legally purchased by adults, and socially used by millions of people.

Nevertheless, the nicotine and tars in tobacco; the ethyl alcohol in beers, wines, and distilled spirits; and even the caffeine in coffee, tea, and cola drinks are drugs. The seriousness of cigarette smoking as a drug-related behavior capable of promoting disease was not widely documented before the *First Surgeon General's Report on Smoking and Health* in 1964. Although many people now acknowledge alcohol as a drug, the nation learned the reality of alcohol abuse when Billy Carter (the brother of one former U.S. president), Betty Ford (the wife of another president), and baseball superstar Mickey Mantle admitted their alcoholism in public.

There is a growing trend to describe drug dependence, alcoholism, and persistent cigarette smoking as "addictive behaviors." These conditions involve some form of participation for short-term pleasure or satisfaction at the expense of long-term unfavorable effects. It is also being increasingly recognized that chemical dependency is one of the most common though undetected "diseases" encountered by modern medicine. To be certain, the many consequences of addiction represent a major public health problem.[5]

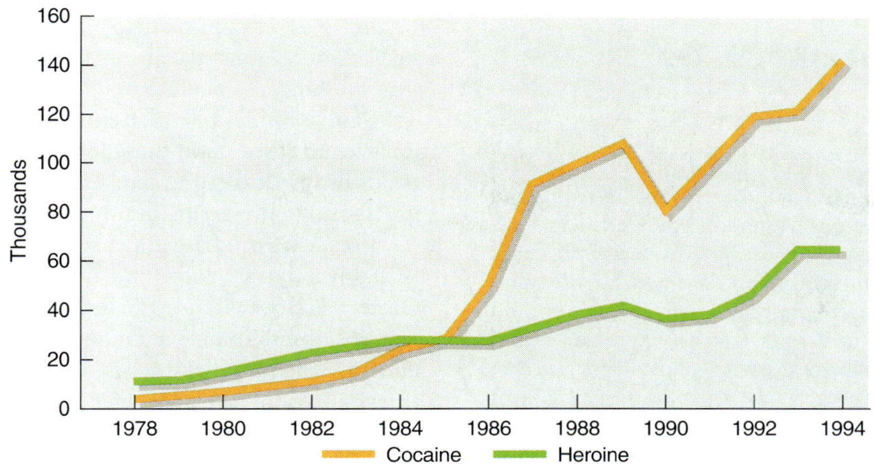

figure 1.1

Cocaine and heroin mentions in drug-related emergency room episodes, 1978–1994.

One indicator of the individual hazard rating associated with psychoactive drugs can be derived from statistics collected by the Drug Abuse Warning Network (DAWN). This information base, monitored by the National Institute on Drug Abuse, collects data from hundreds of hospital emergency rooms and medical examiners located in specific metropolitan and rural areas of the United States.

In one recent year, just over 500,000 Americans were treated in hospital emergency rooms for drug-related problems. Cocaine was a factor in 28 percent (or 142,000) of these emergency visits, while heroin was responsible for 13 percent (or 64,000) of those treated. Episodes involving speed, crank, and other methamphetamine drugs accounted for 17,400 cases.

Attempted suicide was the most commonly reported motive for drug use and was responsible for an estimated 193,000 (or 38 percent) of the 508,000 episodes. Dependence on drugs was the reported motive in 165,000 episodes, or 32 percent; "recreational use" figured in an additional 43,000 (or 8 percent) episodes. Other reasons for going to hospital ER's included unexpected drug reactions (66,000 or 13 percent), and seeking detoxification (52,000 or 10 percent). In some instances, multiple reasons were identified.

U.S. Department of Health and Human Services, 1995; The Drug Abuse Warning Network, National Institute on Drug Abuse and the Office of National Drug Control Policy, 1996.

Drug Use and People Problems

If using drugs and medicines had no long-lasting effects; never impaired physical, mental, social, or spiritual well-being; and always resulted in positive or otherwise health-promoting experiences, there would be no drug problem. But the use of these chemicals can and often does adversely affect humans—from a fetus to the elderly. Drugs and medicines affect people of both sexes and all races, creeds, educational levels, and ethnic and socioeconomic groups. As such, our drug problems basically are "people problems." These problems are based on attitudes and motivations that foster immediate satisfaction of needs and the inability to tolerate pain or frustration. Peer pressure, parent pressure, and the subtle influence of significant others are part of the problem. Living a pressure-filled life of competition, accompanied by the need to succeed at all costs, is also involved, as are conditions of economic deprivation and environmental harshness.

In essence, drug problems lead to many other problems, including

- physical and mental illnesses
- infection with sexually transmitted diseases
- drug addiction or dependency
- adverse reactions and undesired side effects
- premature and sudden deaths
- disrupted family life
- marital discord, often followed by separation or divorce
- aggression
- exploitation of others
- rape
- vandalism and destructive behavior
- impaired performance on the job and in the classroom
- criminal activities that finance an individual's drug supply or "launder" illegal drug profits through financial institutions
- gang-related violence and drug trafficking
- accidents and injuries due to combining drug use with driving or operation of machinery
- imprisonment and institutionalization

One drug, alcohol—America's preferred drug of abuse—is associated with several additional problems, as noted in figure 1.2. Such consequences of alcohol and other drug abuse have led George Gallup, Jr., a noted public opinion pollster, to say:

> America does not have a crime problem. America does not have a problem of job absenteeism and low productivity. America does not have a teenage pregnancy problem. America does not have a problem of broken homes and marriages. America has an alcohol and drug problem.[6]

Basic Definitions

To serve as a foundation for the upcoming chapters in this text, some important terms and concepts are introduced here.

Drug

Any substance that enters the human body and can change either the function or the structure of the human organism is a **drug.** This comprehensive definition of

At Issue

Are we winning the "war on drugs"?

Point: Yes! Despite the recent increase in casual drug use by young people, the national antidrug strategy has made substantial progress since the 1970s. There has been a significant movement away from widespread social tolerance of drug abuse and the use of tobacco cigarettes to the current environment in which the vast majority of Americans strongly disapprove of substance abuse and smoking in public. Furthermore, this majority neither uses illegal drugs nor smokes cigarettes. The numbers of illegal drug users, drinkers, and smokers are much lower now than during the 1980s. Evidence that the war on drugs has been successful is substantial: (1) workplaces are safer and more productive because of drug testing; (2) federal government seizures of drug traffickers' assets now average about $700 million each year; (3) drug treatment programs have improved greatly and are better linked with offender management and drug court programs; (4) adoption of zero tolerance standards has reduced teenage involvement in alcohol-related auto crashes by 20 percent; and (5) additional regulations to restrict smoking have resulted from the increased concern with secondhand smoke of cigarettes and its effects on human health. These facts strongly suggest that we are still winning the on-going war on drugs!

Office of National Drug Control Policy, *The National Drug Control Strategy: 1996* (Washington, D.C.: Executive Office of the President, 1996).

Counterpoint: Not by a long shot! We are not only failing to win the war on drugs; we are losing this pseudowar with its bungling efforts focused so greatly on reducing the supply of drugs. Although younger people are saying no to drugs in larger numbers than ever before, the number of young Americans now using marijuana and other illegal drugs is increasing, and 3,000 youths start smoking for the first time each day. Despite thirty years of increasingly punitive drug policies, illegal drugs are more easily available, drug potencies are greater, drug killings are more common, and drug barons are richer than ever. In addition, the number of drug-related emergency room visits involving cocaine is increasing. If we are winning such an antidrug crusade, why is drug abuse concentrating into those social groups—older and inner-city addicts—who can least afford the problems caused by addiction? While we now spend more on the drug war each year than on private health insurance, unprecedented police power is being concentrated in government, and our court system as well as our prisons are now clogged to the point of breakdown. Is the cost of apprehending, trying, housing, and feeding the drug criminals worth the so-called protection to our society? At best, the war on drugs is really a war on drug users and amounts to tax-supported absurdity. Despite our strictest interdiction efforts, we have not been able to prevent the birth of half a million drug-affected babies in the past few years. The only real success this war has achieved is its inspiration for people to import, grow, manufacture, sell, and use stronger drugs in more dangerous ways. Who says we're winning this war?

Dan Baum, *Smoke and Mirrors: The War on Drugs and the Politics of Failure* (Boston: Little, Brown and Company, 1996).

a drug includes practically all foreign materials—even foods, vitamins, plants, snake venom, air pollutants, and pesticides. In chapter 3, a more specific definition of a drug will be provided, although this basic description will not change.

Medicine

Physicians frequently prescribe drugs to treat or prevent illness. However, when drugs are used in the diagnosis, cure, treatment, and prevention of disease, or for the relief of pain or discomfort, the medical profession typically refers to such drug substances as **medicines.**

Many wonders of modern medical practice are based upon **therapeutics,** the use of drugs in treating and preventing disease and in preserving health.

Prescription drugs, available only by a physician's order, and **over-the-counter** (nonprescription) **drugs** have been successful in relieving many human ailments when used responsibly. Ideally, drugs should be taken for their intended purposes; according to directions; in the appropriate amount, frequency, strength, or manner; and—in the case of prescribed drugs— under the supervision of a physician.

It should be evident that to produce their desired effects, medicines are composed of drugs, but not all drugs are used as medicines.

Drug Misuse

The unintentional or inappropriate use of prescribed or nonprescribed medicine resulting in the impaired physical, mental, emotional, or social well-being of the user is referred to as **drug misuse.** Some individuals consume drugs in excess of recommended dosages or they reduce the standard time interval between doses. Others take prescribed medications without professional consultation or offer their own medicines to others. These are examples of *drug misuse.* Additional drug-misuse practices are listed in box 1.1.

Drug Abuse

Sometimes referred to as substance or chemical abuse, **drug abuse** is the deliberate, continuous use of mind-changing chemical substances (usually for reasons other than legitimate medical purposes) that results in any degree of physical, mental, emotional, or social impairment of the user, the user's family, or society. This comprehensive definition of drug abuse is not based solely on the illegality of the drug that is used, on any specific amount used, time frame of use, or frequency of use. As such, drug abuse does

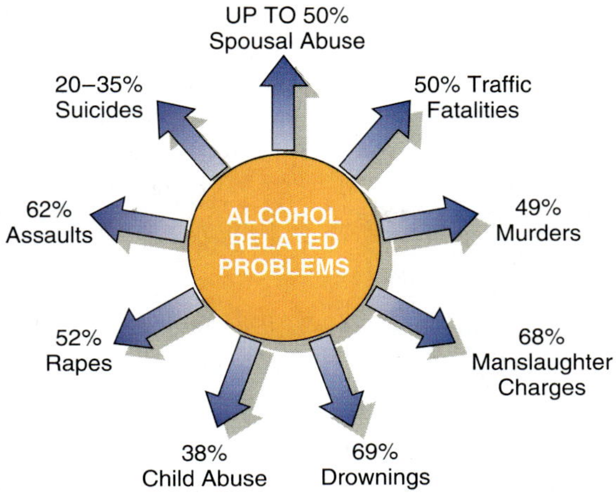

figure 1.2

Americans have a big problem with alcohol, the number one drug of abuse.

Source: Modified from the Office for Substance Abuse Prevention. Data derived from the National Institute on Alcohol Abuse and Alcoholism.

include the unwise use of a legal drug. Many would also consider the use of any legally prohibited drug and the use of any legal drug by underage individuals as additional examples of drug abuse.

A more objective description of drug or substance abuse has been offered by the American Psychiatric Association (APA). According to this organization, substance abuse is a maladaptive or faulty pattern of substance use leading to impairment or distress, with one or more of the following conditions within a twelve-month period:[7]

- Repeated substance use leading to a failure to fulfill one's role obligations at work, school, or home.
- Repeated use of drugs in physically hazardous situations, such as drinking and driving.
- Repeated drug use-related legal problems, such as arrest for disorderly conduct.
- Continued use of a drug despite social or interpersonal problems repeatedly being caused or made worse by the substance.

In essence, drug abuse involves using illegal as well as legal mind-changing drugs that lead to ill effects and undesirable consequences. It also includes the use of legal medicines by healthy people for social convenience or personal pleasure and the use of typically nondrug substances, such as gasoline, to produce druglike effects. Since drug abuse has become the focus of public concern and government action, it has been identified almost exclusively with the **psychoactive** (or psychotropic) **drugs** that primarily affect the human mind. See box 1.2 for the danger signals of drug abuse.

Psychoactive Drug

Often described as a psychotropic (mind-affecting) or mind-altering drug, a psychoactive drug is a chemical substance that changes one's thinking, feelings, perceptions, and behavior. These changes are the result of the drug's action on the human brain. The range of mind-changing, psychoactive drugs includes:

Narcotics—The narcotic analgesics, often referred to as opioids, are powerful painkillers and also produce pleasurable feelings and induce sleep.

Depressants—Also known as sedatives, depressants slow down central nervous system function, relax or tranquilize the person, and produce sleep.

Stimulants—These are chemical substances that usually speed up central nervous system function, resulting in alertness and excitability.

Psychedelics—Sometimes known as mind expanders or hallucinogens, these drugs affect a person's perception, awareness, and emotions, and can also cause hallucinations (completely groundless, false perceptions) as well as illusions (misinterpretations of reality or something imagined).

Marijuana—This intoxicating drug, derived from the hemp plant, can produce depressant and psychedelic effects.

Inhalants—These are volatile nondrug substances that have druglike effects when inhaled. A few inhalants (specifically, amyl nitrite

Box 1.1 Drug Misuse

Some common examples of drug misuse include these:

Taking prescribed or nonprescribed medicines at the improper time.

Discontinuing the use of a prescribed medicine without consulting one's physician.

Failing to recognize, and then not taking appropriate action regarding a "side effect" related to a particular drug or medicine.

Taking at the same time duplicate medications prescribed by different physicians.

Combining alcoholic beverages with depressantlike drugs, such as antihistamines, tranquilizers, or sleeping pills.

Stretching the dose of a particular medicine to make it last longer than the originally prescribed period of use.

Failing to inform your present physician of medicines still being taken but prescribed by your former physician.

Continuing to take medication after the original need for such a drug no longer exists.

Saving old medicines for self-treatment in the future.

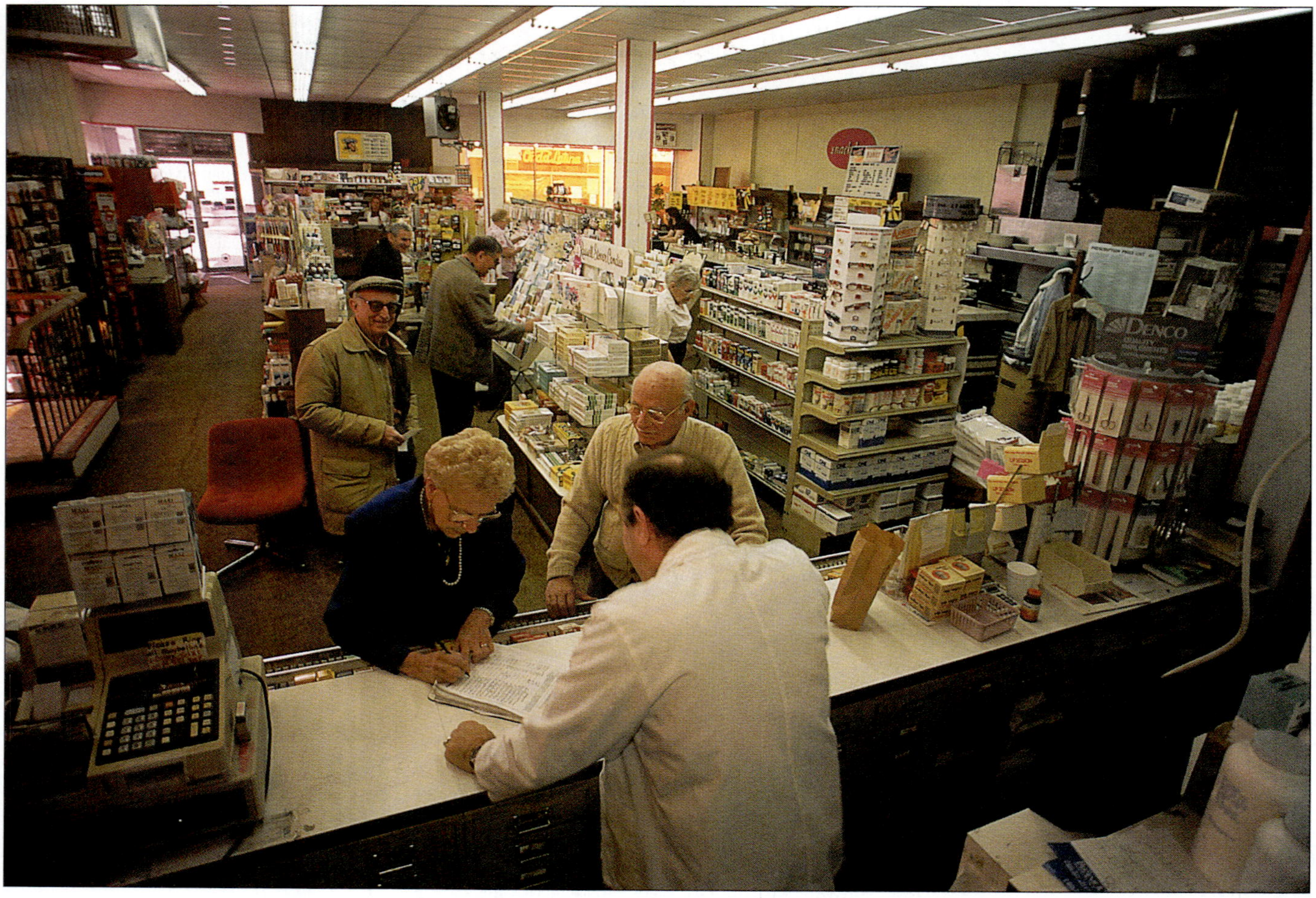

Although over-the-counter drugs are sold in a variety of commercial settings, physician-prescribed medications can be purchased only at a drug store or pharmacy located in a department store, grocery, hospital, or through a mail-order pharmacy service.

and nitrous oxide) do have some medical uses.

Many psychoactive drugs already are integrated into the lifestyle of people who daily consume coffee, tea, beer, cola drinks, cocktails, cigarettes, aspirin, and various sleep-enhancing and alertness-promoting preparations. Some of the psychoactive drugs, such as morphine, barbiturates, and antidepressants, have legitimate medical uses. However, because all mind-affecting drugs have the ability to change mood and behavior, they have a high potential not only for misuse but also for abuse and dependence in the human quest for pleasure or escape from pain.

Drug Classifications

It is possible to classify psychoactive drugs—the major focus of this text—in several ways, as noted in box 1.3. Such classification allows us to learn the common characteristics of a particular group of drugs.

The first major classification groups specific drugs according to their generalized or localized effects on the brain. This is perhaps the most common way of categorizing drugs, and we will use such a classification generally throughout this text for an analysis of various psychoactive drugs.

Generalized central nervous system depressant effect—Drugs in this category are often referred to as "downers" and have a general effect of slowing down, reducing the function of, or depressing excitable brain tissue. Included in this category are ethyl alcohol, barbiturates, nonbarbiturate sedative-hypnotics, minor tranquilizers (antianxiety medications), anesthetics, volatile solvents, and low-dose cannabinoids (marijuana and hashish).

Generalized central nervous system stimulant effect—Sometimes identified as "uppers," the central

Box 1.2 Danger Signals of Drug Abuse

Many people take prescribed drugs that affect their moods. Using these drugs wisely is important for physical and emotional health. But sometimes it is difficult to decide when using drugs to handle stress becomes inappropriate. It is important that your use of drugs does not result in catastrophe. Here are some "danger signals" that can help you evaluate your way of using drugs.

1. Do those close to you often ask about your drug use? Have they noticed any changes in your moods or behavior?
2. Are you defensive if a friend or relative mentions your drug or alcohol use?
3. Are you sometimes embarrassed or frightened by your behavior under the influence of drugs or alcohol?
4. Have you ever gone to see a new doctor because your regular physician would not prescribe the drug you wanted?
5. When you are under pressure or feel anxious, do you automatically take a tranquilizer or drink or both?
6. Do you take drugs more often or for purposes other than those recommended by your doctor?
7. Do you mix drugs and alcohol?
8. Do you drink or take drugs regularly to help you sleep?
9. Do you have to take a pill to get going in the morning?
10. Do you think you have a drug problem?

If you have answered *yes* to a number of these questions, you may be abusing drugs or alcohol. There are places to go for help at the local level. One such place might be a drug-abuse program in your community, listed in the Yellow Pages under "Drug Abuse." Other resources include community crisis centers, telephone hotlines, and the Mental Health Association.

Source: National Institute on Drug Abuse.

Box 1.3 Classification of Psychoactive Drugs

1. Classification according to a drug's effects on the human brain:
   - general depressant
   - local affective depressant
   - general stimulant
   - psychedelic or hallucinogenic
   - narcotic
2. Classification according to a drug's availability with or without a physician's order:
   - prescription
   - over-the-counter
3. Classification as to a drug's relative potential for abuse and dependence as well as acceptability for medical treatment:
   - five schedules as established by the federal Controlled Substances Act of Congress
4. Classification according to a drug's potential for being personal and social hazards:
   - very high hazard rating to a relatively low hazard rating

nervous system stimulants have a general effect of increasing or speeding up the function of excitable brain tissue. Included in this category are the amphetamines, cocaine, caffeine, and nicotine.

Localized affective or limbic center depressant effect—Included in this category are the antipsychotic drugs (major tranquilizers); the antidepressants; and the antimanic drug lithium, used in the treatment of the manic phase of manic-depressive mental illness. These drugs have a localized depressant or modifying effect on the brain's limbic center that controls emotional function. Unlike the central nervous system depressants, the drugs in this category do not slow down the brain's breathing centers.

Psychedelic or hallucinogenic effect—Drugs in this category tend to produce distortion of thought and sensory processes, thereby inducing a psychosis-like state with illusions and hallucinations, often of a visual nature. Lysergic acid diethylamide, mescaline, psilocybin, phencyclidine, and large-dose cannabinoids (marijuana and hashish) are representative drugs in this group.

Narcotic effect—These drugs, the narcotic analgesics, decrease pain by binding to specific receptors (areas) in certain areas of the brain. In this category are the narcotic-agonists—morphine, heroin, opium, as well as methadone, Darvon, and Demerol—which produce pain relief, euphoria, and depression of breathing. The narcotic antagonists, Naloxone, Naltrexone, and Cyclazocine, which block the effects of the agonists, are also in this drug group. When used alone, the antagonists have few or no drug effects.

Drugs used as medicines in the treatment of illness and disease are typically identified as either prescription drugs (requiring a physician's written order) or nonprescription preparations purchased over the pharmacy or store counter without a physician's order. Prescriptions are always required for legitimate medicines in Schedule II, III, and IV, established by the federal government and listed in box 1.3.

However, a classification of psychoactive drugs commonly purchased

table 1.2 Commonly Purchased Over-the-Counter (Nonprescription) Psychoactive Substances

Major Group with Representative Examples	Drug Contents
Alcoholic Beverages	
Beer	Ethyl alcohol, congeners
Wine	Ethyl alcohol, congeners
Distilled spirits	Ethyl alcohol, congeners
Allergy/Cold Relief Medications	
Actifed	Pseudoephedrine hydrochloride Triprolidine hydrochloride
Benadryl	Diphenhydramine hydrochloride
Dimetapp Elixir	Brompheniramine maleate Phenylpropanolamine hydrochloride
Contac Maximum	Phenylpropanolamine hydrochloride Chlorpheniramine maleate
Analgesics (Pain Relievers)	
Advil, Nuprin, Medipren	Ibuprofen
Aleve	Naproxen sodium
Bayer Aspirin, Bufferin	Acetylsalicylic acid
Tylenol, Excedrin	Acetaminophen
Appetite Suppressants	
Acutrim	Phenylpropanolamine hydrochloride
Dexatrim	Phenylpropanolamine hydrochloride
Sleep Aids	
Excedrin PM	Acetaminophen Diphenhydramine citrate
Nytol	Diphenhydramine hydrochloride
Sominex	Diphenhydramine hydrochloride
Unisom	Doxylamine succinate
Stimulants	
No Doz	Caffeine
Vivarin	Caffeine
Tobacco Products	
Cigarettes	Nicotine
Cigars	Nicotine
Pipe tobacco	Nicotine
Chewing tobacco	Nicotine
Snuff	Nicotine

over-the-counter reveals the wide-spread availability of these medications. Such a classification appears in table 1.2. These nonprescription over-the-counter drugs are used to treat minor symptoms, such as drowsiness and sleeplessness, aches and pains, and the relief of allergic reactions. Of course, alcoholic beverages and tobacco products are bought for a variety of reasons and are not usually intended for use as medicines.

An additional classification is suggested by the Comprehensive Drug Abuse Prevention and Control Act of 1970, Title II, more commonly known as the **Controlled Substances Act.** This public law enacted by Congress sorts psychoactive drugs (except for ethyl alcohol, nicotine, and caffeine) into five schedules or categories, based on their actual or relative potential for abuse, their likelihood of causing psychic or physiological dependence, and their current acceptability for medical treatment. This classification is shown in box 1.4.

The last drug classification to be considered here may be interpreted as somewhat controversial. Nevertheless, a consideration of *personal* and *social hazards* associated with drug use, misuse, and abuse is important. These include the potential, inherent hazards of psychological or physical dependence or both; development of tolerance; possibility of irreversible damage to body tissues and disease; likelihood of accidental death or overdose; and predisposition to social dysfunction, recklessness, and self-destructive behavior. An interpretation of one such classification follows:[8]

> *Very high individual hazard rating:* cocaine and amphetamines, ethyl alcohol
>
> *Relatively high individual hazard rating:* sedative-hypnotics, heroin, volatile inhalants, tobacco cigarettes
>
> *Intermediate individual hazard rating:* LSD, PCP
>
> *Relatively low individual hazard rating:* marijuana

Cocaine, alcohol, and tobacco cigarettes are capable of causing serious body-organ or tissue damage. By contrast, there is a somewhat lower potential for heroin either to cause tissue damage or to produce self-destructive behavior. Frequently, heroin users take their narcotic to function normally; but often, like coke users and crack smokers, they commit serious crime to finance their drug-taking behavior. Of course, there are always the real dangers of physical disability or death due to overdose of cocaine and heroin, as noted in figure 1.2. Accidents occurring while a person is under the influence of alcohol, LSD, PCP, and marijuana can also have serious and even fatal outcomes.

In rank-ordering psychoactive drugs according to their inherent *hazard potential to society,* Samuel Irwin originally suggested the following list.[9]

1. Alcohol
2. Sedative-hypnotics
3. Stimulants
4. Heroin
5. Volatile solvents
6. Cigarettes
7. LSD
8. Marijuana

While alcohol is considered here the most potentially hazardous drug to society in terms of its probable misuse and/or

Box 1.4 Selected Psychoactive Drugs and Schedules

In Schedules II, III, and IV, examples of trademark products appear in parentheses.

Schedule I: Substances with a high potential for abuse and dependence. There is no currently accepted medical use in the United States. (Available for research purposes only.)

Heroin

Psychedelics: LSD, mescaline, peyote, psilocybin, DMT, DED, and amphetamine variants: MDA, MDMA, DMA, PMA, STP, DOM, DOB

Phencyclidine (veterinary drug only) and its analogues: PCE, PCPy, TCP

Methaqualone

Marijuana: in spite of recent studies indicating a variety of potential therapeutic uses; and THC, marijuana's active ingredient

Hashish

Designer drugs

Schedule II: Substances with a high potential for abuse, but such drugs have a currently accepted medical use in the United States, often with severe restriction. Abuse may lead to severe psychological or physical dependence. (Usually available by written prescription only, but in an emergency, oral orders may be given to a dispenser. No refills are permitted.)

Opium

Morphine

Codeine

Hydromorphone (Dilaudid)

Meperidine (Demoral)

Cocaine

Oxycodone (Percodan)

Amphetamines

Methylphenidate (Ritalin)

Barbiturates: amobarbital, pentobarbital, and secobarbital

Dronabinol (Marinol), synthetic delta-9-THC

Nabilone (Cesamet), synthetic cannabinoid

Schedule III: Substances with a potential for abuse less than drugs in Schedules I and II. Such drugs have a currently accepted medical use in the United States. Abuse may lead to moderate or low physical or high psychological dependence. (Available by written or oral prescription; five refills in six months with medical authorization.)

Anabolic steroids, although they are not immediately euphoric in their effect

Derivatives of barbituric acid except those listed in another schedule

Glutethimide (Doriden)

Methyprylon (Noludar)

Nalorphine

Chlorphentermine

Phendimetrazine

Paregoric

Tylenol with codeine #4

Schedule IV: Substances with a low potential for abuse relative to drugs in Schedule III. These drugs have a currently accepted medical use in the United States. Abuse may lead to limited physical or psychological dependence relative to drugs in Schedule III. (Available by written or oral prescription; five refills in six months with medical authorization.)

Barbiturates: barbital, phenobarbital

Chloral hydrate

Ethchlorvynol (Placidyl)

Ethinamate (Valmid)

Meprobamate (Equanil, Miltown)

Propoxyphene (Darvon)

Pentazocine (Talwin-NX)

Benzodiazepine antianxiety drugs: (Xanax, Valium, Librium, Ativan, Serax, Dalmane [used as a sleep-promoting sedative], and Tranxene)

Schedule V: Substances with a low potential for abuse relative to drugs in Schedule IV. Such drugs have a currently accepted medical use in the United States and may lead to limited physical dependence or psychological dependence in relation to drugs in Schedule IV. (Availability without prescription depends upon individual state laws.)

Preparations containing limited quantities of certain narcotic drugs used generally for antitussive and antidiarrheal purposes.

Actifed with codeine cough syrup

Lomotil

Parepectolin

Robitussin A-C cough syrup

Triaminic expectorant with codeine

Schedules established by the Controlled Substances Act.
Source: U.S. Drug Enforcement Administration.

abuse and subsequent "harm to others," federal law defines alcohol as legal. However, federal law stipulates that marijuana is illegal even though its potential hazard to society is considered here the lowest of all drugs so ranked in this particular classification. In rank-ordering these drugs, "harm to others" was defined as causing or contributing to social apathy, driving accidents, aggressiveness, and crimes of violence.

Such a classification of drugs is, to be certain, open to criticism and may be described by some as irresponsible or at least controversial. Indeed, law enforcement officials may rank heroin and cocaine as having the greatest adverse effect on society, while social workers may identify alcohol and health educators might focus on tobacco smoking as the top-ranking social drug problem.

After studying the various drugs described in this text, you may want to rerank the psychoactive drugs for their inherent potential for personal and social hazards. However, such a classification does suggest that legalized drugs are not harmless and that under certain circumstances illegal drug use may have minimal risks to the welfare of individual drug takers and the society.

Drug Problems: Health-Related Consequences

The benefits usually associated with using, misusing, and abusing drugs are (1) the experience of some physical or psychological pleasure and (2) the reduction of a frustrating or stressful condition. Often, these benefits are short lived, especially with drug misuse of abuse. There are risks, and hazards that often accompany drug-taking behavior. More deaths, illnesses, and disabilities are due to substance abuse than to any other preventable health condition.[10]

Of the two million deaths in the United States each year, more than one in four is related to alcohol abuse, illicit use of psychoactive drugs, or tobacco use. Many such deaths and other related losses could be reduced significantly by changing people's perceptions, lifestyles, and personal behaviors. Several of these conditions will be explored in later chapters of this text. However, of special concern are the following health-related consequences that may represent an immediate problem for many drug takers.

Delay in Seeking Proper Medical Treatment

Frequent unsupervised use of drugs for a health problem may so effectively mask the symptoms of a disorder or disease that the person believes the condition has been controlled or cured. Therefore, the individual might not seek medical attention early. When such a disorder finally comes to a physician's attention, often little can be done to remedy the problem that has progressed under the protective cover of drugs.

Reduction in Personal Problem-Solving Effectiveness

Using drugs often makes the consumer feel better for a while. However, the underlying causes motivating drug use remain. The ability to use other problem-solving techniques, particularly in interpersonal relationships and identity crises, is often impaired. The techniques may never even be attempted. This is especially true if one is under the influence of certain drugs, such as ethyl alcohol or tranquilizers, on a continuing basis.

Experience of Additional Health Problems

The self-administered use of any psychoactive substance makes the drug taker vulnerable to a number of possible and fairly predictable adverse reactions, including:

1. **Toxic reaction**—A toxic or poisonous reaction accompanies an overdose of any drug. If too much of a chemical substance is taken, a temporary condition of intoxication (poisoning) occurs. This is characterized by a disturbance of function in one or more body-support systems. Intoxication with ethyl alcohol, sedatives, opiates, and even PCP can result in death because of the serious depressant effect these drugs have on the breathing center of the central nervous system.
2. **Panic**—First-time users of marijuana, one of the psychedelics, or even a stimulant often develop fears of losing self-control or of having done physical harm to themselves. Afraid of going crazy, the individuals sometimes exhibit uncontrollable behavior.
3. **Flashback**—After repeated use of psychedelics, a drug user may experience a flashback, the undesirable recurrence of a drug's effects with no recent drug intake (consumption) to explain the alteration of one's sense of time and visual illusions and hallucinations.
4. **Psychopathology**—A psychopathological condition is the occurrence of one or more severe mental disorders, such as major depression, schizophrenia (thought disorder), or bipolar manic-depression. These disorders can occur in a person having a substance-abuse problem. Such an individual may be described as a "dually diagnosed" patient—one who has a mental disorder and a substance-abuse condition. Although there are various forms of this dually diagnosed state, psychoactive substances appear to either unleash or uncover an underlying, preexisting mental disorder or to permanently imbalance the brain's chemistry through years of chronic, toxic effects on the brain.[11] Another form of psychopathology is the organic brain syndrome resulting from physical changes in the brain, sometimes due to long-term poisonous effects of central nervous system depressants, inhalants, and PCP. This syndrome is manifested by confusion, disorientation, and decreased intellectual functioning.
5. **Drug dependence**—Drug dependence is a maladaptive (faulty or inadequate) pattern of substance use leading to observable and

significant impairment or distress. According to the latest edition of the *Diagnostic and Statistical Manual of Mental Disorders* (DSM-IV), at least three of the following conditions must be present for substance dependence to be indicated:

- Developing a tolerance for a drug, thus making it necessary to increase the amount of any substance to achieve intoxication or desired effects
- Experiencing typical withdrawal symptoms when use of a drug is stopped or when using the drug to relieve or avoid withdrawal symptoms
- Taking more of a drug, or using it longer, than intended
- Persistently or unsuccessfully attempting to reduce or control substance use
- Spending excessive time getting and taking a drug and recovering from the drug's effects
- Giving up important social, occupational, or recreational activities because of substance use
- Continuing substance use despite knowing that such use likely causes or makes worse a persistent or recurring physical or psychological problem.

Concepts of drug dependency will be discussed in greater detail in chapter 3.

Use of Adulterated Drugs

When individuals buy "street drugs," they do not always get what they bargained for. Drugs may be mixed, or "cut," with cheaper, inferior, or even more hazardous substances. Most frequently, there is no manufacturing control over the actual composition of the illegal pills, powders, and capsules; there is no standard dosage; and there is little concern on the part of drug sellers for the toxicity of their fraudulent products. Such drug tampering or altering is called **adulteration.**

Typically, street drugs are mixed with other chemicals that mimic or even increase another drug's action.

In many instances, the street drug doesn't even contain the major drug ingredient that the buyer is seeking. Instead, there may be entirely different or possibly similar chemical substances in the adulterated product. Street drugs are often cut with poisons, insecticides, animal tranquilizers, oregano, catnip, milk sugar, or quinine. These items are used to stretch the final product and to increase the seller's profit.

Depending upon what the adulterating substance is, the user stands a high risk of having an unanticipated drug experience or a toxic reaction. There is the added danger that these users may be treated by medical personnel who lack information about the true nature or composition of the consumed drug.

Suicide

Suicide is ranked as the ninth leading cause of death in the United States. Although the highest suicide rate is recorded among persons over sixty-five years of age, the greatest number of suicides occurs among persons fifteen to twenty-four years of age. In this latter age group, self-imposed death is the second leading cause of mortality among white men.[12] At present, an estimated 10,000 American college students attempt suicide each year, and some 1,000 succeed.

Nearly one-third of suicides had been drinking before death, and at least 20 percent were intoxicated at the time of death. It is also estimated that up to 15 percent of single-vehicle traffic accidents have a suicidal intent, with many of those involved having double-indemnity insurance policies.[13] In addition, suicide is one of the more frequent causes of death in long-term heavy drinkers, among whom the rate of suicide is fifty-five times greater than in the general population.[14]

The association between suicide and the abuse of alcohol and other drugs is further highlighted in data from the **Drug Abuse Warning Network** (DAWN), a large-scale drug-abuse data collection system sponsored by the National Institute on Drug Abuse. DAWN records substances linked with drug-abuse episodes reported by emergency rooms and medical examiners in various metropolitan areas of the United States. According to DAWN, suicide was the drug-use motive in 38 percent of emergency room deaths or admissions.

The relationship between drug abuse and suicide is complex and likely involves at least two basic considerations. First, some authorities believe that certain already depressed people use excessive amounts of alcohol or other drugs, especially narcotics and sedative-hypnotics (including the antianxiety minor tranquilizers) as the means or instruments of self-destruction. Second, others emphasize that drugs such as alcohol, cocaine, amphetamines, barbiturates, minor tranquilizers, marijuana, psychedelics, and many nonpsychoactive prescription medicines tend to bring on and intensify psychological depression in individuals who might then develop a fatal despondency that leads to suicide. It is possible that both explanations apply in any analysis of this serious drug-related problem.

HIV Infection and AIDS

Today, **HIV infection** and AIDS are listed as the eighth leading cause of death in the United States. Use of needles to inject certain psychoactive drugs is related to the transmission or spread of **acquired immunodeficiency syndrome (AIDS),** a consideration of this often fatal, but treatable, disease is most appropriate. Medical research has proved that the human immunodeficiency virus (HIV) causes AIDS. A serious, life-threatening illness for which there is no present drug prevention or drug cure, AIDS involves a breakdown of the body's own internal defense system that makes the HIV-infected person more likely to develop certain other diseases that cause death. These "opportunistic" illnesses that overwhelm an individual with a compromised (weakened) immune system include Pneumocystis carinii pneumonia (a parasitic infection of the lungs); Kaposi's sarcoma (a form of cancer of the blood vessel walls visible as blue-violet to brownish skin blotches or bumps); and other yeast, viral, and parasitic infections.

Although the AIDS-causing virus can be spread from an infected mother to her child perinatally (before; during; and after childbirth, through breast-feeding), the major ways of transmitting HIV are through intimate sexual behaviors—involving the exchange of semen, vaginal secretions, or blood—and through exposure to blood or tissues and blood products.[15] Nevertheless, all of these ways of spreading the HIV can be associated with the abuse of alcohol and other drugs.

Perhaps the most obvious relationship between drugs and AIDS is that intravenous (IV) drug users—those who inject illegal drugs directly into their veins—make up the second largest group of people with AIDS in the United States. Female and heterosexual male IV drug abusers account for at least 25 percent of diagnosed cases of AIDS in America. Another 7 percent of such cases occur among homosexual or bisexual males who are also IV drug users. More than 30 percent of AIDS cases are occurring in people with injection-drug use as the major risk factor.[16]

The most dangerous and rapid way to get or give HIV involves the sharing of "dirty" (blood-contaminated) needles and syringes by IV drug users. Frequently, cotton or other materials used as filters, and containers ("cookers") in which a drug is heated and/or dissolved, are also shared. Blood from a previous user most typically lodges in the tip of the hypodermic needle or in the syringe, but it might also be found in other parts of the injection apparatus, collectively referred to as the "works."

Drug injection, whether intravenous or nonintravenous (as seen in skin-popping of heroin or intramuscular injection of bodybuilding steroids), and transmission of HIV are detailed in the following account, which explains why such drug-taking methods are so hazardous.

> During injection, the user may draw his/her own blood into the syringe to mix with the dissolved drug and then inject the blood/drug mixture, a procedure known as "booting." This is done to make sure all traces of the drug are removed from the syringe efficiently. As a result, however, any blood from a prior user which remains in the syringe or in the tip of the needle is injected directly into subsequent users. Traditionally, any cleaning of the syringe or needle involves rinsing them in water or blowing into them. Sterilization equipment is not readily available to users and speed of injection is often paramount in the minds of addicts.[17]

Two factors have been associated consistently with the spread of HIV among intravenous drug users and drug injectors: the frequency of drug injection and the use of "shooting galleries"—places where drug users can rent or borrow injection equipment. Research has also revealed that injecting cocaine alone carries a threefold risk of HIV infection over injecting heroin alone.[18] Such a risk is due to the tendency of cocaine users to inject more frequently than heroin users (cocaine is shorter-acting than heroin), to draw more blood into the syringe to mix with the drug prior to injecting than is done with IV use of heroin, and to use the drug more often in "shooting galleries."[19]

Another area of concern relating drug abuse to HIV infection and AIDS is that alcohol, cocaine, heroin, volatile nitrites, and possibly marijuana are likely to interfere with or suppress various components of the normal immune defense mechanism in the human body.[20] As a consequence, some drug abusers appear to be predisposed to HIV infection or its consequences.[21]

Furthermore, it is believed that the AIDS-causing virus infects and overwhelms an immune system that has been activated, compromised, or challenged. Chemical agents may cause this activation and therefore function as correlated factors (cofactors), but not causal factors, in HIV infection that often progresses to a full-blown case of AIDS.

The last important way in which alcohol and other drugs may affect the spread of HIV and AIDS pertains to the general disinhibition (unblocking) effects of some psychoactive drugs on sexual and risk-taking behaviors. While many believe that alcohol, marijuana, cocaine, and volatile nitrites act as aphrodisiacs—drugs that allegedly increase libido and the enjoyment of sexual behaviors—the use of these chemicals also tends to make people more likely to engage in unwanted and unsafe sexual practices. Without the restraints of conscience, better judgment, propriety, and morality that often serve to control behavior, anything goes—and often does.

The Drug Scene: An Overview

The drug scene is an ever-changing description of the use, abuse, and nonuse of mind-changing drugs across the nation. A variety of sources provide some insight into the drug-using population, psychoactive drug-taking patterns, and attitudes and behaviors that likely contribute to the use of alcohol, tobacco, and other drugs in the United States. General findings from national reports and surveys conducted by health promotion and law enforcement agencies are summarized here.[22] Such information typically focuses on familiar and newer emerging drugs of abuse and the legal, social, or "recreational," drugs so prevalent in our society.

- After nearly thirty years of national antidrug programs, fewer American adults are using illegal drugs on an occasional or nonaddicted basis. At present, the number of illegal drug users—between eleven and twelve million—is almost half of past-month users recorded in the late 1970s and early 1980s. However, illegal drug use among teens has doubled since the early 1990s.
- Males are more likely than females to have used illegal drugs and to have used them in the past month. But American women are closing this gender gap: women are increasingly likely to abuse substances at the same rate as men, and women are starting to smoke, drink, and use illegal drugs at earlier ages than ever before. In comparison with men, women get drunk faster, become addicted quicker, and develop substance abuse-related diseases sooner.
- Certain occupations tend to have higher rates of illegal drug use. Construction workers, food preparation staff, and restaurant wait staff report highest use, while police officers, detectives, administrative support staff, teachers, and child care workers report the lowest rates of illicit drug use.

- Heroin use has increased, especially among young, nonurban, middle-income people. The ability to inhale this drug—a central nervous system depressant and a narcotic—has made it more attractive and its use more acceptable than in the past, when injection was the only method of use. Users of heroin are also beginning first use at younger ages in which smoking and snorting are the preferred routes of administration.
- While cocaine—a central nervous system stimulant—consumption is still high, cocaine and crack use appears to be leveling off or declining in most areas, except in those states near the Mexican border. Although cocaine is often described as the most predominant of mind-changing drugs, with the most diverse composition of users, those who take crack or cocaine hydrochloride appear to be an aging group in their late twenties and early thirties.
- Marijuana, having both sedative and psychedelic effects, continues to be the most commonly used illicit drug in the United States, where it is particularly popular among teens and young adults. In most areas, supplies are plentiful and potency has been increasing.
- Methamphetamine, taken for its stimulant effect, enjoys continued popularity as its use spreads to nearly all areas of the country and to younger drug takers. For many years, use of this drug, also known as speed, crystal, crank, and ice, had been largely confined to the West and the Southwest.
- LSD, the first major psychedelic drug of the 1960s, has been experiencing a renewed popularity and is available in every state. Numerous mail-order sales have created a marketplace where LSD sellers are usually unknown to the buyers. Most users are white, middle-class high school and college students attracted by low prices and the perception that this drug is harmless.
- Rohypnol, a powerful sleeping pill that produces a loss of inhibition and short-term memory, is a prescription drug not licensed for sale in this country. Known as roofies, R-2's, and Mexican valium, Rohypnol has become popular among young people, especially in southern states. In many cases, women have reported being taken advantage of sexually by men who have slipped this drug into alcoholic beverages. Women wake up the next morning knowing they have been raped, but not remembering precisely what has occurred. Consequently, Rohypnol is known as the "date rape" drug.
- Herbal Ecstacy and other "natural drugs" reflect the current romance many Americans have with the natural drug culture and its legal and cheap alternatives to government regulated stimulants. Herbal supplements containing ephedra carry names such as Herbal Ecstacy, Cloud 9, and Ultimate Xphoria.
- So-called "club drugs," including MDMA, Ketamine, 2C-B, psilocybin, and a range of other hallucinogenic drugs, are also increasing in popularity in many areas of the country, particularly at "raves" and dance clubs.
- Alcoholic beverages are consumed by over one-half of the drinking age population. But one-half of users are "light" drinkers who consume no more than 10 percent of the alcoholic beverages sold in the United States.. An estimated twelve to eighteen million people are alcohol dependents (alcoholics). The overall per capita consumption of absolute (pure) alcohol continues its downward turn, due largely to the on-going drop in the use of distilled spirits (hard liquor).
- Tobacco cigarettes are used by over sixty million Americans (including about 4.5 million adolescents) representing a 29 percent national smoking rate. After a significant decline, the number of smokers appears to have leveled off. Now, smoking is up slightly among young adults. By contrast, smoking among teenagers is at its highest level in over a decade, with more than 3,000 young people each day beginning to smoke for the first time.

Hardcore drug use, with its devastating effects on society, is also a major feature of the drug scene. About one in four occasional illegal drug users progresses to chronic drug addiction or dependency. This small minority consumes the majority of illegal drugs and commits a disproportionate number of drug-related crimes. Families and neighborhoods are being devastated by the crime and health consequences that so often accompany drug dependency.

Perhaps the most alarming aspect of today's drug scene is the increasing use of mind-changing drugs by youth, as noted in figure 1.3. In 1991, after almost ten years of decline, the number of individuals trying marijuana for the first time showed a marked increase. Most of these first-time users were young people. Since then, the rate of drug use among youth has continued to climb. With the exception of alcohol, drugs, including stimulants, hallucinogens, and inhalants, are being used increasingly by both teens and preteens. It is marijuana that is used most often!

Many authorities and specialists have attempted to explain this rather gradual rediscovery and growing popularity of illegal psychoactive substances. While there is no one reason for this shift in drug-taking behavior, several likely factors may be responsible for the upward trend in illegal drug use:[23]

1. A new group of teenagers who no longer believe the standard antidrug messages of the recent past.
2. A relaxing of attitudes about the harmfulness and acceptance of drug use, in general, and marijuana, in particular.
3. A dramatic reduction in attention devoted to drug problems in the national news media.
4. Increasing mixed messages sent to youth about drugs and violence. Drugs, drug-taking behavior, and

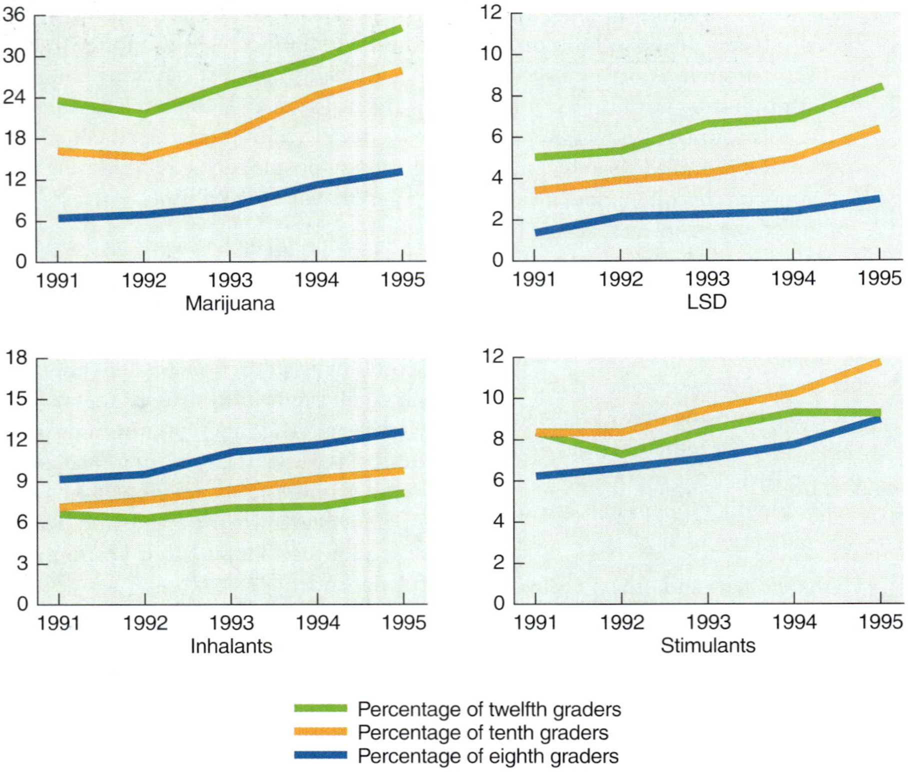

figure 1.3

Adolescent drug use.

In the last few years, use of most illegal drugs has increased among American students in all three grade levels as shown. However, marijuana has shown the sharpest increase. In most instances, these increases began in the early 1990s and reversed a decade or more of decreases in drug usage.

According to the Office of National Drug Control Policy, an estimated 39 million Americans are currently under the age of ten, the greatest number in this age group since the 1960s. If, ten years from now, this group abuses drugs at the same rate as today's youth, drug use will increase by alarming proportions. If drug use increases by the same rate that it has for the past five years, by the year 2000, nearly 1.4 million high school seniors will be using illegal drugs on a monthly basis. The urgent need to reverse drug abuse trends among adolescents is evident.

Source: National Institute on Drug Abuse, The Monitoring the Future Study, *Institute for Social Research, The University of Michigan, 1996.*

violence are too often glamorized or legitimized through powerful messages and images contained in movies, television, music, advertising, and marketing. These persuasive and subtle influences affect youth attitudes and behavior and undermine school and parental efforts to help children make healthy lifestyle choices.

5. Frequent witnessing by youth of their own role models in professional sports and other fields abusing psychoactive substances with few if any unfavorable consequences.
6. The marketing to youth of products that seem to condone or encourage experimentation with illegal substances, such as, an athletic shoe called the "Hemp," temporary tattoos glorifying use of marijuana, and baseball cardlike cards that champion drugs and drug-taking behavior.

The Drug-Crime Relationship

Drugs and crimes are problems that are often closely related in complex ways. Drug-crime relationships are usually expressed as drug-defined offenses, drug-related offenses, and interactional circumstances, as explained in box 1.5.

Drug users report greater involvement in crime and are more likely than nonusers to have criminal records. Moreover, once persons have criminal records, they are more likely than those without such records to report being drug users. In addition, the Drug Use Forecasting (DUF) program of the National Institute of Justice confirms that between one-half and two-thirds of people arrested for major crimes in the United States—including homicide, theft, and assault—were using illegal drugs at the time of their arrest.

The number of crimes typically rises as drug use increases. Criminal activity is as much as two to three times higher among frequent users of cocaine and heroin than among irregular users or nonusers. Not surprisingly, an unusually high proportion of people in drug treatment programs report involvement in serious crimes. Treatment for substance abuse is often required as a condition in the legal processing of criminal cases.

Involvement in crime sometimes precedes drug use, but just as often drug use occurs before involvement in crime. However, frequent use of multiple drugs generally follows involvement in property crime, and its onset may speed up the development of a criminal career.

Frequently, drug users commit violent crimes to get money to buy drugs and support their drug use. However, the connection between violence and illegal drugs, as is seen in homicide, is more typically associated with the distribution and sale of drugs, or drug trafficking disagreements about drug transactions, and getting the competitive advantage over rival dealers, but not with the use of those drugs. However, the violence associated with alcohol is usually committed when either the offender, the victim, or both have used alcohol prior to the criminal event.

Box 1.5 Relationships Between Drug Use and Crime

Drugs and Crime Relationship	Definition	Examples
Drug-defined offenses	Violations of laws prohibiting or regulating the possession, use, distribution, or manufacture of illegal drugs.	Drug possession or use. Marijuana cultivation. Methamphetamine production. Cocaine, heroin, or marijuana sales.
Drug-related offenses	Offenses in which a drug's pharmacologic effects contribute; offenses motivated by the user's need for money to support continued use; and offenses connected with drug distribution.	Violent behavior resulting from drug effects. Stealing to get money to buy drugs. Violence against rival drug dealers.
Interactional circumstances	Drug use and crime are common aspects of a deviant lifestyle. The likelihood and frequency of involvement in illegal activity is increased because drug users and offenders are exposed to situations that encourage crime.	A life orientation with an emphasis on short-term goals supported by illegal activities. Opportunities to offend resulting from contacts with offenders and illegal markets. Criminal skills learned from other defenders.

Source: Bureau of Justice Statistics, U.S. Department of Justice.

Some drugs, particularly alcohol, cocaine, amphetamines, and PCP, increase the likelihood that users will act violently, but this drug-violence relationship is not especially strong, except in the case of alcohol use. Unlike the other psychoactive drugs, alcohol is the only one whose moderate use has been shown to commonly increase aggression in humans. Furthermore, alcohol also increases the likelihood that one will act impulsively, engage in risky behavior, respond violently to events, and be the victim of violent acts.

The Drug Scene: Prospects for the Future

The use of psychoactive drugs and the occurrence of substance abuse and chemical dependency among youth are often used to predict the extent of such problems in the near future. If such a relationship is accurate, then the years ahead will be filled with an abundance of psychoactive drugs and many drug-related problems.

Alcohol, tobacco, and other drug abuse among young Americans is staggering. Although the situation is not close to being solved, the years between 1981 and 1991 witnessed a downturn in the use of most illegal drugs among high school students and young adults. More American youths are choosing a drug-free lifestyle today than did their counterparts of the 1970s. But surveys conducted recently point to some alarming tendencies: increased experimentation once again with illegal drugs and a definite decline in negative attitudes toward or perceived risks of drug use and abuse.

Only the future will tell if the increase in use of specific illegal drugs is a temporary or permanent trend in our drug-using society. Four uncertain factors in predicting drug use and abuse patterns could play a major role in the drug scene of the future.

One factor in the prediction equation is the *role of parents who were drug users* during the 1960s, 1970s, and 1980s. Will they approve, encourage, discourage, or tolerate the use of marijuana, cocaine, alcohol, or some other drug by their children? It appears that many parents who smoked marijuana as teenagers are saying practically nothing about illegal drugs to their children. Expecting that their children will likely experiment with marijuana, some parents may not attach significant or even negative consequences to young peoples' use of mind-changing drugs. Perhaps some of these parents feel somewhat ambivalent about drugs or guilty about their drug use and are therefore fearful of engaging their children in serious conversation about lifestyle choices.

The second factor relates to *organized, national efforts to reduce the supply and demand of mind-changing chemicals,* especially the illegal ones. Some observers believe recent federal government efforts have not been forceful enough in discouraging illegal drug use and have not punished illegal drug users severely enough. Others question why so many schools continue to teach antidrug programs that have been evaluated as totally ineffective in reducing illegal drug usage among young people.

In addition, we are uncertain about the likelihood of success of U.S.A.-sponsored programs to eliminate or reduce the harvest and production of illegal drugs in countries such as Bolivia, Columbia, Mexico, and Thailand. We also do not know if worksite educational efforts and drug-testing programs to detect the use of psychoactive drugs will be effective in permanently lowering drug abuse or discouraging initial use of illicit drugs.

However, we do know that epidemics of drug abuse do not occur spontaneously. Law enforcement officials also know that early recognition of the spiraling stages of drug use can forestall the next likely events in a drug's developing use, if appropriate countermeasures are taken at the local community level.[24]

Also to be considered is a third factor, the *number of individuals who will perceive risks of and develop negative attitudes toward drugs.* The more an individual believes in the personally threatening and socially disrupting aspects of drug use, and the more firmly held those negative biases tend to be, the less likely there will be serious drug use by such a person, even if drugs are available and even with various pressures to use drugs.

The last factor in the prediction equation is the *success or failure of the continuing movement to legalize certain or all presently illegal psychoactives.* Viewing the present drug control strategy as law enforcement gone amok and a masked threat to democracy, some officials strongly support the case for legalizing all mind-altering substances. The citizens of several states have approved the medical use of marijuana. Some people view this as a first step toward the legalization of drugs, while others believe it is an enlightened approach to the management of certain diseases. Officials who oppose the legalization of drugs for any purpose see the drug control strategy as essential to the preservation of a safe, stable, and productive society.

Thus, the battle lines have been formed between those who believe the war on drugs has already been lost and those who maintain that present antidrug measures are working and are necessary to achieve alcohol- and drug-free schools and work environments.

It had been predicted that the 1980s revival of conservatism in national politics and traditional values among the general public would have a dampening effect on attitudes and practices regarding alcohol and drug abuse. The nation experienced a ten-year decline in alcohol and other drug abuse, but such a general trend is reversing among young people. The national commitment to dealing with problems of drug misuse, substance abuse, and addiction will likely continue and remain substantial. However, it is unlikely that the public desire to end drug problems will ever be fully realized. As long as Americans view the pursuit of pleasure and the avoidance of pain through drug use as personal rights, there will probably be serious drug problems in the United States.

Considering demographic data, rising concern for legal liability, the negative reaction to the increase in use of illegal drugs by young people, and the growing importance of health promotion and disease prevention, the author makes the following predictions about future drug policies and drug-taking practices.

1. There will likely be additional restrictions placed on tobacco smoking in public and sales to minors, with a further increase in taxes on both tobacco products and alcoholic beverages. Such actions will likely result in a further decline in the use of both legal drugs—nicotine and alcohol.
2. There will likely be periodic increases in the use of illegal psychoactive drugs, followed by declines in use after countermeasures are once again implemented.
3. There will likely be a limited tolerance of occasional adult use of currently illicit drugs, particularly marijuana. Such tolerance, however, will not be extended to the workplace or to those under the age of majority or to the public use of illegal drugs.
4. There will likely be no widespread legalization of currently illegal psychoactives—except for medical use of marijuana—despite federal and state flirtations with changes in present anti-drug-use laws and penalties.
5. There will likely be even stricter laws to curtail driving under the influence of alcohol, marijuana, and other mind-changing drugs and medicines. Further restrictions on the advertising of alcoholic beverages and tobacco products, along with stronger warning messages on beverage alcohol and tobacco containers, are anticipated. Drug-testing programs to discourage illegal drug use among the military, government employees, the workforce in private-sector business and industry, and among student-athletes could lower the demand for illegal psychoactives.
6. There will likely emerge a renewed national commitment to protect young people from exposure to drugs. This effort will be facilitated by a smaller number of young people in the total population, and by better-informed parents who will be enabled to take part in primary- and secondary-prevention activities. Additionally, there will likely be more effective school- and community-based education and intervention programs.

The drug scene will likely be marked by considerable, though evolving, change. Based upon the popularity of psychedelics in the 1960s; the widespread use of marijuana in the 1970s; the cocaine/crack cocaine epidemic of the 1980s; and the apparent resurgence of marijuana, psychedelics, and high-purity heroin in the 1990s, it is fairly certain that drug fashions will change and change again.

Chapter Summary

1. Widespread and persistent use of mind-changing drugs remains firmly entrenched in America. To counter the continuing personal and social costs of legal and illegal drug abuse, federal, state, and local governments have continued their war on drugs for nearly thirty years.
2. A drug is a substance that can change the structure or function of the body, while a medicine is a drug used in diagnosis, care, treatment, or prevention of disease.
3. Use and abuse of psychoactive chemicals often result in people problems involving physical and mental illness, drug dependency, disruption of relationships and family life, various forms of exploitation, impaired job performance, accidents, and even imprisonment.
4. Drug misuse involves the unintentional or inappropriate use of prescribed or nonprescribed medicine, whereas drug abuse is the deliberate use of chemical substances for reasons other than their intended

medical purposes, resulting in personal or social impairment.

5. Psychoactive drugs change thought, feelings, perceptions, and behavior and are specified as narcotics, depressants, stimulants, psychedelics, and inhalants.
6. Psychoactive drugs may be classified by their general or localized effects on the central nervous system, by their relative degree of medical usefulness and abuse potential, and by their potential for causing personal and social dangers.
7. Drug problems related to the use of psychoactive substances include delay in proper medical treatment; reduction in problem-solving effectiveness; experience of adverse reactions; the use of adulterated drugs; and increased risk of suicide and infection with HIV, the virus that causes AIDS.
8. Adverse reactions or conditions associated with psychoactive drug use are toxic reactions, panic, flashback, psychopathology, and drug dependence.
9. Premature deaths, health care costs, loss of productivity, and expenses related to crime and destruction of property are among the unanticipated consequences of psychoactive substance abuse. One other disturbing consequence of our illegal drug problem is criminal activity, which typically rises as drug use increases. Although complex, drug-crime relationships are expressed as drug-defined and drug-related offenses, and as interactional circumstances.
10. After a ten-year period of reduced illegal drug usage (from 1981–91), the current drug scene is characterized by increased use of nearly all illegal drugs and cigarettes by young people; emerging drugs, such as Rohypnol and natural stimulants; and hard core drug use often marked by addiction.
11. The drug scene of the future will likely be determined by the role of parents who used drugs in their youth; the adequacy of organized, nationwide efforts to reduce the supply and demand of psychoactive drugs; the degree to which people perceive risks and develop negative attitudes toward mind-changing drugs; and the success or failure of the movement to legalize psychoactive drugs.

World Wide Web Sites

University of Michigan Monitoring the Future (survey of drug use among secondary and college students and young adults)

www.isr.umich.edu

Web of Addictions: Fact Sheets (Facts on every psychoactive drug from various research institutions)

www.well.com/user/woa/facts.htm

National Institute on Drug Abuse: National Trends

www.nida.nih.gov/infofax/nationtrends.html

Review Questions and Activities

1. Explain how illegal chemical substances, legally produced medicines, and legal social drugs contribute to the current drug problem in America.
2. Describe our current drug problems as basic "people problems."
3. Distinguish between the following terms: *drug* and *medicine; drug misuse* and *drug abuse.*
4. Identify five major classification groups of psychoactive drugs based on their effects on the brain.
5. Survey class members to determine their use of psychoactive drugs purchased over-the-counter without a prescription. Do any of these OTC medicines have common drug ingredients? (Ask class members to write down the drugs listed on the label.)
6. Classify each of the following psychoactive drugs according to their *effects* on the central nervous system, their *ability to be purchased without a prescription,* the *provisions of the Controlled Substances Act,* and their potential for individual and social harm: beverage alcohol, nicotine in cigarettes, heroin, cocaine, marijuana, amphetamine, and LSD.
7. Identify the major health-related consequences often associated with drug-taking behavior.
8. Define each of the following terms in relation to psychoactive drug use: *toxic reaction, panic, flashback, psychopathology,* and *drug dependence.*
9. Describe the current drug scene in terms of psychoactive drugs used, involvement of young people, and extent of hard-core drug abuse.
10. Based upon your own knowledge and prediction ability, formulate a description of the American drug scene in the year 2005.

References

1. U.S. Department of Health and Human Services. Substance Abuse and Mental Health Administration. *Substance Abuse and Mental Health Statistics Sourcebook, 1998,* edited by Beatrice A. Rouse (Washington, D.C.: GPO, 1998)
2. Robert H. Coombs and Douglas Ziedonis, eds., *Handbook on Drug Abuse Prevention* (Boston: Allyn and Bacon, 1995), xiii.
3. Jill Smolowe, "Choose Your Poison," *Time.* 26 July 1993, 56–57.
4. Preface to "Political Pharmacology: Thinking about Drugs," *Daedalus* 121, no. 3 (summer, 1992): vi.
5. Avram Goldstein, *Addiction: From Biology to Drug Policy* (New York: W. H. Freeman and Company, 1994), 5–9.
6. George Gallup, Jr., as quoted in *Prevention Plus II: Tools for Creating and Sustaining Drug-Free Communities,* Office for Substance Abuse Prevention, DHHS Pub. No. (ADM) 89-1649 (Washington, D.C.: GPO, 1989), 2.
7. American Psychiatric Association, *Diagnostic and Statistical Manual of Mental Disorders.* 4th ed. (Washington, D.C.: American Psychiatric Association, 1994) 182–83.
8. Samuel Irwin, *Drugs of Abuse: An Introduction to Their Actions and Potential Hazards,* 11th ed. (Tempe: Do It Now Foundation, 1995), 29–33.

9. Irwin, *Drugs of Abuse,* 32.
10. Institute for Health Policy, Brandeis University, *Substance Abuse: The Nation's Number One Health Problem,* vol. 8 (Princeton, N. J.: Robert Wood Johnson Foundation, 1993).
11. Darryl Inaba and William Cohen, *Uppers, Downers. All Arounders,* 2d ed. (Ashland, Ore.: CNS Productions, 1993), 322–24.
12. U.S. Public Health Service, *Healthy People 2000: National Health Promotion and Disease Prevention Objectives,* Summary Report (Boston: Jones & Bartlett, 1992), 17. Reprinted from DHHS Publication No. (PHS) 91-50213.
13. Sidney Cohen, *The Substance Abuse Problem Vol. 2: New Issues for the 1980s* (New York: Haworth Press, 1985), 113.
14. Gail Gleason Milgram and the Editors of Consumer Reports Books, *The Facts about Drinking* (Mount Vernon, N. Y.: Consumers Union, 1990), 57.
15. Abram S. Benenson, ed., *Control of Communicable Diseases Manual,* 16th ed (Washington, D.C.: American Public Health Association, 1995), 4.
16. Centers for Disease Control and Health Promotion, "U.S. HIV and AIDS Cases Reported through December, 1995," *HIV/ AIDS Surveillance Report* 7, no. 2 (1996): 10.
17. Don des Jarlais and Dana E. Hunt, "AIDS and Intravenous Drug Use," *National Institute of Justice AIDS Bulletin,* February 1988, 2.
18. Richard E. Chaisson and others, "Cocaine Use and HIV Infection in Intravenous Drug Users in San Francisco," *Journal of the American Medical Association* 261, no. 4 (27 January 1989): 561–65.
19. Dale D. Chitwood and others, "HIV Seropositivity of Needles from Shooting Galleries in South Florida," *American Journal of Public Health* 80, no. 2 (February 1990): 150–52.
20. Barry Stimmel and the Editors of Consumer Reports Books, *The Facts about Drug Use: Coping with Drugs and Alcohol in Your Family, at Work, in Your Community* (New York: Haworth Medical Press, 1993), 271–73; National Institute on Alcohol Abuse and Alcoholism, "Alcohol and AIDS," *Alcohol Alert* no. 15, PH 311 (January 1992): 1–4; Omar Bagasra and others, "Alcohol Intake Increases Human Immunodeficiency Virus Type I Replication in Human Peripheral Blood Mononuclear Cells," *Journal of Infectious Diseases* 167, no. 4 (April 1993): 789–97.
21. Donald I. Abrams, "The Nature of AIDS," in *Acquired Immune Deficiency Syndrome and Chemical Dependency* (Washington, D.C.: GPO, 1988), 3–14; and Rob Roy MacGregor, "Alcohol and the Immune System," in *Acquired Immune Deficiency and Chemical Dependency* (Washington, D.C.: GPO, 1988), 31–41.
22. Office of National Drug Control Policy, *Pulse Check: National Trends in Drug Abuse* (Washington, D.C.: Executive Office of the President, 1996); Office of National Drug Control Policy, *The National Drug Control Strategy: 1996* (Washington, D.C.: Executive Office of the President, 1996); National Institute on Drug Abuse, *The Monitoring the Future Study,* conducted by the Institute for Social Research, The University of Michigan (Washington, D.C.: GPO, 1995); "Substance Abuse News Briefs: Teenage Drug Use Still on the Rise," *Substance Abuse Report* XXVII, no. 1 (1 January 1996): 7; Center on Addiction and Substance Abuse at Columbia University, *Substance Abuse and The American Woman* (New York: The National Center on Addiction and Substance Abuse, 1996); Selected newspaper articles and reports of surveys conducted by the Centers for Disease Control and Health Promotion, the Gallup Poll, the National Institute on Alcohol Abuse and Alcoholism, the National Institute on Drug Abuse, and the National Institute of Justice; and Center on Addiction, *Substance Abuse.*
23. Fred W. Garcia, "Farewell," *Prevention Pipeline* 9, no. 2 (March/April, 1996): 5–7.
24. Marcia Chaiken, "Can Drug Epidemics Be Anticipated?" *National Institute of Justice Journal* no. 226 (April 1993): 23–30.

Chapter 2

The allure of drugs

Origins of drug-taking behavior

KEY TERMS

Agent-Related Etiology
Altered Conscious Experience
Coping
Decreased Awareness
Demographics
Enabling Factors
Endemic Drug Use
Environment-Related Etiology
Etiology
Genetic Predisposition
Host-Related Etiology
Increased Awareness
Modeling
Multifactorial Theory
Peer-Group Influence
Predisposing Factors
Reinforcing Factors
Risk Factor
Social Drug
Youth Rebellion

chapter objectives

After you have studied this chapter, you should be able to do the following:

1. Define the key terms.
2. Discuss the origins of drug-taking behavior in terms of altering emotional states.
3. Distinguish between increased awareness and decreased awareness in relation to use of drugs.
4. Explain how young people are "taught to use and abuse drugs" by adults.
5. Distinguish between youth rebellion and pursuit of recreation as factors motivating drug abuse among young people.
6. Analyze drug-taking behavior according to predisposing, enabling, and reinforcing factors.
7. Explain why adolescents are particularly susceptible to the beginning of drug-taking behavior.
8. Discuss the role of psychoactive drug use in the process of coping and adjusting to stress.
9. Explain drug use as a possible reflection of preexisting personality difficulties.
10. Distinguish between factors of availability and accessibility as they pertain to enabling drug use and abuse.
11. Identify two pharmacological effects of addicting drugs that foster the continuation of drug abuse.
12. Explain the role of drug reinforcers in the pleasure-motivated use of psychoactive drugs.
13. Identify at least five functional aspects of psychoactive-drug-taking behavior.
14. Explain how the following factors could influence drug use: the changing composition of a nation's population; the women's movement; adverse economic conditions; and an emphasis on a natural lifestyle.
15. Describe the influence of the peer group on the use of psychoactive drugs.
16. Identify two possible effects of media drug advertising on the use and abuse of psychoactive substances.
17. Compare and contrast agent-related, host-related, and environment-related etiological factors in drug abuse and drug dependence.

Why People Use and Abuse Drugs

Most behavioral scientists agree that there is no single explanation for drug-taking behavior. While any drug is usually taken or used for some immediate benefit or advantage, it is likely that a combination of several predisposing factors contribute to the use of legal "recreational" drugs and to the illegal and nonmedical use of psychoactive substances.

Drug-taking behavior that occurs again and again despite numerous unfavorable consequences to individuals and society has also confused researchers for many years. There are various educated guesses to explain the continuing use and abuse of mind-altering chemicals that appear to produce many problems. Nevertheless, there is considerable agreement that the factors responsible for beginning nonmedical use of drugs are often quite different from those that produce extended use.[1]

Altered Consciousness

Perhaps the primary reason so many people seek out and take psychoactive drugs is to change their own awareness or conscious experience.[2] Typically, they want to have a good time, feel good, relax, get away from stress, lessen boredom, fit in and be accepted, feel less lonely, relieve emotional and physical pain, seek greater insight, and explore the unknown universe. In some ways, this search for an **altered conscious experience** to feel different may be an acquired motivation similar to the basic drives of hunger, thirst, and even sex.[3]

Although there are many ways to change or alter one's consciousness—praying, exercising, dancing, making love, and skydiving are a few—psychoactive drugs provide an easy and relatively quick way to achieve this goal. The altered consciousness consists of some change in thinking, feeling, perceiving, or behaving. Moreover, this change in awareness is often marked by feelings of euphoria, lightness, self-transcendence, concentration, and energy.[4]

Another reason for drug use and abuse originates in the historical search for pleasure and relief from pain in a harsh environment. Certain drugs serve as popular and readily available agents for temporarily achieving **increased awareness,** a form of psychic stimulation allowing for variations in thought processes, ideas, and even behaviors.

However, others increasingly view the abuse of alcohol and other drugs as having deep social roots. Drug-taking behavior may be an effort to adjust to a variety of environmental challenges, often ending in **decreased awareness.** This state or condition of decreased awareness represents an escape from reality and a desire for total narcosis. Here, too, drugs are convenient agents for changing mood and behavior—to feel less pain, to get relief, to feel nothing.

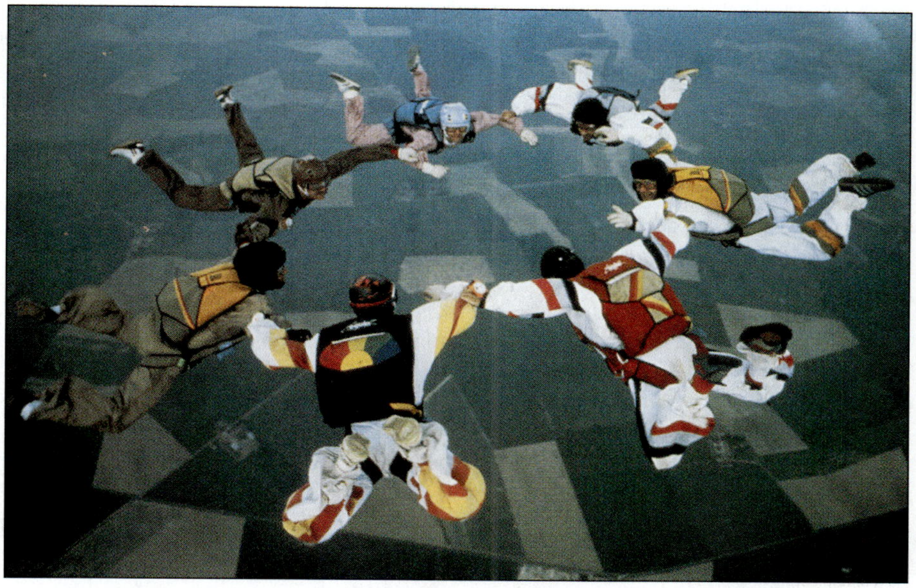

Skydiving, making love, praying and exercising are some of the ways people change or alter their consciousness. Psychoactive drugs also offer an easy and relatively quick way to achieve such a goal, but this form of "flying high" can be potentially more dangerous.

© G. Savage/Vantstadt/Photo Researchers, Inc.

Social Definition of Drug Abuse

America's drug problems are also related to socially defined attitudes, values, and behavioral norms regarding drugs and their perceived usefulness. For example, in America there is no widely held, consistent agreement on the acceptability or unacceptability of drug usage. While millions of people engage in legal alteration of consciousness by drinking, smoking, and pill taking, many others—including these same drug users—adamantly oppose the nonmedical use of illegal drugs. Apparently, approved or "appropriate" drug use is still more closely related "to how a drug is obtained and the purpose for which it is used rather than to its effects."[5]

Before 1960, much of the illegal and nonmedical use of drugs was thought to occur among criminals, the urban poor, and nonwhites. These population groups were considered to be dangerous and a threat to the social and moral order.

When illegal drug use spread to white, middle- and upper-class youths in the early 1960s, the public definition of "appropriate" drug use was changed slightly and temporarily to embrace marijuana. Several states even decriminalized the possession of relatively small amounts of marijuana for an individual's private use. However, with the dramatic increase in recreational illicit drug use during the 1970s, the nation adopted a "zero tolerance" policy in the 1980s and these states have increased the penalties for possession of marijuana.

Such unusual perceptions and interpretations of various drugs, how they are obtained, why they are used, and who uses them are reflected in various social applications: contradictory and unenforceable drug laws, ambiguous messages subtly conveyed about the desirability of altered states of consciousness, and the toleration of social disorganization resulting from legalized drug use.

Perhaps an underlying issue that society must face is whether there is such a thing as responsible drug use as distinguished from irresponsible use and how such responsible use should be defined. Even if this issue and other related ones are ever resolved, the origin of drug problems will likely be found to be as much in the collectively held attitudes and values of society as in the individual drug takers or their psychoactive chemicals.

At Issue

Is intoxication a basic human need?

Point: The human pursuit of intoxication (i.e., drug-induced altered consciousness) is a universal drive as basic as hunger and thirst. People of all ages throughout history have enjoyed altering their consciousness, naturally and chemically, just as little children like to spin around until they are dizzy and disoriented. Some respected scientists believe that humans have a natural need to change their awareness from time to time, in response to a harsh or boring environment, or in an effort to decrease feelings of fatigue, tension, and anxiety. Just as important, intoxication can enhance or enliven our experiences and vitalize our own perceptions. Intoxication can also be a unifying symbol, a temporary condition encouraging solidarity and social relationships with fellow drug users. The desired effects of taking mind-changing drugs can be an exhilarating experience with new and unique psychic characteristics.

Counterpoint: To describe intoxication as a desirable and basic human need is ridiculous and tragic. Such a concept runs counter to the traditions of Western civilization that emphasize the importance of human reasoning, decision-making ability, and the wisdom of maintaining rational control over human behavior. To become intoxicated with drugs impairs these distinctly human abilities. Moreover, there is not a single anticipated effect of intoxication that cannot be achieved through natural highs, including meditation and prayer. Major religions of the world oppose intoxication and drunkenness because such conditions of impairment interfere with the creator-creature relationship. Moreover, there is also potential danger that any drug used continuously to achieve intoxication for whatever reason will impede psychological and spiritual growth and possibly result in drug dependence.

A Drug for Every Ailment

Although drug taking has typically been associated with a rebellion of youth against authority, drug usage is more accurately an imitation of adult behavior. Repeatedly, young people see adults treating their symptoms, using liquor, coffee, tobacco, and various medicines to change their moods; to be comforted; and to escape from pain or other irritations. Thus, the achievement of instant relief through medication and the promises of a happy, painless solution to every problem are not creations of the youth culture. The older generation has set an example with its overflowing medicine cabinets, the suggestion that for every ailment there is a drug to cure it and the basic denial of anxiety, worry, and depression as normal feelings. In effect, suffering and pain have lost their cultural significance. With pain now being so easy to kill, it appears rational to flee from it rather than face it, even at the cost of addiction.[6]

In a true sense, the adult "teachers" have been most effective; the young "students" have learned their lessons well. Increasingly, and with few exceptions, both groups subscribe to the idea that existence without drugs is impossible. We turn to drugs to solve, even if only temporarily, a myriad of internal problems.

Also contributing to this growing reliance on drugs are the technology of the pharmaceutical industry, the subtle compliance of medical practitioners, and the often unreasonable expectations of many patients. Modern drug therapy is characterized by the new "wonder drugs" introduced each year, a vast increase in drug promotion through advertising to physicians and patients, and the tendency of the public and the medical profession to rely on medication for nearly every physical and mental problem. The modern physician's role is to get the right drug to the right patient in time for the medicine to do some good.[7] Recently, media print and television advertising of prescription drugs has created an informed group of consumers who demand specific drugs from their physicians.

Rebellion Against the Establishment Versus Recreational Use

Beginning in the 1960s, drug use among middle-class youth increased substantially and was viewed typically as a "chemical cop-out." This drug use may have symbolized a **youth rebellion** that was a generational process over independence, a common confrontation between parent and child. Adolescents, perceiving adults to be living sterile, pointless, and insignificant lives, sought to be as unlike their parents as possible. This they achieved through the hallucinogenic, mind-expanding drugs in their search for new levels of consciousness, understanding, self-analysis, and communication. Illegal drug use was also an attempt to test parental tolerance, concern, and maybe even interest.

It is unlikely that rebellion against and alienation from parents and authority alone can explain the continued use of illegal and recreational drugs at present. It is fairly certain that much of the drug usage today is motivated by self-indulgence, a desire to feel better, an attempt to escape from boredom or routine, and perceived social pressure. In essence, using drugs for recreation.

Using and Abusing Drugs: A Behavioral Analysis

Why individuals use drugs and abuse chemical substances remains somewhat a mystery. Those who study drug-taking behavior suggest that complex physical, psychological, and social factors interact to convert nonusers into users and experimental users into frequent abusers. One model proposed to explore health behav-

Box 2.1 A Conceptual Model for Analyzing Determining Factors in the Use and Abuse of Psychoactive Drugs

Predisposing Influences (Susceptibility)	Enabling Influences (Facilitation)	Reinforcing Influences (Encouragement)
Attitudes about drugs and the "quick fix"	Availability of drugs	Alteration of consciousness, increased awareness and unawareness
Demographics and sociocultural influences		
Adolescence	Accessibility to drugs	Experience of pleasure
Myths about drugs	Ineffective legal deterrence	Task accomplishment
Personality and coping	Lack of social controls	Social and peer-group pressure
Unique psychological characteristics	Inability to say "no" to experimentation	Advertising and media programming about drug taking
Social changes and conflicts	Effects of addicting drugs: withdrawal, depression, and mental impairment	Family dynamics
Heredity	Actions of the "enabler"	Influence of modeling
Family: psychological aspects	Family interference with treatment of drug abuser	

The three basic categories of determinants (predisposing, enabling, and reinforcing) should not be viewed as separate or discrete influences in the use and abuse of psychoactive drugs. Rather, they might be considered more appropriately as interdependent, interconnected, and even supplementary. As such, the three categories portray drug-taking behavior as the result of many diverse and interrelated factors that initiate and perpetuate drug use and drug abuse. Can you identify additional factors in each category?

iors considers **predisposing, enabling,** and **reinforcing factors.**[8] Such a model will be used in this chapter to analyze various internal and external forces, motivations, attitudes, demographic variables, and influences of individuals and institutions in the use and abuse of psychoactive drugs (see box 2.1).

Predisposing Factors in the Use and Abuse of Drugs

The factors in this category collectively contribute to drug-taking behavior and include the existing knowledge base of individuals, their beliefs, attitudes, and those human characteristics that make them particularly susceptible or inclined in advance to use and abuse drugs.

Demographics and Sociocultural Influences

Demographics Demographics are distinct social characteristics and vital statistics of human populations. They provide a unique insight into various predisposing forces that appear to determine or strongly influence the use or nonuse of alcohol and other drugs. Specific demographics, based on studies of large populations of Americans, are:[9]

Age and gender. Younger people drink and use drugs more often than older people. Males typically drink more often than women at any age level, and men are much more likely than women to abuse psychoactive drugs. However, younger women are rapidly closing this gender gap.

Family structure. Single and divorced people tend to drink more heavily, all things being equal, than married people, however, marital instability does not always lead to increased usage.

Income. The more affluent individuals, in terms of real family income, typically drink more than the less affluent.

Education. Education tends to lower the likelihood that a person would use drugs. College-educated people might be expected to have a lower incidence of substance abuse, yet individuals who finish any educational program—eighth grade, high school, or college—have lower rates of alcoholism than "noncompleters" who begin the next level of education but drop out before finishing the program.

Employment. About 6 percent of employed adults (eighteen years of age and older) currently use drugs, compared with nearly 12 percent of the unemployed. However, because so many more people have jobs, about 71 percent of current drug users are employed.

Sociocultural Influences Whether youth-oriented television, movies, and concerts influence group and individual drug-taking behavior or merely reflect current practices, there is a growing impression that the "drug culture" is staging a return.[10] After more than ten years in which illegal psychoactive drugs were negatively portrayed, musical groups, television programs, movies, and even fashion apparel have recreated a popular culture that once again glorifies and promotes the use of psychoactive drugs.

For example, despite a television advertising ban on tobacco products, scenes of cigarette smoking have increased in programming.

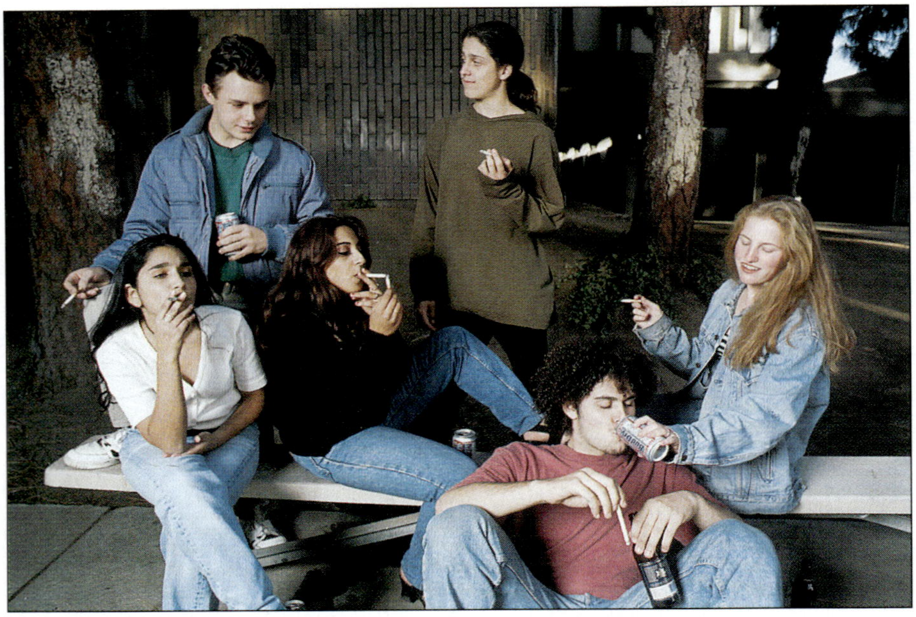

If you look carefully, you can detect two of the so-called "gateway drugs" being used by these young people. The traditional entry substances to drug-taking behavior are being used at increasingly younger ages, often beginning during middle school.

© *Michael Newman/PhotoEdit*

Adolescence

Individuals are not born as drug users and nonmedical use of chemical substances during infancy and early childhood is still considered abnormal, so the initial experimentation and subsequent, more regular patterns of drug use typically occur during adolescence. Moreover, the traditional entry substances to drug taking continue to be tobacco, alcohol, marijuana, and inhalants—the so-called gateway drugs.

Tobacco use usually begins by age fourteen.[11] Almost all first use occurs before graduation from high school. By contrast, most students are between twelve and thirteen years old when they take their first alcoholic drink.[12] It is apparent that the period of greatest risk for beginning the use of tobacco and alcohol is during early adolescence, often when children are entering junior high school. For too many youths, the use of alcohol and other drugs begins during the elementary school years.

Some authorities believe that limited drug use is a "normal part" of growing up because experimentation with numerous chemical substances is commonly reported and experienced among adolescents. For some, early experimental drug use is equated with "coming of age in America," a rite of passage marking one's entry into adulthood and departure from childhood.

Indeed, one study confirms the idea that drug experimentation can be a normal adolescent development and need not lead to long-term catastrophic consequences.[13] The majority of adolescent experimenters do not go on to become drug abusers.

However, other research has demonstrated that the younger persons are when they first use a drug, including alcohol (outside the context of medical treatment and/or limited family or religious rituals), the more likely they are to have alcohol and other drug problems. Consequently, those who first use beverage alcohol in a peer setting at ages twelve to thirteen are far more likely to have drug problems with alcohol than are young people who first use alcohol at age twenty-one.[14]

The teen and preteen years are times of exploring new ideas, fast learning, and risk taking.[15] Young people exhibit an excessive drive in their pursuit of new and novel sensations and stimulation. Experimenting with an expanded range of behaviors and lifestyles is often viewed as part of the natural process of separating from parents and developing a sense of independence and personal identity. At the same time, adolescents tend to develop an increased sense of concern with their own appearance and abilities—described as "adolescent egocentrism." These two conditions make teenagers especially vulnerable to the influences of peer groups.

Young people often accept dares to try the untried, including mind-altering drugs. They are known for their willingness to take risks; they have not yet mastered control over their impulses. Oriented to the here and now, many adolescents look for immediate satisfaction and cannot tolerate frustration. The emphasis is on having fun now, not on the probable or possible future consequences related to using chemical substances.

When confronted with the possibility of adverse effects due to using nonmedical drugs, adolescents tend to be underconcerned with such effects and overestimate their ability to avoid harmful, destructive patterns of drug and alcohol use. They are, after all, "immortal and invulnerable." They may also begin to see the evident contradictions and inconsistencies in the arguments of parents and other authority figures who counsel against the use of mind-changing substances.

In an attempt to prevent alcohol and other drug use among young people, possible risk factors have been studied for many years. **Risk factors** are conditions or characteristics that, when present, increase the probability of psychoactive drug use.

One study indicted that there are risk factors for substance abuse and other delinquent behavior in all areas of an adolescent's life, including the community,

table 2.1 Risk Factors for Adolescent Problem Behaviors

Risk Factors	Adolescent Problem Behaviors: Substance Abuse	Delinquency	Teen Pregnancy	School Drop-Out	Violence
Community					
Availability of drugs	✔				
Availability of firearms		✔			✔
Community laws and norms favorable toward drug use, firearms, and crime	✔	✔			✔
Media portrayals of violence					✔
Transitions and mobility	✔	✔		✔	
Low neighborhood attachment and community disorganization	✔	✔			✔
Extreme economic deprivation	✔	✔	✔	✔	✔
Family					
Family history of the problem behavior	✔	✔	✔	✔	
Family management problems	✔	✔	✔	✔	✔
Family conflict	✔	✔	✔	✔	✔
Favorable parental attitudes and involvement in the problem behavior	✔	✔			✔
School					
Early and persistent antisocial behavior	✔	✔	✔	✔	✔
Academic failure beginning in elementary school	✔	✔	✔	✔	✔
Lack of commitment to school	✔	✔	✔	✔	
Individual/Peer					
Alienation and rebelliousness	✔	✔		✔	
Friends who engage in a problem behavior	✔	✔	✔	✔	✔
Favorable attitudes toward the problem behavior	✔	✔	✔	✔	
Early initiation of the problem behavior	✔	✔	✔	✔	✔
Constitutional factors	✔	✔			✔

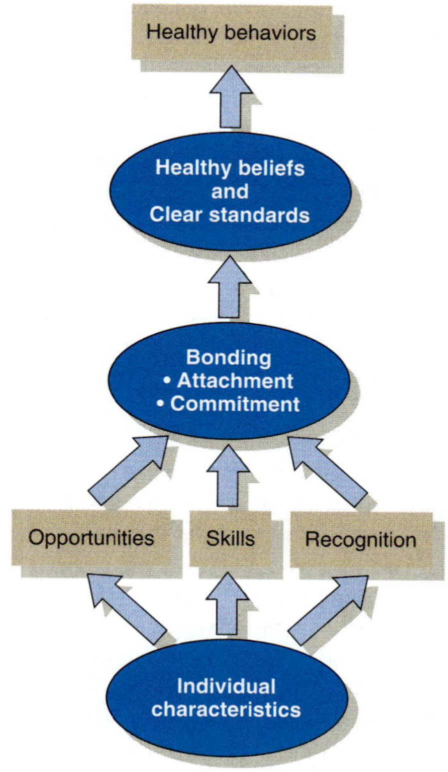

figure 2.1

Protective factors for healthy behavior.

From Communities That Care. © *1990–1999. Reprinted with permission from Developmental Research and Programs, Inc., Seattle, WA, at* www.drp.org.

family, school, peer relationships, and personality characteristics (see table 2.1). Equally important is that there are protective factors in each of these areas, which can be fostered by parents, school personnel, and the community (see fig. 2.1). The presence of any or all of these risk factors does not mean that substance abuse will take place, the absence of these risk factors does not mean that substance abuse will take place, and the absence of these risk factors does not indicate that there won't be substance abuse. In all likelihood, drug use develops from the interaction of multiple personal and environmental factors.[16]

Curiosity

Basic curiosity has attracted many people into the arena of drug use. The potential for partaking in the novel, the possibility for untried delights, and the promise of profound and unpredictable effects have lured many individuals into drug experimentation.

Personality and Coping

Coping is a term for various methods or techniques used to adjust—to accommodate to the demands of stress and daily living without being overwhelmed.

Psychoactive drugs, especially alcohol, tobacco, and marijuana, are often used as a coping method in dealing with problems of personal identity, self-esteem, boredom, family discord, academic pressures, and chronic depression. In some instances, drug abuse is related to asserting independence or more simply a self-indulgent desire for well-being. In fact, various pills, booze, tobacco, and pot appear to resolve these stress-generating problems, at least temporarily.

These drugs, therefore, are convenient tools in the search for relief, escape, love, security, and power.

One of the dangers associated with any drug taken for coping purposes is that its prolonged use tends to undermine self-esteem and personal power. Temporary feelings of enhanced power, confidence, security, and even creativity are assigned to the drug rather than to the self. As the drug is credited for its beneficial effects, drug takers tend to confirm their own personal deficiencies and thereby prolong their dependence on chemicals. Now the drug takers are less powerful than the drug, and their feelings of personal adequacy plunge even lower. This situation results in more drug taking in an attempt to resolve personal inadequacy.

Although the foregoing discussion has dealt with drug use in the search for personal and social adjustment, research also reveals that drug use may be a symptom of personality characteristics. In comparison with those who are not preoccupied with drugs, drug users often display high novelty-seeking tendencies, high risk-taking behavior, and little or no need for praise or approval. Such individuals tend to be impulsive. They like to try exciting and dangerous things and do not worry about the consequences of their high-risk behavior. Moreover, personality factors such as rebelliousness; orientation toward independence; low self-concept; alienation; and a high tolerance of deviance have also been related to drug use, especially among youth.[17]

Despite extensive studies linking various personality traits to a predisposition for heavy alcohol and other drug use as well as for addiction, no general "addictive personality" seems to exist.[18] Each addiction and each drug-use problem is different from the next; each individual's personality and drug-using circumstances differ from the next person's.

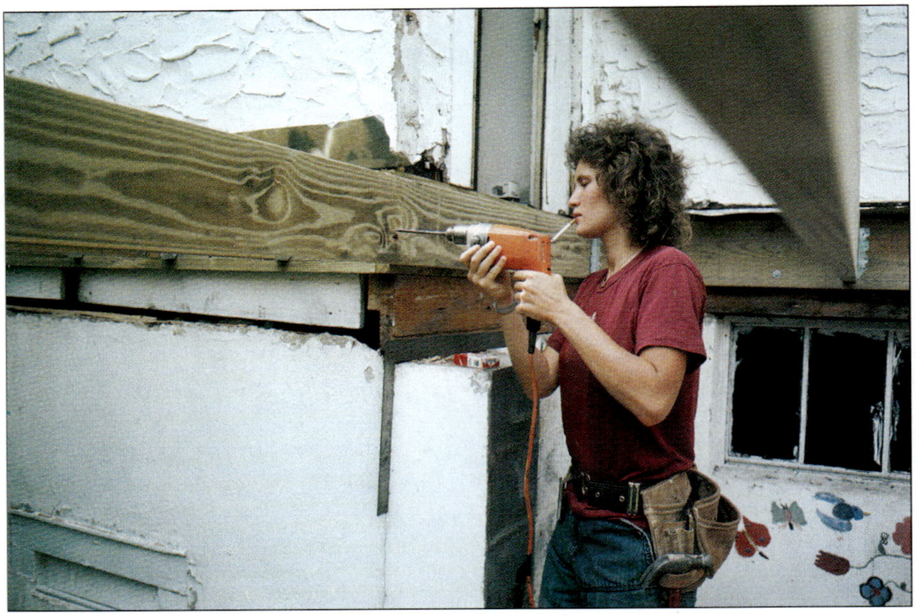

Psychoactive drugs, including tobacco, are often used as a coping method in dealing with the demands of daily living and high-stress jobs. Sometimes, such use leads to involvement in the addiction cycle.

© Richard Hutchings/PhotoEdit

Changes and Conflicts in Society

The use of drugs has been related to their availability. This availability will likely grow as the increase of new medications continues and the reservoir of misused and abused drugs expands with the aid of innovative designer drugs, adulterated substances, diverted pharmaceuticals, and the latest concoctions of "kitchen chemists."

The epidemic use of drugs has evolved into a type of **endemic drug use,** a situation in which a significant yet declining number of people engage in semitolerated forms of drug-taking behavior on a continuing basis. As such, endemic use of alcohol and other drugs will not likely disappear in America, where it has become something of a tradition.[19]

However, as with most social phenomena, drug use will likely persist, decline, or even increase as a consequence of several notable and predisposing forces:[20]

1. *The changing composition of the nation's population.* With fewer young people in proportion to the growing numbers of the elderly, the drug-abuse potential may decline while drug misuse and medication errors increase.
2. *The women's movement.* Females are adopting more behaviors previously defined as masculine. As women smoke more cigarettes and drink more alcoholic beverages, their incidence of lung cancer and alcoholism accelerates. With equality in the realm of socially approved drug use has come the gender-equal penalty of disease.
3. *The possibility of adverse economic conditions.* Declines in economic conditions carry the potential for future epidemics of drug abuse. Although the most recent epidemic began in the relative economic affluence of the 1960s, the upsurge of drug usage coincided with the social protest of the Vietnam War era. Will new economic depressions bring about another increase in illicit drug use? If large numbers of individuals feel alienated from the greater society, because of unemployment and its consequences of depersonalization and dehumanization, they may seek comfort in psychoactive chemicals.
4. *The new emphasis on natural and healthful lifestyles.* As more individuals engage in health-promoting and disease-preventing activities, rates of drug misuse and abuse will likely decline. Fewer drugs will be consumed as negative attitudes toward them emerge.

Confronted by a confusing future, certain to be marked by more change and conflict, individuals respond to such crises with a variety of adjustive responses. Common options include constructive or destructive rebellion, regression and personality disorders, passive acceptance or passive withdrawal, and preoccupation with the experience of the present. Drug taking accompanies and sometimes facilitates such responses. Predictably, psychoactive substances will remain available for various reasons—to promote social interactions; stimulate artistic creativity; enhance physical performance; treat illnesses; relieve pain; escape from boredom and stress; function in religious ceremonies; alter human emotional states; heighten pleasure; and satisfy the human needs to relax, delude, arouse, destroy, and fantasize.[21]

Heredity

Although genetic transmission is not considered a predisposing factor in the initiation of using psychoactive drugs, heredity is thought to play a significant role in alcoholism, one of many drug dependencies and clearly a form of substance abuse.[22] Researchers have established an association between a "dopamine receptor gene" and alcoholism.[23] While this initial association has not yet been supported by other research, such a finding indicates that an abnormality in a specific gene may cause susceptibility to at least one subtype of alcoholism. Although surprisingly strong, this genetic link has not been proven to cause alcoholism. Nevertheless, the development of alcoholism is not only a case of genetics versus the environment; it is definitely one of genetics *and* the environment.[24]

Precisely how **genetic predisposition** combines with environmental influences in the development of alcoholism has not yet been completely determined. The leading explanations center around specific variations in nerve cell or membrane function, sensitivity to alcohol's effects, and brain-wave patterns. Such inherited variations likely result in a neurochemical vulnerability to alcoholism.

While evidence of a genetic component in alcoholism has been established, there is no direct indication that heredity is also a contributing factor in other forms of psychoactive drug abuse. However, genetics may be a determining factor in individual responsiveness to specific mind-changing chemicals and other drugs. Such hereditary influences could explain why some people are more sensitive than other people to drug effects, and therefore more susceptible to certain drug dependencies.

There is also the possibility that some common genetic defect—perhaps a neurochemical deficiency—will be found to be the basis for drug dependencies. If such a susceptibility is inherited, then the absence of the basic neurochemical defect might suggest that some resistance to drug dependence is inherited too.

Enabling Factors in the Use and Abuse of Drugs

In this second category are those factors that enable, facilitate, or make possible drug-taking behavior and substance abuse. Common enabling forces include the availability of both legal and illegal psychoactives, accessibility to various mind-changing drugs, actions of community and government agencies, and various skills or lack thereof possessed by the potential drug user or drug abuser.

Availability

It is often claimed that without drugs there would be no drug use or abuse. Certainly the presence of psychoactive drugs is an important enabling factor that allows people to engage in drug-taking behavior and sustain certain consequences of that behavior. For instance, while there is no evidence in the United States that a greater number of outlets selling beverage alcohol causes new drinking, several studies indicate that a lower minimum drinking age does lead to greater accident and fatality rates among young people who have been drinking and driving.[25]

After a recent ten-year decline in casual use, illegal drug consumption is rising again and such mind-changing chemicals as marijuana, LSD, and amphetamines are plentiful and widely available. Each year billions of gallons of beverage alcohol, billions of tobacco cigarettes, and at least three billion doses of illegal drugs are consumed for nonmedical reasons. Each year American drug problems remain at epidemic levels. Many people believe that whenever the nonmedical use of mind-changing drugs in any society becomes significant, there will likely be significant drug problems.

Accessibility

Until thirty-five years ago, most persons, including the young, could easily obtain only three major psychoactive substances: alcohol; tobacco products; and intoxicating inhalants, such as gasoline and airplane glue. Numerous other legal and illegal substances were available, but use of such mind-changers was usually confined to small population subgroups. Young people did not have money to buy illegal drugs; strict parental supervision did not permit or allow drug usage, though beer drinking and cigarette smoking were often tolerated if not approved; and fear of getting caught by police officials was somewhat higher than today. In brief, most people, especially the young, could not obtain illegal drugs even if they were available.

Growing up safely and soberly is not so simple at present in America. Affluence has made expensive drugs obtainable, and expanded production and distribution have made them more affordable.

Social and Institutional Deficiencies

Among the more subtle enabling factors in drug-taking behavior and substance abuse are the inadequacy of legal deterrence and the absence of drug-use standards or guides. Many people perceive the prohibitions and penalties associated with illegal drug use as largely ineffective. Getting caught is no longer viewed so negatively, rather, it is commonly seen as an unfair intrusion into the private pursuit of pleasure. The person who gets caught is merely unlucky and unfortunate. There is a relatively low risk of getting caught violating most drug-use laws.

In addition, few guidelines have been adopted to bring social controls to drug-taking behavior. There appears to be continuing fear of doing cocaine, especially crack cocaine, but marijuana, smoked and snorted heroin, and LSD have resurfaced as drugs of choice, largely because their methods of use are considered safe ways to avoid transmission of the AIDS virus. Regarding alcohol, there is only a slowly evolving consensus about the meaning of reduced-risk use. Guidelines that discourage heavy consumption of alcohol, reject intoxication, and promote the social use of alcohol (rather than binge drinking to get drunk) have attracted only a minority of youthful drinkers.

Those who promote "responsible usage" of illegal drugs—responsible decisions and actions that could reduce many of the unwanted consequences of taking psychoactives—are criticized for encouraging general use of alcohol and other drugs or, at least, unlawful behavior. The prevailing attitude among the general public is that the individuals who use illegal psychoactives deserve the difficulties they experience, and that they should be punished for criminal activity. Such a belief contributes to many other problems that usually accompany substance abuse—such as the need to build more jails and prisons in which to incarcerate drug offenders, thus raising taxes, and the higher level of HIV transmission that results when needle exchange programs are prohibited, thus increasing government-funded hospital costs for AIDS patients.

Personal and Professional Deficiencies

As research revealed the general ineffectiveness of many drug education programs, it became apparent that many young people started using drugs because they had never acquired skills for dealing with peer pressure or feelings of personal and social insecurity. Children often feel that personal value and significance are measured by group conformity, which frequently includes taking drugs. Young people choose to say "yes" to drugs because of the power of this peer pressure and the perceived rewards of drug use. They probably have the skills to say "no," however, they need to be given more persuasive reasons to do so.

A little-discussed enabling factor that contributes to drug abuse is inadequate physician training and care of patients. Many who experience long-lasting pain, stress, or tension, and many "hidden" or undiscovered alcoholics, are treated with psychoactive therapeutic medications, particularly antianxiety medications and sedative-hypnotics. Without proper medical diagnosis and careful treatment management skills, physicians sometimes unwittingly promote chronic drug dependencies in their patients.

Peculiar Effects of Drugs

Not to be overlooked as a decisive factor in the continuing use of specific psychoactive chemicals is the pharmacology (effects or actions) of drugs. Drug users often persist in the use/abuse cycle because withdrawal symptoms and afteruse depression are too severe to endure. Drugs are taken to avoid the drastic changes in physical functioning and behavior experienced in alcohol withdrawal, to feel normal again in heroin withdrawal, and to escape the posthigh depression found in cocaine addicts deprived of their drug supply.

Others who are mentally impaired by the effects of drugs such as alcohol can no longer evaluate the seriousness of their problem-producing drinking behavior. They continue to drink because they no longer have control over the drug. Now the drug controls the user, and the substance abuse persists.

Enabling Process

In nearly every case of drug abuse, including alcoholism, the drug-dependent individual has a supporting cast of actors and actresses—essentials in most stage plays and theatrical performances. However, in this real-life drama, the supporting cast assumes the role of an *enabler,* who effectively protects the dependent person from the natural and logical consequences of drug abuse and thereby contributes to a worsening of the disease.

Usually, enabling behavior is well-intentioned, sincere, and motivated by a sense of love and loyalty. Fear, shame, and desire for family self-preservation are other motivations behind enabling. Through the enabling process, the many physical, social, occupational, and economic problems that tend to plague the dependent and his or her family are postponed, at least temporarily. But by softening the impact of these problems, and by preventing the occurrence of life crises that might lead the dependent into treatment, the enabler prolongs the disease of drug dependency.[26]

The enabler can be anyone who has a relationship with the dependent, such as child, parent, coworker, friend, neighbor, lover, or roommate. Even physicians, police, and judges sometimes function as enablers. Most frequently, though, the dependent's spouse is the primary enabler.

Enabling practices are many and varied, and they include "covering up" for the dependent's mistakes or negligence; making excuses; lying to protect the dependent; apologizing repeatedly for the dependent's erratic and sometimes bizarre behavior; and gradually taking over the dependent's responsibilities within the family. Additional enabling behaviors focus on denying that drug abuse is a problem; avoiding situations and conflicts that might cause the dependent to use drugs again; minimizing the seriousness of the problems associated with the dependent's drug usage; rationalizing drug use to excuse the dependent's inappropriate behavior; attempting to control the amount of drug consumed; waiting and hoping that the drug problem will go away; and refusing to talk about drug use and abuse.[27]

While these enabling actions may seem irrational and illogical, the enabler most often perceives them as survival tactics. Such activities are rarely labeled as choices or alternatives; enablers often have no alternatives as they view the deteriorating condition of the dependent, the relationship with the dependent, or the family of the dependent. But by their own survival practices, enablers make possible, or facilitate, the continuing use and abuse of drugs. They reduce the likelihood of intervention by someone or some agency; they thereby postpone the dependent's entry into a treatment and rehabilitation program.

Reinforcing Factors in the Use and Abuse of Drugs

The third category of determinants having an impact on drug-taking behavior and

table 2.2 Perceived Desirable and Other Effects, Duration of Effects, and the Drug Enforcement Administration's View of Risk of Dependence of Selected Illegal Psychoactive Drugs

	Short-Term Effects			
Drug Type	Desired	Other	Duration of Acute Effects	DEA View of Risk of Dependence
Heroin	• Euphoria • Pain reduction	• Respiratory depression • Nausea • Drowsiness	• 3 to 6 hours	• Physical—high • Psychological—high
Cocaine	• Excitement • Euphoria • Increased alertness, wakefulness	• Increased blood pressure • Increased respiratory rate • Nausea • Cold sweats • Twitching • Headache	• 1 to 2 hours	• Physical—possible • Psychological—high
Crack Cocaine	• Same as cocaine • More rapid high than cocaine	• Same as cocaine	• About 5 minutes	• Same as cocaine
Marijuana	• Euphoria • Relaxation	• Accelerated heartbeat • Impairment of perception, judgment, fine motor skills, and memory	• 2 to 4 hours	• Physical—unknown • Psychological—moderate
Amphetamines	• Euphoria • Excitement • Increased alertness, wakefulness	• Increased blood pressure • Increased pulse rate • Insomnia • Loss of appetite	• 2 to 4 hours	• Physical—possible • Psychological—high
LSD	• Illusions and hallucinations • Excitement • Euphoria	• Poor perception of time and distance • Acute anxiety, restlessness, sleeplessness • Sometimes depression	• 8 to 12 hours	• Physical—none • Psychological—unknown

Source: Modified from the National Institute on Drug Abuse.

substance abuse is the *reinforcing factors.* Among these are influences that usually encourage the continuation of drug use once it has begun, although they may in some instances be influential in initiating drug use. Specific reinforcing factors are the experience of pleasure or relief of pain resulting from using drugs (as noted in table 2.2); the realization of other beneficial functions of drug usage; the importance of peers in drug-taking behavior; and the impact of media advertising on the nonmedical use of psychoactive chemicals.

Pleasure

According to one theory of learning, behavior is controlled by its consequences. Therefore, an activity followed by a positive event will be strengthened or maintained, while an activity followed by an unpleasant event will be weakened or eliminated.[28] This learning theory (operant conditioning) can also be used to help explain why people use drugs on a continuing basis.

Those consequences that strengthen or maintain drug-taking behavior are referred to as *reinforcers.* When a so-called positive stimulus, such as feeling good or getting high, is added to a marijuana-smoking situation, and when the pleasure and enjoyment serve to maintain the marijuana use the condition is described as *positive reinforcement.* And when a so-called negative stimulus, such as tension or pain, is removed after drinking alcohol this experienced relief also maintains the drinking behavior, and is called *negative reinforcement.* Thus, the consequences of drug-taking can function as either positive or negative reinforcers, both of which serve to maintain or increase the likelihood of repeated drug use (see fig. 2.2).

The varieties of drug-derived fun or pleasure are many. There can be experiences of inner peace, tranquility, joyous delight, relaxation, serenity; kaleidoscopic perceptions; surges of exhilaration; and heightened and prolonged physical sensations. The universality of these pleasurable

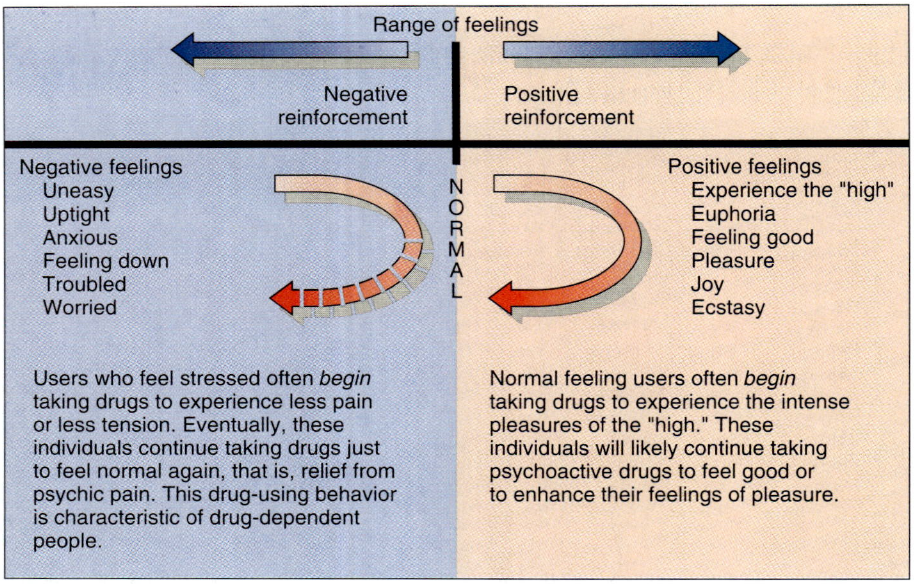

figure 2.2

Reinforcement and drug-taking behavior.

appeals has been acknowledged throughout history as a general explanation for most nonmedical drug use.

For any behavior, the more rapidly a reward or pleasant experience follows the particular activity, and the more often such behavior is rewarded, the stronger the learning or habit becomes. The use of psychoactive drugs is no exception to this general rule. If a drug is injected or inhaled, the reinforcement occurs rapidly, leading to the development of a strong habit. Also, if the drug is short-acting and must be used frequently each day, there are many occasions for reinforcement or learning of drug-taking behavior. If the drug used is one that causes physical dependence, the motivation for repeated use is established firmly because of the fear of the discomfort of withdrawal.[29] Originally taken to experience pleasure, the drug is now used to avoid pain, a powerful motivating force.

Functional Aspects of Using Drugs

Some people persist in the use of psychoactives because these chemicals can help them accomplish certain tasks perceived as desirable. For instance, amphetamines can help students stay awake all night to cram for a test. Stimulants have also been used to extend the performance of truck drivers and improve the physical ability and reaction time of athletes. Painkillers have been most effective in reducing the discomfort of injury and disease. Sedatives help people to achieve a drug-assisted sleep. Tranquilizers calm the anxious person.

Those who seek to improve their sexual performance and enjoyment have often resorted to certain psychoactive drugs for their alleged *aphrodisiac* effects. Cocaine and Ecstasy are chemical substances often believed to be endowed with such hoped-for powers. Alcohol has long been valued as a "sexual enhancer." In practice, however, most people find that Shakespeare's reference to alcohol is more accurate: alcohol provokes and unprovokes lust; alcohol provokes the desire, but it takes away the performance. Too much alcohol prevents a male's erection and a female's orgasmic response.

There is no scientific evidence supporting the belief that marijuana has any physical aphrodisiac effect. Studies suggest that among some males there is a temporary but definite lowering of the male sex hormone in the blood following use of marijuana. A loss of sexual interest is likely. But due to marijuana's effect on one's memory, sense of time, and attention span, some marijuana smokers believe that it increases one's sexual enjoyment. Of course, the socially communicated and strongly held belief in such a positive sexual effect is likely to have psychological substantiation. The placebo effect—believing that something will happen—is most powerful when supported by myth.

LSD and other psychedelic drugs have also been used to search for greater insight, personal understanding, awareness of subconscious thoughts, and creativity—evidence of mind expansion. Some people have turned to drugs to forget the past and escape the present temporarily and to keep going.

Social and Peer-Group Aspects

It is probable that the more popular psychoactive chemicals—alcohol, tobacco cigarettes, and marijuana—are used initially and continually thereafter as **social drugs.** As such, they are vehicles that help people better enjoy the company of others. While the adoption and repeated use of mind-changing drugs are related to their ability to enrich social intercourse, their distribution to others is often a form of social exchange, a learning phenomenon, or a rite of passage.

In recreational or social settings, the power of **peer-group influence** is considerable among friends and acquaintances. This is particularly true for adolescents and young adults who have doubts about their own identity and are concerned with acceptance by others. Often they willingly conform to group norms and participate in activities chosen by their peers. For lonely and emotionally isolated young people in need of belonging to something or someone, the only thing they have to do is smoke, drink, or take other drugs. Thus, drug-using groups are easy to join. Drug taking becomes symbolic of group identification. Coparticipation in an activity that is secret and illegal often fosters a bond of conspiracy that further cements such interrelationships and enables the continuation of alcohol and other drug abuse.

There is widespread agreement that association with alcohol-using and other drug-using peers during adolescence is one of the strongest predictors of adolescent alcohol and other drug use.[30] The influence of peers is especially powerful for beginning the use of tobacco cigarettes and marijuana. When friendship and friendship groups revolve around the use of mind-changing drugs, however, nonusing peers do not generally fit in. Alcohol-using and other drug-using peers are usually intolerant of or uninterested in pursuing friendships with nonusing peers.[31]

Advertising and Media Programming

The promised benefits of taking drugs are familiar. They include a change in pace or emotional state, relief from tension and boredom, a pickup to combat fatigue, the promotion of sleep, or just plain fun. Such benefits also are frequently cited in the appeals of television commercials, as is well known even by preschoolers. Such beliefs are also portrayed on television and in motion pictures where characters drink alcoholic beverages more frequently than people in real-life situations do.

A typical American adolescent is exposed to approximately three thousand acts of drinking per year through television alone, according to the federal Center for Substance Abuse Prevention. These repeated exposures to the modeled behavior of athletes and former athletes, rock stars, television celebrities, and other attractive people are likely to result in behavioral change, if social learning theory is valid. Advertisers are banking on it!

Advertising The invitation to drug use comes not only where over-the-counter and prescription psychoactives, beers, and wines are touted, but also in newspapers and magazines and on outdoor billboards, where distilled spirits and tobacco products are advertised widely.

For many years, the distilled spirits industry voluntarily withheld the advertising of "hard liquors" on commercial television. But such a policy, never applied to cable television, has been reversed. Apparently in reaction to declining liquor sales, Seagram's began advertising one of its Canadian brand whiskies on commercial TV in 1996.

Box 2.2 A Proposal to Limit Alcohol Advertising and Promotional Activities

1. *Develop and implement effective programs for alcohol abuse prevention and education on American college campuses.* Promotional materials encouraging drinking on campus; distribution of free alcoholic beverages for promotional purposes on campus; and sponsorship of any on-campus activity, event, or competition by an alcoholic beverage company would be forbidden.
2. *End corporate welfare for the alcoholic beverage industry.* Tax deductions for advertising and goodwill expenses would be ended, and federal funds would no longer be used to promote the sale or export of American produced alcoholic beverages.
3. *Protect children from alcohol advertising.* Prohibit advertising of alcoholic beverages on audio tape or disc, videotape, video arcade game, computer game, and film. Outdoor advertising of such beverages would be forbidden near any school, playground, or other youth-oriented facility. Severe restrictions on advertising in publications with youth readership and on television between the hours of 7:00 A.M. to 10:00 P.M. would be enforced.
4. *Require more specific rotating warnings on alcohol advertisements* including broadcast, print, billboards, and in-store displays. The new warnings would emphasize alcohol as an addictive drug; dangers of mixing alcohol with over-the-counter, prescription, and other illicit drugs; drinking in relation to high blood pressure, liver disease, and cancer; necessity of driving a car only when sober; danger of drinking while pregnant; and the possibility of fatal alcohol poisoning.
5. *Require truth in alcoholic beverage labeling.* Labels would have to disclose the container's alcohol content by volume, the number of drinks per container, a toll-free telephone number for information on alcohol use and abuse, and a definition of a "drink" as a serving of a malt beverage, wine, or distilled spirit containing 0.6 ounces of alcohol by volume.

(Introduced to the U.S. Congress by Rep. Joseph Kennedy of Massachusetts.) From "Alcohol Advertising," *Monday Morning Report*, June 17, 1996. Reprinted by permission of Alcohol Research Information Services.

By contrast, the tobacco industry is restricted by law from promoting cigarettes and smokeless tobacco on TV.

Health authorities have proposed a ban on television beer ads because of the likely influence of advertising on young and impressionable people. Others have advocated severe restriction or the prohibition of media advertising of alcoholic beverages (see box 2.2). Supporters of such restrictions are particularly concerned about the inappropriate portrayal of drinking while driving or pregnant. The underlying messages of alcohol advertising are that (1) use of these products is risk-free and (2) alcoholic beverages are normal and essential parts of social events. In other words, you can't have a good time unless you drink, and if you drink, you can always have a good time!

Product advertising is often defended as the voice of free choice and the only way manufacturers can win consumers from competing brands. But as critics maintain, the advertising of beverage alcohol also tends to

> glamorize alcohol use and give a one-sided view without providing information about the likely, adverse consequences, such as combining alcoholic beverages with auto racing
>
> associate drinking alcoholic beverages, especially beer, with various professional sports teams and former well-known athletes, supposedly conveying approval of consumption by important role models
>
> recruit new first-time drinkers—including young people—by making sweeter drinks (fruit-flavored wine coolers) that will be more acceptable and pleasing from the first sip, and by the clever use of lovable "party

animals" as the focus of the commercials

target certain groups of people such as minorities, women, and people of color.

convey the message that drinking is the key to fun and sexual success

In the face of declining sales to an ever-declining market of domestic smokers, cigarette makers also advertise widely in the print media, but not on television. Some national and regional sporting events are also supported by manufacturers of tobacco products.

Although a causal link between drug advertising and drug abuse has not yet been established, it is assumed that such ads do influence the heavier use of drugs among the general public. Apparently, the billions of dollars spent each year by alcohol and tobacco manufacturers to promote their products is certain proof that they believe advertising is a cost-effective method of attracting customers. There is a consensus that massive and persistent advertising for over-the-counter drugs and now prescription drugs has taught both younger and older Americans that pills and potions are the answer to just about every health problem—real or imagined.

One observer, who defines addiction as a need for something that gives the feeling of completeness, raises a further condemnation of advertising: We are smart enough not to believe in the ridiculous claims of individual ads, but can we escape their underlying message that only by buying or taking something into our bodies can we be made whole and healthy? Do we have any reasonable complaint about the amount of addiction in society when we teach it every day through sponsored ads in the mass media?[32] Nothing fulfills our love for the quick fix better than drugs—legal as well as illegal.

Television Programming and Movie Scripts Surveys regarding television programs and movies indicate that the average young person will be exposed to thousands of drinking episodes annually and an increasing number of cigarette-smoking instances. Critics of such advertising contend that the

At Issue

Should advertising of alcoholic beverages be banned or restricted?

Point: There is an urgent need to severely limit or ban the advertising of beer, wine, and distilled spirits in all media, but especially on television. Alcohol is currently the leading cause of death for people under the age of twenty-four years. Beverage alcohol kills five times as many Americans as all other illegal drugs combined, and is responsible for at least three million teenagers and young adults addicted to alcohol.

Print ads for alcohol do not reach nearly as many people as television and the typical American youth watches TV an average of 5.3 hours each day, therefore the primary means of appealing to the youth market has become the television commercial. This form of advertising is the key to new, entry-level drinkers. First there was Spuds MacKenzie, the original, lovable party animal for Bud Light beer. Next came the three chirping Budweiser frogs that became more recognizable to elementary school children than Smokey the Bear, Tony the Tiger, and the Mighty Morphin Power Rangers. More recently, two "graduating" dogs—favorite animals of young people—appeared in behalf of Seagram's Crown Royal whisky, the first hard liquor to be advertised on regular television.

Realizing that the average age of young Americans who take their first drink is only thirteen years, it appears that the alcoholic beverage industry wants to get in on the action as soon as possible. But more than products are being sold. Those young people reporting greater awareness to television beer advertising had more favorable beliefs and attitudes about drinking and beer, greater knowledge of beer brands and slogans, and increased intention to drink alcoholic beverages as adults. Whether it's dogs, frogs, or Halloween masks, such marketing practices seem to produce positive results: a new crop of drinkers for each generation.

"Alcohol Advertising," *Monday Morning Report* 20, no. 11 (17 June 1996):1–3.

Counterpoint: Oh, get a life! The proposal to restrict or ban alcoholic beverage ads, especially on television is not only ridiculous, but unconstitutional. While alcohol abuse is a major problem among youths as well as among adults, such a problem will likely continue to exist with or without commercials on television.

Educate, discuss, and debate the merits of drinking. Then let informed people make a free choice. After all, drinking is legal for adults over twenty-one years of age. Moreover, for millions of Americans, beer, wine, and distilled spirits are part of the good life, the American way of life. We should be promoting this, rather than trying to destroy it.

More importantly, however, forbidding or restricting alcohol ads is unconstitutional. Advertising, even vulgar and tasteless, is nonetheless a distribution of information. The free flow of commercial information is indispensable to a free and democratic society. Those who would ban alcohol ads base their argument on the unique character of electronic communications in 1971, when the U.S. Congress forbade cigarette ads on radio and television. Since then, the so-called public airways have been expanded considerably and television no longer holds a monopoly on electronic transmission. It would be unnatural and impossible to control satellite transmissions, telephone conversations, e-mail, faxes, beepers, and cellular phones, therefore, such an attempt at censorship of television advertising would also be impossible and unconstitutional. In the present political environment, attempts to censor one type of product would be a violation of corporate civil rights.

Michael Gartner, "Proposal to Ban Liquor Ads Silly," *USA Today* (2 July 1996): 11A.

frequency of alcohol and cigarette use in television programs and movies exaggerates the prevalence of alcohol and tobacco use in the real population and conveys the impression that everyone is either drinking or smoking, or both.

Many of the circumstances in which drinking is portrayed on television deliver other incomplete and inaccurate messages. Too often, drinking is pictured as consequence free. As described by the Center for Substance Abuse Prevention, it is not uncommon for a television or movie hero to "put a few drinks away" and then rush off in a sports car. No questions asked and no harm done. In addition, television and movie characters frequently use alcohol to reduce tension in uncomfortable or frustrating situations. As a consequence, young people learn the value of "relief drinking"—that alcohol can lessen pain or discomfort.

What viewers do not learn is that in the long run such relief drinking lessens neither discomfort and unhappiness nor frustration. Screenwriters tend to have greater artistic leeway and they are more likely to depict characters who use illegal drugs in a casual and, once again, risk-free manner.

Box 2.3 Families with Little or No Drug Use

Information on the reduction and prevention of drug misuse and abuse can be obtained from studies of those families who rarely or never use drugs. In comparison to drug-using families, the nonusing or low-use families show the following characteristics.

1. Children perceive more love from parents, particularly the father.
2. There is less difference between how parents would ideally like their children to be versus how they actually perceive them.
3. Children are seen as more assertive, although a basic firmness in child rearing is maintained.
4. Parents and their children's friends are compatible.
5. Parents have more influence on their children than do peers and emphasize discipline, self-control, and family tradition.
6. Less approval of drug use is expressed by parents and peers.
7. There is more spontaneous agreement observed in family problem solving.
8. Family members function more democratically or quasi-democratically, with shared authority and better communication.

Source: National Institute on Drug Abuse.

The Family's Influence on Drug Abuse

It is common knowledge that children of smokers tend to smoke themselves. If parents drink and take pills to escape personal problems, to feel better, or to have a "good time," their children may grow up to believe that mind-changing drugs are the appropriate solution to disappointments and other forms of stress. This relationship between parental drug-taking behavior and that of their children is referred to as **modeling.**[33] The reverse is also true. Families who have little or no drug use also serve as models for their children, as noted in box 2.3.

Theories on Drug Abuse and Drug Dependence

The foregoing observations, concepts, and descriptions have provided some insight into the causes, or **etiology,** of alcohol and other drug use and abuse. Numerous etiological factors have been examined within a framework of predisposing, enabling, and reinforcing determinants. However, many scientists and drug-abuse therapists are not satisfied that they know why people continue to use drugs in ways that are often personally and socially destructive. Consequently, researchers have formulated various models and theories that explain, wholly or in part, the underlying causes of drug abuse and drug dependence, sometimes referred to as addiction.

The several theories are categorized under three major public health headings or models, each representing an important though contrasting class of etiological factors. The first heading deals with the so-called *agent,* in this case the psychoactive drug. According to this agent-based model, abuse and dependence have an **agent-related etiology:** psychoactive drugs cause drug abuse and drug dependence or addiction. The basics of this particular theory propose that most everyone who takes one or more psychoactive drugs long enough and in large enough amounts will likely develop drug abuse and/or drug dependence.

In the second major category are theories of **host-related etiology,** which explain drug abuse and drug dependence as the result of some predisposition or unusual condition within the so-called *host,* that is, the person who takes the drug. Whether it is genetics (genetic theory), or faulty metabolism of drugs (biological theory), or failure to have learned appropriate coping skills or having learned addictive behaviors (psychological theory), or the development of a psychiatric disorder, something within the individual makes that person especially vulnerable to drug abuse and/or drug dependence.

The last major category is identified as **environment-related etiology,** including those etiological factors operating in the drug taker's external circumstances, experiences, and interrelational settings. Factors external to the drug taker and other than the drug are considered as forcing the individual into drug abuse and eventually drug dependence. Some of the theories identified in this category are social learning theory (with its emphasis on modeling influences), sociocultural theory, and environmental stress theory (which views individuals as seeking escape from the harshness of their surroundings through mind-changing drugs).

In each of the three categories, some theories focus on specific causative factors or forces. However, many authorities believe that two or more factors from two or more categories interact in complex ways to result in drug abuse and drug dependence. It is probable that heredity and environment combine in some undefined way in a psychologically unique and susceptible individual who uses a psychoactive drug in a particular social setting. From such an intricate combination the conditions of drug abuse and drug dependence develop. Such combination theories are sometimes called **multifactorial** or multifaceted—having many possible causative or contributing factors.

Chapter Summary

1. Drug-taking behavior is likely the result of many interrelated factors. Moreover, a consensus exists that the influences that initiate nonmedical use of drugs are usually different from those that produce extended drug abuse.
2. Alteration of one's consciousness or awareness is probably the primary reason people take psychoactive drugs. Drug use often originates in the search for pleasure or for relief from pain.
3. Youth often take drugs in imitation of adults, many of whom are convinced that an appropriate drug treatment exists for every ailment.
4. Youth rebellion and increased drug use of the 1960s was a rejection of traditional values and a generational conflict between parents and children. By contrast, much of today's drug abuse is likely motivated by the pursuit of recreation and the pleasure principle.
5. An analysis of drug-taking behavior reveals a framework of predisposing influences (that make the individual susceptible), enabling influences (that facilitate initial use and abuse), and reinforcing influences (that encourage continuing drug use and abuse).
6. Predisposing factors in drug-taking behavior include demographics, sociocultural factors, and aspects of adolescence, including experimentation, egocentrism, risk taking, and impulsivity. Low self-esteem and social confidence, the need for peer approval, and the tendency to overestimate the ability to avoid destructive drug use also predispose the adolescent to use of drugs.
7. Basic curiosity about the new and novel predispose people to initiating drug use.
8. Use of psychoactive drugs often reflects basic personality factors and represents attempts to cope with problems of personal identity, self-esteem, boredom, and assertion of independence.
9. Epidemic (sudden increase) and endemic (widespread prevalence over a continuing period) drug use are influenced by changes in the national population, the women's liberation movement, adverse economic conditions, and numerous alterations and conflicts in American society.
10. Enabling factors in drug taking include the widespread availability of psychoactives; accessibility of mind-changing drugs made possible by affluence and parental permissiveness; ineffectiveness of legal deterrence; and lack of social controls, including guidelines for responsible use of drugs. Additional enablers are the lack of motivation to say no to drugs; the mismanagement of patients by physicians; the pharmacology of addicting (dependency-producing) drugs; and the actions of enablers.
11. Reinforcing factors in drug use and abuse are the experience of pleasure and relief of pain, that psychoactive drugs often help people accomplish tasks perceived as desirable, the influence of peer groups, and the impact of drug advertising in the media and television programming.
12. Theories of drug abuse and drug dependence are considered under three major classifications: those that are related to the agent (the drug itself), those that are related to the host (the drug taker), and those that are related to the environment (the sociocultural setting). While these theories provide differing explanations, some authorities now suggest a multifactorial approach to the etiology of drug abuse and drug dependence.

World Wide Web Sites

Partnership for a Drug-Free America

www. drugfreeamerica.org

National Clearinghouse for Alcohol and Drug Information

www.health.org

National Center on Addiction and Substance Abuse at Columbia University

www.casacolumbia.org

Review Questions and Activities

1. Define the term *altered conscious experience.*
2. Distinguish between the concepts of increased awareness and decreased awareness.
3. Explain how socially defined attitudes, values, and behaviors concerning drugs influence the current drug problem.
4. What are some possible effects on individuals and society because of the widely held belief that an effective drug exists for every ailment?
5. Discuss the importance of adult drug-taking behavior, youthful rebellion against the establishment, and the

pursuit of recreation and pleasure in the occurrence of drug abuse in young people.

6. Distinguish among the following terms related to drug-taking behavior: *predisposing factors, enabling factors,* and *reinforcing factors.*

7. Why does experimental use of psychoactive drugs so often occur during the adolescent stage of human development?

8. Explain how psychoactive drugs used as coping mechanisms can result in decreased self-esteem and diminished feelings of personal power.

9. What psychological characteristics commonly describe the individual likely to become preoccupied with drugs?

10. What changes and/or conflicts in society are operating to influence the usage of psychoactive drugs in America?

11. How do the factors of availability and accessibility enable or facilitate drug use and abuse?

12. In what specific ways do the effects of addicting drugs contribute to the continuing use and abuse of psychoactive substances?

13. In what ways are psychoactive drugs reinforcers of drug-taking behavior?

14. Explain how some of the functional uses of psychoactive drugs could lead to serious difficulties.

15. In what specific psychological aspects are young people often vulnerable to the power of peer-group influence in the recreational use of drugs?

16. Survey television, radio, and newsprint media for three days and record the number, type, and relative appeal of drug-related commercials. What message or messages are conveyed in these commercials about drug use?

17. Using the major factors under the categories of predisposing, enabling, and reinforcing determinants, rank-order the causes of or influences on drug use and abuse from the most important to the least important. Compare your rank-ordered list with those of other class members and discuss similarities and differences in the lists.

18. What major factors are used to categorize various theories on drug abuse and drug dependence? Which major category of etiological factors appears to be the most significant causative force?

References

1. H. Thomas Milhorn, Jr., *Drug and Alcohol Abuse* (New York: Plenum Press, 1994), 5–8.
2. Andrew Weil and Winifred Rosen, *From Chocolate to Morphine,* rev. ed. (Boston: Houghton Mifflin, 1993), 14.
3. Ronald K. Siegel, *Intoxication: Life in Pursuit of Artificial Paradise* (New York: E. P. Dutton, 1989), 10, 207–27, 313.
4. Weil and Rosen, *From Chocolate to Morphine,* 15.
5. Frank R. Scarpitti and Susan K. Datesman, "Introduction," in *Drugs and the Youth Culture,* ed. F. R. Scarpitti and S. K. Datesman (Beverly Hills, Calif.: Sage, 1980), 10.
6. Ivan Illich, "Medical Nemesis," in *The Nation's Health,* ed. P. Lee, N. Brown, and I. Red (San Francisco: Boyd & Fraser, 1981), 78.
7. Mark S. Gold, with Michael Boyette, *Wonder Drugs: How They Work* (New York: Simon & Schuster, 1987), 18.
8. Lawrence W. Green and others, *Health Education Planning: A Diagnostic Approach* (Palo Alto, Calif.: Mayfield, 1980), 68–76.
9. "Who Uses What: Drug Use by Occupation," *Substance Abuse Report* 24, no. 8 (15 April 1993): 4; Andrew Treno, Robert Parker, and Harold Holder, "Understanding U.S. Alcohol Consumption with Social and Economic Factors: A Multivariate Series Analysis, 1950–1986," *Journal of Studies on Alcohol* 54, no. 2 (1993): 146–56; and Kathleen Bucholz, "Alcohol Abuse and Dependence from a Psychiatric Perspective, *Alcohol Health and Research World* 16, no. 2 (1992): 197–208.
10. John Leland, "Just Say Maybe," *Newsweek,* 1 November 1993, 51–54.
11. U.S. Department of Health and Human Services, *Preventing Tobacco Use among Young People,* a report of the Surgeon General, executive summary (Atlanta: U.S. Department of Health and Human Services, Public Health Service, Centers for Disease Control and Prevention, Office on Smoking and Health, 1994), 64.
12. Office of the Inspector General, *Youth and Alcohol: A National Survey (Drinking Habits, Access, Attitudes, and Knowledge)* (Washington, D.C.: Department of Health and Human Services and the National Clearinghouse for Alcohol and Drug Information, 1991), 4.
13. Jonathan Shedler and Jack Block, "Adolescent Drug Use and Psychological Health," *American Psychologist* 45, no. 5 (May 1990): 612–30.
14. Robert Dupont, ed., *Stopping Alcohol and Other Drug Use before It Starts: The Future of Prevention,* Office for Substance Abuse Prevention Monograph No.1, DHHS Pub. No. (ADM) 89-1645 (Washington, D.C.: GPO, 1989), 3.
15. Rebecca Razavi, "Risk Taking in Children and Adolescents," *ADAMHA News* 15, no. 3 (May 1989): 9.
16. J. D. Hawkins and D. M. Catalano, *Communities that Care,* Developmental Research and Programs, Inc. (WRP, 1993), Seattle, WA.
17. Bureau of Justice Statistics, *Drugs, Crime, and the Justice System* (Washington, D.C.: GPO, 1992), 22.
18. "Is There an Addictive Personality" *University of California at Berkeley Wellness Letter* 6, no. 9 (June 1990): 1–2.
19. Felicity Barringer, "Youthful Drinking Persists: With Teens and Alcohol, It's Just Say When," *New York Times,* 23 June 1991, 1, 4.
20. Louise G. Richards, "The Epidemiology of Youthful Drug Use," in *Drugs and the Youth Culture,* ed. F. Scarpitti and S. Datesman (Beverly Hills, Calif.: Sage, 1980), 55.
21. Harvey B. Milkman and Stanley G. Sunderwirth, *Craving for Ecstasy: The Consciousness and Chemistry of Escape* (Lexington, Mass.: Lexington Books, 1987), 18.
22. George Vaillant, *The Natural History of Alcoholism* (Cambridge: Harvard University Press, 1983), 63–71; and National Institute on Alcohol Abuse and Alcoholism, *Alcohol and Health: The Eights Special Report to the U.S. Congress* (Rockville, Md.: National Institutes of Health, Public Health Service, 1993), 61–83.
23. Kenneth Blum and others, "Allelic Association of Human Dopamine D2 Receptor Gene in Alcoholism," *Journal of the American Medical Association* 263, no. 15 (18 April 1990): 2055–60.
24. Ting-Kai Li and Jane C. Lockmuller, "Why Are Some People More Susceptible to Alcoholism?" *Alcoholism Health and Research World* 13, no. 4 (1989): 310–15.
25. Steve Olson, with Dean Gerstein, *Alcohol in America: Taking Action to Prevent Abuse* (Washington, D.C.: National Academy Press, 1985), 40–41.
26. Al Mooney, Arlene Eisenberg, and Howard Eisenberg, *The Recovery Book* (New York: Workman, 1992), 501.

27. Louis Krupnick and Elizabeth Krupnick, *From Despair to Decision* (Minneapolis: CompCare, 1985), 24.
28. Michael Lewis and Jane Lockmuller, "Alcohol Reinforcement: Complex Determinant of Drinking," *Alcohol Health and Research World* 14, no. 2 (1990): 98–104.
29. J. Jaffe, R. Petersen, and R. Hodgson, *Addictions: Issues and Answers* (New York: Harper & Row, 1980), 18.
30. Helene White, Marsha Bates, and Valerie Johnson, "Learning to Drink: Familial, Peer, and Media Influences," in *Society, Culture, and Drinking Patterns Reexamined,* ed. David Pittman and Helene White (New Brunswick, N. J.: Rutgers Center of Alcohol Studies, 1991), 177–97.
31. Office of Substance Abuse Prevention, *Prevention Plus II: Tools for Creating and Sustaining Drug-Free Communities* (Washington, D.C.: GPO, 1989), 26.
32. Philip Slater, "Society's Pressure Causes Drug Dependency," in *Opposing Viewpoints: Chemical Dependency,* ed. Claudia B. Debner (St. Paul: Greenhaven Press, 1985), 25.
33. Ruth Maxwell, *Kids, Alcohol & Drugs: A Parent's Guide* (New York: Ballantine Books, 1991), 203–06.

Chapter 3

Pharamacology

Drug actions and interactions

KEY TERMS

Addiction
Autonomic Nervous System
Axon
Biotransformation
Blood-Brain Barrier
Central Nervous System
Cerebellum
Cerebrum
Chemotherapy
Dendrite
Dose
Drug Action
  Activation
  Inactivation
Drug Dependence
Drug-Receptor Interaction
Homeostasis
Hypothalamus
Inhalation
Injection
Medulla Oblongata
Metabolism
Neuron
Neurotransmitter
Peripheral Nervous System
Pharmacology
Physical Dependence
Placebo Effect
Psychological Dependence
Solubility
Synapse
Therapeutic Index
Tolerance
Withdrawal Syndrome

chapter objectives

After you have studied this chapter, you should be able to do the following:

1. Define the key terms.
2. Describe four major methods of drug administration.
3. Describe the basic patterns of drug distribution within the body.
4. Explain the significance of the blood-brain barrier in relation to psychoactive drugs.
5. Discuss the various processes involved in the elimination of drugs from the body.
6. Explain drug activity in terms of the drug-receptor interaction.
7. Name six different ways or actions by which drugs can change cell function.
8. Explain how factors of dose, age, body weight, gender, time, disease, and emotional states could affect drug actions.
9. Describe the general organization of the nervous system in terms of major functions and structures.
10. Distinguish between the central nervous system and the peripheral nervous system with its major subdivisions.
11. Compare the general functions of the sympathetic and parasympathetic divisions of the autonomic nervous system.
12. Explain in detail the various processes involved in continuing a nerve impulse from one neuron to another.
13. Name several neurotransmitters.
14. Identify several parts of the human brain affected either directly or indirectly by psychoactive drugs.
15. Relate several recreational psychoactives and several prescribed medications with specific effects on human sexual function.
16. Distinguish among the following terms: *physical dependence, psychological dependence, tolerance,* and *withdrawal sickness.*
17. Identify several criteria established by the American Psychiatric Association by which to describe a drug-dependent individual.
18. Describe addiction or drug dependence as a process.
19. Explain how each of the following conditions differ from one another: tachyphylaxis, kindling, cross-tolerance, and cross-dependence.
20. Explain four major categories of drug interactions.
21. Identify four factors thought to be responsible for the placebo effect.

Pharmacology

In their search for sustaining foods, prehistoric humans undoubtedly introduced a wide assortment of substances into their bodies. These people sought nourishment, but occasionally they also experienced drowsiness and sleep, intense pleasures, reduction of pain, and sometimes even poisoning and sudden death. While modern Americans may be somewhat more sophisticated about their food intake, many still desire some of the changes in thinking, feeling, and behavior achieved almost accidentally by their ancient counterparts.

With advances in scientific investigation, researchers eventually sought to determine the relation between substances taken into the body and the resulting changes in body function and behavior. Such endeavors have given rise to the scientific discipline of **pharmacology,** the study of the composition, uses, and effects of drugs. Traditionally, the major concern of pharmacology has been the study of drugs intended for medicinal use, such as drugs used to diagnose (specify or determine via examination), prevent, treat, or cure disease. Even when such chemicals were misused and abused, sometimes for recreational purposes rather than for treating disease, the standard description of a drug was considered adequate. However, with the introduction of oral contraceptives in the mid-1950s, pharmacologists had to revise their definition of a drug. The "Pill" was not used in the diagnosis, prevention, treatment, or cure of disease—unless pregnancy was to be considered a disease.

Consequently, pharmacologists have revised their definition of drugs to include *any substance that in small amounts produces significant changes in a person's body, mind, or both.*[1] This newer definition seems more appropriate, especially with the increased use of recreational drugs, street drugs, and designer drugs, many of which never had any intended medical use.

The science of pharmacology has given rise to four major subdivisions recognized as special areas of study and application:

1. *Pharmacokinetics*—the study of what the body does to drugs, including the processes of absorption, distribution, biotransformation and metabolism, and excretion.
2. *Pharmacodynamics*—the study of what drugs do to the body, including the effects of drugs and the mechanisms of their actions.
3. *Pharmacotherapeutics*—the use of drugs in treating diseases. When drugs are used specifically to destroy or weaken invading organisms or to prevent or treat diseases, the treatment is referred to as **chemotherapy.**
4. *Toxicology*—the study of poisons.

Basic concepts from these pharmacology subdivisions will be explained in this chapter or in later chapters dealing with specific psychoactive drugs and prescription and over-the-counter medications.

Box 3.1 Common Routes of Drug Administration with Selected Psychoactive Substances

Oral*—through the mouth.* Pain-relieving tablets of aspirin and ibuprofen, liquid alcoholic beverages, blotter paper impregnated with LSD, psilocybin mushrooms.

Parenteral*—by injection.*

- Intravenous (into a vein). "Mainlining" of heroin, cocaine, and injection of alcohol into a vein.
- Subcutaneous (just beneath the skin's surface). "Skin-popping" of heroin.
- Intramuscular (into a muscle). Injection of slow-absorbing antipsychotic drugs directly into a muscle.

Inhalation*—through the lungs.* Breathing in of smoke containing nicotine from tobacco, or tiny particles of cocaine, crack cocaine, methamphetamine (crank or ice), heroin, tetrahydrocannabinol (THC) from marijuana smoke, and vapors from gasoline, toluene, paint thinner, and butyl nitrite (Rush).

Absorption*—through mucous membranes of the nose and mouth; under the tongue; in the rectum, vagina, and urethra.* Snorting or sniffing of powdered cocaine and crystals of methamphetamine; alcohol enema, insertion of cocaine into the rectum and vagina; and nicotine from chewing tobacco in the mouth.

Transdermal*—through the skin.* Nicoderm skin patch to help quit smoking by preventing tobacco craving and withdrawal.

How Drugs Enter the Body

For a drug to have any more than a superficial effect, like antacids in the stomach or antidandruff shampoos on the scalp, the chemical agent must enter the blood-vascular system. It must be absorbed or transported from the site of administration into the bloodstream, and then distributed by the blood throughout the body to various tissues and fluids. The manner in which the drug is introduced (the route of administration) is an important factor in determining how quickly the drug will be absorbed, chemically broken down or metabolized in the body, and eventually eliminated. In turn, the efficiency of these processes will determine how fast the drug will act, how strong the drug's effects will be, and how long the drug remains in the body and continues to produce some desirable effect.[2]

Although drugs can be administered in several ways, they are usually given or taken *orally* (by mouth), *parenterally* (by injection), or by *inhalation* (breathing in through one's nose, see box 3.1). Other means of introducing drugs into the body are by way of absorption across the mucous membranes of the nose, rectum, and vagina; across the skin barrier (transdermally); and by surgical implantation.

Most commonly, drugs in capsule, tablet or caplet, pill, or liquid form enter the body by way of the mouth. From the mouth, the solid or liquid drug passes into the stomach and eventually into the intestine, where most of the chemicals are absorbed (transferred) into the bloodstream. Oral administration is convenient, permits self-medication, and avoids the physical and psychological discomforts of injection. However, this route of administration is not ideal for all drugs. Absorption is sometimes slowed by the presence of food in the stomach and the excessive movement of the gastrointestinal tract.

Less commonly, drugs can be given *rectally,* that is, through the rectum, the terminal end of the digestive tract. This method is particularly advantageous if the person is unconscious, has difficulty

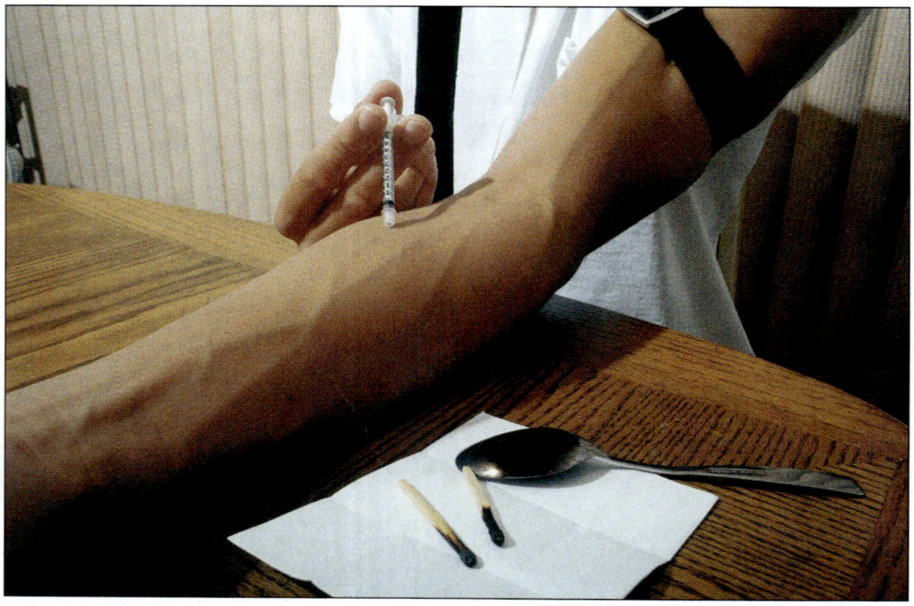

Shooting up heroin. This picture demonstrates the parenteral administration of drugs in which a solution of a chemical substance (heroin) is injected into the bloodstream. The drug abuser is engaging in intravenous injection, a form of parenteral drug use commonly known as "mainlining."

© Tony Freeman/PhotoEdit

in swallowing, or is vomiting. However, drugs administered rectally in the form of a suppository or even an enema may be incompletely and irregularly absorbed.

The term *parenteral* describes the administration of drugs, such as antibiotics, insulin, and anticlotting medicine, into the bloodstream directly or indirectly by **injection,** without having to be absorbed through the digestive tract. This can be accomplished by *intravenous injection* (known as an IV or "mainlining," in which a drug is inserted directly into a vein); *intramuscular injection* or IM (directly into muscle tissue); or *subcutaneous injection* or "skin-popping" (just beneath the skin's surface). On rare occasions, drugs may be injected directly into the peritoneal or visceral cavity of the body and into the cerebrospinal fluid. Each of the more common routes of drug administration has its distinct advantages and disadvantages, as noted in the following list.[3]

Administration of drugs by injection

1. produces a more rapid response than can be obtained by oral or rectal administration.
2. achieves more accurate dosage, because drug destruction in the digestive tract is avoided.
3. bypasses the unpredictable absorption processes occurring in the stomach and intestine.
4. provides insufficient time, in comparison with orally administered drugs, to counteract unexpected drug reactions or accidental overdose. Once given, an injection cannot be recalled.
5. requires sterile conditions to avoid infectious diseases caused by bacteria and viruses that can damage the liver, heart, and other body organs.
6. presents a potentially painful situation for the drug taker, and a life-threatening situation if the virus that causes acquired immunodeficiency syndrome (AIDS) is transmitted by using shared, blood-contaminated needles for intravenous injection.

Inhalants

Certain drugs in mist form can be administered by **inhalation,** in which chemicals are absorbed into the blood by passing through the lungs. Volatile anesthetic gases, paint thinner and gasoline vapors, nonvolatile aerosols, tobacco and marijuana smoke, and the smoke of freebased and "crack" cocaine can pass through the thin membranes of the lungs' air sacs and readily enter the bloodstream.

Inhalation of drugs produces an extremely rapid effect, because chemicals absorbed into the blood from the lungs go directly to the brain and bypass the heart in their initial distribution. As a consequence, volatile gases are the preferred form of anesthetics because their blood levels can be controlled with great precision. This control of dosage is also a major advantage of breathing in drug vapors and drug smoke. Other than volatile gases, the major disadvantage of inhalation is the potential for irritation of and damage to lung tissue.

A variation of inhalation is known as *snorting,* the intranasal administration of drugs. In this route of entry, a water-soluble drug such as cocaine is snorted or sniffed, being absorbed through the moist mucous membranes that line the nasal passages. The drug enters the blood vessels near the surface lining.

While most psychoactive drugs are administered by mouth, rectum, injection, or inhaling, the future of drug use could be changed dramatically by the development and approval of a relatively new drug form. In the 1990s, the U.S. Food and Drug Administration authorized use of a rate-controlled, transdermal drug system—a method by which a drug is absorbed through the skin. Worn on the skin's surface behind the ear or on the arm or chest as small disks or patches, the drug is absorbed directly into the bloodstream at programmed rates.

Each small patch of the transdermal system is composed of four layers, or membranes, that serve as a backing container, a drug reservoir, a rate-of-release controller, and an adhesive that holds the "circle of drug" to the skin. The first drugs to be dispensed in transdermal patches were used to alleviate motion sickness and angina pectoris.

Another method of drug administration is being used after extensive research: nasal sprays that promote the absorption of certain medicines through the mucosa of the nasal cavity (directly into the blood vessels of the nostrils).

Drug Distribution and Elimination

After a drug has been absorbed into the bloodstream, it is widely *distributed* throughout the body. Such dispersal, however, reflects the physical and chemical nature of the drug and its ability to spread or pass through various membranes—cell walls, capillaries, the brain, and the placenta.

This selective ability of a particular drug to spread from areas of high concentration to areas of low concentration is known as its **solubility,** that is, its condition or quality of being dissolved in body tissue.[4] Some drugs are more soluble in body fats, while others are more easily dissolved in water. Most cell membranes contain several fat layers, therefore drugs that are soluble in fat can pass through the membranes rapidly. All psychoactive drugs are soluble in fat, though some dissolve faster than others.[5]

Three patterns of drug distribution or dispersal have been identified in the human body.[6]

1. Some drugs, including blood-plasma substitutes, remain largely within the bloodstream.
2. Other compounds, such as ethyl alcohol and certain sulfa drugs, become almost uniformly distributed throughout every body cell. Alcohol even crosses the placenta and endangers the developing embryo or fetus.
3. Most drugs are unevenly distributed in the body in accordance with their solubility and differential ability to penetrate different membranes of the body.

Although *psychoactive drugs* affect thinking, feelings, and behavior—functions controlled by the nervous system—most of these chemicals will be found outside the brain at any given time, even during states of drug intoxication and poisoning.

The Blood-Brain Barrier

To have a psychoactive effect, a drug must be able to leave the tiny blood vessels (capillaries) supplying the brain and enter the nearby nerve cells. A selective resistance to movement effectively prevents certain substances from entering brain tissue because of the unique, tightly fused cell wall structure of the capillaries in the brain—unlike those in other body parts. This "resistance to the passage of some substances through the brain's capillary walls"—based on drug solubility—is known as the **blood-brain barrier.**[7]

Fat-soluble drugs, such as the general anesthetics, and water-soluble molecules easily cross the blood-brain barrier, as do those drugs already identified as having a psychoactive effect. Heroin crosses the barrier more easily than morphine, due to heroin's greater fat solubility. Though acting as a protector of the brain against certain toxic substances, the blood-brain barrier is neither absolute nor invariable.[8]

Certain disease states modify the permeability of the blood-brain barrier, allowing the entry of penicillin during periods of brain inflammation and trauma. Ordinarily, this common antibiotic cannot easily cross the barrier.

Metabolism and Excretion

As drugs are circulated throughout the body, they undergo processes of *metabolism* and *excretion,* both responsible for the *elimination* of the drugs and the termination of drug action.

The complex chemical changes that alter drugs and convert them to substances that can be eliminated from the body are collectively known as **metabolism.** A special system of enzymes (chemicals that tend to speed up certain body processes) that function mainly, but not exclusively, in liver cells carries out these metabolic reactions. Thus, the liver is a vital body organ that transforms fat-soluble substances to more water-soluble compounds and changes poisonous chemicals to less toxic metabolism by-products. Such complex liver actions that change the chemical or pharmacological properties of a drug by metabolism are referred to as **biotransformation.**

When the recently biotransformed substances are carried by the blood to the *kidneys,* the metabolized drug by-products are *excreted,* or eliminated from the body in the urine. Consequently the kidneys, with their filtering action, are the major route of eliminating biotransformed and toxic substances from the human body. This action of the kidneys helps maintain the body's chemical **homeostasis,** that internal state of constancy or equilibrium necessary for normal functioning.

Although most drugs are excreted by the kidneys, small amounts will also be eliminated via several minor pathways of excretion. These routes include sweat, saliva, gastric secretions, bile, feces, mother's milk, and the lungs. Though several psychoactive substances are absorbed through the lungs, including nicotine, marijuana, and cocaine, only the highly volatile drugs such as anesthetic gases are excreted through the lungs.

Drug Actions

Although there are technical distinctions between **drug actions** and drug effects, this brief description will employ these terms interchangeably.

Drug actions are the result of a chemical interaction with some part of the human organism. Drugs replace body chemicals that are deficient, act against bacteria and other disease-causing agents, or interfere with cellular function. In this text, two major pharmacological actions will be described: (1) those resulting from the use of *structurally nonspecific drugs;* and (2) those associated with *structurally specific drugs.*

A structurally nonspecific drug action results when a particular chemical substance is given or applied in a relatively large dose that forms a thin layer over an entire area of body cells. Examples of such a drug are the anesthetic gases, ethyl alcohol, and antiseptic preparations. An antiseptic, for instance, acts in a nonspecific way on all human cells encountered, as well as on all bacterial cells in a human wound. The antiseptic effectively kills or retards microbial growth.

But, structurally specific drugs produce effects based upon their unique chemical structure. The interaction between such drug molecules and human cells involves small, highly specific areas called *receptors.*

According to major explanations of drug activity, *receptors* or receptor substances are thought to be localized portions on the surface of or within a particular cell, such as the cellular membrane, enzymes, and nucleic acids. It is further presumed that a particular drug must interact with or attach itself to the appropriate receptor in a body cell before any change in cell function occurs.

The **drug-receptor interaction** is often compared with a "lock-and-key" mechanism as illustrated in figure 3.1. According to this concept, the better-fitting drug molecule bonded with the appropriate receptor produces the more desirable effect or action. If the drug binds inadequately to the drug receptor, there is no drug action or effect.

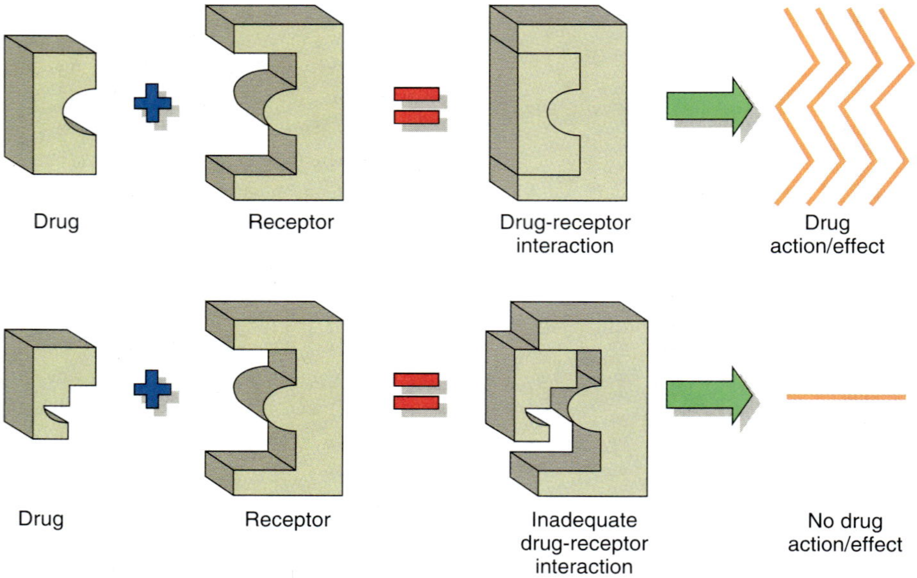

figure 3.1

The drug-receptor interaction.

The body's own natural chemicals, called *neurotransmitters*—discussed later in this chapter—also bind to these receptor sites and initiate a particular response in the cell. If a drug binds to the same site, adds to the effects of the body's own neurotransmitters, and enhances cell response, the drug is referred to as an *agonist.* However, if a drug prevents the body's own natural chemicals from binding to its receptor, and as a consequence blocks a particular cell response, the drug is then identified as an *antagonist.*

Drugs change cell function by one or more of the following specific methods.[9]

1. **Activation**—an increase in the rate of functional activity due to the effect of an agonist drug that stimulates the cell to do something. Cocaine, caffeine, amphetamines, and methylphenidate (Ritalin) tend to speed up central nervous system functions.
2. **Inactivation**—a reduction in the rate of functional activity due to the effect of an antagonist drug that stops, dampens, or depresses certain cellular processes. Ethyl alcohol narcotics, sedative-hypnotics, and tranquilizers slow down or depress the activities of the central nervous system. Low doses of marijuana may also have a depressant effect, a form of inactivation.

   Blocking is a form of inactivation that obstructs or effectively prevents a particular action or response. For example, antihistamine drugs block typical allergic reactions.

   Another form of inactivation, closely related to blocking is known as *inhibition.* This drug action is the likely method by which analgesics stop or reduce pain and psychedelic drugs change cell functions. By interfering with or inhibiting the normal activities of certain chemicals manufactured in the brain, LSD permits the brain to be assaulted by an excessive amount of sensory input. One result of this "sensory overload" is visual hallucinations; another is bizarre behavior related to gross distortion of thought and sensory processes—evidence of the psychedelic effect. At high-dose levels, marijuana sometimes acts as a psychedelic drug, too.
3. *Substitutive*—a temporary replacement of a crucial substance that is not being produced to restore an optimal bodily condition. For example, a hormonal product may be given to a female who cannot produce her own estrogen.

   However, if the body completely loses its ability to produce an important chemical substance, a more permanent substitute or replacement will be made on a continuing basis. The long-term administration of insulin to diabetics is an example of substitutive therapy.
4. *Curative*—a healing or health-restoring action brought on by destroying or preventing the growth of disease-causing organisms. Antibiotics kill bacteria by interfering with the manufacture of bacterial cell walls.
5. *Irritation*—the abnormal excitation of some body part or function. This action may be an exaggerated form of stimulation. Laxatives irritate the large intestine to initiate defecation.

Factors Influencing Drug Actions

In addition to the route of administration, drug distribution throughout the body, and processes of drug metabolism and elimination, the following factors also influence drug responses.

Dose-Response Relationship

The quantity or amount of drug that is taken at any particular time is called the **dose** or dosage. In some instances, the greater the dose, the greater the drug effect or response. However, for other drugs, an increase in dosage beyond the level needed to produce a given response will have little or no effect.

The *threshold dose,* or minimal dose, is the smallest amount of a given drug capable of producing a detectable response. Less than such an amount is known as a *subthreshold dose,* which fails to produce a detectable response. However, drugs are also said to have a *maximum effect,* the greatest response produced by a specific drug, regardless of the dose administered.

The term *median effective dose* is used to express the considerable variation among drugs and the differing responses by individuals to the same dosage of the same drug. Abbreviated as ED_{50}, the median effective dose describes the dosage required to produce a specific response in 50 percent of test subjects. If the response to a particular dose is death, the dosage is identified as the *lethal dose.* That amount of drug that will be fatal for 50 percent of test subjects is then called the *median lethal dose,* or LD_{50}.

In this consideration of dosage, even though all drugs are potential poisons when given in sufficient amounts, even the most deadly poisons are usually nontoxic (nonpoisonous) when given at extremely low dose levels.

When psychoactives or any other drugs are used in the treatment of illness,[10] the dosage must be sufficient to produce a beneficial response without causing adverse effects, including death. Therefore, the aim of drug therapy is to achieve a level of medication in the blood or tissues that lies somewhere between the minimum effective dose and the maximum safe concentration of a drug.

This dosage level is referred to as a drug's *therapeutic range.* For instance, digitalis drugs and the sedative-hypnotic chloral hydrate have a narrow therapeutic range, so the margin of effectiveness and safety is small. By contrast, other drugs such as penicillin and THC (the major psychoactive component of marijuana), have a much wider therapeutic range, and are considered relatively safe.

An index for rating the relative safety of drugs for use in large populations of humans has been identified as the therapeutic ratio, or **therapeutic index** (TI).[11] Sometimes referred to as a drug's standard safety margin, the laboratory therapeutic index is usually defined as the ratio between the median lethal dose (LD_{50}) and the median effective dose (ED_{50}), and is represented by the following: $T.I. = LD_{50}/ED_{50}$.

Nevertheless, a more realistic method of calculating the T.I. in a therapeutic setting with human beings involves the use of the *effective dose in nearly all patients* (ED_{99}) and the *lethal dose in practically no patients* (LD_1). A ratio calculated on the basis of LD_1/ED_{99} yields a more meaningful interpretation of the therapeutic index. The greater this ratio, the safer the medication.

Age

In comparison with so-called average 18- to 65-year-old adults, infants and the elderly usually display more sensitivity to the effects of drugs. Infants tend to have underdeveloped abilities to metabolize and excrete drugs. As a consequence, drug actions within their bodies tend to be prolonged. The elderly, too, are likely to have impaired ability to metabolize and eliminate drugs from their bodies, part of the phenomenon of aging. Poor absorption in some older people is also a factor in reducing the effects of certain drugs. In another instance, one drug has a special reputation for reacting differently in children than in adults. Ritalin, a powerful stimulant for adults, acts as a depressant in hyperactive children.

Body Weight

Giving the same amount of a drug to a 90-pound person and a 200-pound person is likely to produce significantly different results because of the greater concentration of the drug in the blood of the lighterweight individual. Lightweight people usually experience a greater drug effect than heavier people when all other factors, including dosage, are similar. By contrast, the heavier individual with more blood and body fluids to dilute an absorbed drug thus reduces the concentration of the dissolved drug—the amount of the drug contained per unit volume of body fluid.

Gender

Although males and females respond similarly to drugs, females are usually more sensitive to the effects of some drugs than males. This gender difference is often associated with the variable concentrations of proteins, lipids (fats), and water in the human body. For instance, a female who weighs exactly the same as a male and drinks exactly the same amount of an alcoholic beverage as the male will almost always have a higher blood-alcohol level. Such a condition is related to the higher proportion of fat and lower proportion of water typically found in the bodies of females in comparison with the bodies of males. While alcohol is readily soluble in fat, it is even more soluble in water.

Males, on the other hand, tend to have more body fluids or a higher water content in which to dilute the alcohol consumed. As a consequence, females tend to become more intoxicated than males after drinking approximately the same amount of alcohol.

Other gender factors influencing drug effects include the fluctuating levels of female sex hormones during the menstrual cycle. In general, females absorb ethyl alcohol more rapidly during the premenstrual phase of the menstrual cycle. If these females happen to be taking oral contraceptives, however, they are still at considerable risk of intoxication if they drink alcoholic beverages. Simply stated, taking birth control pills tends to slow down the body's ability to metabolize ethyl alcohol. Thus, the drug effects of alcohol would be prolonged beyond the normal, expected period of influence.

Women also lack a stomach enzyme that functions to partially oxidize ethyl

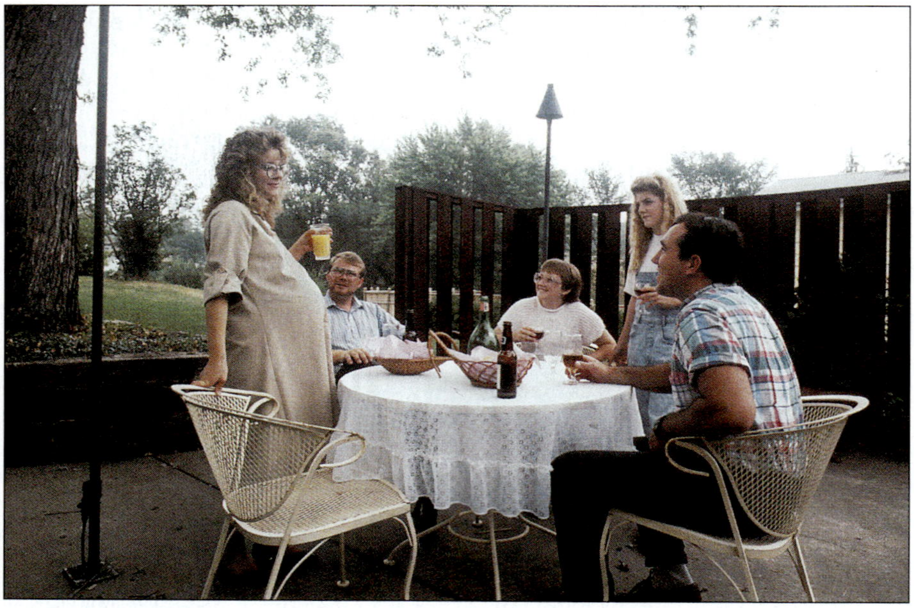

Most psychoactive drugs, including alcohol, can cross the "placental barrier." Recognizing this fact, the pregnant woman in this photo is being good to her baby before it is born by drinking nonalcoholic beverages during her pregnancy.

© James L. Shaffer

alcohol before it enters the bloodstream. Men, who tend to have such a stomach enzyme, are thus able to metabolize equal amounts of alcohol more rapidly than women. Again, females tend to have higher blood alcohol levels than men when they drink the same amount of an alcoholic beverage.

Females should be extremely cautious about taking any drug during pregnancy, because many prescribed and recreational drugs cross the placenta and can then damage the embryo and fetus. At one time the placenta was considered a barrier that prevented toxic substances and harmful organisms from being transferred from the mother to the developing new life form. Today it is known that the "placental barrier" is crossed preferentially by fat-soluble compounds and by those substances having a molecular weight of less than 1,000. Most commonly used drugs, including psychoactive chemicals, have such characteristics and pass readily through the placenta. Rapid transfer of anesthetics, alcohol, barbiturates, cocaine, marijuana, morphine, and heroin occurs from the mother to the embryo or fetus.

Time

The length of time between taking a drug and observing the anticipated effect is referred to as the "onset of action." Some drugs act shortly after entering the body; others may require several hours or even days before their effects become apparent. After the onset of action, drugs will vary in terms of the time required to achieve their maximum effects, as well as the duration of time during which drugs continue to have an effect.

Disease

The presence or absence of a disease condition will often alter a person's response to a drug. For instance, aspirin reduces fever but has no effect in lowering normal temperature. People with impaired liver and kidney function often have difficulty metabolizing and excreting drugs and thus experience prolonged drug effects. Such people are unable to eliminate drugs from their bodies in a normal period. But, when diarrhea exists, some drugs are transported through the gastrointestinal tract so rapidly that drug absorption is significantly reduced.

Mind-Set

Often referred to as the *mind-set,* one's emotional state or climate is recognized as having a potentially significant impact on drug responses. Temperament marked by anger, fear, sadness, joy, or any other emotion can bring about changes in various bodily processes, namely, secretion of gastric juices and hormones, and alteration of blood pressure, heart rate, pulse, and respiration. These bodily processes, in turn, influence drug absorption, distribution, metabolism, and excretion—which can modify the response to a drug.

However, taking a drug and having a particular expectation of that drug's effects also refers to the condition of mind-set. If an individual uses a drug, especially a psychoactive one, in anticipation of "getting high," feeling more powerful or secure, or experiencing a new altered state of consciousness, such a mind-set can and often does result in an exaggerated behavioral response, as expected. This mental predisposition is as important as pharmacology in determining whether the effect of a drug is ultimately perceived as desirable or undesirable, pleasant or unpleasant. For instance, experienced users are often able to get intoxicated on lower-potency marijuana than most first-time users are, presumably because experienced marijuana users expect to do so, while the novice users may be fearful of the drug's effects. Such beginners often have a negative response to the psychoactive drug. Similarly, the use of a fake or inert substance that produces a drug response (the so-called placebo effect discussed later in this chapter) is also based upon a mind-set of trust, belief in a physician's judgment, and expectation of relief.

Environmental Setting

Closely related to mind-set in changing a drug response are the various factors of the *environmental setting.*[12] The environment includes not only the physical place in which a drug is taken but also the psychosocial circumstances surrounding the drug use.

The impact of the environment on drug action can be significant with mind and behavior-altering chemicals. For example, using a psychedelic drug in a controlled laboratory situation or among caring, protective friends will likely result in fewer "bad trips" than would be experienced in "street use" of the same drug or among uncaring drug takers. Also, the effect of drinking alcoholic beverages in celebration of New Year's Eve or an athletic victory may be different from the effect of using the same amount of beverage alcohol in the presence of one's parents, the college dean, or a disapproving loved one.

The influence of environmental setting on drug use was also apparent during the Vietnam War of the 1960s and 1970s. Many American soldiers smoked high-grade heroin, primarily to escape boredom and to help make time pass more quickly. Medical authorities had predicted that most of the soldiers would eventually become addicted. Few did when they returned to the United States. Apparently, the unique environmental setting of Army life in Vietnam shaped this pattern of drug use.[13] When the soldiers left the conflict in southeast Asia, most of them stopped using heroin.

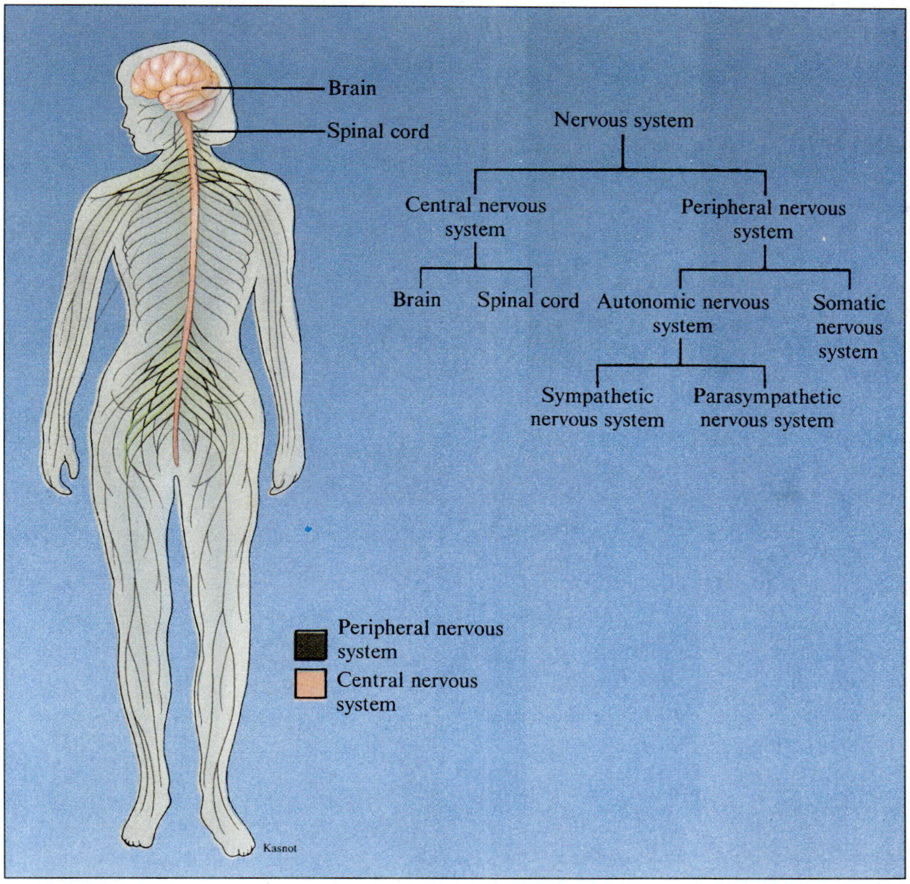

figure 3.2

The nervous system consists of the brain, spinal cord, and numerous peripheral nerves.

From Psychology, *3d edition by Lester M. Sdorow. Copyright © 1995 Wm. C. Brown Communications, Inc. Reprinted by permission of The McGraw-Hill Companies.*

The Nervous System

Although all drugs are capable of producing more than a single response, the so-called psychoactive substances—the major concern of this text—have their primary effect on the human nervous system. Therefore, this descriptive analysis will focus on the structure and function of the nervous system. It will provide a basic understanding of how drugs alter nerve function, mental processes, mood, feelings, consciousness, perceptions, and behavior. Subsequently, a brief consideration will be given to the effects of drugs on other body systems and to the role of chemotherapy in modern medical practice.

Organization of the Nervous System

The nervous system consists of specialized structures that control and coordinate the body's activities. Such functions are conducted in three basic ways: (1) *sensory reception*—the detection of stimuli from within and outside the body; (2) *interconnection*—the transmission of electrochemical messages from one part of the nervous system to another; and (3) *motor response*—the initiation of an appropriate response, such as a muscular contraction or glandular secretion, due to a message sent out to such parts by a nerve center.

As shown in figure 3.2, the nervous system has three major structures: the *brain*, the *spinal cord*, and the *peripheral nerves*. Each of these consists mainly of **neurons,** the functional and structural units of this body system. Neurons are specialized cells that can send electrochemical messages (impulses) to one another and to other cells outside the nervous system.

The nervous system is subdivided into two major parts:

1. The **central nervous system** (CNS) is composed of the brain and the spinal cord. Drugs of abuse and many of the commonly misused drugs have their primary effect on the central nervous system.
2. The **peripheral nervous system** consists of the nerves that branch out from the central nervous system and connect it to other parts of the body, including the extremities. Anatomists and physiologists have subdivided the peripheral nervous system into two additional subdivisions:
    a. The *somatic system*—the cranial and spinal nerves connecting the central nervous system to the skin and the skeletal muscles.

b. The *autonomic system*—the nerves that connect the central nervous system to the organs of the body cavity (the viscera), including the heart, stomach, intestines, and various glands. This subdivision's nerves function involuntarily and automatically without conscious control or effort.

The **autonomic nervous system** is subdivided into two more parts:[14] (1) the *sympathetic division,* which prepares the body for energy-expending activities; and (2) the *parasympathetic division,* which aids in restoring the body to a resting state after an emergency. The parasympathetic division tends to counterbalance the actions of the sympathetic division. These two subdivisions act in opposition to each other—the parasympathetic counterbalancing or opposing the action of the sympathetic—therefore their function is described as *antagonistic.*

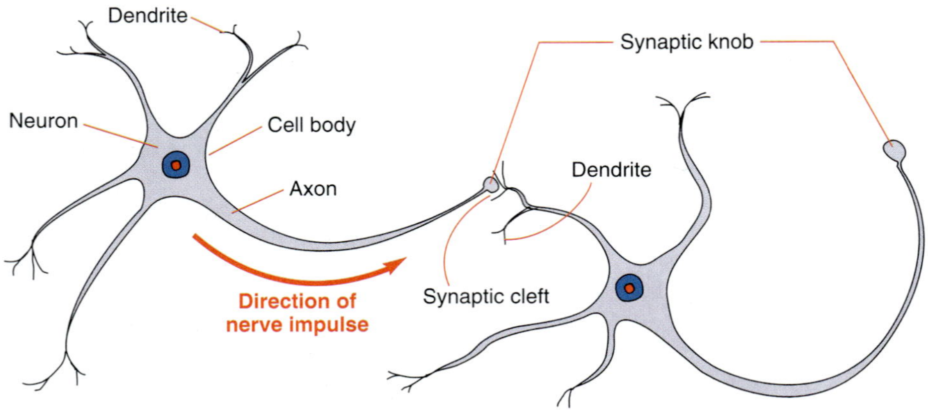

figure 3.3

For an impulse to continue from one neuron to another, it must cross the synaptic cleft at a synapse or junction between two neurons.

The Nerve Cell

As the basic unit of the nervous system, a nerve cell, or *neuron,* is capable of receiving stimuli and transmitting electrical messages or impulses. Depicted in figure 3.3, a neuron consists of a *cell body,* or *soma,* containing a nucleus, granular cytoplasm, and other structures common to body cells.

Extending from the neuron are two types of *nerve fibers.* **Dendrites** are fibers that send nerve impulses toward the cell body; **axons** carry impulses away from the cell body. In general, each neuron has several dendrites but only one axon.

Originating in the dendrite, an electrical impulse is integrated in the cell body and then transmitted down the axon. Transmission of the impulse, known as the *action potential,* is accomplished through the loss of an electrical charge on the nerve fiber's membrane. Although psychoactive drugs do not act primarily on the axon, local anesthetics do, and thus block the transmission of pain impulses to the brain.

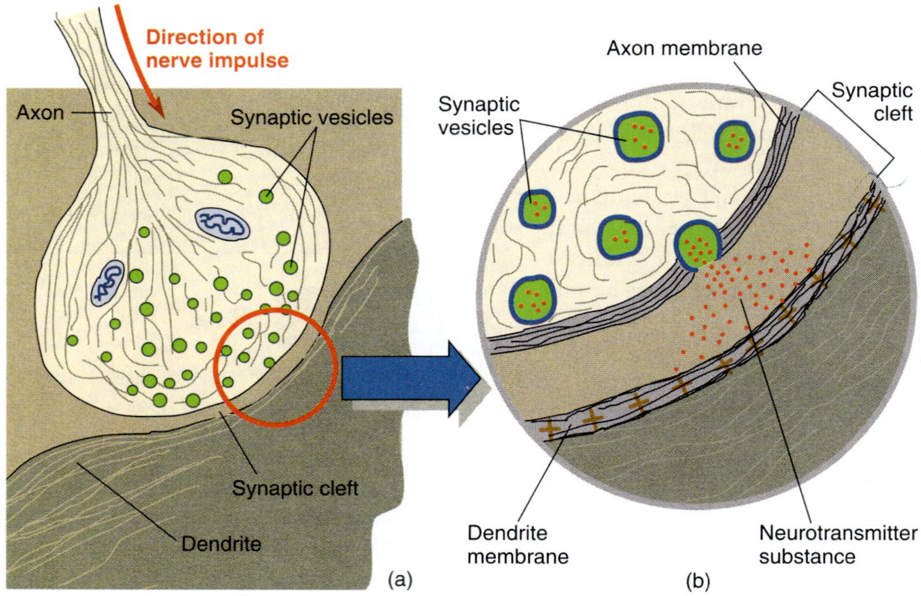

figure 3.4

(a) When a nerve impulse reaches the synaptic knob at the end of an axon, (b) synaptic vesicles release a neurotransmitter substance that diffuses across the synaptic cleft.

The junction between two nerve cells—the meeting place between the axon of one neuron and the dendrites of another neuron—is known as the **synapse.** Before an electrical impulse can be continued from one neuron to the next, it must cross a narrow space or gap named the *synaptic cleft,* illustrated in figure 3.4. The crossing-over process from axon to dendrite is accomplished not by any electrical discharge but by chemical transmission. It is at the synapse that other chemicals, specifically the psychoactive drugs, have their major effect.

Neurotransmitters

Rounded *synaptic knobs* at the ends of axons contain chemical factories called *synaptic vesicles.* These tiny, saclike structures manufacture chemical substances, the **neurotransmitters.** When an electrical impulse reaches the end of an axon, the following sequence of events rapidly occurs.

1. A nerve impulse reaches the synaptic knob.
2. The neurotransmitter substance ruptures from the synaptic vesicles into the synaptic cleft.
3. The neurotransmitter substance diffuses across the synaptic cleft.
4. The neurotransmitter substance reacts with the membrane of the dendrite on the other side of the cleft.
5. Electrical charge is lost on the dendrite membrane.
6. The nerve impulse is reestablished in the dendrite fiber and the transmission of the action potential continues.
7. By special chemical carriers, the neurotransmitter substance is rapidly returned to the synaptic vesicles of its origin for eventual reuse. However, a smaller amount of the neurotransmitter may undergo decomposition by special enzymes. These processes terminate the action of the neurotransmitter substance, until the next impulse reaches the synaptic knob of the axon. Both processes prevent continued stimulation of the dendrite.

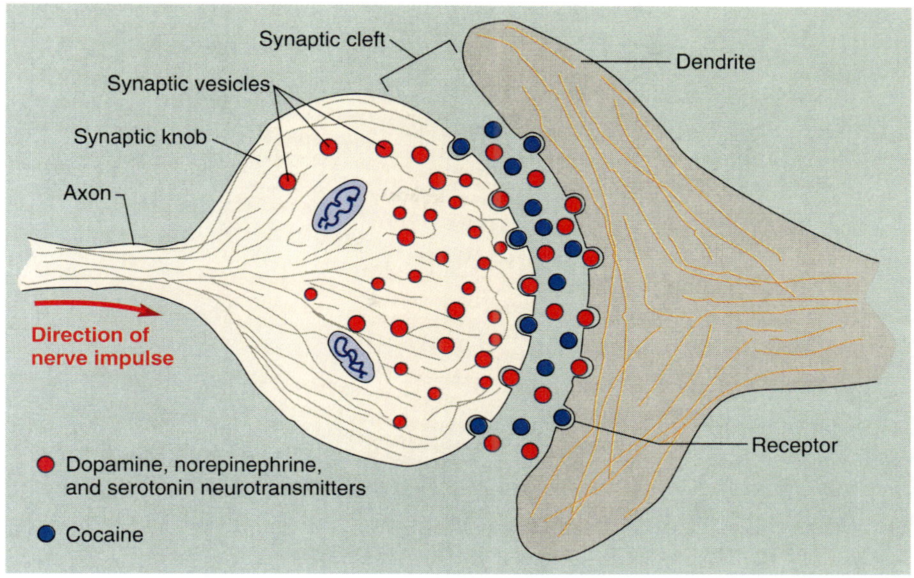

figure 3.5

How one psychoactive drug produces its effects. Cocaine produces its stimulating and euphoric effects by increasing the levels of three specific neurotransmitter substances: dopamine, norepinephrine, and serotonin. The drug, cocaine, binds to its own receptors in the axon's synaptic knob and therefore blocks the re-uptake and reuse of these neurotransmitters. Consequently, the levels of these neurotransmitters are increased in the synaptic cleft and their effect is prolonged as they continue to bind to the receptor sites in the dendrite.

It is through the repetition of these sequential events that a nerve impulse is conducted from one neuron to another. Neurotransmitters function as the chemical signals by which nerve cells send and receive information. The result of such an electrochemical communication is the production of thoughts, perceptions, emotional states, and physical actions.

Many different neurotransmitters are produced by the nervous system.[15] However, only the following are described here in relation to psychoactive drugs:

Acetycholine—an excitatory neurotransmitter (one that triggers a nerve impulse) released by axons both within and outside the central nervous system. It influences heart rate, learning, and memory.

Norepinephrine—one of the catecholamine neurotransmitters in the brain, associated with arousal reactions and moods. It influences sleep, appetite, blood pressure, heart rate, learning, memory, and affective disorders.

Dopamine—another catecholamine neurotransmitter in the brain, associated with body movement. It influences vision, motor control, appetite, euphoria, and schizophrenia.

Serotonin—a brain neurotransmitter associated with regulation of sensory perception, sleep, and body temperature. Alterations in the proper functioning of serotonin have been related to mental illnesses and certain drug-induced hallucinations.

Gamma-aminobutyric acid or GABA—an inhibitory neurotransmitter substance (one that blocks the transfer of a nerve impulse to an adjoining neuron) in the brain. When the normal functioning of GABA is disrupted at the synapses, convulsions may occur. GABA restrains brain activity with a reduction of arousal, aggression, and anxiety.

Other neurotransmitter substances include glycine, histamine, glutamate, adenosine triphosphate, prostaglandins, enkephalins, and endorphins. The latter two chemical substances will be discussed further in the chapter on narcotics.

Drugs and Synaptic Transmission

Some drugs increase the excitability of neurons, whereas others reduce or inhibit such activity. Many psychoactive drugs resemble specific neurotransmitters. As a consequence, these drugs can interact with the receptor sites of various neurotransmitters, either mimicking or blocking the actions of the neurotransmitter they resemble (see figure 3.5).[16]

The results of such psychoactive substance-neurotransmitter interactions

table 3.1 Selected Psychoactive Drugs with Affected Neurotransmitters and General Effects

Psychoactive Drug	Neurotransmitter Affected	General Effect
Atropine from the deadly nightshade plant	Acetylcholine	Sedation, confusion, hallucinations, amnesia
Nicotine	Acetylcholine	Increased alertness
Alcohol and other sedative-hypnotics	GABA	Depression of the central nervous system
Valium	GABA	Decreased level of anxiety
LSD	Serotonin and Dopamine	Inhibits release of serotonin, increases release of dopamine resulting in sense of euphoria
Prozac	Serotonin	Elevation of mood
Cocaine and Marijuana	Dopamine	Intense pleasure, alertness, and increased movement
Cocaine and Amphetamines	Norepinephrine	Euphoria, increased heart rate, constriction of blood vessels, increased blood pressure
Tricyclic antidepressants	Dopamine	Mood elevation

produce the effects typically associated with specific drugs, as noted in table 3.1. Methamphetamine or speed mimics the effects of norepinephrine and results in stimulation and positive emotion, while cocaine mimics the effects of dopamine. Drugs related to LSD and certain antidepressants limit the effects of serotonin, but increase dopamine levels creating a sense of euphoria. Alcohol and the sedative-hypnotics enhance the inhibitory action of GABA, thus contributing to a depressant effect on the central nervous system.

Nicotine mimics or intensifies the effect of acetylcholine, while atropine (a drug that decreases gastrointestinal movements) blocks the action of acetylcholine. The effect of atropine is thus described as anticholinergic; that is, acting against acetylcholine that cholinergic nerve fibers release.

By contrast, certain drugs prescribed to control hypertension (high blood pressure) are described as *adrenergic* blockers because they prevent the release of norepinephrine neurotransmitters from adrenergic nerve fibers or compete with adrenergic, neurotransmitter receptor sites in the heart.

While some neurons produce two or three different neurotransmitters, others release only one neurotransmitter. At least thirty neurotransmitter substances have been identified in the human nervous system. Sometimes, specific neurotransmitters reach a condition of imbalance, resulting in various diseases and disorders, as listed in table 3.2.

The Brain

The brain is the largest and most complex structure in the nervous system. A collection of more than 100 billion neurons (nerve cells) and fibers, the brain is contained within the skull and integrates human behavior into a unified whole. Changes in thought processes, feelings, and behavior resulting from the use of various psychoactive drugs can be more easily understood when one is aware of the major brain structures and their functions.

Among the important parts of the brain are:

1. The *brain stem* with its three components—the medulla oblongata, pons, and the midbrain;
2. The *diencephalon* with its specialized areas—the thalamus, hypothalamus, and the limbic system;
3. The *cerebellum;* and
4. The *cerebrum* (see fig. 3.6).

Brain Stem

The brain stem is the continuation of the spinal cord in the skull and connects the brain with the spinal cord. The parts of the brain stem are made up of many tracts of nerve fibers and special masses of gray matter called nuclei.

Medulla Oblongata

The **medulla oblongata** is the direct upward continuation of the spinal cord within the skull. It is composed of ascending and descending nerve fibers connecting the brain and spinal cord. Located herein are the *vital centers* responsible for controlling breathing (respiration center), blood pressure (vasomotor center), heart rate (cardiac center), contraction of heart musculature, functioning of the gastrointestinal tract, sleeping and waking, behavioral alerting, attention and arousal, coughing, sneezing, swallowing, and vomiting.

Opiates and barbiturates can so severely depress these centers that death may occur, often from respiratory failure. Antihypertensive drugs appear to exert their effect here too, depressing the center controlling the tone of blood vessels.

Pons

The pons is a rounded bulge on the underside of the brain stem that connects the medulla with the midbrain. It contains ascending and descending nerve

table 3.2 Selected Diseases and Disorders Associated with Neurotransmitter Imbalances

Condition	Symptoms	Imbalance of Neurotransmitter in Brain
Alzheimer's disease	Memory loss, depression, disorientation, dementia, hallucinations, death	Deficient acetylcholine
Clinical depression	Debilitating, inexplicable sadness	Deficient norepinephrine and/or serotonin
Epilepsy	Seizures, loss of consciousness	Excess GABA leads to excess norepinephrine and dopamine
Huntington's disease	Personality changes, loss of coordination, uncontrollable dancelike movements, death	Deficient GABA
Hypersomnia	Excessive sleeping	Excess serotonin
Insomnia	Inability to sleep	Deficient serotonin
Mania	Elation, irritability, overtalkativeness, increased movements	Excess norepinephrine
Myasthenia gravis	Progressive muscular weakness	Deficient acetylcholine receptors at neuromuscular junctions
Parkinson's disease	Tremors of hands, slowed movements, muscle rigidity	Deficient dopamine
Schizophrenia	Inappropriate emotional responses, hallucinations	Deficient GABA leads to excess dopamine
Sudden infant death syndrome ("crib death")	Baby stops breathing, dies if unassisted	Excess dopamine
Tardive dyskinesia	Uncontrollable movements of facial muscles	Deficient dopamine

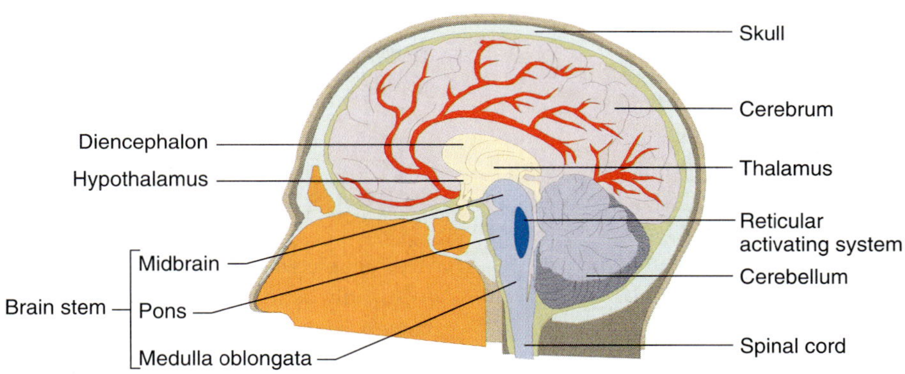

figure 3.6

The human brain with some of the major parts identified.

fibers that relay impulses among the cerebrum, cerebellum, and spinal cord.

Midbrain

Also referred to as the mesencephalon, the midbrain is a short segment of the brain stem situated just above the pons. The midbrain contains bundles of nerve fibers that serve as motor pathways, or neuronal relays, between the cerebrum and lower parts of the nervous system. It also contains visual and auditory reflex centers that control eye and head movements. Psychedelic drugs may induce auditory or visual hallucinations by acting on these reflex centers.

Diencephalon

The diencephalon is the region of the brain located between the large masses (hemispheres) of the cerebrum and the brain stem. The major components of the diencephalon serve as a relay station for sensory impulses and help maintain the internal stability of the body's functioning.

Thalamus

The thalamus is part of the brain located between the cerebrum and the midbrain. In conjunction with the cerebral cortex, the thalamus functions as a central relay station of the brain, where all incoming sensory impulses, except for smell, synapse before being channeled to appropriate regions of the cerebrum. Additionally, it interprets sensations as painful or pleasurable and is associated with temperature and pressure.

Hypothalamus

Another portion of the diencephalon near the junction of the thalamus and midbrain is identified as the **hypothalamus.** It functions to maintain homeostasis by regulating various visceral (body cavity) activities and by linking the nervous system with the endocrine system by ductless glands.

The hypothalamus has several important functions. It controls heart rate, arterial blood pressure, water and electrolyte (chemical) balance, hunger (eating), body weight, movements and glandular secretions of the gastrointestinal tract, sexual behavior, and the synthesis of neurosecretory substances that stimulate hormonal production by the pituitary gland. Also functioning in the regulation of emotions and behavior, the hypothalamus is a prime site of action of many psychoactive drugs.

table 3.3 Functions of the Cerebral Lobes

Lobe	Functions
Frontal lobes	Motor areas control movements of voluntary skeletal muscles. Association areas carry on higher intellectual processes such as those required for concentrating, planning, complex problem solving, and judging the consequences of behavior.
Parietal lobes	Sensory areas are responsible for the sensations of temperature, touch, pressure, and pain involving the skin. Association areas function in the understanding of speech and in using words to express thoughts and feelings.
Temporal lobes	Sensory areas are responsible for hearing. Association areas are used in the interpretation of sensory experiences and in the memory of visual scenes, music, and other complex sensor patterns.
Occipital lobes	Sensory areas are responsible for vision. Association areas function in combining visual images with other sensory experiences.

From *Hole's Human Anatomy & Physiology,* 6th. ed. by David Shier, Jackie Butler, and Ricki Lewis. Copyright © 1993 Wm. C. Brown Communications, Inc. Reprinted by permission of The McGraw-Hill Companies.

Limbic System

Components of the cerebrum interconnected with the thalamus and hypothalamus form a complex area of the diencephalon known as the limbic system. This system functions in the regulation of emotions, including fear, anger, pleasure, and sorrow. As such, it has a significant effect on human behavior, especially those aspects likely to promote survival. Nearly all psychoactive drugs of abuse have some direct influence on the limbic system.

One specialized area of the limbic system is a small structure called the *nucleus accumbens.* This small area is associated with pleasure. As such, it acts as a common brain pathway that drugs follow in rewarding drug-taking behavior. It is likely the nucleus accumbens is also the part of the brain that controls the process of addiction or drug dependency.

Certain tranquilizing drugs, such as Valium and Librium apparently depress or partially inactivate limbic system functions at dose levels below those that depress other brain functions. Rather than behavioral depression, these drugs result in tranquilization with its calming effect and relief of anxiety.

Cerebellum

This structure is a large, convoluted mass of nerve tissue situated below the cerebrum and behind the pons and medulla. The **cerebellum** communicates with other parts of the brain by various nerve tracts.

From a functional viewpoint, the cerebellum serves as a reflex center in coordinating and integrating skeletal muscle movements. Depression of the cerebellum, achieved by ethyl alcohol intoxication, results in loss of muscle coordination, staggering, and loss of balance.

Cerebrum

The largest and most complex part of the brain, the **cerebrum** contains billions of neurons and nerve centers that have sensory, association, and motor functions. The cerebrum coordinates and interprets internal and external stimuli, and it is the site of higher mental functions such as memory and reasoning. Specific regions of the cerebrum perform various functions, as noted in table 3.3.

There is a consensus of opinion that many psychoactive drugs affect cerebral function either directly or indirectly. Stimulants, including amphetamines, increase neuronal activity, sometimes to the point of hallucinations. Depressant-type drugs, such as ethyl alcohol and barbiturates, decrease nerve cell function, thus affecting concentration and perception of stimuli.

Drug Dependence

Most people who use psychoactive drugs do so only as long as the problems and dangers associated with such use do not outweigh the perceived benefits. Most individuals are capable of using mind-changing drugs only occasionally and in moderate amounts. However, some find it extremely difficult or even impossible to control their use. This condition of uncontrolled drug use is usually referred to as **drug dependence** or drug addiction, the heart of the modern drug problem.[17]

Often described as a psychological or physical condition (or both) in which a drug user needs regular doses of a chemical to function normally, drug dependence can occur in an individual who uses a drug periodically or on a continuous basis. Even though drug dependence is not exclusively associated with psychoactive drugs, the term is often used with reference to chemical mood and behavior modifiers.

For many years, the word **addiction** was used to define compulsive use of drug substances, especially the narcotics and alcohol. Even today, the vast majority of people and many drug treatment and rehabilitation specialists use this term to describe drug taking in which the user's behavior is largely controlled by a substance that has a psychoactive effect and whose use is reinforcing. Addiction also involves compulsive use of a drug despite damage to the individual or to society. Furthermore, the drug-seeking behavior can take precedence over other life priorities.[18] Once the addictive state has developed, the drug becomes so important to the addict that he or she is completely uninterested in other people and activities.

In the past, considerable difficulty arose in distinguishing among the several interpretations of *addiction* and its companion term *habituation,* used to describe a drug that was merely habit forming. As compulsive drug use assumed even more varied dimensions with the newer recreational psychoactives, the World Health Organization eventually proposed substituting the more neutral term *drug dependence* for addiction.[19] Variations in drug-abuse terminology include *chemical dependency* and *substance abuse* (or *alcohol and other drug abuse*), more inclusive perhaps than the older terms.

Some authorities use the terms *drug addiction* and *drug dependence* as scientifically equivalent because both refer to the behavior of repeated intake of mind-changing substances. While *addiction* is the word used by the National Institute on Drug Abuse and other organizations when information is provided at a general level, the term *drug dependence* is preferred in the scientific and medical literature.

The Continuum of Drug Use and Drug Dependence (Addiction)

Although many people, including addiction therapists, believe that drug dependence is an either/or condition—it is either present or not—chemical dependence or addiction may be seen more accurately as a continuum or succession from moderate excess to severe, compulsive use. In one sense, drug dependence appears to evolve over time, which varies from one person to another. As a consequence, an individual might be described as abstaining from drugs, using one or more drugs on a social basis, abusing a drug occasionally, abusing one or more drugs on a continuing basis, or being addicted to a drug.[20]

This concept of the evolving or developing nature of addiction views drug usage as a continuum ranging from nonuse to long-term addiction to one or more drugs. The following are the stages of the drug-use continuum:[21]

Total abstinence, or complete nonuse of recreational psychoactive drugs, including alcoholic beverages.

Rare social use, or infrequent recreational use of a psychoactive drug, but without any drug-related problems.

Heavy social use/early problem use of psychoactive drugs in which frequent excessive use is accompanied by the onset of various drug-related problems, including legal, financial, social, occupational, and personal—a condition that might be considered drug abuse.

Heavy problem use/early addiction marked by frequent excessive use in association with drug-related problems, beginning medical complications, and the traditional withdrawal syndrome when unable to continue use of the drug.

Clear-cut drug addiction in which long-term compulsive use is characterized by the classic withdrawal syndrome following abstinence, multiple drug-related problems, various medical complications linked with drug abuse, use of psychological defense mechanisms (rationalization and projection) to explain abnormal drug use, and the possibility of death resulting from alcohol and/or other drug dependence.

As these stages or levels demonstrate, drug use can be classified according to various intensities and patterns, of which drug dependence or addiction is viewed as one extreme on the drug-use continuum (see fig. 3.7).

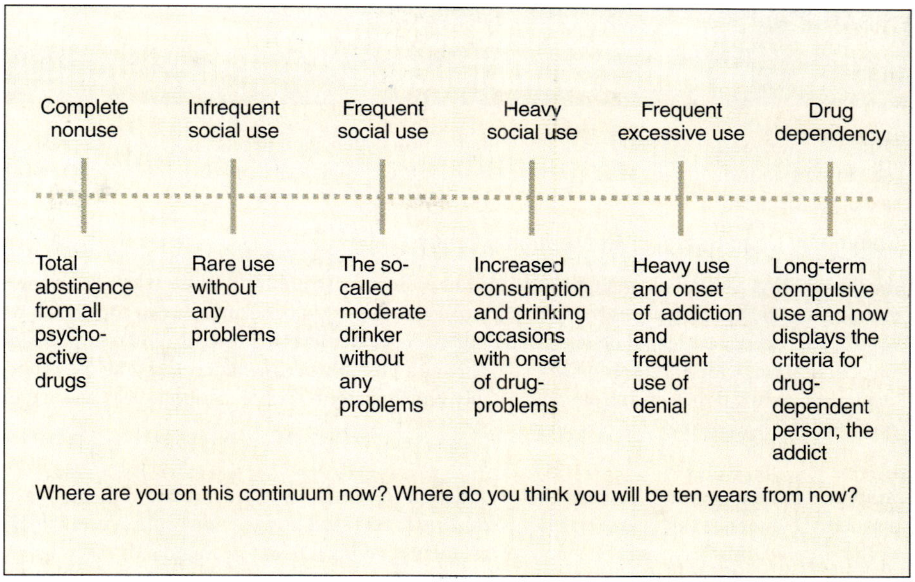

figure 3.7

The drug nonuse, use, abuse, and dependency continuum.

Modified from Harold Doweiko, Concepts of Chemical Dependency, *2nd. ed. Pacific Grove, Calif.: (Brooks/Cole Publishing Company, 1993) 11–13.*

Box 3.2 Drugs and Sex: Selected Drugs and Their Possible Effects on Human Sexual Function

Drugs of abuse and frequently prescribed medications, identified here, can have undesirable effects on normal sexual functioning. Such drugs may impair an individual's sexual arousal, disrupt the sexual desire process, interfere with one's sexual performance, and therefore block sexual satisfaction.

Commonly Used Social or Recreational Drugs

Alcohol or ethyl alcohol in small doses tends to lessen sexual inhibitions, but in larger amounts it often reduces the male's ability to achieve erection and delays or reduces the female's experience of orgasm. Serum testosterone levels tend to decrease as blood alcohol levels increase, resulting in decreased sexual desire among males. At higher levels of intoxication, women tend to experience lowered levels of vaginal vasocongestion, which will inhibit sexual desire and possibly performance. Chronic use often leads to impotence, and among long-term alcoholics, sexual desire disappears. Eventually, the long-term female alcoholic may also experience menstrual disturbances, infertility, and a possible loss of secondary sex characteristics.

Amyl and *butyl nitrite* are inhalants that produce a brief "high" and also tend to enhance the sensation of orgasm. Due to its relaxation of the ringlike muscles around the anus, amyl nitrite has been used frequently by homosexual drug users.

Psychedelics, such as LSD, have been reported as greatly increasing sexual desire and performance as well as producing asexual and nonerotic experiences. MDA, the so-called "love drug," may stimulate feelings of warmth and desire for communication, prerequisites for sexual interaction. Some MDA users remain motionless, however, during their drug experience.

Depressants, such as the sedative-hypnotics, tend to lessen inhibitions, may increase sexual desire, but may also produce inability to achieve erection, ejaculation, and orgasm in moderate to large doses.

Stimulants, specifically cocaine and amphetamines, are often considered aphrodisiacs, because they force the release of dopamine and norepinephrine neurotransmitters that are linked with natural sexual excitement. Cocaine may heighten sexual arousal and delay orgasm in fairly low doses. High-dose use, however, seems to correlate with high-risk sexual practices, while prolonged use often results in decreased sexual desire, erectile and ejaculation difficulties in the male, and anorgasmia (inhibited orgasm) in the female. Amphetamines typically increase sexual desire and delay orgasm in low doses, but high-dose use or prolonged use tends to have a negative impact on sexual performance and satisfaction.

Marijuana users experience varied effects, including relaxed sexual inhibitions, increased sexual pleasure, no impact whatsoever on sexual drive or performance, and also negative feelings about sexual function. Erectile problems, lowered testosterone levels, disruption of normal sperm production, and—in the female—vaginal dryness, have been reported. Enhanced sexual awareness is experienced more often when both parties are under the influence of marijuana.

Stimulants, such as amphetamines, may either increase or decrease sexual desire and tend to reduce potency. Cocaine may heighten sexual arousal in fairly low doses, and delay orgasm, but regular use often results in decreased sexual desire.

Opioids, the narcotic analgesics, tend to impair sexual desire, performance, and satisfaction, and may even temporarily decrease female fertility, delay ejaculation, and reduce erections and orgasms during high-dose use. However, pain experienced by females during intercourse may be reduced.

Prescription Drugs

Antabuse, or disulfiram, an aversive drug used to deter abusive drinkers from alcoholic beverages, may cause reduced potency.

Cimetidine (Tagamet), a frequently prescribed antiulcer drug, may cause impotence and enlarged breasts in males and decreased sexual desire in females.

Conjugated estrogens (Premarin) can produce feminization, including loss of sexual desire, impotence, enlarged breasts, and shrinkage of the testes.

Guanethidine (Ismelin), used in treating hypertension (high blood pressure), prevents ejaculation. Other antihypertensives, such as clonidine (Catapres), may cause impotence in males or loss of sexual desire in females and males.

Continued

Levodopa (Larodopa), a drug used in treating Parkinson's disease, may be responsible for increased sexual desire in some men and women

MAO inhibitors, including phenelzine (Nardil), used in treating psychological depression, may cause impotence.

Major tranquilizers, specifically thioridazine (Mellaril), sometimes cause ejaculatory problems.

Minor tranquilizers, the antianxiety drugs such as Valium and Librium, may reduce sexual desire and impair ejaculation.

Oral contraceptives may cause a reduction in sexual desire among some women.

Tolbutamide (Orinase), an oral antidiabetic medication, may cause prolonged, painful erections in some males.

Over-the-Counter Drugs

Aspirin can induce impaired spermatogenesis (formation of sperm), leading to reduced fertility in males.

Vitamin A in excessive dosages can result in menstrual disorders.

Vitamin C in doses of 1 gram or more can also impair spermatogenesis.

Ibuprofen may delay the onset of menstruation by as much as fourteen days.

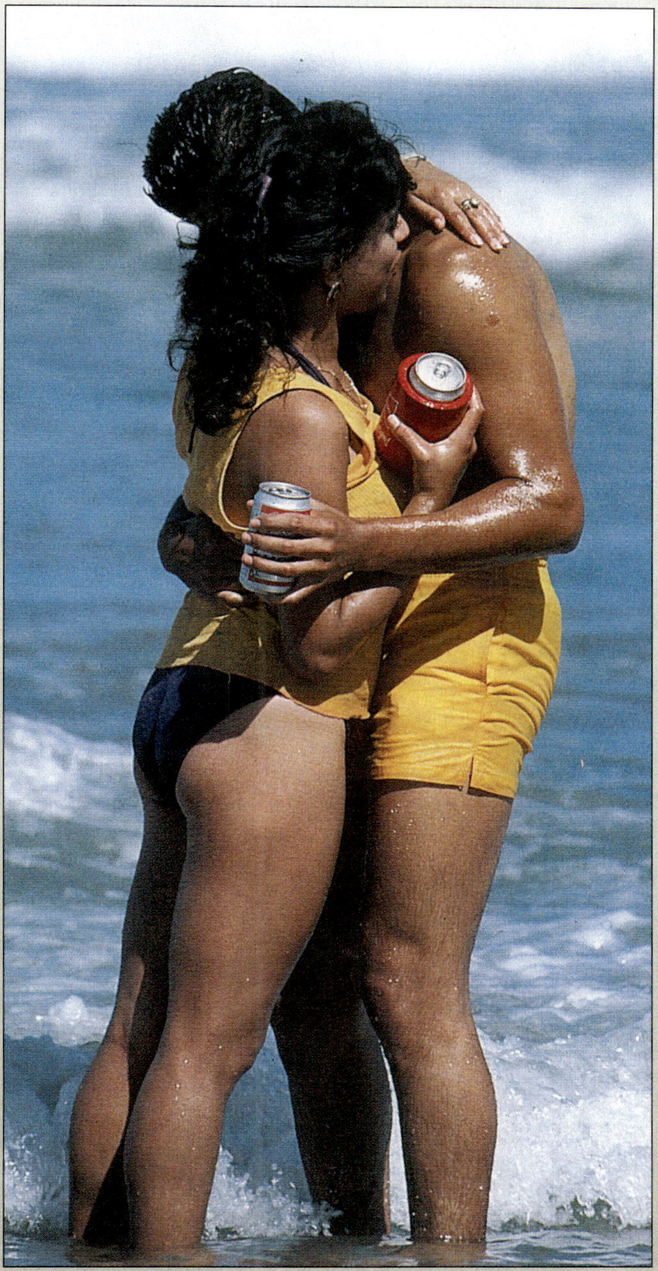

The romantic link between alcohol and sex is greatly exaggerated. While small amounts may provoke sexual desire, larger amounts may spoil the capacity to perform or respond.

© Bob Daemmrich/The Image World

Sources: Harold Doweiko, *Concepts of Chemical Dependency,* 2nd. ed., pp. 401–410, Brooks/Cole, Pacific Grove, Calif., 1993; and James Rybacki and James Long, *The Essential Guide to Prescription Drugs,* pp. 1115–1120, Harper Perennial, New York, 1996.

Criteria for Psychoactive Drug Dependence

It is apparent that no single pattern of drug dependence fits all drugs or drug takers. While all psychoactive chemicals can produce a psychological dependence with repeated use, this particular condition is markedly present in the narcotic opioids, but only mildly present in caffeine and marijuana. With heroin, there is considerably more tolerance than in alcohol abuse, but there are more severe withdrawal symptoms associated with alcohol than are usually present with the narcotic drug. To account for such variations, a single multifactorial category of substance dependence disorders has been proposed by the American Psychiatric Association. This category includes all major drugs of abuse, including caffeine.

According to the American Psychiatric Association's official diagnostic handbook, the *Diagnostic and Statistical Manual of Mental Disorders* (DSM-IV), substance dependence is a maladaptive (faulty or nonproblem-resolving) pattern of drug use leading to clinically significant impairment or distress characterized by three (or more) of the following criteria, occurring at any time in a twelve-month period:[22]

- *Tolerance,* distinguished by either of the following:
  - There is a need for markedly increased amounts of the drug substance to achieve intoxication or the desired effect.
  - There is a markedly diminished effect with continued use of the same amount of the drug.
- *Withdrawal,* specified by either of the following:
  - Characteristic withdrawal syndrome (combination of symptoms) develops when use of the drug has been stopped.
  - The drug substance is often taken to relieve or avoid withdrawal symptoms. (These criteria might not apply to marijuana, other cannabis preparations, hallucinogens, and phencyclidine.)
- *Impaired control*
  - The chemical substance is often taken in larger amounts or over a longer period than the drug taker intended.
- *Desire to quit or unsuccessful attempts to control*
  - There is a persistent desire or unsuccessful efforts to cut down or control substance use.
- *Time spent using drugs*
  - A great deal of time is spent in various activities needed to acquire the drug substance (including theft), to take the substance (as in chain-smoking), and recover from the drug's effects.
- *Neglect of activities*
  - Important social, occupational, or recreational activities are given up or reduced to seek or take a drug.
- *Drug use despite knowledge of problems*
  - Use of a drug continues despite knowledge of having a persistent or recurring physical or psychological problem caused or made worse by substance use. For instance, cocaine use continues despite an individual's awareness of cocaine-induced depression, or drinking of alcoholic beverages persists despite recognition that an ulcer has been made worse by repeated alcohol consumption.

While preoccupation with drug use, the evolving "love affair" between drug taker and drug substance, and the occurrence of drug-related problems can be observed by others, and therefore documented, only the drug abuser experiences several other aspects. These aspects deserve a more thorough analysis, especially psychological dependence, tolerance, physical dependence, and the withdrawal syndrome.

Psychological Dependence

A nonspecific term, *psychological* or *psychic dependence* refers to drug dependence without any physical complications. An individual who develops **psychological dependence** on a particular drug has a strong desire to repeat the use of that drug either occasionally or continuously for emotional reasons. The persistent drug taking is related to the reinforcing or rewarding effects of the drug.

Although the body does not require the drug in a physical sense, the person has an intense craving or compulsion for it to maintain drug-induced pleasure and a feeling of well-being, to achieve a maximum level of functioning, to reduce tensions, or to dull reality. When drug seeking becomes compulsive and a regular behavioral pattern, psychological dependence has reached its peak. Deprived of the drug, the user will typically experience a period of readjustment, accompanied by some degree of anxiety, irritability, and restlessness. No physical complications follow the discontinuance of drug usage.

An individual may be psychologically dependent on a drug without being physically dependent on that drug. The opposite is also true: It is possible to be physically dependent on a drug without being psychologically dependent, although such occurrences are relatively rare and almost always involve the administration of a physician-prescribed narcotic analgesic in a medical facility. However, such a distinction between psychological and physical dependence might not be relevant, because long-term users of drugs producing only psychological dependence act and function in much the same way as addicts of drugs that produce physical dependence.[23]

While psychological dependence is a characteristic of all drugs of abuse, the condition is often considered insignificant in comparison with physical dependence. Such is not the case! In chronic drug use, psychological dependence is increasingly viewed as more serious and more difficult to deal with than physical dependence.[24]

Tolerance

An altered physiological state, **tolerance** develops with the repeated use of almost all drugs.[25] This condition is usually defined as a decreased response to the effects of a drug. As a consequence of this reduced sensitivity, the dosage must be increased to achieve the desired effects.

The onset of tolerance may be rapid or gradual, depending upon the drug used. However, this condition is not an all-or-none phenomenon, because a person may develop a tolerance to one aspect of a particular drug's action but not to another. Also, tolerance can accompany psychological dependence upon a drug without the occurrence of physical dependence. Nevertheless, the need to increase the dosage is more often seen in conjunction with the latter condition.

Usually the degree of tolerance varies with the drug and with other circumstances. Psychedelic drugs produce an extremely high tolerance rapidly, while a high tolerance to the opioids and amphetamines also develops but at a much slower pace. A somewhat lower and more variable degree of tolerance develops with the repeated use of alcohol, nicotine, and marijuana.

Theories that explain the mechanisms of physiological or tissue tolerance may appear both contradictory or complementary. One major theory holds that tolerance is the result of alterations in how a drug is processed in the body after repeated doses are taken. Changes occur in the normal processes of drug absorption, distribution, metabolism, or elimination. For instance, the liver and other body organs destroy or break apart the drug substance more quickly due to a process called *enzyme induction* or excrete it more efficiently. As a result, less of the drug reaches the site of its action. Another contrasting theory is based on the reduced sensitivity of nerve-cell receptor sites that takes place over a long period of drug taking. This represents a form of cellular or tissue adaptation in which reaction to the drug is diminished. It is also possible that the nerve cells (neurons) create additional receptor sites to accommodate the increased dosage of a drug.

In some instances, there is a condition known as *tachyphylaxis* or *acute tolerance*, which is an extremely rapid development of tolerance after only one or a few doses of the drug. LSD, amphetamines, and cocaine tend to show rapid development of tolerance, especially when large doses are used for short periods. This phenomenon may be due to the rapid exhaustion of a neurotransmitter or an accelerated loss of receptor sensitivity.

According to Sidney Cohen, the condition of *kindling* may be thought of as the exact opposite of tolerance.[26] In this form of "reverse tolerance," drug takers can become more sensitive to the effects of a drug, rather than less sensitive. Analogous to igniting a wood fire, the so-called *kindling effect* spreads slowly at first, then suddenly erupts in a symptom compared to a briskly burning blaze. For instance, in cocaine use, the brain may become sensitive to the drug after repeated average doses, so that even low amounts of the stimulant may bring on seizures.

After long-term heavy use of alcohol, another example of "reverse tolerance" may also be evident. A liver damaged by the buildup of fat and the assaults of hepatitis and/or cirrhosis may no longer be able to metabolize effectively any alcohol consumed. Consequently, even small amounts of beverage alcohol result in elevated blood alcohol levels and the rapid experience of intoxication.

One additional concern with tolerance is the development of *cross-tolerance,* a condition in which the reduced pharmacological response to one drug results in a lessened response to another drug. Cross-tolerance, however, typically occurs among drugs belonging to the same class or related classes of chemical substances. For example, an individual tolerant to morphine is also tolerant to all other narcotic drugs, including heroin and methadone. However, such a person will not have a tolerance to alcohol and barbiturates, which belong to another class of psychoactive drugs.

Physical Dependence

An altered physiological state, physical or physiological dependence is induced by the frequent use of a drug and results in unwanted and adverse physical symptoms—the withdrawal syndrome—when drug use has stopped. Often described as a condition of physical need, **physical dependence** is presumed to have existed only when withdrawal symptoms occur.

The causes of this physical need are the temporary and compensatory changes in the cells of the nervous system. These changes in cellular functioning permit the nerve cells to work in their accustomed fashion in the presence of a particular chemical substance and take place over several weeks or months. Thus physical dependence is a state of functional adaptation to a drug in which the presence of a foreign chemical becomes "normal" and necessary. In other words, the absence of a drug would constitute an abnormality, and the presence of a drug is required for normal function.

Often considered as the most hazardous aspect of drug abuse, physical dependence is likely to develop with continuing use of narcotics, barbiturates, minor tranquilizers, ethyl alcohol, and cocaine, and to a lesser degree with nicotine, caffeine, marijuana, and the amphetamines. Only use of the psychedelics and volatile inhalants does not result in physical dependence.

Cross-dependence is a condition in which a person who is physically dependent on one drug can prevent withdrawal symptoms by using other drugs in the same pharmacological class or a closely related drug class. For example, methadone can be substituted for heroin and prevents the occurrence of withdrawal when heroin use is discontinued. In general, those drugs that exhibit cross-tolerance will likely demonstrate cross-dependence to one another.

Withdrawal Syndrome

As mentioned, the condition of physical dependence is revealed only when drug use is discontinued. If the drug is removed abruptly, "normal" cell function is disturbed, resulting in hyperexcitability (overactivity) or hypoexcitability (underactivity) of the nervous system.

Typically, when a person who is physically dependent on a central nervous system depressant (alcohol, barbiturates, or narcotics) stops using the drug, the *withdrawal symptoms* in evidence are restlessness, overactivity of the nervous system, and agitation—an uneven or disturbed form of stimulation. Withdrawal symptoms that occur after long-term use of cocaine, a central nervous system stimulant, are marked by psychic depression and uncontrolled drowsiness and excessive sleep. These drastic alterations in physical function and behavior, experienced after drug

Box 3.3 Drug Interactions *Double Trouble*

Drug interaction is the phenomenon that occurs when one or more drugs present in the body alter the actions or effects of another drug present in the body at the same time. When drugs are taken in combination, the effects usually fall into one of the following categories.

Independent

Drugs taken together may work independently of each other, that is, neither one affects the drug actions of the other.

Antagonistic

Drugs taken together may interact so that the effect of either or both agents is blocked or reduced. The interaction "equation" is represented as 2 + 2 = 3.

An antagonistic interaction is likely to occur when the antibiotic tetracycline is taken at the same time with penicillin, another common antibiotic medication. Tetracycline reduces the effectiveness of the penicillin and may prolong an infection.

Another antagonistic drug interaction involves the combination of barbiturates and oral contraceptives. The headache remedy tends to reduce the effectiveness of the oral contraceptives.

The narcotic antagonist naloxone counteracts the effects of heroin or morphine overdose.

Additive

Drugs taken together may interact so that the net effect of the combination is the sum of the effects of the individual substances. The interaction "equation" may be represented as 2 + 2 = 4.

An additive effect is produced by the simultaneous consumption of two barbiturates, such as phenobarbital and secobarbital.

The interaction of narcotic analgesics with the phenothiazines (major antipsychotic drugs) may result in either an additive effect or a potentiated drug interaction.

Potentiating or Synergistic

Drugs taken together may interact so that the effects of two substances in combination is greater than merely additive. This phenomenon may occur when one drug that has no specific unfavorable effect by itself increases, enhances, or potentiates the undesirable effect of a second drug by altering its distribution, its conversion into other chemicals, or its excretion from the body. Such a drug interaction is described as *potentiating* and its interaction "equation" may be represented as 0 + 1 = 3.

In a synergistic drug interaction, the effect of the second drug may be intensified or multiplied by the effect of the first drug, or the duration of the second drug's action may be prolonged beyond normal expectation. The synergistic interaction "equation" may be represented as 1 + 3 = 7.

In potentiating and synergistic drug interactions, the user does not experience the effects of both drugs as they would function alone. Rather, the combined effects of the two drugs are much greater than the sum of their parts.

An example of a potentiating drug interaction involves the use of a prescribed ulcer medication, Tagamet, together with alcoholic beverages. The antiulcer drug tends to increase blood-alcohol levels and may make drinkers more drunk if they do consume alcoholic beverages.

The following are some of the more dangerous combinations that can result when psychoactive drugs are taken together with other types of drugs or medication. These drugs should never be combined without the consent and supervision of a physician:

Barbiturates in combination with tranquilizers, alcohol, drugs for high blood pressure, stimulants, cortisone, painkillers, diuretics, anticonvulsants, or birth control pills

Tranquilizers in combination with barbiturates, antihistamines, alcohol, drugs for high blood pressure, stimulants, antidepressants, or painkillers

Stimulants in combination with barbiturates, tranquilizers, beer, drugs for high blood pressure, antidepressants, anticonvulsants, drugs for diabetes or digitalis

Antidepressants in combination with tranquilizers, alcohol, drugs for high blood pressure, stimulants, diuretics, anticoagulants, or asthma spray

Source: National Clearing House for Alcohol Information, as modified, National Institute on Alcohol Abuse and Alcoholism, Department of Health and Human Services.

use is terminated, are known collectively as the classic **withdrawal syndrome,** *withdrawal sickness,* or the *abstinence syndrome.* Usually, the syndrome consists of symptoms broadly opposite to the drug's usual effects and produces a kind of "rebound" effect.[27]

Common signs and symptoms of the withdrawal syndrome may include watery eyes, runny nose, yawning, perspiration, restless sleep, irritability, loss of appetite, insomnia, tremors, nausea, vomiting, stomach cramps, diarrhea, elevation of heart rate and blood pressure, pain in muscles and bones, muscle spasms, convulsions, anxiety, depression, suicidal tendencies, and occasional psychotic episodes.

While the process of withdrawal can be painful and in some instances results in death, it nevertheless permits the nerve cells to return to their predrugged state and reduces the level of tolerance that has developed. Sometimes, especially with heroin and other narcotics, a type of "prolonged" abstinence or withdrawal may be experienced in which elevated blood pressure, heart rate, and intense cravings suddenly recur many months and even years after the original withdrawal process. Similar to post-traumatic stress, the prolonged withdrawal phenomenon is possibly activated by exposure to particular sights, sounds, or odors. These stimuli cause the former addict to experience memories of the original withdrawal syndrome and the severe cravings for the drug. This rather strange condition may be the basis for relapse—the return of a person who has undergone withdrawal to the addictive or drug-dependent state.

With increasing frequency, multiple-drug dependence—evidence of polydrug abuse—is being reported by physicians and hospitals. In such cases, the individual goes through a series of withdrawal syndromes from each abused drug.

Another potential hazard of polydrug abuse is drug interaction (see box 3.3).

The Placebo Effect

One of the more unusual aspects of pharmacology is the **placebo effect.** Derived from the Latin word meaning "I will please," a *placebo* is a preparation or treatment that has no specific effect on a patient's illness. Many view a placebo as a fake medicine, an inert substance that has no pharmacologic effect, such as a sugar pill or an injection of sterile water. Such nonmedicated items are administered for their psychological effect.

Placebos are often used to test the effectiveness of new medicines. In clinical trial experiments, one group of patients receiving a new drug is compared with another group given an identical-looking placebo. This type of drug effectiveness testing is known as a *single-blind study.* When the identity of the medicine—placebo or active form—is withheld from both the test subjects and the evaluators, the drug testing design is called a *double-blind study.* If the active test drug fails to achieve better results than those obtained through the use of a placebo, the test drug is considered ineffective.

Surprisingly, placebos can have a positive and even beneficial effect on many patients in certain circumstances. Placebos have been recorded not only as reducing pain, but also as healing ulcers, relieving hay fever, coughing, and elevated blood pressure, and enhancing physical performance. On the average, about one-third of individuals receiving placebos are helped.

The precise mechanisms of a positive placebo effect are not well understood, especially because no specific drug response is anticipated. Most believe that the placebo response arises from the person's unique mental set and predisposition or from the entire environmental situation in which the inactive substance is taken.[28] It is now apparent that the patient's faith, beliefs, and expectations regarding the placebo, the physician's enthusiasm, and the context in which the substance is taken are powerful elements in placebo-induced and in drug-induced responses.

Other factors that may explain how nonmedicines sometimes work have been proposed, including:

- Increased production of endorphin neurotransmitters, morphinelike chemicals within the human body that act on neuron receptors in the central nervous system to deaden pain.
- Activation of the body's immune system, a complex of biochemical processes that provide resistance to specific diseases.
- The patient's anxiety level, rather than gullibility or suggestibility. As the level of anxiety or free-floating fear increases, one's chance of responding favorably to a placebo increases.

As research into the positive placebo effect continues, some scientists believe that it can be used ethically as a powerful tool to enhance the benefits of modern medical practice.

Chapter Summary

1. Pharmacology is the study of the composition, uses, and effects of drugs.
2. Since the introduction of chemical agents that have no relation to treating diseases, a drug is now defined as any chemical that affects living processes.
3. Drugs are most frequently administered orally, parenterally, and by inhalation.
4. After absorption, drugs are distributed in various patterns, metabolized and biotransformed by the liver, and excreted chiefly by the kidneys.
5. Structurally specific drugs interact with localized portions of cells, the receptors, to change cell functions.
6. Drugs can change cell function by activation, inactivation, substituting, curing, and irritation.
7. Dosage, age, body weight, gender, time, disease, mind-set, and the environmental setting can affect drug actions within the human body.
8. The nervous system consists of the central nervous system (brain and spinal cord) and the peripheral nervous system, subdivided into the somatic and autonomic nervous system.
9. The sympathetic and parasympathetic subdivisions of the autonomic nervous system act in an antagonistic manner.
10. As the basic unit of the nervous system, the neuron consists of a cell body, one axon, and several dendrites.
11. An electrical impulse is transmitted from the axon of one neuron to the dendrite of another neuron by chemical substances, the neurotransmitters.
12. Psychoactive drugs interacting with neurotransmitters have their major effect on the synapse, the junction between nerve cells, especially those in the specialized structures of the brain.
13. Major characteristics of drug dependence include various undesirable behaviors related with persistent drug use or abuse, such as increasing preoccupation with a drug, inability to fulfill common roles due

to drug abuse, and not being able to stop drug use, as well as psychological and physical dependence, the development of tolerance, and the experience of withdrawal symptoms.

14. Drug interactions are categorized as independent, antagonistic, additive, and potentiating or synergistic.
15. A placebo is a nonmedicated preparation that has no specific pharmacologic effect on a patient's illness.

World Wide Web Sites

Society for Neuroscience

www.sfn.org/briefings

Neurosciences on the Internet

www.neuroguide.com

Review Questions and Activities

1. State the definition of pharmacology and distinguish among its four major subdivisions.
2. Explain the following terms as related to drug administration: *oral, absorption, parenteral,* and *inhalation.*
3. What are the patterns of drug distribution in the human body?
4. Describe the processes involved in the elimination of drugs from the body.
5. What is a drug receptor?
6. Distinguish among the following drug actions: activation, inactivation, substitutive, curative, and irritation.
7. Define threshold dose, median effective dose, maximum effect, and lethal dose.
8. How do factors such as age, body weight, disease, gender, and emotional states affect drug actions?
9. Identify the major parts and functions of the nervous system.
10. Define the following terms: *neuron, cell body, axon, dendrite, synapse,* and *synaptic cleft.*
11. How is a nerve impulse transmitted from one neuron to another?
12. What is the significance of the following: acetylcholine, norepinephrine, dopamine, serotonin, GABA?
13. What possible effects could psychoactive substances have on the functions of the medulla oblongata, midbrain, cerebellum, hypothalamus, limbic system, and cerebrum?
14. What are some possible effects of using psychoactive drugs on human sexual function?
15. How do the following characteristics of drug dependence differ from one another: psychological dependence, physical dependence, tolerance?
16. In what way can addiction or drug dependence be viewed as a continuum?
17. What criteria have been established. by the American Psychiatric Association to describe a drug-dependent individual?
18. Distinguish between an additive drug interaction and a potentiating drug interaction.
19. Explain how a placebo could have a positive effect on a patient.

References

1. Andrew Weil and Winifred Rosen, *From Chocolate to Morphine,* rev. ed. (Boston: Houghton Mifflin, 1993), 9.
2. Diana Fishbein and Susan Pease, *The Dynamics of Drug Abuse* (Boston: Allyn and Bacon, 1996), 52–53.
3. Robert Julien, *A Primer of Drug Action,* 7th ed. (New York: W. H. Freeman and Company, 1995), 11–12.
4. Christina Dye, *Drugs and the Body: A New Way to Understand Psychoactive Chemicals and Ourselves* (Tempe, Ariz.: Do It Now, 1989), 11–13.
5. Ibid., 13.
6. William Creasey, *Drug Disposition in Humans: The Basic of Clinical Pharmacology* (New York: Oxford University Press, 1979), 33–34.
7. John Hole, *Human Anatomy and Physiology,* 6th ed. (Dubuque, Iowa: Brown & Benchmark, 1993), 674.
8. Leslie Benet, Deanna Kroetz, and Lewis Sheiner, "Pharmacokinetics: The Dynamics of Drug Absorption, Distribution, and Elimination," in *Goodman & Gilman's The Pharmacological Basis of Therapeutics,* 9th ed. (New York: McGraw-Hill, 1996), 10.
9. John Fried and Sharon Petska, *The American Druggist's Complete Family Guide to Prescriptions, Pills, and Drugs* (New York: Hearst Books, 1995), 7–8.
10. Roberta Morgan, *The Emotional Pharmacy* (Los Angeles: Body Press, 1988), 32–37.
11. Bertram Katzung, ed., *Basic Clinical Pharmacology,* 4th ed. (Norwalk, Conn. Appleton & Lange, 1989), 24.
12. Tibor Palfai and Henry Jankiewicz, *Drugs and Human Behavior* (Dubuque, Iowa: Brown & Benchmark, 1991), 94.
13. Weil and Rosen, *From Chocolate to Morphine,* 25.
14. David Shier, Jackie Butler, and Ricki Lewis, *Hole's Human Anatomy & Physiology,* 7th ed. (Dubuque, Iowa: Times Mirror Higher Education Group, Inc., 1996), 426–432.
15. Floyd Bloom, "Neurotransmission and the Central Nervous System," in *Goodman and Gilman's The Pharmacological Basis of Therapeutics,* 9th ed. (New York: McGraw-Hill, 1996), 275–84.
16. Gesina Longenecker, *How Drugs Work: Drug Abuse and the Human Body,* (Emeryville, Calif.: Ziff-Davis Press, 1994), 19–21.
17. Lester Grinspoon and James Bakalar, *Drug Abuse and Addiction: The Harvard Medical School Mental Health Review* (Boston: Harvard Mental Health Letter, 1993), 2.
18. C. Everett Koop, *The Health Consequences of Smoking: Nicotine Addiction: A Report of the Surgeon General* (Washington, D.C.: GPO, 1988), iv, 7.
19. N. B. Eddy and others, "Drug Dependence: Its Significance and Characteristics," *Bulletin of the World Health Organization* 32 (May 1965): 721–33.
20. Harold Doweiko, *Concepts of Chemical Dependency,* 2d ed. (Pacific Grove, Calif.: Brooks/Cole, 1993), 12–13.
21. Ibid.
22. American Psychiatric Association, *Diagnostic and Statistical Manual of Mental Disorders,* 4th ed. (Washington, D.C.: American Psychiatric Association, 1994), 181; and "DSM-IV Makes Changes in Substance-Related Disorders," *Substance Abuse Reports* 25, no. 15 (1 August 1994): 4–5.
23. Erich Goode, "Addiction and Dependence," in *Drugs in American Society,* 4th ed. (New York: McGraw-Hill, 1993), 28–34.
24. Robert O'Brien and others, *The Encyclopedia of Drug Abuse,* 2d ed. (New York: Facts on File, 1992), 257–58.
25. Grinspoon and Bakalar, *Drug Abuse and Addiction,* 4.
26. Sidney Cohen, *The Chemical Brain: The Neurochemistry of Addictive Disorders* (Irvine, Calif.: CareInstitute, 1988), 60.
27. O'Brien and others, *Encyclopedia of Drug Abuse,* 308. Julien, *A Primer of Drug Action,* 45–46; and
28. Palfai and Jankiewicz, *Drugs and Human Behavior,* 91–94.

Part Two

The Depressants

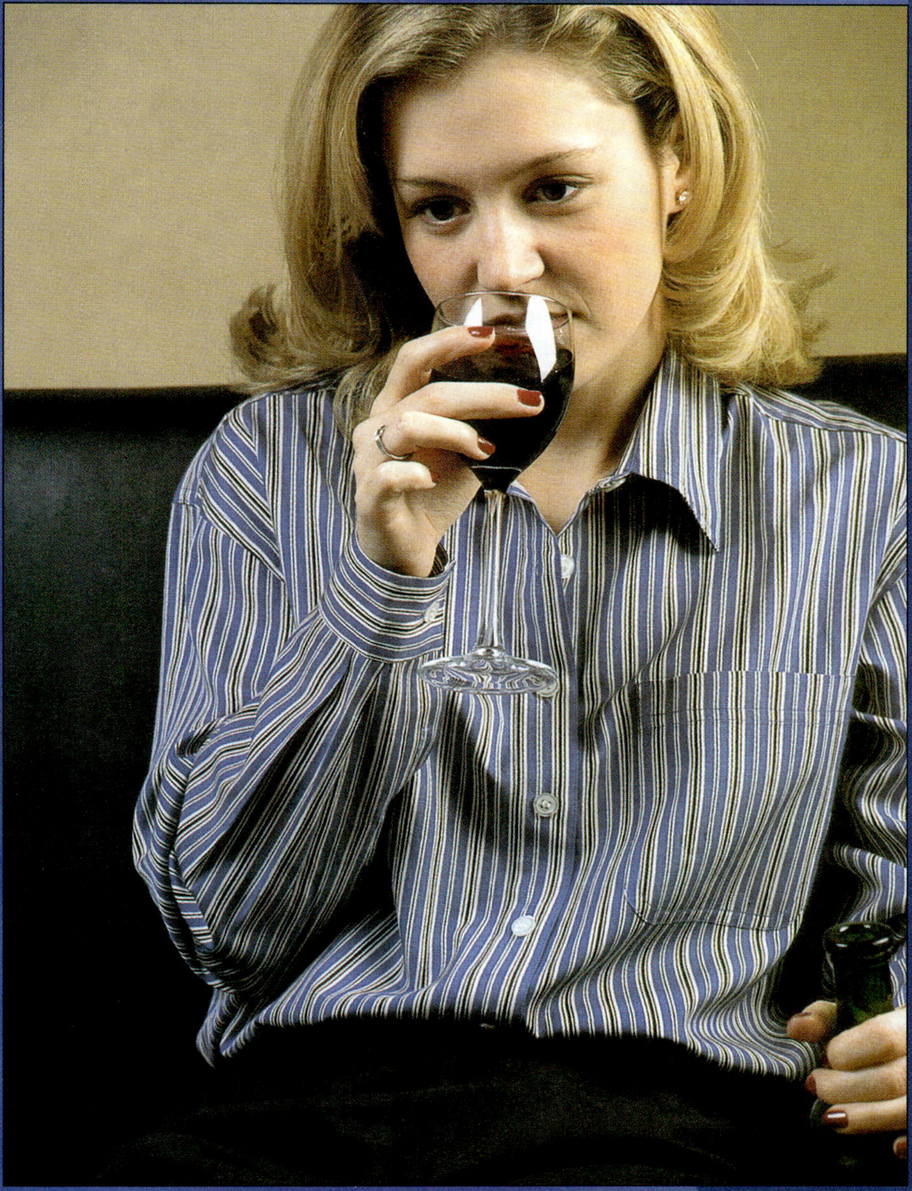

Questions of concern

1. When will the costs of alcohol abuse and alcoholism outweigh the perceived benefits of alcoholic beverage consumption?
2. Why are narcotics so frequently thought of as "devil drugs," the worst of abused psychoactive substances?
3. Wouldn't a tranquilized society be more peaceful and stable than our current tension-filled and stressful society?

Chapter 4

Alcohol: America's drink-drug

KEY TERMS

Absorption
Abstinence
Alcohol States of Consciousness
Ambivalence
Beer
Binge Drinking
Bioavailability
Blood-Alcohol Concentration
Bootlegging
Breathalyzer
Congeners
Distilled Spirits
Distribution
Equivalent Amount
Hangover
Intoxication
Moonshining
Oxidation
Pseudostimulation
Rapid Eye Movements
Social Drinking
Standard Serving
Temperance
Wine

chapter objectives

After you have studied this chapter, you should be able to do the following:

1. Define the key terms.
2. Identify the major factors and organizations in American society that led to the beginning of the historical period known as Prohibition.
3. Explain how faulty attitudes about drinking and the condition of ambivalence regarding alcohol use have contributed to various alcohol problems in our society.
4. Describe the recent drinking scene in the United States in terms of users and nonusers, amount consumed by various drinking groups in the drinking-age population, and the annual per capita consumption of pure alcohol.
5. Relate the alcohol use pattern known as binge drinking to personal, social, and academic problems on many college campuses.
6. Explain why alcohol use and especially heavy drinking are so prevalent among many American college students.
7. Identify several techniques of so-called "social drinking" that might tend to reduce the risks associated with using alcoholic beverages.
8. Name at least five perceived benefits associated with using alcohol for purposes of an altered consciousness and discuss the implications these perceived benefits might have for alcohol education and prevention.
9. Compare the three major classes of beverage alcohol in terms of production, relative alcohol content, and the amount of alcohol per typical serving.
10. Identify at least five factors that can influence the absorption of ethyl alcohol.
11. Describe the process of alcohol oxidation.
12. Explain the phenomenon of intoxication in relation to blood-alcohol concentration, central nervous system depression, and gender differences in oxidizing alcohol.
13. Distinguish between the four alcohol states of consciousness.
14. Discuss the impact of mind-set and emotional setting on intoxication.
15. Identify short-term effects of alcohol on sensation and perception; emotions; sleep; motor skills; sexuality; and the function of the kidneys, heart, blood vessels, and liver.
16. Identify long-term effects of heavy alcohol consumption on the gastrointestinal system, the liver, nutritional status, the nervous system, the endocrine system, mental functions, the cardiovascular system, skeletal muscles, and the development of certain cancers and specific infectious diseases.
17. Compare and contrast four basic alcohol-drug interactions in terms of possible consequences and the potential for harm.

Alcohol in Society

For centuries people have used beers, wines, and distilled spirits. Having originated spontaneously in nearly every culture, the phenomenon of drinking persists because individuals apparently like the effects it produces. Unlike tobacco and marijuana cigarette smoking, the use of alcoholic beverages has been an established custom in America for more than three hundred years. Most people consider alcohol a social beverage; too few recognize it as a "drink-drug" with great potential for serious abuse.

Drinking has long been viewed as a source of desirable, temporary mood modification and conviviality, on the one hand, and as a significant factor in personal and social disorganization, disease, and immorality, on the other. These contradictory effects have given rise to a somewhat ambivalent attitude toward alcohol use.

Americans spend more than $92 billion each year on beverage alcohol. In purchasing a variety of perceived benefits and pleasures, they pay over $13 billion in alcohol revenues or taxes, which amounts to only a small fraction of the federal budget—considerably less than 1 percent. Through alcohol abuse and alcohol dependence, they also generate a yearly expenditure of at least $166 billion.[1] This total estimated annual cost of national alcohol-related problems reflects expenditures for death expenses, reduced productivity in the workforce, lost employment, motor-vehicle crashes, crime, welfare programs, incarceration, and treatment and rehabilitation services.

All states provide for the legal sale and consumption of beverage alcohol. However, specific restrictions controlling its manufacture; availability; and the time, place, occasion, and qualifications for drinking persist. For example, over 200 counties in 17 states allow "package" or container sales only, and another 400 counties in 15 states prohibit all sales of alcoholic beverages. Also, all states have a 21-year-old minimum drinking age, though a few have considered adopting a lower age limit again. Some state officials and the alcohol beverage industry want Congress to repeal the federal requirement that states receiving federal highway funds must mandate a 21-year minimum purchase age for beer, wine, and distilled spirits.

Despite the widespread availability and legal use of beverage alcohol, two illegal activities continue—**moonshining** (illicit production of distilled spirits) and **bootlegging** (secret and unlawful transportation and sale of beverage alcohol). The former practice is usually undertaken to avoid paying high federal and state taxes on distilled liquors. The latter is an attempt to make money by selling alcoholic beverages without having a state liquor license.

While drinking may still be considered a social norm, for the vast majority of Americans—nondrinkers and light, infrequent drinkers—alcohol use is not an important part of their lives. Only one-third of the total drinking-age population consumes about 90 percent of alcoholic beverages sold in the United States.[2]

At Issue

Isn't a drinking age of 21 years inconsistent with the general age of majority at 18 years?

Point: Setting any particular drinking age is not only arbitrary but illogical. But setting age 21 years as the minimum drinking age is unrealistic and largely unenforceable because all other legal privileges and responsibilities are conferred at age 18. Americans can vote in national elections, serve in the military, sign contracts, and marry without parental consent when they are 18 years old. By setting an older drinking age, we treat young adults like children. Some young people can engage in responsible, nonproblem use of alcohol at age 16, while many individuals over 35 years of age routinely display their immaturity when consuming alcohol. The whole "drinking age" controversy is ridiculous!

Counterpoint: Not really. Quite simply, too many 18- to 20-year-olds cannot handle the right to drink alcoholic beverages. A more reasoned response to this issue is provided by the National Highway Traffic Safety Administration, which maintains that there is nothing inconsistent in saying that a person may be ready to accept and responsibly exercise a particular right or privilege at one age, but may not be qualified for a different right or privilege until a later age. Neither is it unfair to say that the person in question may not be the best judge of whether he or she is ready for a new privilege. Isn't it logical to state that an 18-year-old may be sufficiently mature to carry out a military service obligation, but at the same time may not be ready to handle drinking responsibly? After all, young people entering the military receive extensive training by experts and live in a well-regulated and highly disciplined environment. The situation is not comparable to purchasing and consuming a six-pack of beer.

Historical and Cultural Aspects

Whether by accident or by intent, beverage alcohol has played more than an inconsequential part in our national history. The earliest immigrants brought their own drinking attitudes and practices to their new homeland. According to legend, the Puritans landed at Plymouth Rock because their beers and victuals were running low. Contrary to popular belief, these early settlers considered alcohol as the "good creature of God," and beers and wines became normal parts of family life and festive occasions. It was also during the colonial period that many a Yankee fortune was amassed by manufacturing rum from supplies of West Indies molasses. The rum was then traded for slaves in Africa, giving rise to the infamous "trading triangle" of molasses, rum, and African slaves. New England traders and shippers had discovered a flourishing business.

Box 4.1 The Eighteenth Amendment to the United States Constitution

1. After one year from the ratification of this article the manufacture, sale or transportation of intoxicating liquors within, the importation thereof from the United States and allterritory subject to the jurisdiction thereof for beverage purposed is hereby prohibited.
2. The Congress and the several states shall have concurrent power to enforce this article by appropriate legislation.
3. This article shall be inoperative unless it shall have been ratified as an amendment to the Constitution by the legislatures of the several states, as provided in the Constitution, within seven years from the date of the submission hereof to the states by the Congress.

This article was proposed in the Congress by resolution on December 18, 1917. It was then declared ratified by three-fourths of the states on January 16, 1919, and went into effect one year later, on January 16, 1920. This constitutional amendment ushered in the so-called "noble experiment" known as the Era of National Prohibition.

From Temperance to Prohibition to Repeal

Early attempts to promote **temperance** were part of a moral crusade by several Protestant churches. Initially their aim was not abstinence but *moderation* in the use of beer and wine. People were actively discouraged from drinking whiskey and rum—popular distilled spirits. However, by the late 1830s this movement had evolved into a campaign for *total* **abstinence** from alcoholic beverages. The temperance movement gradually switched from education and moral persuasion to political organization and the power of the ballot box to realize its goal. Leaders of this social and moral reform movement sought to legally repress the liquor trade and prohibit the sale of alcoholic beverages.

Eventually the Prohibition Party, the Anti-Saloon League, and the Women's Christian Temperance Union were successful in their campaign to establish nationwide prohibition by amendment to the federal Constitution. This effort was extraordinary, because as the major force supporting prohibition, the women of America, had not yet been granted the right to vote.

Passing Congress with the necessary two-thirds majority, the Eighteenth Amendment to the U.S. Constitution was submitted to the states for ratification. By the end of 1918, the needed thirty-six states had ratified the amendment that prohibited the manufacture, sale, or transportation of intoxicating liquors used for beverage purposes. The Volstead Act, passed in 1919, provided the amendment's enforcement. The constitutional amendment went into effect in January 1920 and ushered in the so-called Prohibition Era, America's "noble experiment." What was considered only immoral before was now also illegal (see box. 4.1).

The nearly fourteen-year period of national Prohibition (1920–33) was not particularly successful in eliminating the evil and harmful effects of "demon rum" and other alcoholic beverages from America. The Volstead Act was inadequately enforced, and organized crime grew into a vast network engaged in smuggling "bootleg booze." Ethnic minorities representing millions of drinkers felt that their natural folkways had been unjustly suppressed. Many who would never dream of violating other laws casually visited "speakeasies" or contracted with bootleggers to obtain their alcohol.

After both drinkers and nondrinkers began to question the government's right to make moral judgments, and at the height of the Great Depression, America decided to end the noble experiment. Introduced by Congress, the Twenty-First Amendment to the U.S. Constitution repealed the Eighteenth Amendment and ended national Prohibition in December 1933. Thirty-six states had ratified the amendment in less than ten months. Other than federal taxation and production standards, the control of manufacture, distribution, and sale of alcoholic beverages reverted to the states.

Attitudes Toward Drinking

Many alcohol specialists believe that attitudes about alcohol and drinking are at the core of our present alcohol problems. In effect, our "stupid thinking" about beverage alcohol contributes to our national "stupid drinking." Myths about alcohol still prevail—that everyone drinks; that drinking is sophisticated; that drinking is an essential part of a happy and successful life and the essential ingredient of a successful party; that alcohol use improves thought and creativity; and that boozing is a necessary element of masculinity. Until such faulty perceptions are modified, efforts at promoting less-destructive drinking practices are not likely to be successful.

Although most Americans are identified as drinkers, there remains a strong disagreement about the significance of alcohol in terms of use and nonuse. Such conflict between the closely coexisting value structures of permissiveness and abstinence generates a considerable degree of confusion and mixed feelings regarding alcoholic beverages and their effects upon human behavior, health, and society.

There is no consensus of opinion on the goodness or badness of drinking. There is no standard of moderation or agreement as to what constitutes responsible drinking. There are no strict controls for social use of alcohol or against abuse of alcohol. We often laugh at drunks who overdose on alcohol, but we rarely think that the person who has overdosed on sleeping pills or who has had a psychotic reaction to LSD is funny.

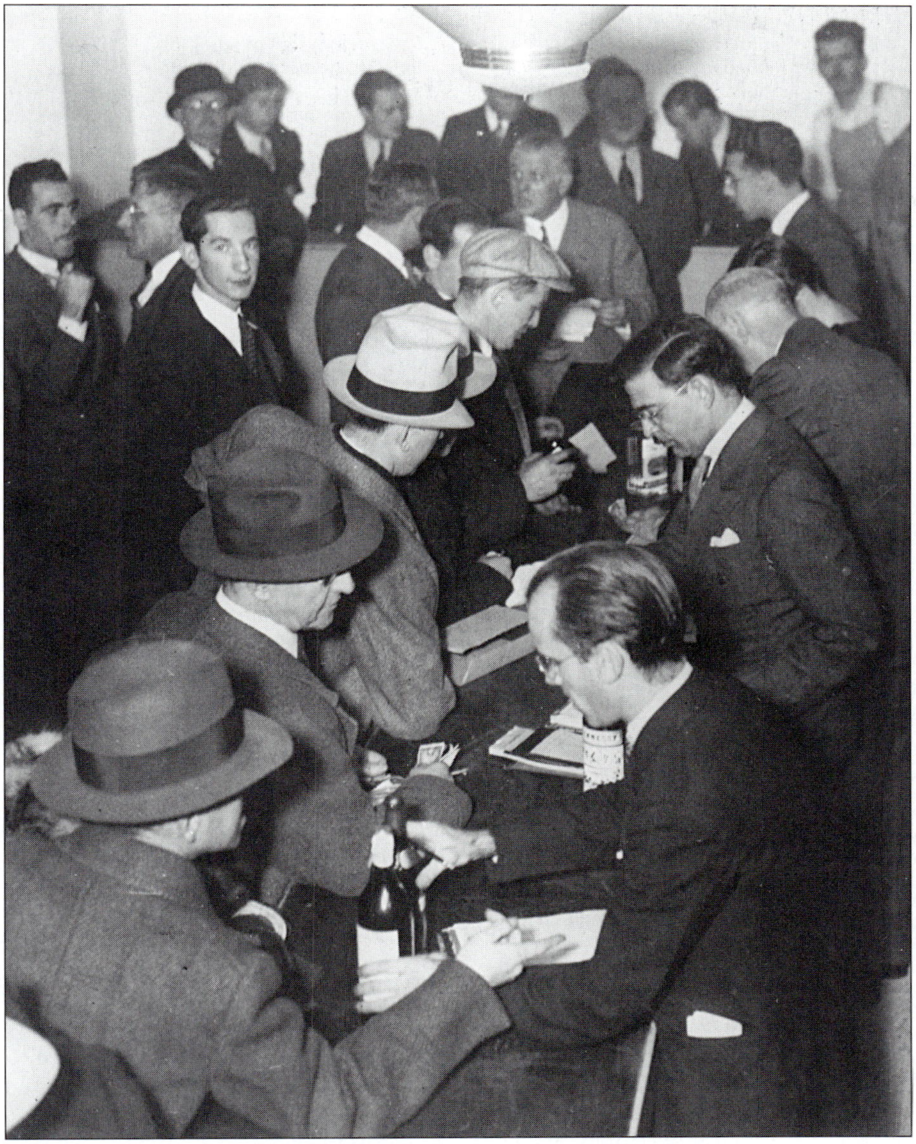

A "speakeasy" during Prohibition. Although the eighteenth Amendment forbade the manufacture, sale, and transportation of intoxicating liquors, some people could buy various alcoholic beverages at secret clubs and meeting places, if they spoke the proper password at the entrance door.

The Bettmann Archive

(Does our reaction to intoxicated people subtly encourage drunkenness?)

Although heavy use of alcohol in combination with escape drinking—the use of alcohol to escape reality—often sets the stage for problem drinking, many Americans tend to associate heavy consumption with manliness, admire the individual who can hold his or her liquor, and largely approve of escape drinking when confronted with personal problems. And when junior gets drunk we thank God that he was not involved with dope or one of those hard drugs.

Although national prohibition ended sixty-five years ago, the temperance movement, Prohibition, and repeal may have been responsible for a number of beliefs and attitudes that contribute to our present alcohol problems.[3] The following are examples.

> Drinking is immoral. It is disapproved by many churches and often linked with gambling and illicit sex.
>
> Nice women do not drink. The alcoholic female, therefore, is to be condemned more than the alcoholic male.
>
> At one time, the sale of alcoholic beverages was illegal, but many people broke the law. Perhaps this is a factor in the continuing disrespect for drinking laws today.
>
> The federal government once said that buying beverage alcohol was illegal. Now the government permits such purchases. Does the government know what is best for its citizens?
>
> All drinking is the same. Therefore, little or no distinction is made between alcohol use and alcohol abuse. Many people do not recognize any differences among various drinking patterns, such as social drinking, occasional excessive drinking, progressive excessive drinking, and chronic alcoholic drinking.
>
> The alcoholic will eventually lose his or her job, his or her family, and self-respect, and will end up as a skidrow bum. The stereotype of the alcoholic as a "down-and-outer" was born, and now we fail to detect the alcoholic in the early stages of problem drinking because the individual still has a job and a family.

Ambivalence and the Drinking Society

Such moralistic and contradictory attitudes create a good deal of confusion about what is acceptable drinking behavior. Some people feel uncomfortable about drinking and some feel uncomfortable about not drinking.

In a society with such mixed feelings and cultural **ambivalence**—the perception of both positive and negative aspects occurring in the same thing at the same time—many alcohol-related problems, including alcohol abuse and alcohol dependence, are likely to exist. The contrasting and often contradictory nature of our attitudes and practices regarding alcohol become apparent in several areas of concern:

1. The different moralities of alcohol use, as reflected in different religious denominations. ("Drinking is evil." "Alcohol is a gift of God.")
2. The varying reactions of individuals to inebriation. These range from disgust and contempt to admiration and hilarity.
3. The conflict over the major focus in alcohol education. Shall it be on abstinence, moderation, or alcoholism?
4. The confusion about the nature of alcoholism. It is variously described as alcohol dependence, a disease, a personality defect, a form of self-indulgence, a lack of will power, a personal health problem, and a sociolegal problem.
5. The difficulty in reducing public intoxication. The standard procedure of arrest, jailing, and release, followed soon by the rearrest, jailing, and release of the same person (the "revolving-door routine") does not appear to reduce the incidence of public intoxication or alcoholism. Such punitive measures will not give way to treatment and rehabilitation until society perceives chronic alcohol abuse and alcohol dependence (alcoholism) as both a health problem and a drug problem.

In this ambivalent, drinking society, with its mixed feelings about alcohol use and nonuse there are many contradictions regarding drinking behavior. Perhaps there would be less ambivalence if this drinking behavior were viewed as less of a moral issue and more of a health issue.

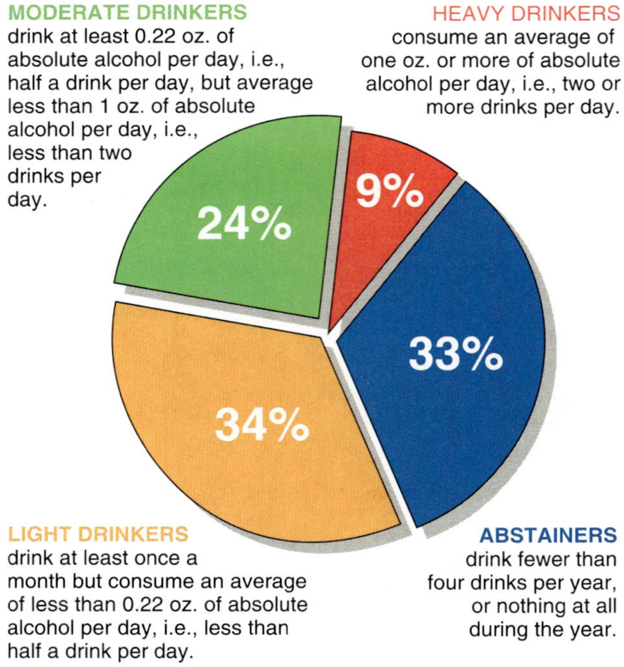

figure 4.1

American drinking practices. Most of the drinking-age population in the United States either abstains from alcohol use or drinks very little. It is also apparent that significant numbers of individuals move from one drinking category to another over a period of years. Some former drinkers become abstainers, and some nonusers eventually become drinkers.

Source: National Institute on Alcohol Abuse and Alcoholism.

Drinking Today

Polls by various organizations suggest that drinking behavior is normal, and abstinence or nonuse of alcoholic beverages is abnormal. With about 111 million people who drink just over two gallons of absolute (pure) alcohol per person each year, one might conclude that most Americans drink a lot of alcohol and that our society consumes more alcoholic than nonalcoholic beverages.

But most surveyed drinkers vary considerably in terms of age, gender, education, geography, and especially in terms of amount consumed and frequency of use. In reality, the vast majority of our national drinking-age population of light, infrequent drinkers (34 percent of the total) and abstainers or nonusers (another 33 percent) consumes no more than 10 percent of alcoholic beverages sold in the United States (see fig. 4.1). So-called moderate drinkers (24 percent of the total) consume nearly 25 percent of alcohol sold, while heavy drinkers (just 9–10 percent of the drinking-age population) drink nearly two-thirds of alcoholic beverages—the equivalent of 12–14 standard drinks a day per heavy drinker. This latter consumption level often indicates alcohol addiction.

For most Americans in the drinking age population, alcoholic beverages play an insignificant role or no role in their lives. It is also evident that if the heavy drinkers in our drinking society were to moderate their consumption to only two drinks each day, many breweries, wineries, and distilleries would be in Chapter 11 bankruptcy.

Perhaps such a moderation trend has already begun. Americans now consume six times the amount of nonalcoholic beverages as they do of beer, wine, and distilled spirits. With beer sales flat and use of distilled spirits falling, the consumption of pure (absolute) alcohol per person each year appears to be declining (see fig. 4.2).

An analysis of several studies reveals the following general statements that describe the patterns of alcohol use in our society today:

- Younger adults tend to drink more than older adults.
- There are more male drinkers than female drinkers.

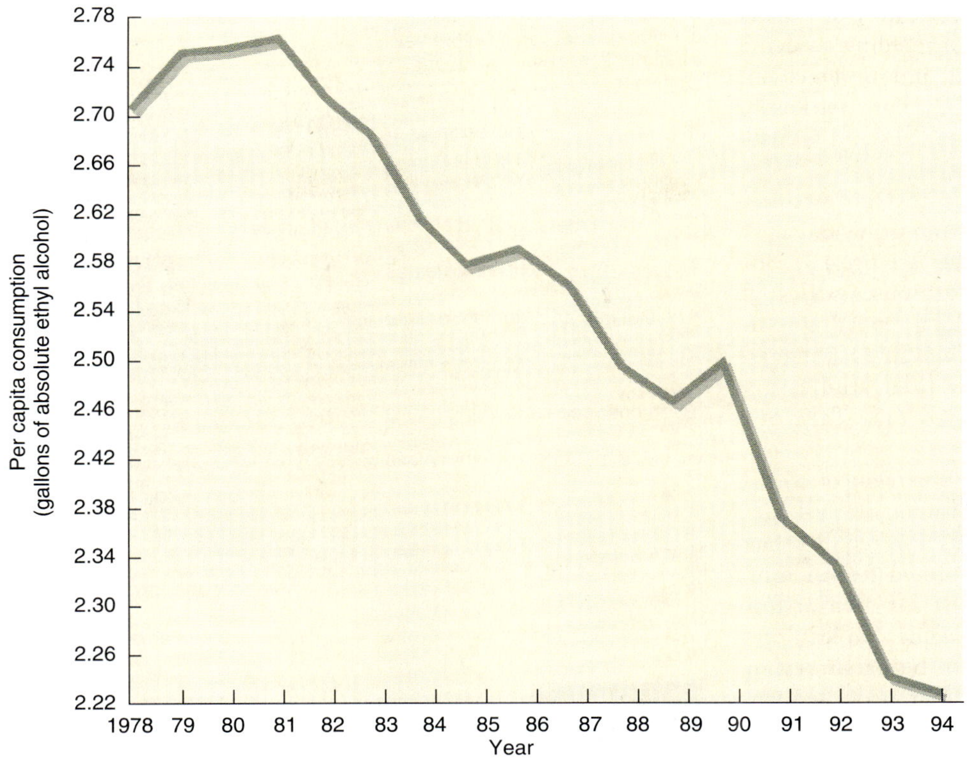

figure 4.2

Recent pattern of per capita consumption of pure (absolute) alcohol in the United States from 1978 through 1994.

Notice the peaking of total alcohol consumption in 1979–81, with the subsequent continuing decline. Researchers have advanced several reasons to explain the steady decline in the apparent use of alcoholic beverages, including:

1. **Increased public awareness regarding the personal and social risks associated with alcohol use and abuse, and especially risks based on the widely held misconception that distilled spirits or hard liquor are more hazardous than beer and wine in relation to alcohol-impaired driving and crashes; Fetal Alcohol Syndrome, and alcoholism.**
2. **Changing demographics with an increase in the proportion of the American population over sixty years of age in which consumption is relatively low.**
3. **The rather conservative cultural climate that has existed for the past fifteen to twenty years, with an associated decrease in the social acceptability of heavy drinking.**
4. **Changes in drinkers' tastes that have moved away from distilled spirits, especially the brown ones, and toward beverages with lower alcohol content, such as beers and wines.**
5. **Increasing concern among individuals about overall health, wellness, and fitness.**

Source: National Institute on Alcohol Abuse and Alcoholism and the Alcohol Research Information Service.

- There are more female light drinkers than male light drinkers.
- More men are heavy drinkers than women.
- There tends to be more drinking among the employed than the unemployed.
- The north central region of the United States has a greater percentage of heavy drinkers than other national regions.
- The southern region of the United States has a greater percentage of abstainers than other national regions.
- The greater the family income, the more likely the adults will drink.
- There is more heavy drinking among those earning less than the poverty level than those who earn above the poverty level.
- A greater percentage of those who are widowed abstain than those who are married, divorced, or never married.
- But more widowed and divorced men are heavy drinkers than those who are married or never married.

Drinking Among College Students

One of the more studied American populations of drinkers is college students. While the percentage of these students who drink on a daily basis has declined recently, there is still a great amount of alcohol use connected with college life. Alcohol is not only the most widely used mind-changing drug on and around campus, it is also the one drug that causes the most problems, including academic failure, dropping out, and unwanted and unprotected sexual behavior contributing to unplanned pregnancies and sexually transmitted diseases.

Many other undesirable consequences can result from using and abusing alcohol in college (see fig. 4.3). Students who live on campuses with high levels of binge drinking report more incidences of assault, unwanted sexual advances, and having their studies disturbed or having to take care of a drunken student.

While almost 88 percent of college students have used alcohol, nearly 40 percent of these students also reported having "binged" (consumed five or more drinks in one sitting for men or four drinks in a row for women) at least once within two weeks of being surveyed.[4] **Binge drinking** is often associated with residence hall damage, and, increasingly, with other forms of violent behavior, including sexual aggression and assault, fights, and alcohol-impaired driving. On many campuses, binge drinking has become a common pattern of alcohol consumption among students who confine their use of alcoholic beverages to weekends, on which occasions they tend to drink heavily and with the intention of getting drunk.

A massive study of 56,000 students at seventy-eight colleges across the United States revealed that those who drink the most alcohol typically wind up with the lowest grades (see fig. 4.4). In addition, students at smaller colleges were found to consume even more alcohol than those attending larger institutions of higher learning.[5] Other findings revealed that more than one-third of students admitted to driving while intoxicated at least once; more than one-quarter said they had experienced blackouts (a classic symptom of alcohol dependence); and just over one-fifth of students claimed they suffered from a hangover at least six times during the previous year.

Why is there so much heavy drinking among college students? As in the general population, heavy drinking and related alcohol problems may be associated with an impulsive personality,

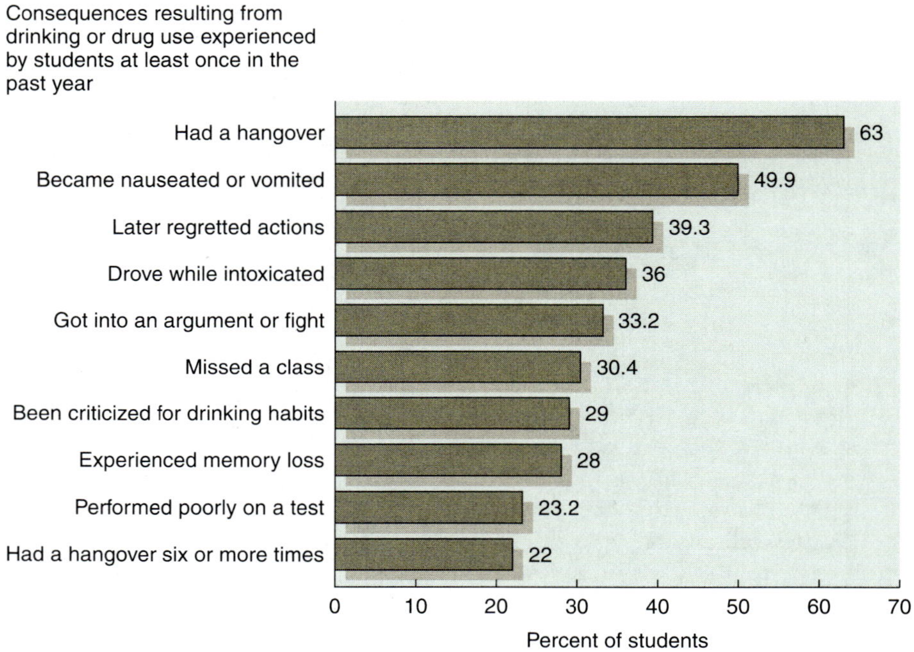

figure 4.3

Consequences of college students' alcohol and other drug use.

Source: Center for Substance Abuse Prevention

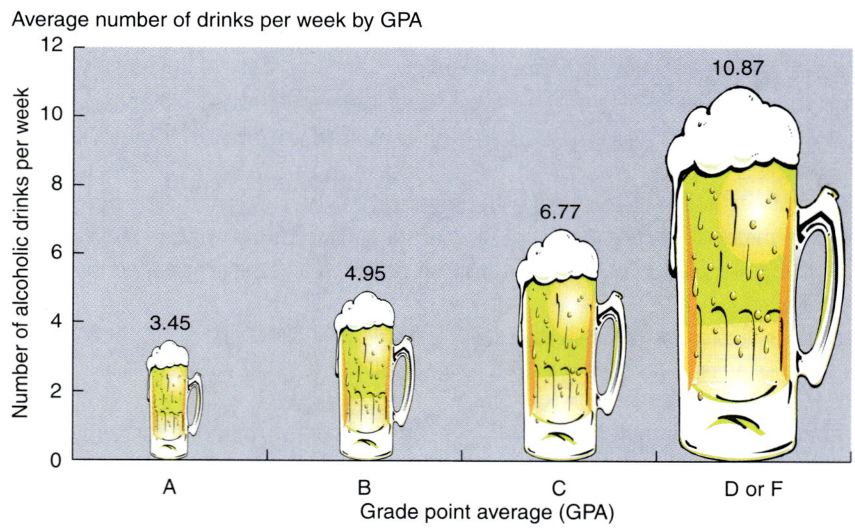

figure 4.4

Poor grades linked to alcohol use by college students. Students who reported D and F grade point averages consumed an average of eleven alcoholic drinks per week, while those who earned mostly As consumed only three drinks per week, according to a survey of 56,000 college students. The survey, "Alcohol and Drugs on American College Campuses: A Report to College Presidents," was conducted by researchers from Southern Illinois University at Carbondale (SIUC) and the College of William and Mary in Virginia. It is the largest survey ever of college drinking habits and their consequences.

Source: Center for Substance Abuse Prevention

psychological problems of depression or anxiety, and a positive family history of alcohol abuse. However, some unique factors may also influence drinking behavior in college.[6]

First, students often perceive their peers' drinking levels to be higher than their own and higher than than they actually are. These exaggerated perceptions of others' drinking are in turn linked with greater individual consumption of alcohol.

Second, many students appear to have deeply held expectancies that alcohol will loosen inhibitions or promote relaxation. Such positive expectancies are often related to increased consumption and tend to predict changes in drinking behavior by college students and others as well.

Third, despite the number of alcohol-related problems experienced, many students apparently relate their drinking to their degree of social acceptance. Those who binged once or twice each week reported more perceived intimacy in their relationships with others than those who did not binge drink. Being accepted and feeling approved by one's peers are powerful motivators to use and sometimes overuse alcohol.

Fourth, students who consider parties or athletics important to the college experience and those who drink to get drunk appear most likely to binge drink or to drink more heavily.

Fifth, drinking in groups and serving oneself may promote higher levels of alcohol consumption. In one particular instance, college students at bars tended to drink more beer when in groups and when ordering pitchers than when alone and when ordering only glasses or bottles.

It appears that college students' consumption of alcohol is influenced significantly by the social behavior and drinking of those around them. But college students may also tend to drink more than their noncollege counterparts because of a unique environment that promotes heavy consumption.[7]

- Many college and university customs, norms, and traditions seem to encourage specific dangerous alcohol use practices and patterns.
- College students and university campuses are particularly heavily targeted by the advertising and promotions of the alcoholic beverage industry, especially beer producers. Off-campus bars also lure student drinkers with discounted pitchers of beer or other specials that reward increased consumption.
- College students tend to drink more recklessly than others and to engage in "drinking games" and other dangerous drinking practices.

As college students mature and begin to take personal responsibility for making healthy lifestyle choices, they often learn that getting drunk does not need to be a rite of passage, and hangovers are not a prerequisite for graduation.[8]

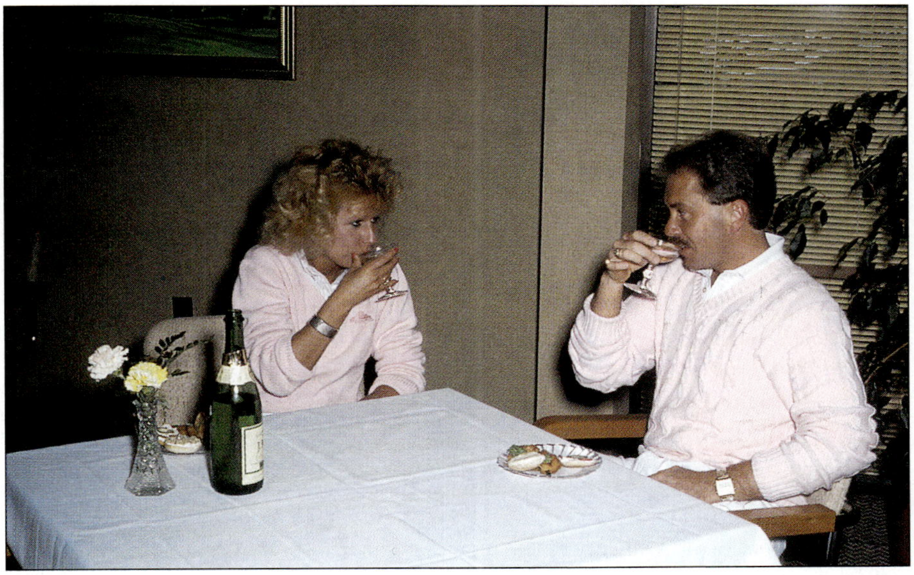

Drinking that tends to promote interpersonal relationships and feelings of camaraderie is often referred to as social drinking, while dietary drinking describes the use of alcoholic beverages as compliments to certain foods or as basic ingredients in special food dishes. This couple seems to combine the two types of drinking.

© James L. Shaffer

Personal and Social Uses of Alcohol

For many people, there will probably always be the need for an adaptive mechanism—a means of altering an individual's inner being of feelings and perceptions in relation to his or her surroundings.[9] Alcohol serves that function well.

Social Drinking

By definition, drinking is the consumption of beverages containing ethyl alcohol. From a sociological viewpoint, drinking is described as a particular group's customary way of using beverage alcohol. Such a custom is learned by other members of that group and is continued by the group because drinking serves to promote interpersonal relations and to enhance feelings of camaraderie and solidarity (see box 4.2). The pleasure derived from drinking is primarily reciprocal; that is, drinking by one of the group brings satisfaction to the other drinkers. Alcohol is seen as the "social lubricant" in which many inhibitions are lowered. For Americans, this form of learned drinking behavior—**social drinking**—is the common way of using alcoholic beverages.[10]

Ritualistic Drinking

Ritualistic use of alcohol is seen in religious ceremonies wherein wine is sacred and drinking is an act of communion.

Box 4.2 What Is Social Drinking?

Social Drinking Is	Social Drinking Is Not
A glass of wine to enhance a meal	Three fast martinis before lunch
A drink or two while you are having fun	Having a drink to have fun
Sipping and eating	Gulping drinks on an empty stomach
Using alcohol as a beverage	Forgetting what you did while drinking
Drinking and talking with friends	Drinking and worrying alone
Never having to say you are sorry for what you did while drinking	Showing off how much you can hold
Knowing when to say when	Using alcohol as a problem solver

Where does social drinking end and problem drinking begin? There is no simple answer. However, here is one good description: *If you need a drink to be social, that's not social drinking!*

Source: *Social Drinking*, Operation Threshold, United States Jaycees, 1975. Funded by the National Institute on Alcohol Abuse and Alcoholism.

Other cultural ceremonies—celebrating birth, birthdays, engagements, marriages, anniversaries, good fortune, sometimes even death—are also traditionally celebrated with alcoholic beverages.

Dietary Drinking

For some, alcohol is an essential part of one's dietary intake, a complement to certain foods or, like cooking wine, a basic ingredient in special food dishes. When alcohol is served along with meals and integrated with routines of family living, the risks of excessive use and intoxication are considerably diminished.

Drinking for Altered Consciousness

There is little doubt that the major reason so many people use alcoholic beverages is to change their conscious experience.[11] This alcohol-induced state of awareness is usually perceived as a sensation of feeling better, feeling less bad, or just feeling different. Alcohol can produce a tranquilizing effect that reduces tension and anxiety. Stressful situations are often more easily tolerated, irritations of daily living seem to diminish, and relaxation is often promoted or enhanced. In some instances, drinking may provide a pleasant and relatively safe way to feel "high" or even powerful with one's peers or strangers.

Although thoughts of power, aggression, and even sexual conquest tend to increase regularly with increased drinking among men, female social drinking is sometimes related to enhancing or increasing traditional aspects of femininity, such as personal warmth, lovingness, expressiveness, and affectionateness. However, heavy use among females has sometimes been associated with attempts to escape temporarily from gender-role conflict.[12]

According to Sigmund Freud, an early twentieth-century researcher in the emerging field of psychology, drinking was one way of *satisfying hidden dependency needs* that adults are forbidden to express. As such, alcohol abuse could express a secret desire for support and care from others, while maintaining an appearance of adult sophistication and independence—qualities often linked with alcohol use.

A more contemporary explanation of using and abusing alcohol focuses on the basic motivation of *satiation* or *excessive satisfaction.*[13] Drinking becomes an antidote or countermeasure for psychic pain. Psychologically, binging on alcohol is an attempt to cut off negative feelings by reducing stimulation from both the internal and the external environment. As such, alcohol works as a stress reducer.

Research also suggests that the desire for *altered states of consciousness* or intoxication (i.e., being influenced by a drug's effects) is an acquired motivation similar to the innate drives of hunger, thirst, and even sex.[14] Accordingly, humans have a natural need to change their awareness from time to time, in response to environmental stressors or just plain boredom, or in an effort to decrease feelings of fatigue, tension, and anxiety. This concept values intoxication for its alleged ability to enliven daily experiences, vitalize one's perceptions, and serve as a unifying symbol that encourages solidarity or unity among fellow drinkers.

Unfortunately, millions of drinkers use alcohol to produce *unawareness* (narcosis) exclusively. They do not wish to return to reality but seek a hiding place from the world in a bottle. Frequent drinking for narcosis only is the type that often leads to alcohol dependency and reduced life expectancy.

Thus, alcohol can serve a variety of personal and social uses. Some of these are less problem producing than others.

Alcoholic Beverages

The term *alcohol* usually denotes a specific chemical compound, ethyl alcohol. One of several chemicals in the "alcohol family," ethyl alcohol is a thin, clear, colorless fluid with a mild, aromatic odor and pungent taste. It is capable of being mixed with water in all proportions, is diffusible through body membranes, and is the essential and characteristic ingredient of beverage alcohol. Ethyl alcohol is also present in many nonprescription medications (see table 4.1) and often is used in the preparation of chemical detergents, flavorings, and fragrances. When added to gasoline, ethyl alcohol improves the octane rating; mixing 10 percent ethanol with 90 percent gasoline produces the motor fuel gasohol.[15]

The ethyl alcohol contained in beverages is derived from certain grains and fruits by the process of fermentation. In this natural chemical process, yeast cells act on the sugar content of fruit juice or another sugary substance and convert the

table 4.1 Selected Nonprescription Medications That Contain Ethyl Alcohol

Type of Medication	Alcohol Content (%)
Antidiarrhea medication	
Immodium A-D	5.25
Pepto Diarrhea Control	5.25
Astringent	
Witch hazel	14.00
Internal analgesic	
Excedrin PM liquid	10.00
Tylenol Adult Extra Strength liquid	7.00
Vitamin preparation	
Centrum	6.60
Mouthwash preparation/dental rinse	
Cepacol	14.00
Listerine	26.90
Plax	8.50
Scope	16.60
Toothache/cold sore/canker sore remedy	
Anbesol	70.00
Orajel Mouth-Aid	70.00
Zilactin Medicated Gel	80.00
Cough/cold/allergy medication	
Benadryl cold liquid	10.00
Cheracol Plus cough syrup	8.00
Comtrex	20.00
Contac Severe Cold	18.50
MediFlu	19.00
NiteTime Relief (Plus)	25.00
Nyquil	25.00
Tylenol Max Strength Cough	10.00

Source: Author's analysis of nonprescription medications available for sale in drug stores, department stores, and groceries.

sugar to carbon dioxide and ethyl alcohol. The following chemical equation represents the fermentation process:

$$\underset{\text{glucose (sugar)}}{C_6H_{12}O_6} \xrightarrow{\text{(Yeast)}} \underset{\text{ethyl alcohol}}{2\,C_2H_5OH} + \underset{\text{carbon dioxide}}{2\,CO_2}$$

Fermentation continues until all the sugar has been acted upon by the yeast cells or until the fermenting mixture contains about 14 percent alcohol by volume. At this point, the concentration of ethanol is sufficient to cause the multiplying yeast cells to die and fermentation ends.

Rarely does one consume pure alcohol. Intake is accomplished in the form of alcoholic beverages. By law, alcoholic beverages include any beverage in liquid form that contains not less than one-half of one percent (0.5 percent) of ethyl alcohol (ethanol) by volume and are intended for human consumption.[16]

These alcoholic beverages are usually classified by their method of production and are specified as:

1. *Fermented beverages* produced through fermentation alone. There are two basic kinds of fermented beverages: wine, the result of fermentation of grape or other fruit juices; and malted beverages or beers, brewed principally from cereal grains and malted barley.
2. *Distilled spirits* produced by the distillation of any alcohol-containing mixture, such as, a wine or distiller's beer from a fermentation process. Any of the several types of distilled spirits is referred to as *hard liquor* or *liquor.* A so-called hard liquor contains at least 40 percent alcohol by volume with the designation of 80 proof.

Wine

Made from the fermented juice of grapes or other fruits, **wine** typically has an alcohol content of 10 to 14 percent by volume. There are five basic types of wines: red, white, and rosé, and sparkling wines or champagne, which contain carbon dioxide (all referred to as table wines); and dessert or cocktail wines (with alcohol contents ranging from 15 to 24 percent). The higher alcohol content of the dessert wines, such as sherry, port, Madeira, and the vermouths, is the result of adding *neutral high-proof spirits* (ethyl alcohol) or brandy to a table wine.

Although the original "light" wines with reduced caloric value did not prove to be popular, "wine coolers" became an overnight success. Syrupy sweet, fruity beverages with little or no alcohol taste, wine coolers are blends of red or white wine, fruit juice, carbonated water, and sugar. They typically contain from 1.5 percent to 6.0 percent alcohol by volume. Such concoctions proved popular among junior and senior high school students, who consumed about 35 percent of wine coolers sold in the United States shortly after their introduction to the market.[17]

Beer

Including the regular and the newer low-calorie "light" varieties with less alcohol, **beers** are derived from cereal grains—barley, rye, corn, and wheat. The process of beer making is referred to as brewing and includes the conversion of cereal broth starch to a fermentable sugar, fermentation, and storage. The resulting product contains from 3.6 percent to 6 percent alcohol by volume, though the typical alcohol content of popular beers is about 4 percent to 4.5 percent—characteristic of the traditional "regular beers."

Light beers, by contrast, contain fewer calories per serving. The alcohol content is usually about 3.2 percent by volume, but may be as high as 4.7 percent. Reflecting perhaps the increased health consciousness of Americans and the growing awareness of alcohol abuse, the newer "low-alcohol beers" contain about 1.8 percent of ethyl alcohol. So-called nonalcoholic beers are "near beers" that contain less than 0.5 percent alcohol by volume. These products are referred to as "brews"—not beers—because they would have to contain a higher alcohol content to be considered a beer, according to federal government regulations.[18] Nevertheless, the National Council on Alcoholism and Drug Dependence warns that the new brews may have sufficient alcoholic content to trigger a response among recovering alcoholics that could lead to a relapse into problem drinking.

After brewing, the resulting clarified fluid is carbonated and bottled or canned. Besides water and alcohol, beer contains minute substances called **congeners,** as do all alcoholic beverages. Common congeners are dextrins, maltose, certain soluble minerals and vitamins, organic acids, acacia or gum arabic, salts, and carbon dioxide. Some of these are added to preserve, stabilize, enhance flavor, and produce or promote foaming.

Most American beers are lager beers and have a light color and a relatively low alcohol content of 4.0 percent to 4.5 percent by volume. Malt liquor has a delicate, aromatic flavor and between 5 percent and 6.9 percent alcohol content, though some versions have been brewed with an alcohol content of 9.5 percent. Malt beverage "coolers" have a much lower alcohol content, ranging from 3.2 percent to 4.8 percent. More bitter than malt liquor are ale, stout, and porter—high-powered beers with "full-bodied" taste and an alcohol content of 6 to 7 percent by volume.

One variant in the ever-expanding beer family is a concoction named "ice beer." This particular beer is brewed at an extremely cold temperature. This innovative marketing gimmick of brewers has an alcohol content equal to that of many malt liquors—between 5 and 6 percent. Another variant is Twisted Lemon Alcoholic Drink, a clear lemonade-flavored malted beverage. This new generation beverage is advertised as a refreshing alternative to beer, wine, and liquor on all occasions.

Distilled Spirits

Whiskey, vodka, gin, and brandy are **distilled spirits** and are made from fermented mixtures of cereal grains or fruits that are heated in a still. Rum, another distilled spirit, is derived from molasses, and tequila is made from the fermented juice of the cactuslike century plant, the mescal.

Alcohol has a lower boiling point than other substances in the fermented mixture, therefore ethyl alcohol boils off first when the mixture is heated. The invisible vapors or spirits are cooled and condensed. These distilled fluids have a relatively high alcohol content, along with some water and flavoring ingredients. The alcohol content of such distilled beverages, ranging from 40 to 50 percent by volume, is indicated by the term *proof.* Proof is twice the percentage of alcohol by volume. Thus, a whiskey labeled 90 proof contains 45 percent alcohol by volume.

Another type of distilled spirits is liqueur, a sweet alcoholic drink made by mixing or redistilling spirits with or over fruits, flowers, plants, nuts, beans, seeds, or cream. These flavoring agents impart their essence to the particular liqueur, such as Creme de Cacao (cacao is a vanilla bean), Kahlua (coffee), and Cointreau (orange).

In an attempt to increase market share, distillers also market a "mixed-drink cooler," or "breezer," a fruit-flavored beverage containing about 4 percent alcohol by volume. This product resembles a wine cooler, but the added alcohol is a distilled spirit. Such a mixture amounts to a diluted mixed drink.

An even more recent liquor entry is the alcoholic lemonade drink, often referred to as "alcopop" or "sweet liquor-spiked soda."[19] Sold under the youth-appealing names of Hooper's Hooch, Two Dogs Lemonade, Mrs. Pucker's Alcoholic Orangeade or Citrus Brew, and Hucker's Alcoholic Cola, these "alcoholic soft drinks" began slipping into America during test marketing in the mid-1990s. These drinks are 30-proof, sweet-tasting alcoholic drinks, and may be the liquor industry's response to declining sales of distilled spirits. The controversy surrounding these alcoholic soft drinks is the fear that they have been designed to appeal to children and the perception that there is such a thing as "safe alcohol."

Equivalent Servings

The major types of alcoholic beverage—beer, wine, and distilled spirit—differ as to alcohol content. Nevertheless, a typical serving of any one beverage contains approximately the same amount of ethyl alcohol as does a typical serving of any other alcoholic beverage, though specific servings vary in terms of volume (see box 4.3).

Referred to as the **equivalent amount,** this quantity of alcohol is about 0.6 ounce, a little over one-half ounce of ethanol. Thus, people who drink a **standard serving** of an alcoholic beverage—defined as one 5-ounce glass of table wine, one 12-ounce wine cooler, one 12-ounce can or bottle of regular beer, or one shot glass of "hard liquor" with 1.5 ounces of 80 proof whiskey or an equivalent distilled spirit—consume approximately the same amount of ethanol. In terms of typical servings, then, distilled spirits are not "stronger" or "harder" than beer or wine. Beer and wine coolers are not insignificant or harmless beverages.

There are, however, limitations to the concept of "equivalence" in servings of alcoholic beverages. The typical serving of beer is predetermined at the brewery at the time of canning or bottling, but the typical servings of wines and distilled spirits tend to vary according to the person who pours them. Sometimes mixed drinks or cocktails—combinations of one or more of the major types of distilled spirits with or without flavorings, soda, fruit juice, or water—contain two or more shots of hard liquor. In these instances, then, the equivalency rule does not apply!

Box 4.3 Alcohol Equivalencies and Drinking

Drinkers beware: Watch for wine glasses that hold more than five oz., A dessert wine in place of a table wine, a higher alcohol content beer or ale or a "lite beer" instead of a regular beer, a higher proof distilled spirit as a substitute for 80 proof liquor, and "canned cocktail" containing six oz. of vodka or gin martini—considerably more than one shoot in a mixed drink.

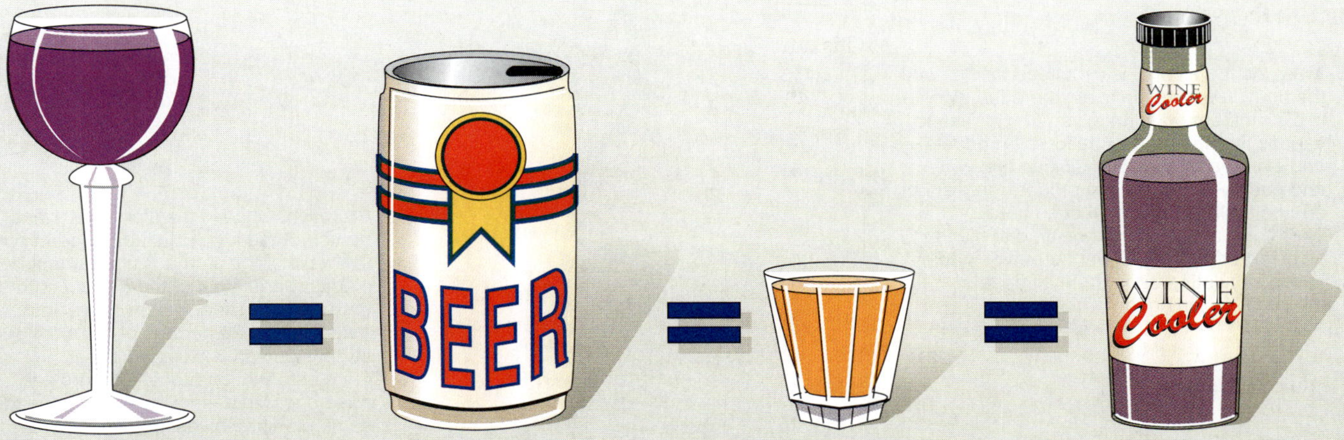

1 glass of wine	1 can or bottle of beer	1 shot glass with distilled spirits	1 bottle of wine cooler
5 oz. of table wine	12 oz. of beer	1.5 oz. of whiskey/other hard liquor	12 oz. of wine cooler
12% alcohol by volume	4.5% alcohol by volume	40% alcohol by volume or 80 proof	5% alcohol by volume
5 x 0.12 = 0.6 oz.	12 x 0.045 = 0.54 oz.	1.5 x 0.4 = 0.6 oz.	12 x 0.05 = 0.6 oz.

Alcohol Within the Body

As it enters the body, alcohol is subjected to three basic body processes—absorption, distribution, and oxidation. These processes are described in this section. The relatively small amount of ethyl alcohol that is not oxidized is eventually eliminated unchanged in the urine, sweat, and breath. However, there is no scientific basis for the belief that intoxicated people can urinate, sweat, or breathe themselves sober! (See fig. 4.5.)

Absorption

Once the beverage is swallowed and conveyed to the stomach, the process of **absorption** begins. Unlike other foods, alcohol requires no digestion and passes readily through the walls of the gastrointestinal tract, where tiny blood vessels pick up the alcohol. About one-fifth of the total alcohol consumed is absorbed in the stomach. The major site of absorption, however, is in the small intestine. A number of factors can influence absorption.

1. *Concentration of alcohol.* The greater the concentration of alcohol in a beverage, the more rapid will be the rate of absorption. Given the same quantity of alcoholic beverages, two ounces of whiskey will produce a higher blood-alcohol level or **blood-alcohol concentration** than two ounces of beer. (Blood-alcohol level or concentration is the ratio of alcohol present in the blood to the total volume of blood, expressed as a percentage.)
2. *Amount of alcohol.* The more alcohol consumed at any one time, the longer the absorption period will be.
3. *Rate of drinking.* Rapid consumption through gulping a drink will likely result in an elevated blood-alcohol level. Drinking in small, divided amounts prevents high concentrations of alcohol because less is available for absorption.
4. *Amount of food in the stomach.* The presence of food in the stomach delays the absorption of alcohol, especially when milk products and foods high in protein are consumed before drinking. Diluted by the food contents, alcohol is retained for a longer period in that body organ where absorption occurs more slowly than in the small intestine.
5. *Body weight.* The more a person weighs, the lower will be the blood-alcohol level. Heavier people have more body fluids in which the alcohol is diluted.
6. *Body chemistry and emotions.* During the premenstrual phase of the menstrual cycle, females tend to absorb alcohol more readily. If

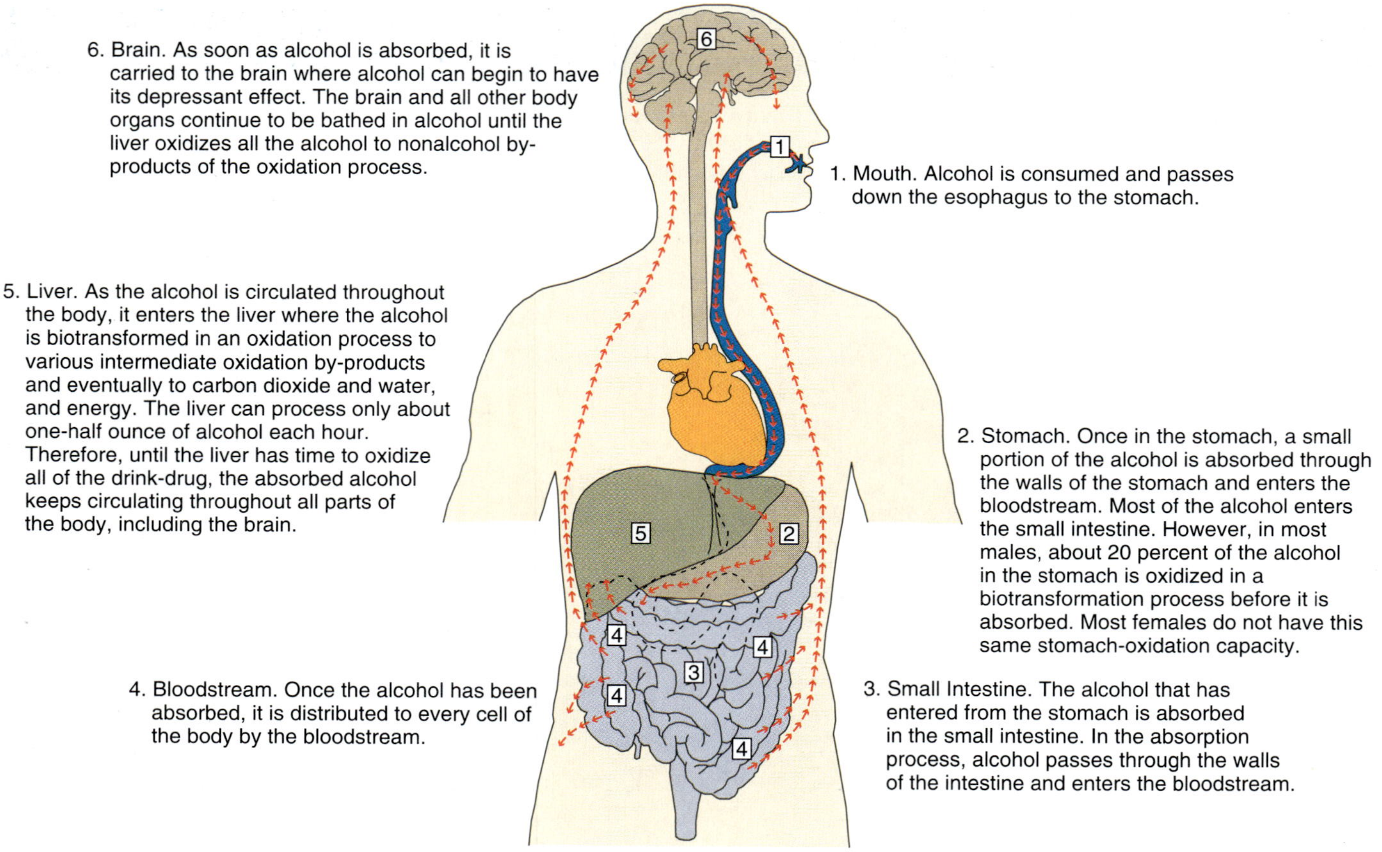

figure 4.5

The pathway of alcohol in the human body.

Source: Modified from the National Institute on Alcohol Abuse and Alcoholism

women are taking oral contraceptives (birth control pills), they also will absorb alcohol more rapidly. Unique patterns of body functioning may determine individual reactions to alcohol. Anger, fear, stress, nausea, the condition of the stomach tissues, and even fatigue have been identified as factors affecting the emptying time of the stomach.

Distribution

Having passed through the capillary walls of the small blood vessels in the intestines, the alcohol is now circulated to all parts of the body. Eventually it is distributed evenly in the body's fluids and cells, achieving a concentration proportionate to the water content and blood supply of the organ or tissues in question. The **distribution** of alcohol continues a general dilution process begun when the beverage was consumed. Regardless of the original alcohol concentration, the blood-alcohol level (or concentration) rarely exceeds 0.60 percent. At this level, nearly all drinkers would likely be dead. The moderate drinker's blood-alcohol level approximates only a few hundredths of 1 percent by comparison.

Oxidation

Most of the alcohol consumed, absorbed, and distributed—between 90 percent and 98 percent—is combined eventually with oxygen.[20] This process of **oxidation** involving biotransformation eventually results in the formation of water and carbon dioxide and the production of heat and energy.

First, a special gastric enzyme (alcohol dehydrogenase) breaks down about 20 percent of the alcohol in the stomach before the alcohol enters the bloodstream.[21] This "first-pass" metabolism of ethyl alcohol appears to be more effective in males than in females, but less effective in alcoholics than in nonalcoholics (see box 4.4).

After the remaining alcohol passes into the bloodstream, the process of oxidation continues in the liver. There, alcohol dehydrogenase enzyme also acts as a catalyst in changing more of the alcohol into acetaldehyde, a toxic substance. Very rapidly this by-product is further oxidized to acetic acid in a chemical process occurring within the liver and other organs. Authorities disagree as to the site of the third phase of oxidation, in which acetic acid is changed to water and carbon dioxide, the process yielding about seven calories of energy per gram of alcohol.

Box 4.4 Why Women Can't Hold Their Liquor Like Men

It has been known for many years that females tend to be more vulnerable than males to the effects of alcohol. Such a gender difference traditionally has been related to the overall smaller body size of most females and the lower proportion of water in the bodies of women in comparison with men's bodies. As a consequence, females have less body fluid and a lower water content in which to dilute any alcohol consumed. Women, therefore, become more intoxicated than men after drinking the same amount of beverage alcohol.

Studies suggest yet another factor that tends to make alcohol even more risky for women than for men.[a] According to American and Italian scientists, women are also more susceptible to alcohol's effects because they have less of a protective stomach enzyme that breaks down (oxidizes) a portion of the alcohol consumed before it enters the bloodstream. Men tend to produce higher amounts of gastric alcohol dehydrogenase than women, and as a result, men do not get as tipsy as women on the same number of drinks.

Women have less of the gastric (stomach) enzyme than men, therefore females will absorb up to nearly 30 percent more alcohol into the bloodstream than males of the same weight who have drunk an equal amount of beverage. Therefore, when women of average size drink one serving of beverage alcohol, it will have nearly the same effects as two drinks for average-size men.[b]

Other findings of the studies indicate the following:

Women who drink small amounts of alcohol may be more adversely affected than men in their ability to drive and perform other similar tasks requiring close attention and coordination.

Drinking on a full stomach is more desirable than consuming alcohol on an empty one. Food in the stomach delays the absorption of alcohol, so the gastric enzyme has more time to oxidize some of the alcohol before it enters the bloodstream or passes into the small intestine where absorption occurs more rapidly.

The lower amount or total absence of the stomach enzyme may also explain why women alcoholics tend to experience more liver damage than do alcoholic men. The livers of females work harder to break down alcohol and thus become subject to more wear and tear on that particular body organ.

[a]Mario Frezza et al., "High Blood Levels in Women: The Role of Decreased Gastric Alcohol Dehydrogenase Activity and First-Pass Metabolism," *The New England Journal of Medicine* 322, no. 2 (11 January 1990): 95–99.

[b]Anastasia Toufexis, "Why Men Can Outdrink Women," *Time*, 22 January 1990, 61.

While the rate of alcohol oxidation varies from person to person due to size of liver, enzyme activity, diseases of the liver, and certain drug reactions, the average rate of disposition is estimated to be one-third of an ounce of pure ethyl alcohol or two-thirds to three-fourths of an ounce of whiskey per hour, or the equivalent in beer or wine. This is fairly constant for each person. Individuals are advised to consume no more than one serving of beverage alcohol per hour because of the liver's limited oxidation capacity.

Activities to increase the oxidation rate of alcohol have not been successful, except in experiments with intravenous administration of fructose and dialysis of the blood. These are rarely available to the vast majority of drinkers. The use of black coffee, cold showers, stimulant drugs, and exposure to fresh air have no significant effect on increasing alcohol oxidation. The intoxicated person may be more alert but is still drunk and still impaired! Time is the only practical thing that will sober up an individual who has consumed too much alcohol.

At extremely high blood-alcohol levels, another liver enzyme system, the so-called microsomal ethanol oxidizing system (MEOS), becomes activated.[22] After long periods of heavy alcohol consumption, the MEOS appears to increase its activity significantly, allowing for greater oxidation of ethyl alcohol. Such a function allows some alcohol-dependent individuals to drink extremely large amounts of alcohol without apparent effect.

Intoxication

The most noticeable consequences of alcohol use pertain to changes in thinking, feeling, and behaving. Such alterations of feelings and conduct are caused by the action of alcohol on the central nervous system, specifically the brain, and are in direct proportion to the *blood-alcohol level (BAL)* or *blood-alcohol concentration (BAC)*.

Most drinkers who have a relatively low BAC from taking one drink in an hour will experience only mild effects, such as slight changes in feeling, heightening of existing moods, and little impairment of mental function, if any. However, definite impairment begins in a BAC zone ranging from 0.03 percent to just below 0.10 percent. As the BAC increases, the degree of mental inefficiency increases. Feelings of relaxation and sedation are experienced, and the control of voluntary muscles declines in the performance of fine motor skills. These changes are manifestations of alcohol's *progressive, depressant action* on the brain, as represented in table 4.2.

Functional impairment increases rapidly and more noticeably after the BAC reaches 0.10 percent and takes several forms: decreased inhibitions, less efficient vision and hearing, unclear speech, difficulty in performing gross motor skills, deterioration of judgment, and a general feeling of euphoria. Studies reveal that with a BAC between 0.10 percent and 0.15 percent, about 65 percent of drinkers display definite signs of physical and mental impairment. At a BAC of 0.20 percent, nearly all drinkers display profound and obvious signs of intoxication—difficulty in walking and

table 4.2 Alcohol Intoxication: Progressive States of Impairment with Increasing Blood-Alcohol Concentrations (BAC)

BAC	Possible Effects of Alcohol
0.01%	Usually mild effects, if any; slight changes in feeling; heightening of moods.
0.03%	Feelings of relaxation and slight exhilaration; minimal impairment of mental function.
0.06%	Mild sedation; exaggeration of emotion; slight impairment of fine motor skills; increase in reaction time; poor muscle control; slurred speech.
0.09%	Visual and hearing acuity reduced; inhibitions and self-restraint lessened; increased difficulty in performing motor skills; judgment is now clouded.
0.10%	Legal evidence of driving under the influence of alcohol in most states.
0.12%	Difficulty in performing gross motor skills; blurred vision; unclear speech; definite impairment of mental function.
0.15%	Major impairment of physical and mental functions; irresponsible behavior; general feeling of euphoria; difficulty in standing, walking, talking; distorted perception and judgment.
0.20%	Mental confusion; decreased inhibitions; gross body movements can be made only with assistance; inability to maintain upright position; difficulty in staying awake.
0.30%	Severe mental confusion; minimum of perception and comprehension; difficulty in responding to stimuli; general suspension of sensibility.
0.40%	Almost complete anesthesia; depressed reflexes; state of unconsciousness or coma likely.
0.50%	Complete unconsciousness or deep coma, if not death.
0.60%	Death is most likely now, if it has not already occurred at somewhat lower BACs following depression of nerve centers that control heartbeat and breathing. Such a person is "dead drunk."

Source: From *Health: The Science of Human Adaptation*, 5th ed. by Charles Carroll. Copyright © 1991 Wm. C. Brown Communications, Inc. Reprinted by permission of The McGraw-Hill Companies.

speaking and irresponsible and often antisocial behavior.

Intoxication is a temporary state of mental chaos and behavioral dysfunction resulting from the presence of ethyl alcohol in the central nervous system. Alcohol is being consumed faster than it can be oxidized. Like other sedatives, it has a depressant action on the various control centers in the brain, and it interferes with the transmission of nerve impulses at the synapse. As the brain becomes more anesthetized, the drinker has difficulty maintaining an upright position, experiences dulled perception and minimal comprehension, and finally loses consciousness. If the BAC exceeds 0.60 percent, the drinker's brain becomes so depressed that breathing and heartbeat cease, and death results.

Mechanism of Impairment

Traditionally, it has been thought that the higher brain centers of the cerebral cortex that control judgment and inhibit or restrain behavior are depressed first. Then, as the presence of alcohol in the central nervous system increases, paralysis of the lower brain centers, including the medulla, occurs and results in poor coordination, confusion, disorientation, stupor, coma, or death.

Later research indicates that the nerve cells within the brain's "arousal centers" of the reticular activating system are extremely sensitive to the depressant effect of alcohol. Such depression tends to induce a state of disinhibition (unrestrained behavior) and mild euphoria, accompanied by talkativeness, animated feelings, noisy behavior, increased levels of activity, and expansiveness of the personality. These changes in behavior and mood are usually referred to as **pseudostimulation**—apparent, yet false or deceptive, stimulation. However, as the level of alcohol in the neurons increases, the cerebral cortex also becomes depressed and the state of disinhibition and euphoria ceases.

Alcohol and States of Consciousness

Intoxication produces an altered state of consciousness in individuals. Behavioral and biological differences suggest, however, that the period of mood and behavior modification is not a unitary or single state. Rather, the duration of alcohol effects is a time composed of several different states of consciousness, depending on whether the blood-alcohol concentration is increasing (the ascending limb of the blood-alcohol curve) or decreasing (the descending limb of the blood-alcohol curve).[23]

Four **alcohol states of consciousness (ASC)** during intoxication have been identified.[24]

ASC-1: the time of alcohol absorption and increasing blood-alcohol concentrations, characterized by talkativeness, laughter, motor incoordination, impaired performance on various cognitive, motor, and sensory tasks, and poor memory

ASC-2: the time beginning after the peak blood-alcohol concentration has been obtained and the blood-alcohol level is declining, during which the drinker becomes quiet and tired, but impaired performance is beginning to improve

ASC-3: the time beginning about halfway between peak blood-alcohol concentration and zero blood-alcohol level, in which the individual feels confident that he or she is perfectly sober, yet a detectable blood-alcohol concentration is still present

ASC-4: the time during which all traces of alcohol have disappeared from the body, but for up to thirty-two hours after drinking, positional alcohol nystagmus (PAN) eye movements can be detected in which the eyeballs involuntarily oscillate laterally, vertically, or in a rotary manner

Psychological Aspects of Intoxication

While the presence of alcohol in the central nervous system is the basis for intoxication, the psychological makeup of the drinker and the psychological atmosphere of drinking are important factors influencing intoxicated behavior.

The drinker's emotional makeup or temperament has been labeled as the *mind-set.* This factor is important in producing behavioral reactions accompanying alcohol use and any drug use. A person who drinks with the expectation of getting "high" will often display a form of "psychological intoxication" before "physiological intoxication" is possible. The author recalls an incident in which a nonalcoholic fruit drink was served to several people at a party. Before the beverage was consumed, the adult guests, most of whom were infrequent or light drinkers, were told that vodka had been added to the drink, but no taste would be detected. The results were amazing! After just a few sips, some of the guests claimed they felt warmer; a few mentioned the feeling of dizziness; the conversation became more animated; and the activity level of several guests increased markedly. This situation is a good example of the psyche's influence on the body.

Not only the individual's mind-set but the *emotional climate* or *setting of drinking* also sets the stage for certain behaviors. Imagine the excitement that surrounds a victory celebration of an athletic contest or the completion of an academic semester. The psychological atmosphere of these events predisposes drinkers to somewhat boisterous, excessive, and even bizarre behavior. The same individuals consuming the same amount of beverage in a more controlled, restrained setting would likely behave in a more mature way.

For many years, law enforcement officials have determined whether individuals were intoxicated by using field sobriety tests, such as the nystagmus gaze test for variations in the visual tracking of objects, the walk-and-turn test, and the one-leg stand. However, because the mood or mind-set of the consumer, along with the psychological atmosphere of drinking, will likely influence the drinker's responses to alcohol, estimating the degree of impairment by observation has proved unreliable.

Therefore, chemical tests for an objective evaluation of intoxication have been developed and involve the determination of alcohol levels in the blood and the breath. The tests are based on the constant proportion between alcohol concentrations in blood and in the breath. Several breath analysis instruments are available, namely, the *alcosensor, alcometer, drunkometer, intoximeter,* and *Breathalyzer.* The **Breathalyzer,** along with newer high-technology modifications of this device, is being used increasingly by law enforcement officials to identify, alcohol-impaired drivers.

Short-Term Effects of Alcohol

Specific body parts and functions can be influenced directly or indirectly by alcohol. Short-term effects include the following:

Sensation and Perception

Decreases in visual and hearing acuity.

Altered sensitivity to odors and taste.

Reduced sensitivity to pain due to the masking of fatigue.

An appearance that time passes more rapidly.

Underestimation of the speed of moving objects.

Increased sensation of thirst, possibly due to shifting of water from within the body's cells to the spaces between the cells.

Emotions

Feelings of elation.

Decreased fear.

Increases in risk-taking behaviors.

Emphasis on aggressive humor more than nonsense humor.

Reduced inhibitions.

Sleep

Induced sleep because of alcohol's depressant effect on the brain. But regular use over time deprives an individual of **rapid eye movements (REM)** or dreaming sleep, resulting in anxiety, tiredness, and impaired concentration.

Kidneys

Increased urinary output due to the *diuretic effect* of alcohol on the pituitary gland. Alcohol blocks this gland's production of a special chemical substance, the antidiuretic hormone. Without this hormone, which regulates the reabsorption of water before it is voided, the urine volume is increased, but not to the point of dehydration.

Heart and Blood Vessels

Temporary increases in heartbeat and blood pressure.

Dilated peripheral blood vessels in arms and legs. This blood vessel expander effect leads to a loss of body heat while producing a feeling of added warmth.

Constriction of the arteries supplying the heart.

Liver

An accumulation of fat cells that are considered the forerunners of other liver diseases is often associated with prolonged use of alcohol.

Motor Skills

Impairment of most types of performance, although individual susceptibility varies at BAC of 0.10 percent or below.

Increased swaying.

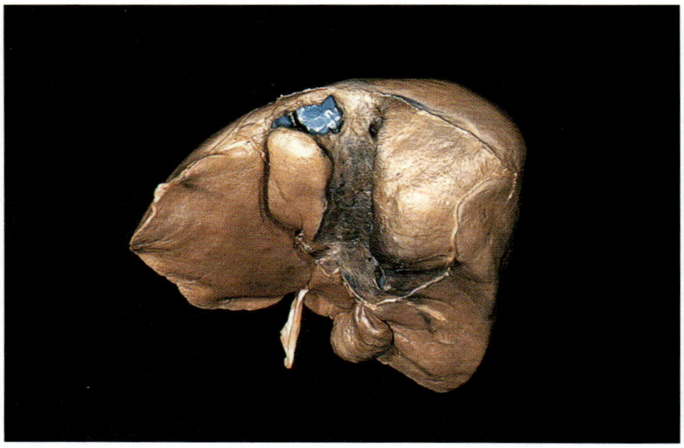

Healthy liver

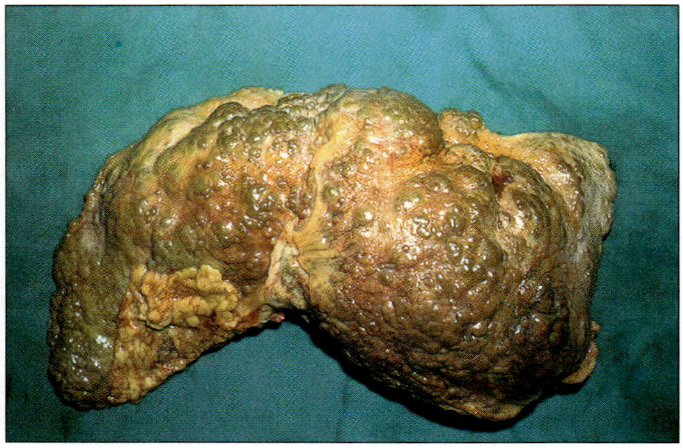

Cirrhotic liver

figure 4.6

A healthy liver compared with a cirrhotic liver. In comparison with a normal, healthy liver, an alcohol-induced cirrhotic liver is, shriveled and hardened. Many functioning liver cells have been replaced by scar tissue, which interferes with important actions of this organ. The "average" cirrhotic individual has been drinking heavily for ten to twenty years.

Photographs courtesy of Emmanuel Rubin, M.D.

Interference with sensorimotor coordination, as in tracking a moving object.

Hangover

Temporary, acute physical and psychological distress following excessive consumption of alcoholic beverages. The experience known as a **hangover** has been related to the amount of *congeners* (nonalcohol components) in beverage alcohol; the type of food eaten and liquor consumed; various emotional influences and expectations; the impact of physical factors, including loud and dark drinking environments; and physical factors, especially fatigue. Nausea, gastritis, headache, and anxiety experienced during a hangover are painful reminders of disrupted body functions that could not be felt while one was intoxicated. A hangover is the body's reaction to excessive drinking and represents a pronounced withdrawal syndrome from relatively large amounts of alcohol. Despite some innovative hangover cures, the only effective cures have been the use of analgesics for headaches and the healing powers of time.

Sexuality

Small doses of alcohol may facilitate sexual activity by helping one to overcome a lack of confidence or feelings of guilt. But while alcohol may provoke desire, larger amounts may spoil the capacity to perform or respond (see box 3.2).

Long-Term Effects of Alcohol

Prolonged, heavy consumption of alcoholic beverages can result in one or more tragic, often life-threatening consequences:

Gastrointestinal system disorders and diseases—These include irritation and inflammation of the esophagus, stomach, small intestine, and pancreas.

Liver disorders and diseases—These involve altered functions in the largest and most chemically complex body organ. Alcohol is now recognized as having a direct, toxic effect on liver tissue, the *hepatotoxic effect.* The trauma consists, first of all, of a fatty liver; which is reversible if drinking ceases. If heavy consumption persists, the fatty liver condition may develop into a chronic inflammation of liver tissue known as *alcoholic hepatitis,* which can be fatal. In some cases, this condition may evolve into *alcoholic cirrhosis,* characterized by the shriveling and hardening of the liver, in which functioning liver cells are replaced by scar tissue. Such disease can develop in spite of adequate dietary intake. The incidence of alcoholic cirrhosis is one indicator of the extent of alcohol abuse and alcoholism. Presently, alcoholic cirrhosis ranks among the twleve leading causes of death in America (see fig. 4.6).

Hypoglycemia—This is a serious condition in which blood-sugar levels are lowered beyond the normal range. Chronic drinking usually places considerable stress on the liver, thus interfering with the body's ability to produce glucose (blood sugar) and to store it as glycogen. The poor nutritional status of many alcoholics causes the glycogen reserves to be depleted, predisposing such individuals to the development of hypoglycemia when food is not eaten for twenty-four hours or more. The brain and spinal cord, which govern basic life processes, depend upon glucose for proper functioning, therefore hypoglycemia brings about a physiological crisis that can be damaging to the body and result in death.

Nutritional deficiency—This is one of the most common yet most undetected problems associated with long-term alcohol use. Alcohol interferes with the nutritional process by adversely affecting digestion, storage, use, and excretion of nutrients.[25] Alcohol is highly caloric, therefore some alcoholics take in as much as 50 percent of their total daily calories from alcohol. While taking in the "empty" calories deficient in vitamins, minerals, essential amino acids, and essential fatty acids, heavy drinkers often decrease their intake of nutrients from other food sources. Diminished appetite, vomiting, and diarrhea also contribute to nutritional imbalance.

Heavy consumption also disrupts normal processes of digestion by causing gastritis (inflammation of the stomach lining), stomach ulcers, and intestinal lesions or sores. These conditions interfere with proper transport, absorption, and activation of vitamins and minerals. The result of maldigestion (improper digestion); malabsorption (inadequate absorption) of nutrients; altered metabolism of nutrients by the liver; and interference with the flow of bile, a digestive fluid, in the gallbladder is *malnutrition* (see fig. 4.7). In turn, this unbalanced or inadequate nutritional state contributes to certain brain diseases, liver disease, pancreatitis, abnormal fetal development, suboptimal health, anemia, convulsions, and malfunction of the small bowel. Though severe malnutrition may be relatively rare, the effects of the subtle nutritional disturbances become more significant as intake of alcohol increases.[26]

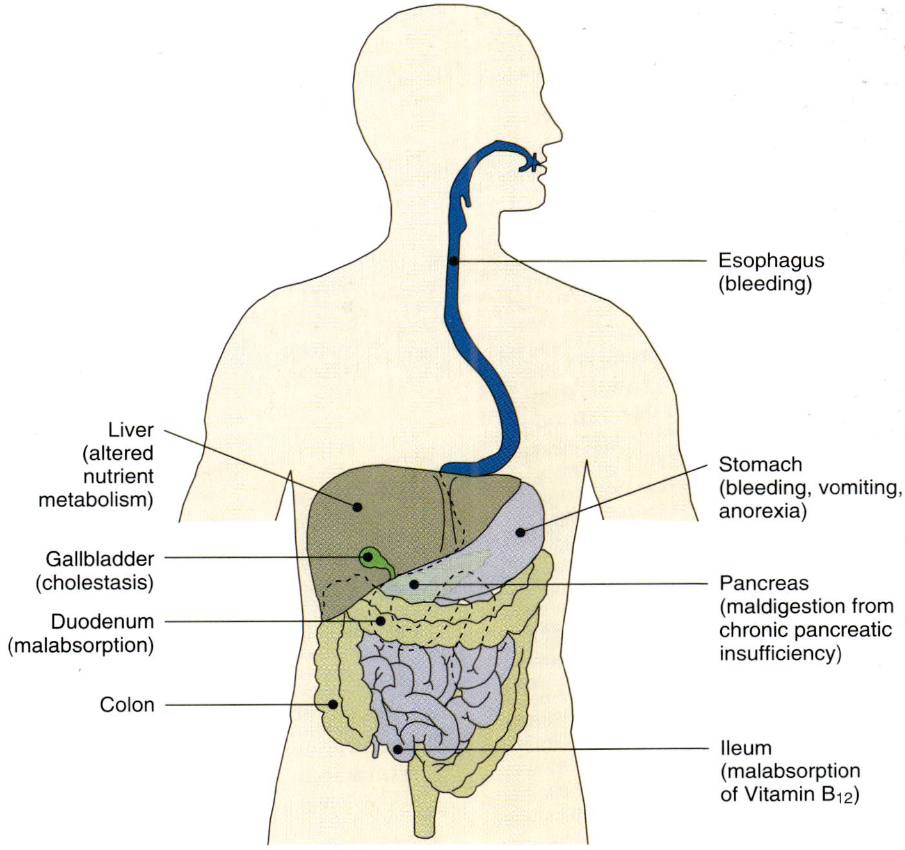

figure 4.7

The human digestive system with various mechanisms of malnutrition.

Source: National Institute on Alcohol Abuse and Alcoholism. Illustration by Alexander Tucker, art director for Alcohol Health & Research World, *Vol. 13, No. 3 (1989): 206.*

Nervous system diseases—Often combined with malnutrition, these surface as impairments of normal nerve cell functioning and cognitive deficits, especially those of problem solving, abstract thinking, concept shifting, psychomotor performance, and difficult memory tasks.[27] For the most severe alcoholics, serious organic impairments of brain function are common complications. Two such mental disorders are *dementia* associated with alcoholism and *alcohol memory disorder*. These disorders are not mutually exclusive, and aspects of each often coexist in the same patient. When linked with alcoholism, dementia surfaces as a deterioration of intellectual abilities and a disintegration of behavior and personality, but without a clouding of consciousness. By contrast, alcohol memory loss disorder, often called Korsakoff's psychosis or Wernicke-Korsakoff syndrome, is described as short-term memory impairments and behavioral changes that occur without clouding of consciousness or general loss of intellectual abilities.

Wernicke's syndrome—Related to thiamine (part of the vitamin B complex) deficiency, this syndrome is characterized by total bewilderment and disorientation, paralysis of the motor nerves of the eye, rhythmical oscillation of the eyeballs, loss of muscular coordination, and diseases of the peripheral nerves. *Korsakoff's psychosis,* often seen in conjunction with Wernicke's disease, includes severe amnesia, the recitation of imaginary experiences, and remarkable personality alterations. Chronic alcohol consumption has also been associated with numerous impairments of the central nervous system and the peripheral nervous system. In addition to these manifestations of alcohol's *neurotoxic effect* (poisonous to nervous tissue) are the occurrence of tolerance and physical dependence, as described in chapter 3.

Endocrine system disorders—These especially affect the hypothalamus, pituitary, and gonads. The production and release of certain chemical regulators (hormones) are altered significantly. In males, these changes result in decreased libido, impotence, and infertility. [28] Such functional difficulties common to male alcoholics are related to reduced testosterone levels, breast enlargement, loss of facial hair, and a wasting away of the testes.

Among women, heavy alcohol consumption is associated with menstrual cycle disorders and high rates of gynecological and obstetrical surgery.[29] Frequently reported conditions include amenorrhea (stoppage of menstruation), anovulation (absence of ovulation), irregular menstrual cycles, and early menopause. Even moderate alcohol use in women may contribute to the risk of infertility associated with ovulatory problems or endometriosis (abnormal displacement of the uterine lining to various locations in the pelvic cavity and elsewhere in the body).[30]

Mental disorders—Usually occurring as part of the alcohol withdrawal syndrome, these are identified as alcohol psychoses; alcoholic hallucinosis; and affective disorders, including disturbances of mood, accompanied by a full or partial manic or depressive syndrome. Alcoholics often have high levels of depression, and alcohol can increase depression.

Cardiovascular diseases—These affect the heart and blood vessels and are common in patients who have been chronic alcoholics for more than ten years. Long-standing use of substantial amounts of alcohol contributes to cardiomyopathy (disease of the heart muscle) and premature heartbeats or total loss of rhythmic beating in the heart's upper chambers.

Heavy drinking, often defined as consuming more than three cocktails or three glasses of beer or wine daily, is related to a 40 percent increased risk of high blood pressure. Middle-aged women and men who drink even more are likely to experience a 90 percent greater risk. Alcohol is also associated with phlebitis (inflammation of the veins) and varicose (unnatural and permanently distended) veins. In addition, research indicates that heavy drinkers are more than three times as likely as nondrinkers to have a stroke or cerebral vascular accident (CVA).[31] This increased risk pertains only to hemorrhagic stroke, in which small blood vessels in the brain rupture or burst. Moreover, this risk is independent of hypertension or high blood pressure. Light and moderate drinkers, by comparison, are more than twice as likely to have such strokes.

In contrast with long-term, heavy consumption, drinking only one or two servings of beer, wine, or distilled spirits daily appears to have a protective effect against heart attack among some drinkers.

Extensive data suggest that alcohol's beneficial effect is due in large part to an increase in blood levels of total high-density lipoprotein (HDL) and both subfractions, HDL_2 and HDL_3. (Lipoprotein is a combination of a blood lipid, or fat, and a protein substance that transports or carries fats in the blood, including cholesterol and triglycerides.)[32]

In a major study, one alcoholic drink was defined as a twelve-ounce glass of beer, or its equivalent in wine or distilled spirits. Individuals who consumed more than one, but fewer than three, drinks per day reduced their heart attack risk by half.

Despite this favorable aspect of moderate alcohol use, drinking any amount of alcohol can have risks for some people, as noted earlier in this section. In terms of ethyl alcohol, the difference between daily small to moderate amounts and large quantities may be the difference between preventing and causing disease.[33] There are other, safer ways of raising HDL levels, including regular exercise and the replacement of saturated fat with monounsaturated fats in one's diet. Encouragement of alcohol use to reduce the likelihood of the occurrence or recurrence of heart disease seems unwise without medical supervision. Even moderate drinking poses serious risks—hypertension (elevated blood pressure), alcohol-related auto accidents, and fetal damage in pregnant women.

Myopathy—This is an abnormal condition or disease of muscular tissues, characterized by muscle weakness, cramps, and wasting away of skeletal musculature.

Cancer—Cancer, or uncontrolled cell growth, is frequently observed in patients who are alcohol dependent or who have alcohol-related cirrhosis. Heavy drinking increases the risk of developing cancer of the tongue, mouth, throat, esophagus, and liver, and is often associated with cancer of the pancreas, large intestine, and rectum. Though still controversial, research suggests that alcohol may also increase the risk of breast cancer in women as much as two times in comparison with women who do not drink.

There is little doubt that heavy drinking is related significantly to many types of malignant cancer. But the precise mechanism of alcohol's involvement remains somewhat a mystery. Studies of laboratory animals have failed to show that pure ethyl alcohol is carcinogenic (cancer-causing) in and of itself.

Consequently, it is believed that some of the congeners or other contaminants in alcoholic beverages may be the culprit in drinking-related cancers. Alcohol may prove to be more of a cocarcinogen: a

table 4.3 Alcohol-Drug Interactions

Drugs	Possible Effects of Combining These Drugs with Alcohol
Anesthetics	
Diprivan	Increases dose required to induce loss of consciousness.
Ethrane and Fluothane	Increases the risk of liver damage.
Antibiotics	
Isoniazid	Decreases availability of this drug in the bloodstream, thereby reducing its effect.
Rifampin	Decreases availability of this drug in the bloodstream, thereby reducing its effect.
Anticoagulants	
Coumadin	Enhanced availability with acute drinking, and increased risk for hemorrhages. Reduced availability with chronic drinking and lessened protection from the consequences of blood-clotting disorders.
Antidepressants	
Tricyclics	Increased sedative effect usually, but chronic drinking can decrease availability of other tricyclics.
Monoamine oxidase inhibitors	One drink may create a dangerous rise in blood pressure.
Antidiabetic medications	
Orinase	Prolonged availability by acute drinking; decreased availability by chronic drinking.
Antihistamines	Intensified sedation effect caused by some antihistamine drugs.
Antipsychotic medications	
Thorazine	Increased sedative effect resulting in potentially fatal breathing difficulties. Liver damage possible with chronic drinking.
Antiseizure medications	
Dilantin	Increased availability and increased risk of drug-related side effects; decreased availability by chronic drinking, which reduces protection against seizures.
Antiulcer medications	
Tagamet and Zantac	Possible increase in the availability with a low dose of alcohol.
Cardiovascular medications	Dizziness or fainting upon standing up by acute alcohol consumption.
Inderal	Decreased availability by chronic drinking, thereby reducing the drug's effect.
Central nervous system stimulants	
Cocaine	No interactions reported.
Amphetamines	Blocked or reduced CNS depressant effect.
Nicotine	Possible cocarcinogenic effect when smoker also drinks alcohol.
Disulfiram (Antabuse)	Flushing of skin; throbbing in head and neck; nausea; vomiting; breathing difficulties; sweating; and in severe reactions there may also be serious cardiovascular and respiratory problems, convulsions, and death.
Narcotic pain relievers	Enhanced sedative effect of opioids and alcohol, thereby increasing risk of death from overdose.
Darvon	Increased availability with increased sedative effect due to a single dose of alcohol.
Nonnarcotic pain relievers	
Aspirin, ibuprofen, and naproxen sodium	Worsening of gastrointestinal bleeding and inhibited blood clotting. Aspirin may increase availability of alcohol, thereby increasing the effects of a given dose of alcohol.
Acetaminophen	Liver damage because of alcohol's activation of the enzymes that biotransform this pain reliever.
Oral contraceptives	Prolonged elevation of blood-alcohol levels with slowed rate of elimination from the body.
Psychedelics	
Cannabis	Additive effect with increased impairment of mental and motor functions.
LSD	Questionable trigger of flashbacks.
Sedatives and hypnotics (sleeping pills)	
Benzodiazepines	Severe drowsiness, increasing risk of household and auto accidents.
Dalmane	Impaired driving ability with low doses of alcohol.
Ativan	Depressed heart and breathing functions.
Barbiturates	Increased availability and prolonged sedative effect with acute drinking. Decreased availability with chronic drinking. Increased sedative effect in the brain, sometimes leading to coma or fatal respiratory depression.

Source: The National Institute on Alcohol Abuse and Alcoholism

promoter, or a vehicle bearing a causal agent. For instance, alcohol appears to interact with tobacco to increase the risk of certain cancers and with the condition of cirrhosis to increase the development of liver cancer.

Infectious diseases—These, particularly pneumonia and tuberculosis, are common to alcohol abusers. The neglect of nutrition, impairment of lung clearance and phagocytosis (a process whereby white blood cells ingest and digest specific bacteria), and decreased immune response mechanisms make alcohol abusers prone to respiratory infections.

Alcohol-tobacco interactions—People who are heavy drinkers also tend to be heavy smokers. The combination of these two drugs significantly increases the risks of developing cardiovascular and lung diseases and cancer of the mouth, throat, or esophagus. In addition, youths who smoke are three times more likely to use alcohol, and smokers are ten times more likely to become alcoholics.[34]

Alcohol-drug interactions—Mixing alcoholic beverages with other drugs can have unpleasant and even fatal effects. The effects of alcohol-drug interactions can range from the relatively minor drowsiness that comes with mixing a cocktail with an antihistamine all the way to loss of consciousness and death.

How much a person is affected by the combination of alcohol and certain prescription drugs, as well as over-the-counter drugs, depends on: body size, weight, age, sex, health status, genetic makeup, and the person's ability to process or change consumed substances before their elimination from the body.

Alcohol can influence the effects of another drug by altering its **bioavailability,** that is, the extent to which an administered drug dose reaches its site of action or the drug's activity within the body, measured by levels of that particular drug in the blood. Typical alcohol-drug interactions appear in table 4.3.

Chapter Summary

1. Continuing a long-term custom, most Americans use alcoholic beverages as a legally and socially approved form of drug taking. But for a majority in the drinking age population, alcohol plays a relatively minor role or no role in their lives.
2. The "temperance movement" began as a promotion of moderate use of beverage alcohol and evolved into a moral crusade aimed at mandating abstinence by law.
3. Enforcement of national Prohibition began in 1920 after passage of the Eighteenth Amendment to the U.S. Constitution. After nearly fourteen years, the "noble experiment" ended when the Twenty-First Amendment was approved in 1933, repealing the provisions of the Prohibition amendment.
4. The emotional legacy of Prohibition and the conflict between permissive use and abstinence have generated a cultural ambivalence toward alcohol. This condition, in which both positive and negative aspects of alcohol are perceived jointly, has contributed to numerous alcohol problems.
5. Drinkers differ considerably in terms of age, gender, education, and geography, but especially in amount consumed and frequency of use. Abstainers and light and moderate drinkers consume only a little over one-third of alcoholic beverages sold, while heavy drinkers—only 9 percent to 10 percent of the drinking age population—consume nearly two-thirds of such beverages.
6. Many college students drink alcoholic beverages, but nearly 40 percent engage in binge drinking, a pattern of excessive use that frequently leads to many personal, social, and academic problems on and around campus. Unique factors influencing college drinking include exaggerated perceptions of peers' alcohol use, positive expectancies, need to be accepted and approved by others, drinking in groups or serving oneself, and living in a pro-use environment heavily targeted by advertisers and the alcoholic beverage industry.
7. Patterns of alcohol use range from nondrinking to chronic (long-term) alcoholic drinking. General uses of beverage alcohol include social, ritualistic, dietary, and the perceived benefits of altered consciousness—variations in thoughts, feelings, and behavior. Alcohol-induced changes in one's consciousness may result in tranquilization, perceived stress reduction, feelings of powerfulness, enhancement of feminity, satisfaction of dependency needs, increased awareness, and increased unawareness.
8. Alcoholic beverages are classified as fermented beverages (beers and wines), and distilled spirits, each type having varying amounts of ethyl alcohol. However, a typical, standard serving of any one beverage contains about 0.6 ounce of pure alcohol, known as the equivalent amount.
9. Once an alcoholic beverage is consumed, it undergoes processes of absorption, distribution, and oxidation. If intake of alcohol exceeds the body's ability to eliminate it, the blood-alcohol concentration will increase. As BACs increase, the depressant effect of alcohol is manifested as intoxication, a temporary state of mental chaos and behavioral dysfunction.
10. The duration of alcohol effects is a time composed of several different states of consciousness, depending on whether the blood-alcohol concentration is increasing or decreasing. Behavioral reactions accompanying intoxication are influenced by the drinker's mind-set and the emotional climate of drinking.
11. Short-term effects of alcohol are evidenced in alteration of sensation, perception, emotions, sleep, and motor skills, and in changes in

kidney, heart, blood vessel, liver, and sexual functions. A hangover is a possibility following excessive consumption.

12. Long-term effects of alcohol consumption, often heavy and prolonged intake, can develop into gastrointestinal disorders, liver diseases and dysfunction, nutritional deficiency, diseases of the nervous system, endocrine system disorders, mental disorders, cardiovascular diseases, certain cancers, and numerous undesirable and possibly fatal alcohol-drug interactions.

World Wide Web Sites

Rutgers University Center for Alcohol Studies

www.rci.rutgers.edu

National Institute on Alcohol Abuse and Alcoholism

www.niaaa.nih.gov

The Higher Education Center for Alcohol and other Drug Prevention

www.edc.org/hec/

Review Questions and Activities

1. Survey class members anonymously to determine their patterns of alcohol use or nonuse. Then, compare the results with the national percentages listed in the textbook. Try to explain any differences or similarities.
2. What is the difference between moonshining and bootlegging activities?
3. Identify the historical factors that led to the adoption of national Prohibition in the United States.
4. State the provisions of the Eighteenth Amendment to the U.S. Constitution.
5. Describe how the emotional legacy of the Prohibition Era has contributed to modern alcohol problems.
6. Name four manifestations of cultural ambivalence as related to alcohol use in America.
7. Describe the current drinking age population of the United States in terms of use and nonuse of alcoholic beverages, relative amounts of beverages consumed, and the annual per capita consumption of ethanol over the past ten years.
8. Relate the pattern of alcohol use known as binge drinking to personal, social, and academic problems among college students.
9. How does drinking for increased awareness differ from drinking for increased unawareness?
10. Compare and contrast the range of alcohol percentages found in beers, wines, and distilled spirits. Do you think most drinkers care about the amount of alcohol in their alcoholic beverages? Explain your response.
11. Ask several nonclass friends or adult family members to define a standard drink and to estimate how much pure (absolute) alcohol is present in various alcoholic beverage servings. What conclusions can be based on the results of your survey? Do you think most drinkers are fairly knowledgeable about the amount of alcohol they drink?
12. Name several factors that influence the absorption of alcohol.
13. What is meant by the term *blood-alcohol concentration?*
14. What are the various intermediate and end by-products of alcohol oxidation?
15. Why can't women hold their liquor like men?
16. Explain the various changes likely to occur as an intoxicated person's blood-alcohol concentration increases from 0.03 percent to 0.30 percent.
17. What is the relation of pseudostimulation to alcohol intoxication?
18. How does alcohol state of consciousness number one differ from ASC-2?
19. Name several short-term and potential long-term effects of alcohol consumption on physical and mental health status.
20. Why does nutritional deficiency often develop in a heavy drinker?
21. Identify four different, specific ways in which undesirable or unanticipated alcohol-drug interactions are likely to occur.

References

1. U.S. Department of Health and Human Services. Substance Abuse and Mental Health Administration. *Substance Abuse and Mental Health Statistics Sourcebook, 1998,* edited by Beatrice A. Rouse (Washington, D.C.: GPO, 1998).
2. "1994 in Review: The Battle for Stomach Share," *The Bottom Line on Alcohol in Society* 16, no. 4 (winter, 1995): 15–28.
3. National Institute on Alcohol Abuse and Alcoholism, "Influences of American History and Popular Media on Drinking Practices in America," in *Planning a Prevention Program* (Washington, D.C.: GPO, 1978), 95–96.
4. National Institute on Alcohol Abuse and Alcoholism, *"College Students and Drinking,"* no. 29, *Alcohol Alert,* no. 29, (July, 1995), 1–4.
5. Cheryl Presley and Philip Meilman, *Alcohol and Drugs on American College Campuses, A Report to College Presidents* (Carbondale, Ill.: Southern Illinois University, 1992), 3–5.
6. National Institute on Alcohol Abuse and Alcoholism, *Alcohol Alert,* no. 29, (July, 1995), 2–3.
7. Lewis Eigen, *Alcohol Practices, Policies, and Potentials of American Colleges and Universities,* Office for Substance Abuse Prevention, DHHS Pub. No. (ADM) 91-1842 (Washington, D.C.: GPO, 1991), 30.
8. Donna Shalala, "Message from the Secretary of Health and Human Services," *Alcohol Alert: College Students and Drinking,* 1.
9. Ronald K. Siegel, *Intoxication: Life in Pursuit of Artificial Paradise* (New York: Dutton, 1989), 10.
10. David Pittman and Helene Raskin White, *Society, Culture, and Drinking Patterns Reexamined* (New Brunswick, N.J.: Rutgers Center of Alcohol Studies, 1991), 175.
11. Andrew Weil and Winifred Rosen, *From Chocolate to Morphine,* rev. ed. (Boston: Houghton Mifflin, 1993), 14.
12. Marian Sandmaier, *The Invisible Alcoholics: Women and Alcohol Abuse in America* (New York: McGraw-Hill, 1980), 91.
13. Harvey B. Milkman and Stanley G. Sunderwirth, *Craving for Ecstasy: The Consciousness and Chemistry of Escape* (Lexington, Mass.: Lexington Books/D.C. Heath, 1987), 18.

14. Siegel, *Intoxication*, 10, 207–27, 313.
15. *World Book Encyclopedia* (Chicago: World Book, 1992), 335.
16. Robert Lipinski and Kathleen Lipinski, *The Complete Beverage Dictionary* (New York: Van Nostrand Reinhold, 1992), 10.
17. U.S. Department of Health and Human Services, Office of the Inspector General, *Youth and Alcohol: A National Survey—Drinking Habits, Access, Attitudes, and Knowledge* (Washington, D.C.: National Clearinghouse for Alcohol and Drug Information, 1991), 6.
18. "Looks, Smells, Tastes Like Beer," *Bottom Line on Alcohol in Society* 10 (1990): 26–28.
19. "California Becomes the Battleground for Alcopops—TGIF, Hooper's Hooch and More . . . ," *The Bottom Line on Alcohol in Society,* 17, no. 2 (summer, 1996): 40–46.
20. William Hobbs, Theodore Rall, and Todd Verdoorn, "Hypnotics and Sedatives; Ethanol," chap. 17 in *Goodman & Gilman's The Pharmacological Basis of Therapeutics,* 9th ed. (New York: McGraw-Hill Health Professions Division, 1996), 361–96.
21. Mario Frezza and others, "High Blood Alcohol Levels in Women: The Role of Decreased Gastric Alcohol Dehydrogenase Activity and First-Pass Metabolism," *New England Journal of Medicine* 322, no. 2 (11 January 1990): 95–99.
22. Nancy M. Lee and Charles E. Becker, "The Alcohols," chap. 22 in *Basic and Clinical Pharmacology,* 4th ed., ed. Bertram Katzung (Norwalk, Conn.: Appleton & Lange, 1989), 278–79.
23. Theodore Rall, "Hypnotics and Sedatives; Ethanol," chap. 17 in *Goodman and Gilman's The Pharmacological Basis of Therapeutics,* 8th ed., ed. A. G. Gilman and others (New York: McGraw-Hill, 1990), 371.
24. Ben Morgan Jones and Marilyn K. Jones, "States of Consciousness and Alcohol: Relationship to the Blood Alcohol Curve, Time of Day, and the Menstrual Cycle," *Alcohol Health and Research World* 1, no. 1 (fall, 1976): 10–15.
25. National Institute on Alcohol Abuse and Alcoholism, "Alcohol and Nutrition," *Alcohol Alert,* no. 22, (October 1993), 1–3.
26. Charles Lieber, "Alcohol and Nutrition: An Overview," *Alcohol Health and Research World* 13, no. 3 (1989): 197–205.
27. National Institute on Alcohol Abuse and Alcoholism, "Alcohol and Cognition," *Alcohol Alert* no. 4 (May 1989), 1–2.
28. Mary Emanuele and others, "The Effects of Alcohol on the Neuroendocrine Control of Reproduction," chap. 5 in *Alcohol and the Endocrine System,* Research Monograph No. 23 (Bethesda, Md: National Institute on Alcohol Abuse and Alcoholism, 1993), 89–116.
29. Nancy Mello, Jack Mendelson, and Siew Teoh, "An Overview of the Effects of Alcohol on Neuroendocrine Function in Women," chap. 7 in *Alcohol and the Endocrine System,* Research Monograph No. 23 (Bethesda, Md: National Institute on Alcohol Abuse and Alcoholism, 1993), 139–69.
30. Francine Grodstein, Marlene Goldman, and Daniel Cramer, "Infertility in Women and Moderate Alcohol Use," *American Journal of Public Health* 84, no. 9 (September, 1994): 1429–32.
31. Richard Donahue and others, "Alcohol and Hemorrhagic Stroke: The Honolulu Heart Program," *Journal of the American Medical Association* 255, no. 17 (2 May 1986): 2311–14.
32. J. Michael Gaziano and others, "Moderate Alcohol Intake, Increased Levels of High-Density Lipoprotein and Its Subfractions, and Decreased Risk of Myocardial Infarction," *New England Journal of Medicine* 329, no. 25 (16 December 1993): 1829–34.
33. Ibid.
34. National Institute on Alcohol Abuse and Alcoholism, "*Alcohol-Medication Interactions.*" *Alcohol Alert,* no. 27, (January, 1995), 1–4.
35. National Institute on Alcohol Abuse and Alcoholism, "*Alcohol and Tobacco,*" *Alcohol Alert,* no. 39, (January, 1998), 1–2.

Chapter 5

Alcohol abuse and alcoholism

KEY TERMS

Alcohol Abuse
Alcohol Dependence
Alcoholics Anonymous
Alcoholism
Antabuse
Blackout
Blood Alcohol Concentration (BAC)
Co-Dependence
Craving
Delirium Tremens
Detoxification
Dry-Drunk Phenomenon
Fetal Alcohol Effects
Fetal Alcohol Syndrome
Loss of Control
Naltrexone
On-The-Job Absenteeism
Problem Drinking
Revolving Door Routine
Withdrawal Symptoms
Zero-Tolerance Limits

chapter objectives

After you have studied this chapter, you should be able to do the following:

1. Define the key terms.
2. Explain the difficulty in defining or identifying a drinking problem.
3. List the major criteria used for determining the existence of alcohol abuse on the part of a drinker.
4. Relate the following contributing factors to worksite problem drinking: cultural, social control, alienation, and work stress.
5. Compare common alcohol countermeasures used to reduce or prevent "public intoxication" and "driving under the influence" of alcohol.
6. Tell what is meant by "property offenses" and "public order offenses" and explain why they might be associated with alcohol abuse.
7. Describe the role of alcohol use and abuse in the following types of accidental injuries and fatalities: falls, drownings, fires, and automobile crashes.
8. Explain how the following factors contribute to the increased risk of crashing in an alcohol-related auto accident: blood alcohol concentration, youthfulness, gender, and use of certain medications.
9. Identify at least five specific alcohol countermeasures and discuss how they might help reduce the epidemic of alcohol-impaired driving.
10. Describe in detail the three principal features of Fetal Alcohol Syndrome.
11. Relate each of the following potential mechanisms of damage to FAS and FAE: maternal nutrients, hormonal deficiencies, local growth factor, and prostaglandin.
12. Discuss alcohol abuse and alcoholism as a family disease in relation to non-alcoholic spouses, children of alcoholics, and the condition of co-dependence.
13. Compare and contrast the following definitions of alcoholism: disease of alcohol dependence, Jellinek's species or types of alcoholism, and the American Psychiatric Association's substance dependence disorder.
14. Discuss the possible causes of alcoholism in terms of the agent (ethyl alcohol), the host (the drinker), and the environment (the psychosocial/cultural setting in which drinking occurs).
15. Describe several of the anticipated signs and symptoms that commonly occur in each of the four developmental phases of alcoholism.
16. Name the three general stages of alcoholism treatment and rehabilitation.
17. Compare the effects of Antabuse and Naltrexone when used as drug therapy in the treatment of alcoholism.
18. Distinguish among each of the following therapies for alcoholism: psychotherapy, family therapy, behavioral therapy, and transactional analysis.
19. Explain the basic nature and operational processes of Alcoholics Anonymous.
20. Describe several ways an individual can reduce problem drinking behavior.

Problem Drinking

Most people believe that when some individuals consume alcoholic beverages, the consequences of excessive or inappropriate use can result in undesirable, difficult situations or conditions often labeled as problems. Although the vast majority of drinkers are not problem drinkers or alcoholics and have never been arrested for public intoxication or "driving under the influence," our society tends to focus more attention on these perplexing and sensational complications than on promoting "rules of nondestructive drinking"—the right and wrong places to drink, people to drink with, types and amounts of beverages to drink, and activities to pursue while drinking.[1]

Trying to identify an alcohol-related problem seems fairly simple. In reality, this task often proves to be complicated.[2] For instance, some people view drinking as a problem and would feel endangered if alcoholic beverages were present in their homes. For others, driving under the influence of alcohol is a real problem, but others would see this behavior as problematic only if they were caught by police officials. Still others would view teenage drinking as not only illegal, but also problem-producing. However, some teens and many adults view heavy drinking as appropriate in many situations or as a demonstration of a prized skill—the ability to hold more booze than anyone else.

The task of defining a problem depends upon many things, including one's perspective of values and priorities; degree of relationship to the drinker; extent of injury or damage experienced; and society's judgment of drinking in relation to custom, law, or threat to the common good. Frequently, alcohol problems are defined easily and accurately by impartial observers who claim they know a problem when they see it. Sometimes those severely afflicted with mental and physical harm by others' problem drinking see the difficulty in their minds, but not in their hearts. To acknowledge the existence of the problem would be too embarrassing or too threatening to a relationship established in love. All too often, problem drinkers are the last to admit to a personal or social crisis due to drinking. They are in denial and blame others for their own predicaments (see box 5.1).

As you study the various alcohol-related concerns in this chapter, determine what criteria are being applied to define them as significant problems.

Problem Drinking and Alcohol Abuse

Most experts agree that **problem drinking** is any use of beverage alcohol that results in some type of damage or harm to the drinker, the drinker's family, or the drinker's community. As such, problem drinking is **alcohol abuse,** because the consumption of alcoholic beverages

Box 5.1 Do You Have An Alcohol Problem? Are You An Alcoholic? Take the Short Michigan Alcoholism Screening Test (SMAST)

Screening tests have been formulated to identify individuals who may have a particular health problem but whose symptoms have not yet become highly visible. One of the more frequently used screening tests for alcoholism is the Michigan Alcoholism Screening Test (MAST). Originally developed by Melvin Selzer, the first MAST had twenty-four items. A revised list of thirteen questions, typically self-administered, is now used with a high degree of effectiveness by clinicians.

1. Do you feel you are a normal drinker? (By normal we mean you drink *less than* or *as much as* most other people.)
2. Does your wife, husband, a parent, or other near relative ever worry or complain about your drinking?
3. Do you ever feel guilty about your drinking?
4. Do friends or relatives think you are a normal drinker?
5. Are you able to stop drinking when you want to?
6. Have you ever attended a meeting of Alcoholics Anonymous?
7. Has drinking ever created problems between you and your wife, husband, a parent, or other near relative?
8. Have you ever gotten into trouble at work because of drinking?
9. Have you ever neglected your obligations, your family, or your work for two or more days in a row because you were drinking?
10. Have you ever gone to anyone for help about your drinking?
11. Have you ever been in a hospital because of drinking?
12. Have you ever been arrested for drunken driving, driving while intoxicated, or driving under the influence of alcoholic beverages?
13. Have you ever been arrested, even for a few hours, because of other drunken behavior?

Scoring and evaluation of the SMAST: An answer to any of the questions that corresponds to the following responses is assigned a value of one point:

1. No, 2. Yes, 3. Yes, 4. No, 5. No, 6. Yes, 7. Yes, 8. Yes, 9. Yes, 10. Yes, 11. Yes, 12. Yes, 13. Yes.

In individuals who score two points, alcoholism is suggested; in those who score three or more points, alcoholism is assessed.

"Short Michigan Alcoholism Screening Test" from *Journal of Studies on Alcohol,* vol. 36, 1975. Reprinted by permission of Melvin L. Selzer, M.D., F.A.C.P.

results in some degree of physical, mental, or social impairment to either the user or someone else.

Problem drinkers can be moderate or light drinkers who occasionally drive after excessive alcohol use and cause accidents. Problem drinkers include those who engage in drinking to become intoxicated and those who drink when such intake would worsen an existing medical condition. Some problem drinkers even engage in the so-called "sport" of competitive consumption to see who can hold more liquor faster.

While the undesirable consequences of alcohol use would be described as the abuse of alcohol, the term alcohol abuse has been given more specific and personalized meaning. According to the American Psychiatric Association, alcohol abuse is a maladaptive or faulty pattern of alcohol use leading to significant impairment or distress, with one or more or the following criteria or conditions occurring within a twelve-month period:[3]

- Repeated drinking leading to a failure to fulfill major role obligations at work, school, or home
- Reoccurring drinking in situations in which alcohol use is physically hazardous
- Recurrent alcohol-related legal problems
- Continued alcohol use despite having persistent or recurrent social or interpersonal problems caused or made worse by the effects of alcohol

In each of the conditions used to describe alcohol abuse, alcoholic beverages are consumed on a continuing basis, in other words, repeatedly, despite an ongoing social, occupational, psychological, or physical difficulty. Here are some examples of alcohol abuse according to the criteria:

1. A college student engages in heavy, binge drinking nearly every weekend during fall and spring semesters. Often beginning on Thursday evening and lasting through Sunday, these binge weekends are followed by missing Monday classes and quizzes due to severe hangovers. His scholarship is endangered by falling grades.
2. A woman repeatedly drives her car while intoxicated and is routinely arrested for this offense and sometimes for disorderly conduct or resisting arrest.
3. A man continues drinking alcohol though his physician has told him that alcohol is making his duodenal ulcer worse.
4. A pregnant woman persists in drinking throughout her pregnancy, though such an alcohol use pattern endangers her baby before it is born and results in frequent arguments with her husband.

In the next five sections of this chapter, various alcohol-related problems or alcohol abuse will be examined in relation to fulfilling one's role obligations in the workforce, involvement with the law and legal authorities, physically hazardous consequences of using alcohol, and the disruption of social and interpersonal relations as seen in family living.

Alcohol Abuse and Work Performance

Contrary to the widely held belief that problem drinkers are too disabled to hold jobs, most alcohol abusers and alcohol-dependent individuals are employed, despite serious work-related and/or interrelationship difficulties. Today, an estimated 7.4 percent of full-time workers and 5.9 percent of part-time workers engage in heavy drinking—five or more drinks per occasion on five or more days in the past thirty days.[4] This amount of alcohol use can and does have serious, adverse consequences in job performance, a fact recognized by most employers and many employees.

Almost 60 percent of the economic costs associated with alcohol abuse and alcoholism are directly or indirectly related to reduced productivity and lost employment. Some specific findings will help explain the huge expenses associated with alcohol abuse in the workplace:[5]

- Absenteeism among alcoholics or problem drinkers is 3.8 to 8.3 times greater than normal. These employees use three times as many sick benefits as other workers, and they are five times more likely to file a a workers' compensation claim.
- Nonalcoholic members of alcoholics' families use ten times as much sick leave as members of families in which alcoholism is not present.
- Up to 40 percent of industrial fatalities and 47 percent of industrial injuries can be linked to alcohol consumption and alcoholism.

Drinking and Job Behaviors

Impaired work performance is not an early indicator of alcohol abuse, but develops over time as part of the progressive nature of alcoholism. Reduced productivity is typically marked by lower quantity and lower quality of work, putting off tasks, neglecting details, more sporadic work pace, and making mistakes or errors of judgment.[6]

Another element contributing to reduced performance is absenteeism. In most instances, physical presence is essential for job performance, but absences from work tend to increase as drinking problems worsen. Problem drinkers often arrive late for work and leave early, a common experience with lower-status occupations. But among high-status problem drinkers, there is less "off-the-job" absenteeism. Professional, managerial, and other "white-collar" employees arrive at work, but once there, tend to display more **on-the-job absenteeism,** defined as frequent disappearances from the work station, lengthy breaks from assigned tasks, sleeping on-the-job, and accomplishing nothing of substance.[7] Further complicating on-the-job absenteeism and contributing to impaired job performance are hangovers and alcohol withdrawal distress, characterized by increased nervousness or jitters, more edginess or irritability, red or bleary eyes, neglecting details, and making more errors in planning and evaluation activities.

Impaired work performance results in more on-the-job accidents. This oc-

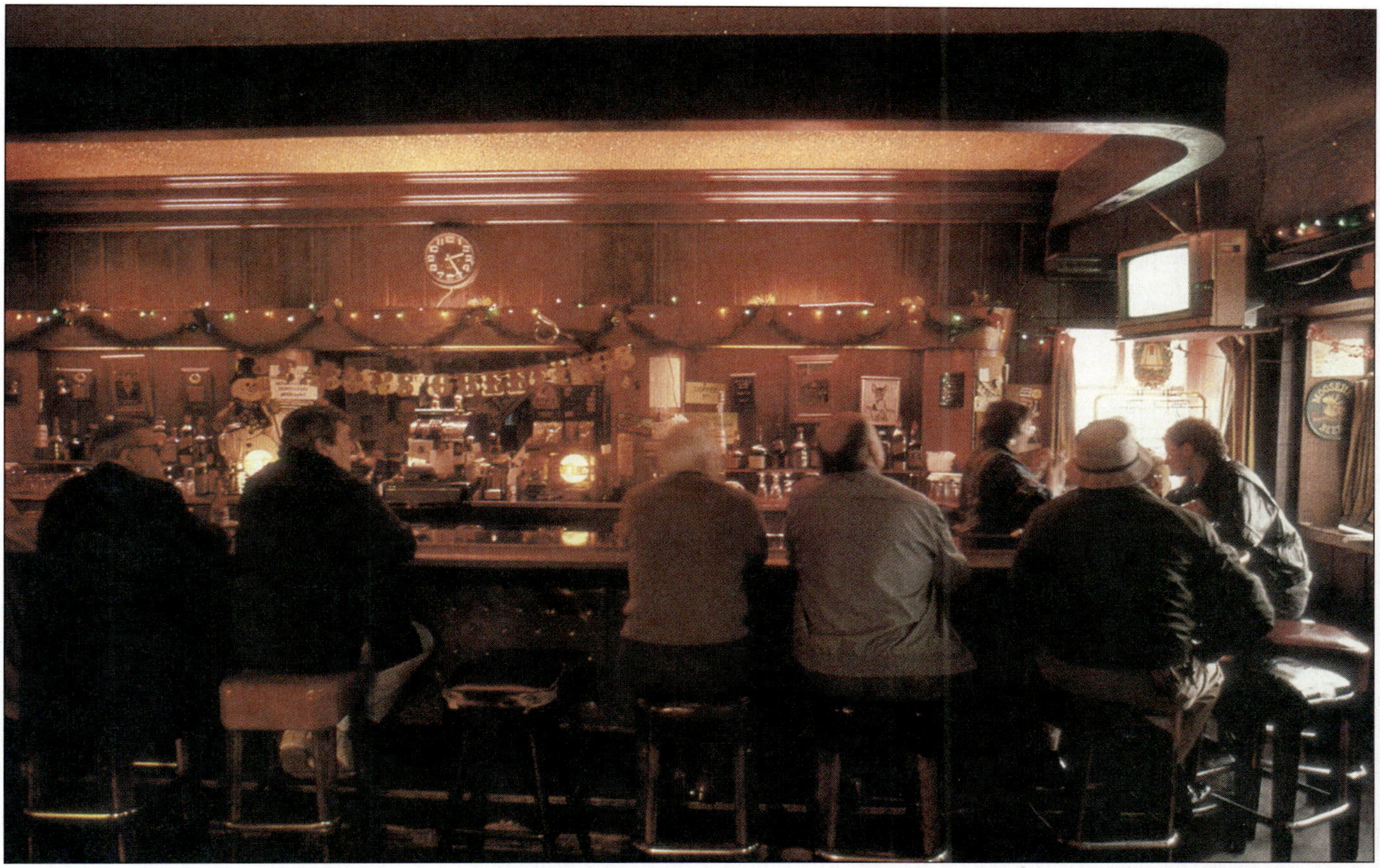

Gathering for drinks at the end of a workday can become a ritualized part of a workplace culture, and for some, can lead to problem drinking.

© Peter Menzel/Stock Boston

curs mostly in early stage alcoholismic, younger problem drinkers who have nearly twice as many such accidents as nonalcoholic workers.[8] Older alcoholics typically have fewer on-the-job accidents, because they take special precautions to prevent such occurrences. They stay home, slow down work assignments, or manage to be transferred from dangerous jobs. Sometimes they even drink alcohol to reduce hand tremors and mistakes that could lead to accidents.

Work Related Factors and Alcohol Abuse

While there is no clear evidence that the workplace causes alcohol abuse or alcoholism, research suggests that one's working environment can encourage problem drinking.[9] Four major contributing factors or perspectives of the worksite are emphasized: cultural, social control, alienation, and work stress.

From a "*workplace cultures perspective,*" both administrative and occupational subcultures contain beliefs about what is and is not acceptable drinking behavior. In some work organizations abstinence may be the norm, while in others there may be support for heavy drinking. Some units of the United States military service still maintain drinking rituals. Other organizations may confine such excessive drinking practices to specific departments, while certain occupational groups, such as longshoremen and construction workers view heavy drinking as a normal, conforming standard.

From a "*social control perspective,*" work roles with little or no supervision, little or no interdependency with others, and work roles with little visibility or those that call for frequent geographic mobility and shift changes tend to loosen individual ties to the workplace, and therefore may allow the development of undetectable alcohol problems. By contrast, work roles that lack creativity, variety, and independent judgment sometimes give rise to feelings of powerlessness. According to this "*alienation perspective,*" dissatisfied employees who feel they cannot achieve their full potential through their job learn to relieve feelings of helplessness through drinking.

The final consideration of work-related risk factors for alcohol abuse is categorized as the "*work stress perspective.*" Here the focus is on workplace experiences translated into life strains. Workplace stressors include the harshness of the working environment, changes in job description or functions, increased machine pacing, monotony, boredom, lack of control over work processes, work overloads, inequality of pay, and job complexity. Many labor experts support the concept that there is a strong relationship between workplace stressors and the development of drinking problems.

Alcohol-Related Law Violations and Violence

Usually, alcohol abuse is associated with criminal law violations and violent crimes in two ways: the infraction of laws dealing with the distribution, sale, and purchase of alcoholic beverages; and the violation of laws related to the behavioral effects of drinking. Only the latter will be described here, as the former violations will be examined in chapter 15.

Public Intoxication

Although arrests for public intoxication or drunkenness still number over 700,000 annually, many states and local communities have, in effect, decriminalized this behavior. During the 1980s, most states enacted their versions of the model Uniform Alcoholism and Intoxication Treatment Act. Under provisions of this act, the former criminal offense of public intoxication is considered a public health problem, and the public drunk is seen as physically sick and in need of medical care. Detoxification and aftercare are the preferred treatments.

Despite this more enlightened approach to public drunkenness, law enforcement officials still spend an enormous amount of time and resources in dealing with this alcohol-related problem. In some areas, the old **revolving door routine**—arrest for drunkenness, brief incarceration in jail, release, and then rearrest with the next episode of public intoxication—still persists. In many others, the new doors of the detoxification unit revolve as rapidly. Without aftercare, lacking in many locations, neither "revolving door" approach has made a significant contribution to treatment and rehabilitation of the alcohol-dependent individual.

Driving Under the Influence

All states have adopted driver blood-alcohol concentration (BAC) limits because so many people combine the use of alcoholic beverages and the operation of a motor vehicle. Operating a vehicle while having a BAC over the given limit is illegal, because drinking alcohol impairs a wide range of driving skills.

To reduce the annual slaughter of more than 17,000 Americans who die in alcohol-related crashes, law enforcement agencies have implemented various strategies to apprehend alcohol-impaired drivers. Nearly 1.4 million drivers are arrested each year for such an offense. Specific legal sanctions, such as driver's license suspension and court-ordered alcoholism treatment, have been designed to reduce rearrest for driving under the influence of alcohol. Of the several deterrent techniques targeted at the drinking-and-driving population, the most effective means has been a combination of license suspension and interventions, such as education, psychotherapy/counseling, and some follow-up activities.[10]

Alcohol-Related Crimes of Violence

Information on the precise role of alcohol abuse in criminal behavior is still limited and often confusing, despite the apparent association between alcohol consumption and violent events. Although the relationship is evident, whether alcohol plays a direct, causal role in such destructive episodes remains unclear.[11] While problem drinkers and alcoholics have criminal records far greater than those expected in the general population, it has not been determined whether drinking excessively leads to criminal activity, whether alcohol abuse is a contributing factor in such behavior, or whether involvement in crime leads to drinking. Another possibility, is that drinking and criminal activity are coincidental; that is, people engaging in crimes happen to be drinking at the time of their illegal behaviors.

Nevertheless, law enforcement officials are likely to encounter an enormous number of alcohol-related criminal offenses, even when public intoxication and "driving under the influence" are excluded from the total. For instance,

- alcohol is involved in high percentages of homicide and assault offenders,
- nearly three-fourths of arrested violent offenders have been drinking,
- prisoners with drinking problems have higher assault rates than prisoners without drinking problems, and
- approximately half of rape offenders have been found to be drinking at the time of the offense (see box 5.2).[12]

Though not considered violent crimes, property offenses (burglary, auto theft, fraud/forgery/embezzlement, larceny, stolen property, arson, destruction of property, and trespass) and public order offenses (weapons, obstructing justice, vagrancy, commercialized vice, rioting, habitual offender, nonsupport or abandonment, and contributing to the delinquency of a minor) are frequently committed by individuals who use alcohol just before perpetrating these crimes. About 40 percent of convicted persons charged with property offenses used alcohol before the offense, and nearly 33 percent of public order offenses involved alcohol use just prior to the crime.

Despite that excessive drinking does play a role in the occurrence of violence, most drinking occasions are not followed by violent acts; violent problem drinkers act violently only occasionally, and violent offenders and others tend to blame drinking for the violence, often as a way to excuse or lessen responsibility.[13]

The exact role of drinking in criminal and victim behavior has been explained as: (1) a disinhibitor of aggressive behavior; (2) an intensifier of anger or enhancer of violence; (3) a" trigger" for aggressive behavior in a culture that approves and glamorizes violence; and (4) a relaxation of social norms and behavioral expectancies during drinking. Intoxication may make an individual particularly vulnerable to many crimes, especially robbery, assault, and rape. It is probable that alcohol's distortion or impairment of knowing, perceiving, and judging abilities (cognitive skills), and the resulting misinterpretation of interpersonal cues and communications, increase the likelihood of violent behavior.

Box 5.2 Some Facts on Alcohol-Related Violence

Violence threatens the health of thousands of American families, and at least 2.2 million people are victims of violent injury each year. Alcohol abuse is consistently found to be associated with suicidal and interpersonal violence. Therefore, efforts to prevent the problems of alcohol abuse should be included into violence prevention programs.

Homicide

The United States ranks first among industrialized nations in violent death rates.

About 50 percent of homicides are committed by drinking assailants, and between 40 and 60 percent of homicide victims are drinking at the time of this criminal act.

One study of homicide victims found that over half had blood-alcohol concentrations of 0.10 percent or greater. In addition, most domestic homicides are preceded by episodes of family violence.

Sexual Assault

In one study, more than half of the convicted rapists were drinking at the time of their offense.

Another study of students at a southwestern university revealed that over half of victims and perpetrators of sexual assaults had been drinking at the time of the assault.

A survey of high school students discovered an alarming attitude regarding drinking and sexual exploitation: 39 percent of males and 18 percent of females believed it is acceptable for a male to force sex, if the female is "stoned" or drunk.

Domestic Violence

Between 2 and 4 million individuals are physically battered each year by partners, including husbands, former spouses, boyfriends and girlfriends, and lovers.

Alcohol is a strong and consistent correlate of marital violence, with alcohol present in at least 50 percent of incidents of wife beating.

Rates of domestic violence are nearly fifteen times higher in households where husbands are described as "often drunk" as opposed to "never drunk."

Women are often battered by their partners during pregnancy.

Whether celebrating the joy of victory or mourning the agony of defeat, many American male football fans under the influence of alcohol tend to vent their emotions on their wives and girlfriends in the form of physical battering. Recent Super Bowl contests have been occasions of greatly increased numbers of wife-beating cases.

Adults who abuse alcohol are more likely than others to physically, sexually, or emotionally abuse their own children.

Source: Data derived from publications of the Center for Substance Abuse Prevention.

Alcohol-Related Accidents

An accident is usually defined as a particular occurrence in a sequence of events that results in unintended injury, death, or property damage. Unintentional injuries, resulting from accidents, are a leading cause of death in the United States and kill nearly 100,000 people a year.[14] Such injuries are also major causes of disability. Motor vehicle crashes account for approximately half of deaths from unintentional injuries, while deaths from falls rank second, followed by deaths from poisoning, drowning, and residential fires.

According to the National Institute on Alcohol Abuse and Alcoholism, alcohol may also increase the severity of trauma incurred in accidents.[15]

Falls

The most common cause of nonfatal injuries and the second leading cause of fatal accidents, falls account for nearly 13,000 deaths a year. At least 17 percent and up to 53 percent of these accidents are associated with alcohol use. The risk for falling for those with blood-alcohol levels of 0.05 to 0.10 percent is three times greater than for those who are not drinking. Moreover, the risk of falling for those with blood-alcohol concentrations of 0.16 percent or higher is about sixty times greater than for those who are not drinking.

Drownings

Drowning ranks as the third leading cause of injury death in the United States. Alcohol is involved in about 38 percent of such accidents involving intoxicated swimmers. Studies have also revealed that between 17 percent and 31 percent of boaters who drowned had consumed alcohol.

Fires

Fires and burns are the fourth leading cause of injury deaths in the United States. In one instance, 64 percent of persons whose deaths were related to fire had blood-alcohol concentrations greater than or equal to 0.10 percent, the blood alcohol level indicative of "driving under the influence of alcohol" in most states.

Other statistics indicate that:[16]

- About one-quarter of aviation deaths resulting from private airplane crashes have involved alcohol,
- One-fifth of people killed in hang gliding accidents in a recent year had detectable blood-alcohol levels,

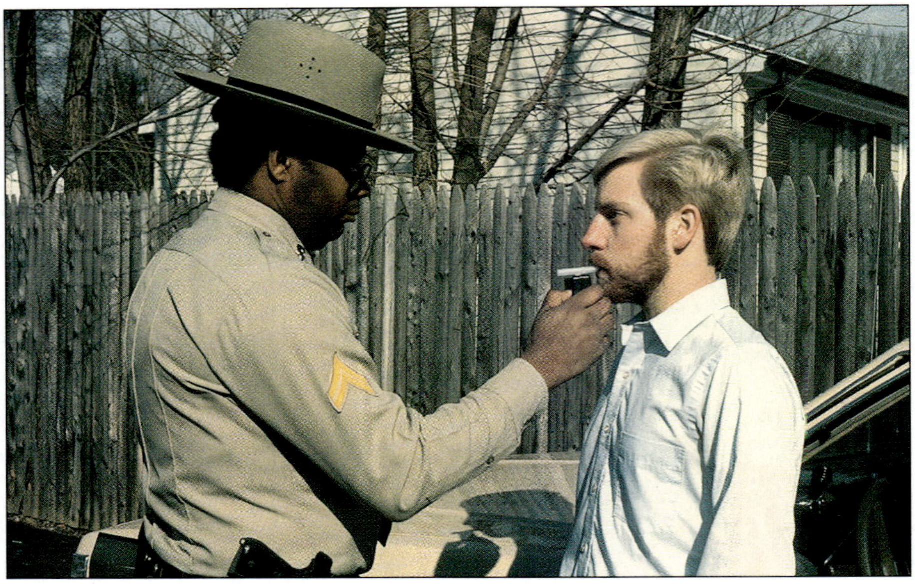

Most people arrested for driving under the influence of alcohol are not considered heavy drinkers; two out of three have never been arrested before for the same offense.

© Stacy Pick/Stock Boston

- Nearly one-quarter of nonfatal bicycle injuries involved alcohol during a recent year, and
- While there is no legal level of intoxication for pedestrians, more than one-third of such individuals over the age of fourteen killed on American highways in one recent year had blood-alcohol levels of 0.10 percent.

Alcohol-Impaired Driving and Auto Crashes

With an arrest rate of one intoxicated driver for every 95–100 licensed drivers, alcohol-impaired driving has become a major violent crime. In the United States, traffic crashes continue to be a leading cause of death for every age group between six and thirty-three years of age.[17] Of these crashes, about 41 percent are alcohol-related, that is, caused by someone's excessive consumption of alcohol combined with operating a car, motorcycle, truck, or bus. This figure represents a slight increase after a decade of decline from 1986, when more than 52 percent of traffic deaths were alcohol-related.[18]

According to the National Highway Traffic Safety Administration, alcohol-related motor vehicle crashes claim about 17,200 lives each year—equivalent to two Americans killed every hour of every day for a year. Most victims of these fatal crashes (about 66 percent) are drinking drivers, drinking pedestrians, and drinking bicyclists. The other 33 percent are nondrinking drivers, nonoccupants (primarily pedestrians and bicyclists), and passengers. In addition to alcohol-related traffic deaths, another half-million people—one person every minute—sustain injuries as a result of alcohol-related crashes: These include permanent brain damage, spinal cord injuries, lost or permanently deformed limbs, blindness, and impotence—lifetimes crippled with severe disability.

An analysis of statistics from the National Highway Traffic Safety Administration and the Behavioral Risk Factor Surveillance System further describes the dimensions of alcohol-impaired driving in the United States.

- Nearly two out of five Americans will be involved in an alcohol-related crash in their lifetime.
- Most people who drink and drive are not heavy drinkers, but moderate and light drinkers. Nevertheless, one-third of those arrested each year for driving under the influence of alcohol have been arrested before for the same offense.[19]
- The prevalence of drinking and driving is highest among men, young adults, and divorced or separated people.
- Drinkers who prefer beer are more likely to drive after drinking and to believe that driving while intoxicated is less serious than do drinkers who prefer wine or liquor.
- A much higher percentage of fatal crashes on weekends (62 percent) than on weekdays (39 percent) involve a driver with a detectable blood-alcohol level.
- A much higher percentage of fatal crashes at night (70 percent) than during the daytime (23 percent) involve a driver with a detectable blood-alcohol level.
- Even though the minimum legal drinking age is twenty-one years in all states, more than one-third of fatally injured drivers under twenty-one had known blood-alcohol concentrations of 0.01 percent or above.
- The amount of alcohol consumed by people arrested for driving under the influence is usually very high. On the average, their BACs register the pure-alcohol bloodstream equivalent of ten to twelve drinks in a four-hour period, or BACs greater than 0.15 percent.

Factors Influencing Crash Risk

The **blood alcohol concentration** or **BAC** is the proportion of alcohol to blood in the body, expressed as a percent. This BAC is the first and most important factor that influences the risk of involvement in an alcohol-related car crash. Studies consistently show that the likelihood of being involved in a crash and the probability of a driver's causing the crash increase as the blood-alcohol concentration increases.

In the area of traffic safety research, the BAC represents the percentage of alcohol in deciliters of blood. (A deciliter is a metric unit of volume equal to 3.39 fluid ounces.) For example, 0.10 percent BAC is the equivalent of 0.10 grams of alcohol per deciliter of blood. Accordingly, a 160-pound man will have a BAC of approximately 0.04 percent one hour after consuming two 12-ounce beers or two other standard drinks on an empty stomach.

All states now specify driver BAC limits, although such limits vary by state. As of 1997, most states maintained a BAC limit of 0.10 percent for drivers age twenty-one and older. However, more than a dozen states have already reduced the limit to 0.08 percent. For drivers younger than twenty-one years, twenty-nine states and the District of Columbia have reduced the BAC limit further to 0.02 percent or lower, thus establishing what is known as **zero-tolerance limits.** Nearly all states will probably adopt these lower BAC limits for young drivers because of federal incentives.

Various skills involved in driving an automobile are not all impaired at the same blood-alcohol concentration.[20] First, with a BAC of 0.02 percent or even lower, a driver's ability to divide attention between two or more sources of visual information can be diminished. Second, significant impairment in eye movements, glare resistance, visual perception, reaction time, certain types of steering tasks, and several other aspects of psychomotor performance begins at a BAC of 0.05 percent or slightly higher.

According to the National Institute on Alcohol Abuse and Alcoholism, the risk of a single-vehicle fatal crash for drivers with BACs between 0.02 and 0.04 percent is estimated to be 1.4 times higher in comparison with drivers who have not consumed any alcohol. For those with BACs between 0.05 and 0.09 percent, the risk is 11.1 times higher, while those with BACs between 0.10 and 0.14 percent the risk is increased by 48 times. For those with BACs at or above 0.15 percent, the crash risk is estimated to be 380 times higher (see fig. 5.1).

BACs above 0.10 percent are not characteristic of social drinking. For instance, to reach a BAC of 0.15 percent within two hours after eating, a 160-pound man would have to consume nine to ten servings of hard liquor or their equivalencies in beer or wine, within one hour. The same drinker would reach the same BAC with one-third less quantity, if the alcohol were taken on an empty stomach.

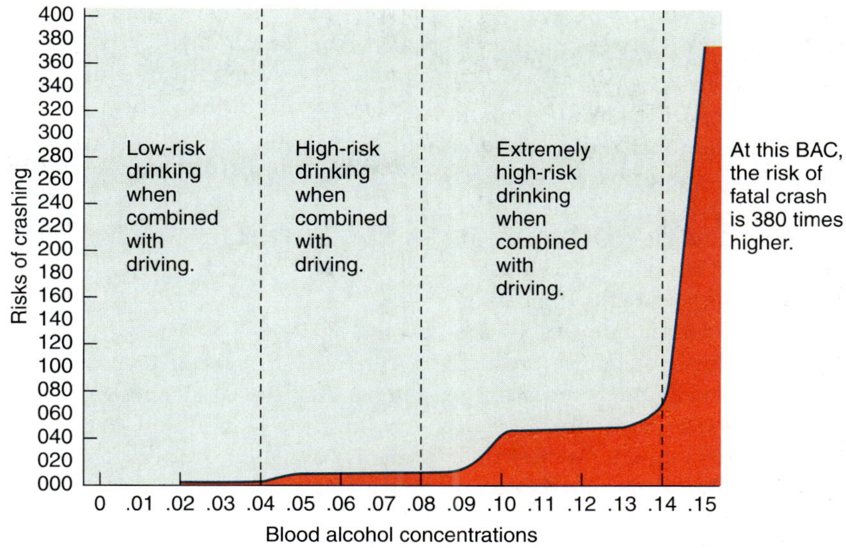

figure 5.1

Drinking and highway safety: Risk of involvement in a single-vehicle fatal crash for drivers with elevated blood alcohol concentrations (BACs). The risk of a single-vehicle fatal crash for drivers with BACs between 0.02 and 0.04 percent is nearly 1.4 times higher in comparison with drivers who have not consumed any alcohol. As the BAC rises, so does the risk of involvement in a fatal crash. At 0.08 percent BAC, the risk is 11 times higher, but at 0.10 percent BAC, the risk has increased to 48 times higher.

Source: Data derived from the National Institute on Alcohol Abuse and Alcoholism.

Other factors also contribute to an increased risk of crashing in an alcohol-related auto accident:[21]

- Youthfulness. Young drivers are at greater risk for alcohol-related crashes than older drivers, because young drivers are inexperienced not only in driving, but also in drinking and in combining these two activities. Despite that young drivers are less likely than adults to drive after drinking, their crash rates are considerably higher than those of all other groups, even at low and moderate BACs. For young drivers, especially, any drinking is too much for safe driving.[22]
- Gender. Nearly twice as many male drivers involved in fatal motor vehicle crashes had BACs of 0.01 percent or greater, in comparison with female drivers. However, the crash risk may be greater for females than for males at BACs ranging from 0.05 to 0.09 percent.
- Combining medications with alcohol and driving. The use of certain medications in combination with alcohol increases the risk of crashing. Alcohol tends to multiply the adverse effects of sedatives, tranquilizers, codeine, antidepressants, most antihistamines, certain cardiovascular medications, and some antipsychotic medicines on the various skills of driving.

Alcohol also has a potentiating effect on injury once a.crash happens.[23] In a crash of a given severity, those vehicle occupants who have been drinking alcohol are likely to sustain greater injury than those who have not been consuming alcohol. When alcohol is present, the general difference in probability of serious injury or death from a crash is about twofold. However, in certain types of crashes, the differences between those with and without alcohol are more than fourfold.

Mechanisms of Impairment

The connection between drinking and alcohol-impaired driving is more complex than a mere depressant effect on the brain. It is commonly recognized that many of those who drink and drive do not display the obvious signs of intoxication: reporting double vision, giving evidence of slurred speech and/or bloodshot eyes, and inability to walk a straight line. Yet they are under the influence of alcohol. Slightly impaired judgment, reduced tolerance to glare, underestimation of speed and distance, drowsiness, a false sense of security, slower reaction time, narrowed peripheral vision, a lessening of depth perception, a reduction of cue-taking, an inflated ego, and undue expansion of aggression all take their toll on the driver's ability.

Also affected at BACs as low as 0.01 to 0.02 percent are three essential driving skills: tracking, information processing, and attention sharing.[24] A relatively difficult psychomotor task, tracking or steering is a driver's ability to maintain a vehicle within lane limits and in the correct direction, while monitoring the driving environment for other important information.

Information processing involves a person's ability to interpret and integrate complex sensory information. Alcohol-impaired drivers require more time to read street signs or recognize and respond to traffic signals than the non-impaired. Such drivers look at fewer sources of information, acquire less total sensory input from the driving environment, and tend to restrict their vision to the center of the roadway.

The third essential driving skill adversely affected by even small amounts of alcohol is attention sharing, the ability to divide one's awareness between two or more sources of visual and/or sound information. In driving, two major tasks must be performed at the same time—maintaining a vehicle in the proper lane and direction and monitoring the driving environment for vital information, including vehicles, traffic signals, pedestrians, and various road hazards. But the alcohol-impaired driver, confronted with the need to divide his or her attention between the tasks, tends to favor one task over the other. Typically, alcohol-impaired drivers restrict their vision to the center of the visual field and fail to observe important events in the driving environment. Divided attention deficits often begin in the 0.02 BAC range, the lowest blood-alcohol level that can be reliably measured.

Countermeasures

To reduce alcohol-impaired driving and the annual toll of alcohol-related auto crashes, the federal and state governments have proposed, enacted, and implemented various actions and policies referred to as countermeasures. Organizations of citizens along with schools and other agencies have also taken significant steps to curb the alcohol-impaired driver. For instance, the National Highway Traffic Safety Administration and the United States Congress set a BAC of 0.10 percent as indicative of driving under the influence of alcohol. This concentration of blood alcohol was eventually adopted by most states as *prima facie* (sufficient) evidence of intoxication while operating a motor vehicle.

Several states have since lowered this original BAC limit to 0.08 percent. Research indicates that this lower limit has reduced overall the proportion of fatal crashes involving drivers at 0.08 percent or higher by 16 percent. There were also 18 percent fewer crashes involving drivers who had BACs higher than 0.15 percent. If all states were to adopt 0.08 percent as their legal blood alcohol limits, between 500–600 fewer fatal crashes would occur each year.[25]

Over the past several years, many states also enacted so-called "per se" (by or in itself) laws that make it unlawful to drive with a blood-alcohol concentration of 0.10 percent or higher, regardless of evidence of alcohol-impaired driving behavior. Numerous states are adopting lower "per se" limits of 0.08 percent or less.

Recognizing that in most people driving skills are adversely affected beginning at a BAC of 0.05 percent, some states are discussing the desirability of setting even lower "per se" limits. You might benefit by determining your consumption limits now.

Under provisions of the Commercial Motor Vehicles Safety Act of 1986, Congress authorized the U.S. Department of Transportation (DOT) to set new limits for alcohol use by truck and bus operators.[26] In 1989, the DOT adopted a BAC limit of 0.04 percent for commercial drivers, commercial shippers, and aviators, while other authorities have proposed for the same groups a zero-tolerance or zero alcohol standard level; that is, any amount of alcohol in the blood would be disallowed. Until individual states also adopt such limits, their application will not be effective. However, some states have already adopted the zero-tolerance standard for teenage drivers; these states suspend the driver's licenses of teenagers found operating a motor vehicle with any detectable blood-alcohol level. Several states have also enacted laws that revoke the driver's licenses of those under twenty-one years of age who commit any drug offense.

The safest policy is not to drive after drinking. If you do drink and then drive, know and stay within your personal limits as well as the legal limits. You can help promote the health and welfare of those who drive on the highways by keeping an intoxicated person from driving. Car keys should be calmly yet firmly taken away from such a person if he or she insists on operating a motor vehicle. If possible, arrange for someone else to drive the drunk person's car, and take the person home yourself, call a taxi, or have the individual stay overnight. Remember, friends do not let friends drive drunk!

Until recently there has been a general public indifference about solving the drunk-driving problem. Many people still believe that drinking-and-driving behavior is acceptable until the drunk driver causes an accident that harms another person. Such an attitude remains the biggest obstacle to solving the drinking-driver problem.

For more than thirty years, outraged parents and friends of young victims of alcohol-impaired drivers have formed action groups that lobby and influence legislators, police, prosecutors, and judges to "crack down" on drunk drivers. Several organizations, such as Mothers Against Drunk Drivers (MADD), have been successful in lobbying for tougher drunk-driving laws and dealing with sentencing violators.

Continuing its efforts MADD has been a major force in reducing drunk driving, raising the drinking age in all fifty states, advocating the rights of those victimized by drunk drivers, and promoting "designated driver" programs. Designated drivers are peer-volunteers who agree not to consume alcoholic beverages at a party so they will be able to safely transport alcohol-impaired individuals back to their residences without endangering other drivers.

An ever-increasing number of driving-while-intoxicated (DWI) countermeasures are available to help end the national epidemic of alcohol-impaired driving. Following are specific countermeasures various federal and state commissions have proposed. Has your state or local community adopted any of them?

- Reduction of the blood-alcohol concentration indicating "driving under the influence" (DUI) or "driving while intoxicated" (DWI) from 0.10 percent or 0.08 percent to 0.04 percent.
- Establishment of a limit of 0.00 percent BAC (true zero tolerance) for drivers under the age of twenty-one.
- Enforcement of "dram shop acts"—either by formal statute or by judicial decision or precedent—that impose liability for damages on social hosts, including fraternities and sororities, who furnish alcoholic beverages to their guests.
- A ban on open containers of alcoholic beverages in motor vehicles.
- Adoption of a "sobriety checkpoint" program—now determined to be constitutional by the U.S. Supreme Court—in which all motorists in a specific area are stopped without selection or discrimination and observed for obvious signs of intoxication. If such signs are apparent, the motorists are asked to take a breath test, usually at the site of the checkpoint.
- Confiscation of a driver's license on the spot (administrative license revocation) for those who are found to have equaled or exceeded the legal BAC limit. License suspension or permanent revocation might follow such action.
- An automatic charge of vehicular homicide imposed for death or serious injury occurring while driving under the influence of alcohol.
- A ban on "plea bargaining" in cases of driving under the influence. In effect, the plea-bargaining process drops charges against a defendant for one serious criminal offense in exchange for an admission of guilt to another, lesser offense. This common legal practice would be forbidden in DUI cases.
- Mandatory jail sentences for driving on a suspended or revoked driver's license.
- Use of preliminary roadside breath tests (or newer saliva tests) to screen potential drunk drivers at the site of apprehension, prior to administering more sophisticated breath analysis tests to confirm the original findings.
- Provision of a system in each state to fund comprehensive alcohol-impaired-driving programs and drinking-and-driving education in worksites, communities, health care agencies, and schools.
- Reduction of the availability of beverage alcohol by eliminating "happy hours" and other reduced-price promotions, limiting hours and density of sales outlets, and requiring impaired-driver prevention training of sellers and servers.
- A matching of alcoholic beverage ads with an equal number of pro-health and pro-safety messages.
- Restrictions on certain advertising and marketing practices, especially those that appeal to "underage" young people. This action would ban the use of sports figures and other youth role models from promoting beer and forbid breweries from sponsoring rock concerts and sporting events.
- Increased excise taxes on alcoholic beverages, and equal taxation of beer, wine, and distilled spirits, based on alcohol content.

Prenatal Alcohol Abuse

Ethyl alcohol is widely recognized as a powerful **teratogen,** a drug capable of interfering with the development of an embryo and fetus and responsible for one or more birth defects. Moreover, alcohol is associated with a wide range of adverse effects in children of women who drink during pregnancy.

Despite the growing awareness that drinking can lead to serious birth defects, nearly one in five women continue to use alcoholic beverages after learning they are pregnant.[27] This behavior places their children at risk for the harmful effects of prenatal alcohol exposure, the leading known environmental cause of mental retardation in the Western world.

Fetal Alcohol Syndrome

For many years it has been observed that children of alcoholic mothers have been born alcohol dependent or physically addicted to alcohol; that is, they experience withdrawal signs and symptoms at birth. Although physicians and laypeople have long suspected that drinking could affect the unborn in even more insidious and permanent ways, it was not until 1973 that pediatrician David W. Smith discovered a direct association between drinking alcohol and birth defects.

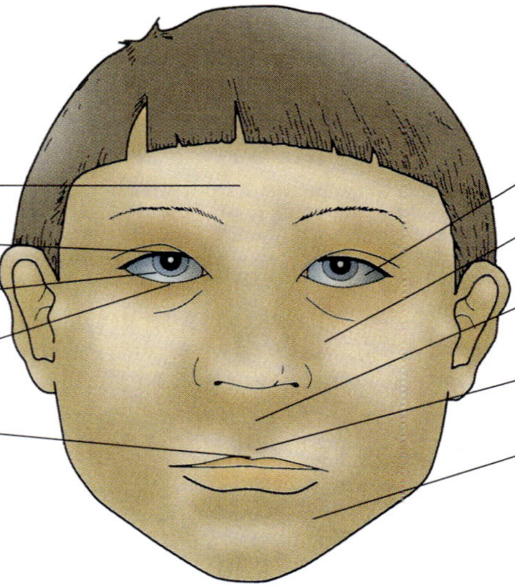

figure 5.2

Frequently occurring facial and head characteristics as seen in children with the Fetal Alcohol Syndrome typically present a "pushed-in-face" effect.

The evidence of medical research suggests the existence of a common pattern of birth defects and mental retardation among some children born of alcoholic women or those who drank excessively during pregnancy. These structural and functional abnormalities have been identified as **fetal alcohol syndrome (FAS).** While all of the defects related to prenatal exposure to alcohol have not yet been established, we know the following:

- Alcohol can be toxic to the fetus, independently of the effects of malnutrition.
- Adverse effects of prenatal exposure to alcohol exist along a continuum, with the complete FAS syndrome at one end of the spectrum and incomplete features of FAS, including more subtle mental and behavioral deficits, on the other.
- Harmful effects of prenatal alcohol exposure on child development can vary from child to child and depend primarily on the pattern and extent of alcohol exposure prior to birth.
- FAS may vary with the race, income, and drinking history of the mother, as well as her medical status and other socioeconomic factors.
- After a woman gives birth to a child with FAS, the probability that her subsequent children will have FAS is about 70 percent.

Principal Features of FAS

The main features associated with fetal alcohol syndrome are grouped into three major categories:[28]

Growth deficiency—Alcohol-exposed infants tend to be smaller in weight, length, and head circumference. Some studies indicate that such growth deficits persist well into childhood. Such children are often only about 65 percent of normal birth length and 38 percent of normal birth weight.

Central nervous system damage—The most commonly observed problem is mental retardation. Difficulty with learning, attention, memory, and problem solving are common, along with incoordination, impulsive behavior, and speech and hearing impairments.

Sometimes these problems in learning skills and psychomotor development persist beyond infancy and are clearly recognizable in preschool-age children.[29] Adolescents and even adults also display the same mental abnormalities originating before birth.

Head and facial abnormalities—The most frequently observed characteristics are shortness of the palpebral fissures (the slits between the opposed lids of the closed eyes); a short, upturned nose with an underdeveloped ridge between the base of the nose and the upper lip; a sunken nasal bridge; folds on the inner aspect of the eyelids; a thin upper lip; an underdeveloped midface; and growth retardation of the jaw. While these abnormalities are individually subtle, jointly they characterize a distinctive face, as noted in figure 5.2

Other major and minor malformations of the human body may also be present among the FAS patient population. There is likely to be an increase in abnormal structures of various organ systems, including cardiac (heart), urinary, genital, and skeletal systems (e.g., peculiar palmar creases), and limited joint movements of the fingers and elbows.

Fetal Alcohol Effects or Alcohol-Related Birth Defects

Developmental effects of prenatal alcohol exposure that are less severe than FAS are classified as **fetal alcohol effects (FAE)** or alcohol-related birth defects (ARBD). Children of alcohol-abusing or alcoholic mothers may display signs in only two of the three defining categories of FAS. Less severe clinical findings include low birth weight, subtle behavioral problems, abnormalities of the mouth or heart, and evidence of mild neurological difficulties. This category of alcohol-exposed individuals is undoubtedly much larger, less easily identified, and often more problematic in terms of social behavior than children with full FAS.

Mechanism of Impairment

Nearly 5,000 infants—one in every 750—are born with FAS every year. An estimated 36,000 newborns are affected by FAE in any one year. Yet the precise manner by which alcohol consumption contributes to harmful fetal and neonatal growth and development has not been fully established. It is likely that much of the trauma occurs early in the first trimester of pregnancy, when harmful exposure to alcohol affects fetal organ development and results in related, major birth defects. At this time, when signs of pregnancy are few and many women are not yet aware they are pregnant, any drinking is perilous.[30]

In addition to the direct toxic effect of alcohol on fetal tissues, other possible mechanisms of alcohol-related damage include the following:[31]

- Alcohol may interfere with the *delivery of maternal nutrients,* such as, essential amino acids and glucose to the fetus. As such, delays in development and defects in fetal organs are the result of poor nutrition in the fetus.
- Alcohol consumption may be associated with *deficiencies of various hormones*—chemicals produced by and released from maternal and fetal glands that influence the formation, development, and regulation of fetal tissues.
- Continued exposure of the fetus to alcohol may interfere with the *function of local growth factors*—chemical substances in the fetal body that influence cell division, differentiation, migration, and protein synthesis.
- During exposure of the fetus to alcohol in the uterus, there is an increase in the production of *prostaglandins.* These tissue chemicals are linked with the constriction of blood vessels in the uterus, placenta, and the fetus, resulting in a lack of oxygen and eventually tissue damage and retarded growth.
- During maternal drinking, alcohol's direct action on the blood vessels of the placenta and umbilical cord reduces the delivery of oxygen to the fetal tissues. *Reduced oxygen levels* can then lead to stoppage or delays in cell division and growth which in turn result in faulty development and malformations in various fetal tissues and organs.

Alcohol's possible effect on the father's sperm cells prior to fertilization has also been investigated for its possible contribution to FAS or FAE. Although ethyl alcohol might interfere with male reproductive function, there is no firm evidence that paternal alcoholism accounts for the specific congenital defects seen in FAS or FAE.

Although no one knows how much alcohol is too much and therefore damaging to the developing embryo and fetus, the FAS risk for human infants seems to increase markedly when the mother's daily consumption is three ounces (six drinks) or more. Between 30 and 40 percent of infants born to women who consume this amount have some FAS defects.

However, the severity of the syndrome might be related more closely to how much is drunk at one time during pregnancy than to frequency of drinking. Binge drinking of more than five drinks on any occasion and drinking during the first two months of pregnancy are two of the strongest maternal predictors of later neurobehavioral deficits among their children.[32]

Prevention of FAS and FAE

In 1981, the U.S. Food and Drug Administration issued its first official, written warning on alcohol and pregnancy. This advisory declared that even women who drank as little as one ounce of alcohol (the amount contained in about two glasses of table wine) twice a week during pregnancy experience significant increases in spontaneous abortion and giving birth to smaller babies or infants with birth defects. Alcoholics and heavy drinkers are more likely to give birth to babies with severe FAS.

In advising expectant mothers and those considering pregnancy that they may be harming their unborn children by drinking even small amounts of alcohol, the Food and Drug Administration and many physicians reject the concept of safe or moderate drinking during pregnancy. Until the exact amount of alcohol that might be safe is known, most medical authorities recommend abstinence from alcohol during pregnancy and breastfeeding, pending confirmation of alcohol's role in relation to fetal development.[33]

The Family and Problem Drinking

According to the American Psychiatric Association, one of the criteria for diagnosing alcohol abuse is a repeated pattern of drinking resulting in failure to fulfill major role obligations. Nowhere are the devastating results of this failure more evident than in the family setting, where the abuse of alcohol often results in a serious psychological, social, and physical disorder that many consider a family disease.

The family and marital interactions of alcohol-abusing people have become a growing field of research, especially in the area of violence. The role of alcohol in violence is not well understood, although personal violence is frequently associated with alcohol consumption by the offending perpetrators. Alcohol is present in one-half of incidents of domestic violence.[34] The most common pattern of such violence includes drinking by both husband and wife. However, the majority of drinkers, even heavy drinkers, never engage in violent behavior. Also, drinking by victims is neither an excuse for nor a direct cause of spousal abuse, but such alcohol use may contribute to their own increased risk of victimization.[35]

In addition, alcohol abuse by the husband, wife, or both could indirectly contribute to family violence by complicating already existing economic and child-care difficulties.

Nevertheless, police records and victimization survey responses recorded by the National Institute on Alcohol Abuse and Alcoholism typically indicate somewhat higher rates of alcohol involvement among offending assailants than among their victims.[36] Moreover, the rate of physical violence significantly increases when male partners increase their alcohol consumption.[37]

When spouse abuse is absent from the marital relationship, problem drinking typically afflicts the couple with some type of sexual problem that often threatens the marriage. Such problems include loss of libido or sexual interest among both males and females, inhibited sexual excitement, impotence in males, and anorgasmia (lack of orgasmic response) in females. Chronic, excessive use of alcohol diminishes sexual performance and sexual desire.

Parents with alcohol problems also have a high potential for neglecting and abusing their children. Alcohol abuse is a contributing factor in about one-third of child-abuse cases, including sexual abuse. There appears to be an alarming similarity between child abusers and alcohol abusers. Among these shared characteristics are low self-esteem, low tolerance for frustration, impulsive behavior, difficulty in experiencing pleasure, and a lack of understanding of the needs and abilities of infants and children. Child-abusing families, like alcohol-abusing families, often share social isolation from friends and neighbors and tend to have parents who were abused as children.

Children of Alcoholics

It is estimated that there are 29 million Americans who may be designated as *children of alcoholics* (COAs). Nearly 7 million of them are under eighteen years of age, and almost 3 million of this group will likely develop alcoholism, other drug problems, and/or other serious coping problems.[38] Moreover, about half of COAs will likely marry alcoholics and are thus at risk of re-creating the same types of stressful and unhealthy families in which they grew up.

There is no doubt that all children are affected adversely by family alcohol abuse and suffer negative consequences. However, the larger proportion of COAs seem to function fairly well and do not develop serious problems during childhood or adulthood. Apparently many COAs make positive adjustments to their family's alcoholism and other alcohol-related problems.

Many children of alcoholics, however, are at an extremely high risk for developing alcohol and other drug problems, and often live with overwhelming tension; stress; and, especially, fears.[39] Some have high levels of anxiety and depression, others do poorly in school, and still others experience problems with coping. Among the most frequently observed differences in COAs are deficits in mental functioning: in perception, reasoning, intuition, and the process of gaining knowledge. While these children tend to achieve lower scores, they nevertheless test within normal ranges for intelligence and knowledge of specific academic subject.[40] However, they often experience school problems, repeat grades, fail to graduate from high school, and require referrals to school counselors and psychologists.

When COAs were first identified as a special population with unique needs and problems, a standard group of symptoms—the *COA syndrome*—was formulated to describe children of alcoholics:[41]

- Toleration of bizarre behavior displayed by parents as normal and acceptable
- Inability to trust others
- Difficulty in expressing inner feelings
- Experience of depression and increased risk for mental illness
- Development of guilt feelings for supposedly causing a parent's alcoholism
- Loss of self-esteem and perception of self and family as oddities
- Feeling of helplessness in controlling oneself and life's events
- Belief in a magical person who will eventually save the child from harm
- Development of an inward life focus to escape from the turmoil of the home

In addition, COAs were commonly observed assuming one of the following distinctive coping roles within the family system.[42]

The family hero or caretaker, who is successful at home and at school.

The scapegoat, who is something of an angry rebel and is often involved in unapproved social behavior.

The lost child who withdraws to the background, never causes trouble, has no opinions, feels unimportant, and isolates himself or herself from others.

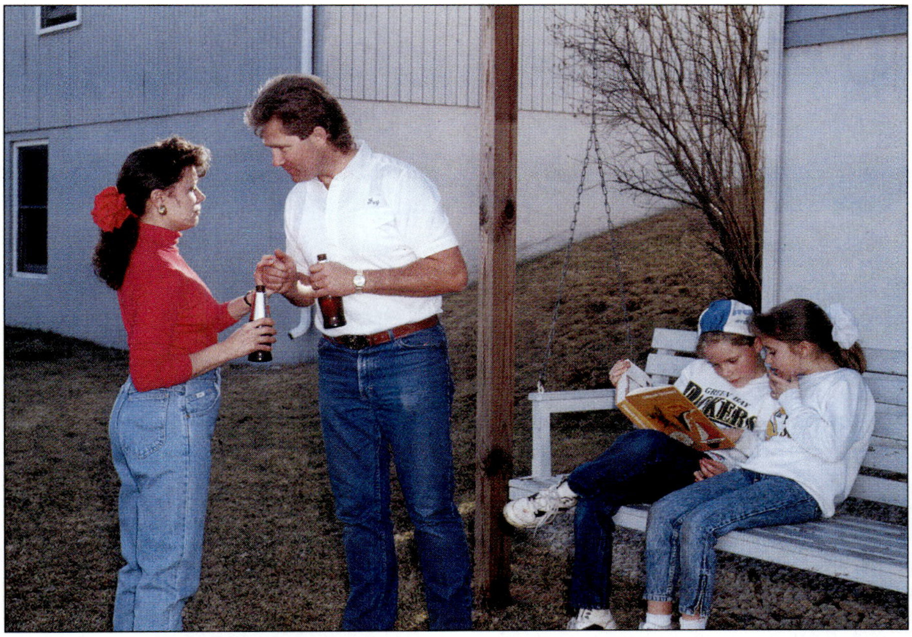

Children of alcoholic parents appear to develop coping skills when their families become endangered by a problem drinker. However, the children are at increased risk for experiencing various psychological problems as well as for alcoholism.

© *James L. Shaffer*

The mascot, who manages to defuse explosive and tense situations, often through humor, by focusing attention on himself or herself.

Critics of the theory of the COA syndrome have contended that many children of nonalcoholic though strongly dysfunctional families—those marked by other drug use, sexual or physical abuse, and ncest—also share some of the same characteristics as COAs. Although the uniqueness of the COA syndrome may be abandoned, the pain created within a child who grows up in an alcoholic home is still acknowledged as significant and serious. The revised COA syndrome appears to include the following characteristics:[43]

- A greater likelihood of becoming an alcohol or other drug abuser
- A strong predisposition toward having psychiatric symptoms as an adult
- A moderately significant increased risk for marital difficulties
- More impulsive behavior as a child
- Delayed language development, fine motor coordination, and sociability
- A higher incidence of cognitive (mental) disorders as a child

Co-Dependence

For the past several years, the term **co-dependence** has been used to describe the unusual coping mechanisms, attitudes, and behaviors that family members sometimes develop in response to a problem-drinking parent, spouse, child, or sibling. Co-dependence is the foundation of the COA syndrome and may also serve as the basis for the behavior of adult children of alcoholics.

The so-called co-dependent learns to cope with the existence of problem drinking in a family member and appears to overlook or minimizes the seriousness of family dysfunction. The nonproblem drinker or nondrinker frequently tolerates the drinking behaviors of a loved one and sometimes cooperates in the elaborate cover-up of making excuses and rationalizing to explain alcohol-abuse situations and their consequences.

Unwittingly, the co-dependence of family members tends to promote problem drinking by delaying any attempts at intervention that are needed to get the alcohol abuser into treatment and rehabilitation. Co-dependency is increasingly viewed as a preoccupation and extreme dependency (emotionally, socially, sometimes physically) on another person or on a substance (such as alcohol, drugs, nicotine, or sugar) or on a behavior (such as working, gambling, or sexual acting out).[44]

However, the most important characteristic of co-dependence is commonly identified as "*external referenting.*" This is a condition in which a person perceives herself or himself as having meaning or significance only in relation to what is outside of the self, or external sources.[45] Lacking intrinsic meaning or self-worth, the external-referenting co-dependent will do almost anything to maintain a relationship, including total psychological self-abandonment.

The chances of interacting with a relative or friend who drinks too much are not remote because alcohol abuse is so pervasive. At least four other people are affected by the disturbing behavior of each of America's problem drinkers and alcoholics. From yet another perspective, then, there are nearly 50 million people who are sharing alcohol problems and who are potential helpers in assisting those who are close and who drink to excess. Some ideas for coping with these relatives and friends are listed in box 5.3.

Alcoholism

In this section, alcoholism will be described in terms of various definitions, prevalence, possible causes, signs and symptoms, and treatment and evaluation.

Overview

The most prominent and extreme form of problem drinking is **alcoholism.** Considered a complex illness or disability, alcoholism is more than just alcohol abuse, though it almost always involves the

Box 5.3 What to Do When Someone Close to You Drinks Too Much

With knowledge, compassion, and patience, the person with "someone close who drinks too much" can play a key role in his or her turnabout, treatment, and recovery from problem drinking.

Such help is usually given in three stages:

1. Learn about the illness of alcoholism and various sources of treatment.
2. Guide the "someone close" to treatment.
3. Support the person during and after treatment.

While waiting for the "right time" for medical and psychological intervention and treatment, the following do's and do not's are recommended for the person who knows someone close who drinks too much.

Do

Try to remain calm, unemotional, and factually honest in speaking with the problem drinker about his or her behavior and its day-to-day consequences.

Let the problem drinker know you are reading and learning about alcoholism and attending Al-Anon or Alateen.

Discuss the situation with someone you trust—a clergyperson, social worker, friend, or some individual who has experienced alcoholism either personally or as a family member.

Establish and maintain a healthy atmosphere in the home, and try to include the alcoholic member in family life.

Explain the nature of alcoholism as an illness to the children of the family.

Encourage new interests and participate in leisure activities that the problem drinker enjoys. Encourage him or her to see old friends in nondrinking situations.

Be patient and live one day at a time. Alcoholism usually takes a long time to develop, and recovery does not occur overnight. Try to accept setbacks and relapses with calm and understanding.

Refuse to ride with the alcoholic person if he or she insists on drinking and driving.

Do Not

Attempt to punish, threaten, bribe, preach, or try to be a martyr. Avoid emotional appeals that may only increase feelings of guilt and the compulsion to drink.

Allow yourself to cover up or make excuses for the alcoholic person or shield the person from the realistic consequences of his or her behavior.

Take over his or her responsibilities, leaving the person with no sense of importance or dignity.

Hide or dump bottles, or shelter the problem drinker from situations where alcohol is present.

Argue with the alcoholic person when he or she is drunk.

Try to drink along with the problem drinker.

Accept, above all, guilt for another's behavior.

Source: National Institute on Alcohol Abuse and Alcoholism.

recurrent use of beverage alcohol that contributes to a variety of personal and social problems. Alcoholism is more appropriately considered as the disease of **alcohol dependence.** The alcohol-dependent person typically displays four fundamental characteristics: (1) tolerance; (2) withdrawal; (3) **loss of control** over drinking; and (4) **craving** for alcohol.[46]

- *Tolerance* is a condition in which, after continued drinking, consumption of a constant amount of alcohol produces a lesser effect or increasing amounts of alcohol are necessary to produce the same effect.
- *Withdrawal* is the experience of various symptoms—the so-called withdrawal syndrome including anxiety; agitation; tremor; elevated blood pressure; and, in severe cases, seizures—that usually occur six to forty-eight hours after the last drink is consumed. The experience of withdrawal indicates the presence of physical dependence, the physical need for continued alcohol consumption.
- *Loss of control* is the inability of an alcohol-dependent person to limit alcohol use on any drinking occasion or the inability to limit with any consistency the duration and amount of drinking or the consequences of consuming alcoholic beverages.
- *Craving* is the intense, overwhelming, and prolonged desire to experience the rewarding mental state of euphoria that eventually establishes alcohol-seeking behavior.

Society in general and until recently, even the medical profession have had considerable difficulty in understanding and defining alcoholism. Over the past two centuries, many differing and even conflicting concepts of alcoholism have emerged. Some of these remain—alcoholism is a sin, a vice, a personality weakness, a bad habit, willful misconduct—and add to confusion and controversy about the precise nature of this psychoactive substance dependence disorder.

It was not until 1946 that E. M. Jellinek proposed the modern disease concept of alcoholism and described the condition as *any use of beverage alcohol that causes any damage to the individual drinker, to society, or both.* Known as the "father" (originator) of the disease concept of alcoholism, Jellinek later identified several *species* or types of alcoholism:[47]

> *Alpha alcoholism*—an entirely psychological reliance on alcohol to relieve physical and psychic pain. There is no loss of control or inability to abstain.
>
> *Beta alcoholism*—a type of alcoholism in which severe medical complications occur, such as nerve irritations, gastric disturbances, and cirrhosis of the liver. There is neither physical nor psychological dependence. No withdrawal symptoms are manifest.
>
> *Gamma alcoholism*—the most prevalent form of alcoholism seen in America. It is characterized by psychological dependence, physical dependence, tolerance, loss of control, and withdrawal symptoms.
>
> *Delta alcoholism*—the predominant form of alcoholism in France. It is similar to the gamma type except that instead of loss of control, there is inability to abstain.

Later, the American Medical Association defined alcoholism as "an illness characterized by significant impairment that is directly associated with persistent and excessive use of alcohol."[48] Manifested as drug dependence, alcoholism involves a progressive preoccupation with drinking, leading to physical, mental, or social dysfunction.

In 1990, the American Society of Addiction Medicine and the National Council on Alcoholism and Drug Dependence adopted a revised definition of alcoholism that gives greater consideration to basic behavioral changes symptomatic of the disease.[49] Earlier, the two organizations emphasized biological tolerance and physical dependence, which appear when the disease has already adversely affected behavior.

According to the revised definition, alcoholism is a *primary, chronic disease* with genetic, psychosocial, and environmental factors influencing its development and manifestations. The disease is *often progressive* and *fatal.* It is characterized by continuous or periodic *impaired control over drinking, preoccupation with the drug, alcohol, use of alcohol despite adverse consequences,* and *distortion in thinking,* most notably *denial.*

Following are brief explanations of the major terms in this lengthy definition:

> *Primary* means that alcoholism as an addiction is not a symptom of some underlying disease state, but is a distinct disease condition separate from other physical or emotional disorders often associated with the alcoholismic state.
>
> *Chronic* refers to the long-term duration of the alcoholismic state. Once this condition has developed, an individual remains an alcoholic and is not likely able to resume controlled drinking.
>
> *Disease*—a condition of distress, uneasiness, or any departure from health—suggests that alcoholism is an involuntary disability that places those affected at a disadvantage in relation to those who are not alcoholismic.
>
> *Progressive* indicates that alcoholism moves through various stages of development the longer it persists and tends to worsen over time.

At Issue

Is alcoholism really a disease?

Point: Most surveyed Americans and the following prestigious health organizations consider alcoholism a disease that requires medical treatment: the American Medical Association, American Psychiatric Association, American Psychological Association, World Health Association, and National Council on Alcoholism and Drug Dependence. Those who live with alcoholics, as well as experienced alcohol treatment specialists and recovering alcoholics, also tend to view alcoholism as a disease. The "disease concept" more appropriately explains than does the "behavior disorder concept" why alcoholics so frequently mistreat and abuse the people they love the most. Moreover, the disease model is helpful in convincing alcoholics to admit their alcohol problems and in getting them treated effectively. Alcoholism's cause or causes remain largely unknown, and signs and symptoms of pathological alcohol consumption vary considerably from one alcoholic to another, yet alcoholics are typically "diseased," or not at ease. They are usually not at ease with themselves, their families, or with society.

Counterpoint: Considering alcoholism as a disease has no scientific basis whatsoever. Alcoholism is better described as a "behavior disorder" or habit that is under considerable voluntary control of the drinker. There is no typical pattern of drinking behavior, which actually ranges widely from one problem drinker to another. If alcoholism were a disease, signs and symptoms would be similar among those affected, there would be no ability to control alcohol consumption on a temporary basis, and there would be no environmental or social factors considered as precipitating the condition. Additionally, there is no precisely identified cause of alcoholism that applies to all alcoholics, and labeling people as diseased only serves to excuse the continuance of the condition and remove any element of self-respect from problem drinking. Thus, alcoholism may be considered a symptom of some underlying personality or mental depression. It certainly isn't a disease!

Fatal describes the ultimate outcome of alcoholism, death, unless intervention and/or treatment stops the progressive nature of the disease. Premature death may come from overdose and physical complications of the brain, liver, and heart, as well as by alcoholism-related suicide, homicide, and motor-vehicle accidents.

Impaired control identifies the alcoholic's inability to limit alcohol use on any drinking occasion or the inability to limit with any consistency the duration of the drinking episode, the amount consumed, and/or the behavioral consequences of drinking.

Preoccupation highlights the exaggerated attention and all-consuming expenditure of energy given to acquiring alcohol, using alcohol, and experiencing the effects of alcohol.

Adverse consequences are those alcohol-related impairments in physical health; psychological functioning; interpersonal relationships; occupational roles; and legal, financial, or spiritual problems.

Denial, an integral part of the disease and an obstacle to recovery, includes not only a refusal to acknowledge the seriousness of drinking-related problems, but also a full range of psychological maneuvers or processes aimed at reducing awareness that alcohol use is the cause of, rather than the solution to, an individual's problem.

table 5.1 Criteria for Alcohol Dependence Established by the American Psychiatric Association and Adapted by the National Institute on Alcohol Abuse and Alcoholism to Focus Solely on Alcohol.

	Criteria
Symptoms	A. Alcohol dependence is a maladaptive pattern of alcohol use, leading to clinically significantly impairment or distress as manifested by three or more of the following occurring at any time in the same 12-month period:
Tolerance	(1) Need for markedly increased amounts of alcohol to achieve intoxication or desired effect; or markedly diminished effect with continued use of the same amount of alcohol
Withdrawal	(2) The characteristic withdrawal syndrome for alcohol; or alcohol (or a closely related substance) is taken to relieve or avoid withdrawal symptoms
Loss of Control	(3) Persistent desire or one or more unsuccessful efforts to cut down or control drinking
	(4) Drinking in larger amounts or over a longer period than the person intended
Neglect of Activities	(5) Important social, occupational, or recreational activities given up or reduced because of drinking
Time Spent Drinking	(6) A great deal of time spent in activities necessary to obtain alcohol, to drink alcohol, or to recover from its effects
Drinking Despite Problems	(7) Continued drinking despite knowledge of having a persistent or recurrent physical or psychological problem likely to be caused or exacerbated by alcohol use
Duration Criterion	B. No duration criterion separately specified. However, three or more dependence criteria must be met within the same year and must occur repeatedly as specified by duration qualifiers associated with criteria (example, "often," "persistent," "continued")
Criterion for Subtyping Dependence	With physiological dependence: Evidence of tolerance or withdrawal (example, any of items A 1 or A 2 above are present)
	Without physiological dependence: No evidence of tolerance or withdrawal (example, none of items A 1 or A 2 above are present)

Source: National Institute on Alcohol Abuse and Alcoholism, *Alcohol Alert: Diagnostic Criteria for Alcohol Abuse and Dependence,* no. 30, PH 359 (October 1995), 5.

Yet another definition is offered by the American Psychiatric Association (APA). This professional organization views alcoholism as a *substance dependence disorder* characterized by a faulty, problem-producing pattern of alcohol use leading to significant impairment or distress. Specific criteria or symptoms used to identify this disorder include tolerance, withdrawal, impaired control, neglect of activities, time involved with drinking, and drinking despite physical or psychological problems caused or made worse by using alcohol (see table 5.1).[50]

Alcoholism appears to be one of those "equal opportunity" illnesses affecting millions of individuals without respect to race, color, creed, sex, ethnic group, marital status, geographical location, or socioeconomic standing. Nevertheless, studies have revealed some unusual variations in the prevalence of this disabling condition.

1. Approximately 5 to 7 percent of adults—about 10 percent of adult drinkers—are likely to be alcohol-dependent at some point in their lives. Several million additional adults and perhaps as many as 3 million teenagers have serious drinking

problems or experience adverse personal or social problems due to alcohol abuse.

2. In the past, alcoholics have tended to be thirty-five to fifty-five years old. However, an alarming increase in adolescent-onset alcoholism has been noted. Factors frequently cited for this increase in teenage alcohol dependency include the easy availability of beverage alcohol; the toleration of drunkenness by parents; the growing use of alcohol to cope with the pressures and conflicts of adolescence; exposure to parental problem drinking patterns; and the emphasis in alcohol advertisements on youth drinks, such as "pop wines," or wine-coolers. Furthermore, statistics indicate that males in their late teens and early twenties have the highest incidence of alcohol-related problems and problem drinking behaviors.
3. Alcoholism is involved in at least one-fourth of admissions to general hospitals. The medical and social costs run to tens of billions of dollars per year—more than the cost of cancer and respiratory diseases combined. Among males aged twenty-five to forty-four years, alcohol abuse is a major factor in four of the leading causes of death—accidents, homicide, suicide, and alcoholic cirrhosis of the liver.
4. Contrary to popular belief, alcoholics are not always drinking uncontrollably and are not even always drinking. Many alcohol-dependent individuals seem to be either abstinent or drinking without symptoms in any given month of alcohol use.
5. Less than 5 percent of alcoholics are found on skid row. Most manage to hold jobs and maintain homes where they are sheltered or tolerated by a spouse and children. The stereotyped image of the alcoholic as the skid-row inebriated bum often deceives the "respectable" alcoholic and his or her family into minimizing the seriousness of problem drinking. Alcoholism is an illness that can occur in people in all walks of life (see figure 5.3).

Possible Causes of Alcoholism

Without alcohol, there would be no alcoholics. However, most people who use beverage alcohol do not develop into problem drinkers. Therefore, while alcohol is a necessary factor in alcoholism, it is not the sole causative agent. Additionally, alcoholism does not result from drinking a particular alcoholic beverage. Furthermore, though many alcoholics share common personality disorders, no well-defined "alcoholic personality" has been identified. It is probable that such behavioral difficulties are the result, rather than the cause, of alcohol abuse.

Alcoholics display such varying backgrounds and characteristics, and so many possible causative factors have been proposed, that some authorities believe many alcoholisms or forms of alcoholism exist rather than a single disorder.[51]

Research has questioned some long-held ideas about the causes of alcoholism. Nevertheless, physical or biological factors, family origin, ethnic differences, and susceptible personality types are recognized as powerful factors in the development of alcoholics. Though research may yet reveal a single cause, many authorities argue for a multicausal or multifaceted origin of alcoholism, and focus on "nature" (hereditary, biological, physical) factors and "nurture" (psychosocial, cultural, environmental) factors.[52] Several of these factors are described in the following sections dealing with

- the agent (ethyl alcohol),
- the host (the person in whom alcoholism develops), and
- the environment (the psychosocial and cultural setting in which alcohol dependence occurs).

The terms *agent, host,* and *environment* are often used to categorize factors or possible causes in the development of any disease or disorder.

Agent-Related Causative Factors

In this category are those properties or characteristics of ethyl alcohol that might contribute to alcohol dependency.

1. Alcohol is a central nervous system *depressant-type drug.* As such, it is capable of altering consciousness and producing a calming and tranquilizing effect.
2. As a *relatively fast-acting drug* in inducing an altered state of consciousness, alcohol carries an increased potential for abuse.
3. In addition to being a central nervous system depressant, ethyl alcohol is also a *psychomotor agitant.* This latter drug effect is usually unrecognized until the calming effect of alcohol has worn off. Then the shaking, tremors, and nervousness that accompany withdrawal are considered evidence of the effect of the "uneven stimulant" and sufficient to cause the drinker to resume his or her alcohol intake.
4. Related to the foregoing factor, alcohol is a psychoactive *drug capable of producing physical dependence* that is *manifested by withdrawal symptoms.* One of the factors maintaining alcohol dependence is the discomfort of withdrawal.

Alcohol-dependent individuals, as noted previously, tend to abuse alcohol to avoid withdrawal and to feel normal again.

Host-Related Causative Factors

This category includes those factors associated with the individual drinker, the so-called host. The drinker presents a unique combination of genetic, biochemical, and psychological forces that somehow predispose that host to alcoholism.

1. *Heredity* is now considered a major predisposing causal factor in many cases of alcoholism. There is no doubt that alcoholism runs in families, even when children are separated from their alcoholic parents and reared by nonalcoholismic adoptive parents. The evidence for such an important genetic influence on alcoholism risk is compelling.[53] Moreover, this

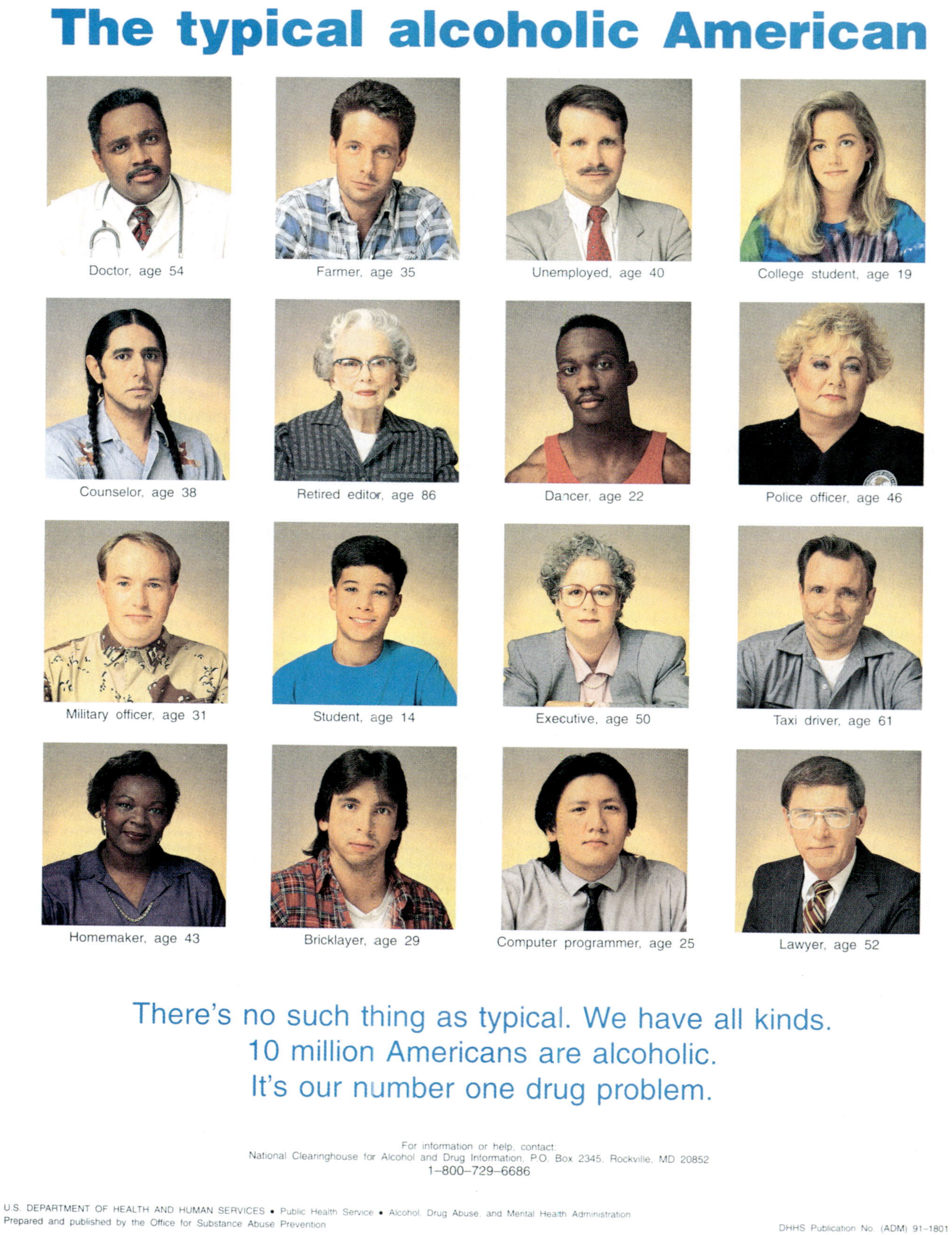
The typical alcoholic American
Doctor, age 54
Farmer, age 35
Unemployed, age 40
College student, age 19
Counselor, age 38
Retired editor, age 86
Dancer, age 22
Police officer, age 46
Military officer, age 31
Student, age 14
Executive, age 50
Taxi driver, age 61
Homemaker, age 43
Bricklayer, age 29
Computer programmer, age 25
Lawyer, age 52
There's no such thing as typical. We have all kinds.
10 million Americans are alcoholic.
It's our number one drug problem.
For information or help, contact:
National Clearinghouse for Alcohol and Drug Information, P.O. Box 2345, Rockville, MD 20852
1-800-729-6686
U.S. DEPARTMENT OF HEALTH AND HUMAN SERVICES • Public Health Service • Alcohol, Drug Abuse, and Mental Health Administration
Prepared and published by the Office for Substance Abuse Prevention
DHHS Publication No. (ADM) 91-1801

figure 5.3

U.S. DEPARTMENT OF HEALTH AND HUMAN SERVICES • Public Health Service • Substance Abuse and Mental Health Services Administration Prepared and published by the Center for Substance Abuse Prevention

U.S. Department of Health & Human Services.

influence appears as strong in women as in men.[54] Two major types or classifications of alcoholism based on genetic predisposition have been identified, and are:[55]

- *Type I or Type A alcoholism* occurs in both males and females, requires the presence of a genetic and an environmental predisposition or trigger, displays only a weak family history of problem drinking, begins later in life after years of heavy drinking, and can take on either a mild or severe form.
- *Type II or Type B alcoholism* affects mainly sons of male alcoholics, is influenced strongly by a genetic predisposition but only weakly by environmental factors, often begins in early adolescence or early adulthood following impulsive behavior and childhood conduct problems, is characterized by moderate severity, and is usually associated with criminal behavior.

Possibly, rather than a specific "alcoholism gene," a genetic predisposition might involve multiple genetic factors that combine with a heavy-drinking environment to produce an increased risk of consuming large quantities of alcohol.[56] Some drinkers might be disabled from adequately judging the effects of alcohol. Consequently, such individuals might become drunk before they know what is happening to them.[57]

This unusual response or "level of reaction" to alcohol may also be an early predictor of future alcoholism, but not in the exact manner one would expect. Most people would assume that the person who becomes intoxicated rapidly is more likely to develop serious drinking problems, especially alcoholism. However, research indicates that if young adult males have a high tolerance for alcohol and can therefore drink large amounts without getting drunk, these drinkers are the ones more likely to develop alcoholism than those who become intoxicated easily.[58] Moreover, sons of alcoholics tend to have this higher tolerance for alcohol at age twenty, indicating once again the significance of genetic influences in the development of alcoholism.

The precise mechanism involved in this predisposition to tolerance is not yet known. It is possible the abnormal reaction to alcohol intake is influenced by one or more physical factors that interfere with alcohol's metabolism or chemical processing in the human body.

2. Alcoholism, especially the early-onset type beginning before age twenty, may indicate a *deficit in or lack of serotonin,* a neurotransmitter that regulates mood, aggression, and impulses. Atypical levels of certain other neurotransmitters may also play a role in predisposing an individual to alcohol dependence.

3. Another theory proposes that alcoholics have a *shortage of endorphins,* the body's pain-relieving and euphoria-producing chemicals manufactured by the brain. Abnormal alcohol consumption might make up for this endorphin deficiency.

4. *Unusual brain electrical activity,* revealed by analysis of electroencephalographic (EEG) patterns, has been found among alcoholics and children of alcoholics. Such findings do not tend to occur in nonalcoholics, and they suggest that the brains of alcoholics and those at risk of becoming alcoholic process information differently from the nonalcoholismic population. These variations in brain electrical activity might serve as "markers" or indicators of a predisposition to alcohol dependence before such a condition develops.

5. Certain *biochemical differences* might also play a role in the development of alcoholism. Faulty enzyme systems that function in the metabolism of ethyl alcohol and acetaldehyde may account for considerable differences in how people process and eliminate alcohol. For instance, many Japanese and Chinese exhibit an intolerance to alcohol, sometimes referred to as the "Oriental flushing phenomenon," based on an absence or low amount of aldehyde dehydrogenase. After small amounts of alcohol are consumed, such individuals often display a cutaneous (skin) flush (reddening) on the face and upper body, and experience unpleasant feelings of warmth and queasiness.

6. While the so-called alcoholic personality has been largely discounted as a factor in alcoholism, two personality types appear to be somewhat susceptible to alcohol abuse—the mostly male "antisocial personality" and the "borderline personality," found usually in females. Though most alcoholics display neither personality type, an underlying common problem of controlling impulses may be the basis for each.

7. Another popular theory often used to explain the basis of alcoholism has been related to an individual's *unique reaction to stress.* Alcohol is used as an escape or relief from various forms of psychological distress, especially loneliness, anxiety, depression, frustration, insecurity, unhappiness, and sometimes guilt. Some individuals might also drink to self-medicate their panic attacks.

Environment-Related Causative Factors

Psychosocial and cultural forces have a significant influence on the development of alcoholism. Frequently identified factors in this category include the following:

1. The *availability and accessibility of alcoholic beverages* determine if ethyl alcohol is the "drug of choice." Widespread promotion of this legal psychoactive substance, its relatively low cost, and its general social acceptability combine to make alcohol the most abused drug in the United States.

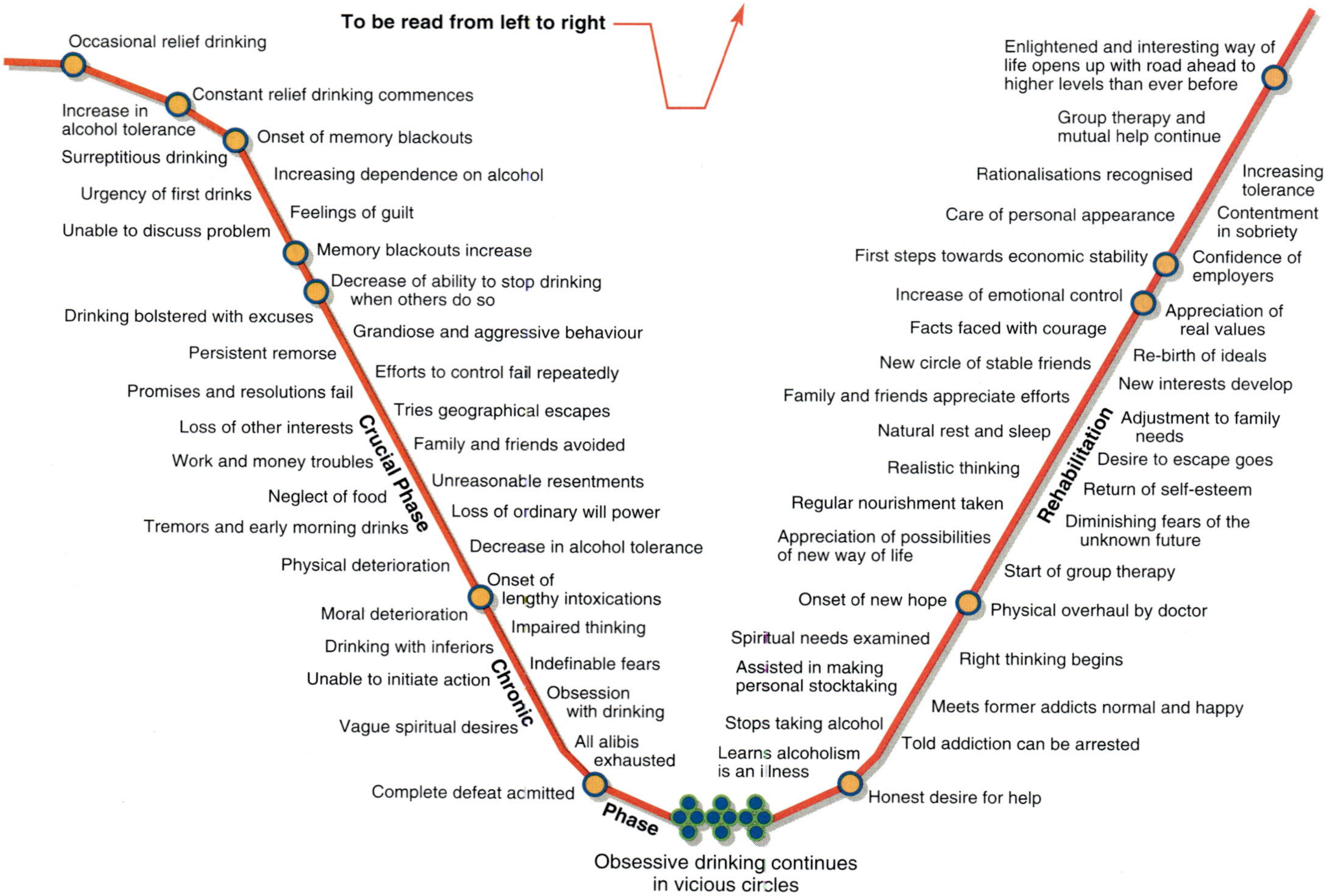

figure 5.4

A chart of alcohol addiction and recovery.

From "Group Therapy in Alcohol" by Max Glatt, as appeared in The British Journal of Addiction, *vol. 54, no. 2. Copyright © Max Glatt. Reprinted by permission of Dr. Glatt and the National Council on Alcoholism and Drug Dependence.*

2. The *absence of clear guidelines for nonabusive alcohol use* in certain populations, the existence of ambivalent attitudes, and conflicting values regarding alcohol often lead to general confusion as to what constitutes acceptable drinking behavior. Unwittingly, our *culture may be encouraging alcoholism* by accepting "relief drinking," by promoting drinking unrelated to family activities and mealtime and by tolerating and perceiving intoxication as funny or manly.
3. *Learning theory* also suggests that children who see parents using alcohol to solve or escape from daily problems will adopt such drinking habits. In addition, children who are given alcohol may be subtly encouraged to drink to gain adult approval and learn that alcohol is only a social beverage rather than a potentially dangerous thing.
4. According to some behavioral scientists, when society permits a large gap to develop between expectations or goals and the means for achieving them, many people express their *alienation* through retreatism and rebellion, as represented in alcoholism. If society labels alcoholism as *deviant behavior,* those so labeled become forced by society into playing a deviant role.

Signs and Symptoms of Alcoholism

Better known than the causes of alcoholism are the signs and symptoms, often described in a series of developmental phases or stages. E. M. Jellinek first established the following four-phase description based on his analysis of recovering alcoholics: (1) the prealcoholic phase; (2) the prodromal or early-warning phase; (3) the crucial phase; and (4) the chronic phase. This initial description was later refined and expanded by other alcoholism and drug dependence specialists, including Great Britain's Max M. Glatt, who depicted the development of and recovery from alcoholism in chart form (see fig. 5.4).

The general phases of alcoholism are identified and explained as follows:

Phase 1: During this initial contact-with-alcohol phase, the evolving alcoholic drinks first for social reasons, but eventually changes the motivations for consumption to include those of anticipated stress reduction and relief from psychological tension or pain. Soon the developing alcoholic seeks out drinking occasions, begins to increase consumption (dose), becomes defensive about his or her intake, and typically associates with new drinking partners who accept the heavier drinking behavior and more frequent intoxication. During this phase, alcohol and drinking become significant parts of daily living s.

Phase 2: In this phase, the alcoholic tends to drink in secret to hide the consumption level and develops several of the early warning signals, such as feelings of guilt about drinking; lying about drinking behavior when confronted by others; an extremely pleasant response to alcohol; drinking before joining others in drinking situations; drinking due to worry, tiredness, or depression; the need for increased intake to produce desired effects (tolerance); and the experience of alcohol-induced amnesia, the **blackout** or memory blank-out. Soon there is no social motivation for drinking. What began as a trend earlier is now the exclusive motivation for intake of alcohol—the expectation of euphoric relief.

Eventually, the alcoholic is preoccupied with procuring a source of alcohol and begins to drink alone, inventing occasions for imbibing if none exist. Intake increases rapidly as guzzling becomes the norm. Sometimes the drinker is unable to abstain. More often, the alcohol abuser cannot control drinking once it has begun, evidence of the loss of control phenomenon—inability to determine with any consistency the duration of drinking or the amount consumed.

A physiological dependency is now established, and if denied a regular dose, the alcoholic will experience **withdrawal symptoms** or the withdrawal syndrome—restlessness, tremulousness or involuntary shaking of the body; insomnia; feelings of depression and anxiety; loss of appetite; mental confusion; and hallucinations and seizures (convulsions; typically occurring within six to eight hours after the last drink. The term **delirium tremens** denotes the intensification and most severe form of the withdrawal symptoms, which usually follow heavy drinking that has lasted over an extended time. Characterized by vivid and terrifying hallucinations, complete disorientation and confusion, and severe agitation with almost continuous motor activity, this medical emergency usually develops between forty-eight to ninety-six hours after the last drink. Fortunately, only a small minority of individuals undergoing withdrawal experience delirium tremens.

Phase 3: Now there is an intensification of all forms of alcohol abuse experienced earlier—more solitary drinking, avoidance of family and friends, and an increase in memory blackouts and passouts. When sober, the alcoholic may regret what was said or done while drinking. To prove that he or she still has everything under control, the drinker will often attempt to restrict personal consumption by going "on the wagon" (an abrupt cessation of drinking). Usually such action is only temporary, excessive intake is resumed, and morning drinking becomes the norm in an attempt to stabilize one's chaotic life. Sometimes a form of reverse tolerance develops as a result of liver damage. In such an instance, the alcoholic appears to be easily intoxicated on a small dose that would rarely have affected behavior earlier in the disease. A series of physical, mental, and social changes now occurs in the alcohol-dependent individual. These may include nervous and gastrointestinal disorders, cirrhosis of the liver, malnutrition, the overuse of defense mechanisms to justify drinking, and a general deterioration in interpersonal relationships. Chain-drinking and extended "benders" are characteristic of this phase of the illness. Hospitalization for alcoholism or an alcohol-related problem is frequently required during this phase.

Phase 4: Progression to this stage usually develops after a number of years of excessive intake. Drinking bouts often last for several days at a time. When the alcoholic gets the "shakes" in the morning upon awakening, more alcohol is consumed to quiet the "nervous" condition. The person is drunk on important occasions and has increasing numbers of blackouts and passouts. Completely oriented around alcohol, the alcohol abuser displays a complete ethical breakdown, unreasonable fears, increased reverse tolerance, and loss of motor coordination. At this point, alcoholics drink to live and live to drink. The medical complications may be so severe that either institutionalization or death occurs unless there is some form of intervention.

Not every alcoholic experiences all of the foregoing signs and symptoms. Moreover, there is great variation in the order in which the abnormal behaviors occur. Also, while alcoholism is a devastating disablement, it tends to display a somewhat inconsistent symptomatology; that is, the alcoholic does not always behave the same way with regard to alcohol. Especially in phase 2 or 3, the alcoholic may enter a stage of remission—a temporary, periodic absence of symptoms—during which time he or she does not get drunk after starting to drink. This phenomenon should not be viewed as a complete cure, because another characteristic of alcoholism is the tendency to have a *relapse,* a return to problem-causing alcohol use. Consequently, the prevention of relapse is an important part of the alcoholic's recovery.

Treatment and Rehabilitation

Modern therapies for alcoholism are usually considered in three general stages: (1) **detoxification;** (2) provision of *medical care* for health problems related to heavy alcohol consumption; and (3) *changing the long-term behavior* of the alcohol abuser so that destructive drinking patterns are discontinued.

Detoxification is the process of "drying out," or ridding the body of alcohol, in which the alcoholic experiences the withdrawal syndrome. Sometimes medications are administered to prevent convulsions and produce a healthy appetite and sound sleep. Nutrient-rich diets and high-strength vitamins are often prescribed, along with the provision of encouragement and emotional support. This stage can require several days.

However, unless the destructive behavior pattern of the alcoholic is altered significantly, the individual runs a high risk of repeated, uncontrolled drinking episodes. Relapses are common and are often fueled by the **"dry-drunk" phenomenon.** This term denotes the alcoholic's state of mind when he or she is not drinking. The dry-drunk syndrome is characterized by a lack of insight, pomposity in personal behavior, an exaggeration of self-importance, an overestimation of one's abilities and intelligence, insensitivity to the needs and feelings of others, a rigid judgmental outlook, tense impatience, and a constant dissatisfaction with life.[59] This behavior must be altered if recovery from alcoholism is to be accomplished to any appreciable degree.

Common treatment approaches, applied in a variety of therapeutic settings, include the following:[60]

Drug therapy or pharmacotherapy—the use of drugs in the treatment of a a disease or disorder. Three major types of drugs are used in alcoholism treatment: *alcohol-sensitizing* or *aversion drugs, anticraving medications,* and *psychiatric medicines.*

One of the first drugs to be used with alcoholics is a deterrent agent that tends to discourage people from resuming drinking once they have stopped. Known as disulfiram (**Antabuse**), this alcohol-sensitizing substance interferes with alcohol oxidation and prolongs the presence of toxic acetaldehyde in the body. If alcohol is consumed, the patient experiences a series of severe physical effects—flushing of the skin, throbbing head and neck, pulsating headache, breathing difficulty, nausea, copious vomiting, sweating, thirst, chest pain, rapid heartbeat, fainting, marked uneasiness, weakness, inability to remain upright, blurred vision, and confusion.[61]

Use of this drug provides the alcoholic with the motivation to avoid drinking. Thus, the taking of Antabuse is a form of *aversion therapy,* treatment that helps a patient stay away from some potentially harmful substance or practice.

Naltrexone, a drug sometimes used in the treatment of opioid addiction, is an example of an anticraving medication. Approved by the Food and Drug Administration, naltrexone is marketed under the brand name of ReVia. This medication helps reduce the craving for alcohol in many abstinent patients and stops the reinforcing effects of alcohol in many patients who do drink. The latter effect often enables patients who consume a small amount of alcohol to avoid full-blown relapse and lessens their chances of returning to heavy drinking. Naltrexone works by blocking certain opioid receptors in nerve cells and presumably reduces the pleasurable sensations associated with drinking alcoholic beverages.

Several psychiatric drugs have been used in treating alcoholics, especially during the withdrawal syndrome. Preferred medications are the benzodiazepines, such as Valium, which tend to subdue the racing sympathetic nervous system and help prevent seizures. Buspirone (BuSpar), another antianxiety drug, has shown a limited effect on curbing alcohol craving and consumption among anxious alcoholics. Antidepressants, such as imipramine and, also tend to decrease alcohol consumption in those alcoholics whose co-occurring depression improved in response to this medication.[62]

Psychotherapy A purposeful conversation between two or more people through which trained therapists help clients achieve greater self-understanding and objectivity in viewing others, and more maturity in the resolution of personal problems. Such a process involves intense self-analysis for the purpose of modifying attitudes, emotional states, and behavior. In addition to individual psychotherapy, there are the self-expressive psychodrama and group therapy, with its feature of mutual support.

Family Therapy A form of psychotherapy based on the proposition that disturbed relationships among various family members may have contributed to or resulted from the destructive drinking of one family member. This form of treatment emphasizes family interactional factors, in addition to individual problems of the alcohol abuser, and proposes changes in the communication patterns of family members. As such, all family members are treated as a unit, rather than isolating the alcoholic and treating that person apart from his or her family.

Behavioral Therapy A general form of psychotherapy is based on the application of human learning theories in a clinical setting. Behavioral therapists emphasize changing the coping patterns of alcohol-dependent individuals rather than changing the underlying causes of self-destructive alcohol abuse.

Some behavioral therapies focus on assertiveness training and improving communication skills and problem-solving methods.

Transactional Analysis A form of group therapy that examines in depth the various verbal exchanges between people. This therapy denies the disease concept of alcoholism. The transactional analyst refuses to participate in the "games" alcoholics play, thus leaving

Box 5.4 The Twelve Steps of Alcoholics Anonymous

1. We admitted we were powerless over alcohol—that our lives had become unmanageable.
2. Came to believe that a Power greater than ourselves could restore us to sanity.
3. Made a decision to turn our will and our lives over to the care of God as we understood Him.
4. Made a searching and fearless moral inventory of ourselves.
5. Admitted to God, to ourselves, and to another human being the exact nature of our wrongs.
6. Were entirely ready to have God remove all these defects of character.
7. Humbly asked Him to remove our shortcomings.
8. Made a list of all persons we had harmed, and became willing to make amends to them all.
9. Made direct amends to such people wherever possible, except when to do so would injure them or others.
10. Continued to take personal inventory and when we were wrong promptly admitted it.
11. Sought through prayer and meditation to improve our conscious contact with God as we understood Him, praying only for knowledge of His will for us and the power to carry that out.
12. Having had a spiritual awakening as the result of these steps, we tried to carry this message to alcoholics and to practice these principles in all our affairs.

them without an incentive to play them. Furthermore, the therapist assigns responsibility for alcoholic behavior to the patient, and tries to instill positive expectancy and hope in the individual problem drinker.

Alcoholics Anonymous

One of the most successful approaches in recovery from alcoholism. **Alcoholics Anonymous (AA)** is a fellowship of problem drinkers who want help in maintaining sobriety. Founded in 1935 by two alcoholics who were unable to achieve an alcohol-free lifestyle individually, AA began when these two joined together to stay sober through mutual support.

Voluntary membership involves an emotional commitment that the alcoholic is powerless over the control of alcohol and that only "a power greater than the self"—AA's concept of God as we understand him—can restore soundness of mind.

The famous "Twelve Steps" of AA express the philosophy and recovery process of this international association. Offering hope of recovery from alcoholism is an essential feature of Alcoholics Anonymous. Such hope is provided by example and supportive interrelationships with other members of this self-help fellowship.

Each person is expected to become involved with the Twelve Steps of AA, an ongoing process that "twelve-steppers" refer to as "working the program . . ." (see box 5.4). The word "alcohol" appears only in the first step. This one reference underscores AA's belief that the main work in recovery is a restructuring of the alcoholic's life.[63]

The Twelve Traditions of AA are the operational principles of the fellowship and express the importance and significance of the group in relationship to its membership, nonmembers, and society in general.

At present, Alcoholics Anonymous has an estimated membership in excess of 1.5 million people in 114 countries around the world. Patterned closely after AA are the Al-Anon family groups for spouses and friends of recovered and recovering alcoholics and Alateen groups for children of alcoholics. For more information about Alcoholics Anonymous, contact:

Alcoholics Anonymous World Services (AA)
475 Riverside Dr.
New York, NY 10163

Secular Alternatives to Alcoholics Anonymous

Women for Sobriety (WFS), the first major alternative to AA was founded in 1975 by a woman who had difficulty recovering from alcoholism within the traditional Alcoholics Anonymous framework. She established this new version of AA, because the original fellowship had been designed primarily for men, and, in her opinion, did not work well for women alcoholics. In mixed groups, men tended to dominate discussion resulting in feelings of intimidation and frustration among women. Consequently, the small groups of WFS focus on the creation of self-esteem—something these recovering female alcoholics had never achieved. Though similar to informal AA discussion groups, WFS meetings forbid the use of caffeine, sugar, and tobacco. For more information about Women for Sobriety, contact:

Women for Sobriety (WFS)
P.O. Box 618
Quakertown, PA 18951

Secular Organizations for Sobriety (SOS) This is also known as Save Our Selves and is the largest of the "nonreligious" alternatives to AA. While there is no structured recovery program for alcoholics, the Suggested Guidelines for Sobriety place great emphasis on overcoming denial and at the same time making sobriety the most important priority in one's life.

Sponsored by the Council for Democratic and Secular Humanism, the meetings of Secular Organizations for Sobriety resemble the informal discussion meetings of AA. However, there is no reference to the spiritual or religious undercurrents prevalent in Alcoholics Anonymous. For more information on Secular Organizations for Sobriety, contact:

Secular Organizations for Sobriety (SOS)
P.O. Box 5
Buffalo, NY 14215

Rational Recovery Systems (RRS) or Rational Recovery (RR) This was established in opposition to AA's concepts of "a higher power," and "once an alcoholic, always an alcoholic." Based on rational-emotive therapy as developed by Albert Ellis, RRS activities teach people how to become emotionally independent from alcohol and organizations dealing with alcoholism. Members promote the belief that the individual problem drinker has sufficient power to overcome addiction and ought not rely on spiritual aspects of recovery commonly expressed in Alcoholics Anonymous. For more information on Rational Recovery Systems, contact:

Rational Recovery Systems (RRS)
P. O. Box 100
Lotus, CA 95651

The Intervention Process

A desirable element of any treatment program is the alcoholic's or the drug abuser's willingness to cooperate with those who can help. This willingness is not usually present at first and is often difficult to achieve. A relatively new process, referred to as *intervention,* can be implemented to help alcoholics and other drug abusers identify their need for making lifestyle changes and for seeking help for their drug problems. Intervention helps a drug-dependent person become aware of and motivated to take the path to recovery. The intervention process is described more fully in chapter 15 as a secondary prevention technique.

The therapies described are offered through many individuals and groups in numerous types of facilities. There are enlightened physicians; community mental health centers; pastoral counseling programs in churches; and general hospitals offering emergency medical services, inpatient care, and outpatient care through clinics.

There are also specialized hospitals that treat only alcoholism and drug abuse and their associated health problems; mental hospitals that provide residential care; Veterans Administration hospitals; and "halfway houses" where recovering alcoholics receive semicustodial care while adjusting to independent living after institutionalization.

Experience has indicated that when treatment and rehabilitation services are coordinated within a job-related or employer-sponsored alcoholism program, recovery rates are considerably higher than ordinarily achieved in other settings. If an alcoholic can remain abstinent and symptom free for five years, then relapse is relatively rare.[64]

Reduction of Problem Drinking

Parents Who Drink and Their Children

Research indicates that Italians, Orthodox Jews, Greeks, Spaniards, Chinese, and Lebanese use alcohol regularly and in quantity, yet tend to have relatively few alcohol-related problems. These cultures have long histories of low-risk drinking and share certain common practices in their use of alcohol. Perhaps Americans who drink should consider and adopt these "immunizing" practices.

The children are exposed to alcohol early in life, within a strong family or religious group.

Parents present a consistent example of moderate, low-risk drinking.

The beverage is viewed mainly as an accompaniment to food and is usually taken with meals.

The beverages commonly used are wine and beer.

Drinking has no moral connotation. It is considered neither a virtue nor a sin.

Drinking is not viewed as proof of adulthood or virility.

Abstinence is socially acceptable.

Excessive drinking or drunkenness is not condoned.

Alcohol use is not the prime focus for an activity.

Most important, there is wide agreement among members of the group on these "ground rules" of drinking.

Host and Hostess Responsibilities

The American house party is another setting in which responsible decisions about alcohol use can help reduce problem drinking. The host and hostess can decide what drinking atmosphere will prevail. Party responsibilities, formulated by the National Institute on Alcohol Abuse and Alcoholism, appear in box 5.5.

For Those Who Drink

Alcohol abuse is everyone's problem. Whether nonuser, moderate or social drinker, or alcoholic, everyone is directly or indirectly affected by alcohol abuse. Whether alcoholism is perceived as a personal threat or not, and whether drinking is viewed as good or bad, the most important thing to remember is that ethyl alcohol is a drug with the potential for adverse drug effects, even when used in social settings.

Social drinking is usually "moderate or low-risk," but the limits of appropriateness are likely to vary from one drinker or drinking group to another. Consequently, promoting so-called responsible drinking behavior may be less than adequate as a method of reducing alcohol problems and

Box 5.5 Party Responsibilities for Hosts and Hostesses

The home setting	Provide seats for all, plan for people movement and keep the lights on.
The bartender	Choose a bartender of known discretion. The eager volunteer may turn out to be a pusher who uses the role to give every glass an extra "shot."
Pace the drinks	Serve drinks at regular, reasonable intervals. The length of the interval will depend on whether the guests are enjoying the company or the drinks more. A drink-an-hour schedule means good company prevails.
Don't double up	Many people count and pace their drinks. If you serve doubles, they'll be drinking twice as much as they planned. Doubling up isn't hospitality; it's rude.
Don't push drinks	Let the glass be empty before you offer a refill. And then don't rush, especially if someone comes up empty too fast. When a guest says "no, thanks" to an alcohol drink—don't insist.
Push the snacks	Do this while your guests are drinking, not after. This is important because food slows down the rate at which alcohol is absorbed into the bloodstream. It also slows down the rate at which people drink.
Serve nonalcoholic drinks, too	One out of three adults chooses not to drink. Occasional drinkers sometimes prefer not to. Offer a choice of drinks besides alcohol—fruit and vegetable juices, tea, coffee, and soft drinks.
Offer more than drinks	When guests focus on the drinks, the party is slipping. Stir up conversation. Share a laugh. Draw out a guest talent. A good host or hostess has more to give than food and drinks.
Serving dinner	If it's a dinner party, serve before it's too late. A cocktail hour is supposed to enhance a fine dinner, not compete with it. After too many drinks, guests may not know what they ate or how it tasted.
Set drinking limits	When a guest has had too much to drink, you can politely express your concern by offering a substitute drink—coffee, perhaps. This is a gentle way of telling a guest that he or she has reached the limits you have set for your home.
Closing the bar	Decide in advance when you want your party to end. Then give appropriate cues by word and action that it's time to leave. A considerate way to close the drinking phase is to serve a substantial snack. It also provides some nondrinking time before your guests start to drive home.

Source: National Institute on Alcohol Abuse and Alcoholism.

alcohol abuse. In a similar manner, urging drinkers to "party sensibly," "know their limits," and "know when to say when" may sound like good advice. But these recommendations have been criticized as lacking in specificity and dealing with generalities that cannot be applied easily.

By contrast the "Zero-One-Three" strategy offers straightforward, unambiguous guidelines for moderate or low-risk drinking. Included are specific, short, and easy-to-apply principles for conducting moderate drinking behavior. Both nondrinkers and drinkers are considered, and the message "It's always OK not to drink" is reinforced in the "Zero-zero alcohol" portion of the safety promotion concept (see fig. 5.5).

In addition, the following suggestions are also offered for those who wish to preserve alcohol use as a nondestructive part of social functions, to avoid the mental chaos of intoxication, and to minimize the risks of alcoholism.

1. Integrate alcohol use with leisure activities, eating, and social functions.
2. Conduct drinking among friends or within the family setting, where social controls are more likely to function.
3. Pace your consumption of alcohol by sipping drinks and becoming involved in conversation. Take your second drink no sooner than one hour after the first. Do not drink fast!
4. Avoid drinking on an empty stomach. Eat ice cream, meat, eggs, or cheese, or drink milk or cream before ingesting alcohol, and also eat while you drink.
5. Dilute distilled spirits with water to retard alcohol absorption; always use plenty of ice cubes; and beware of unfamiliar drinks with unknown alcohol content.
6. Drink in well-lighted, quiet places. Dark and noisy places produce tenseness, which in turn may give rise to overdrinking.
7. Deliberately avoid beverage alcohol when confronted with problems or the need to relax.
8. Watch carefully your personal drinking pattern for early signs and symptoms of problem drinking. Remember, if you need a drink to be social, that is *not* social drinking!

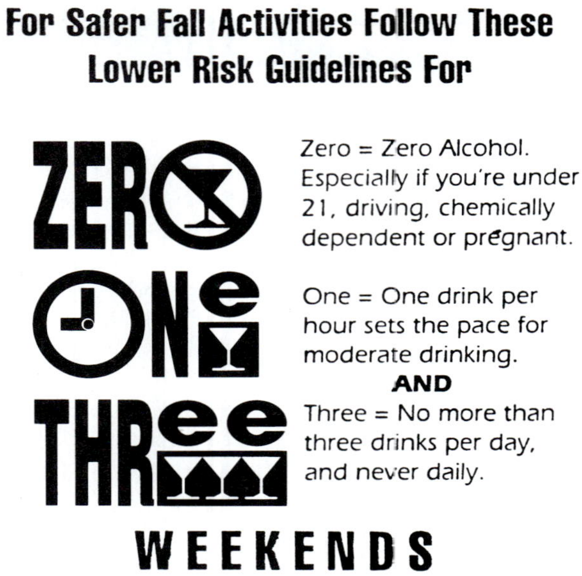
For Safer Fall Activities Follow These Lower Risk Guidelines For
ZERO
Zero = Zero Alcohol. Especially if you're under 21, driving, chemically dependent or pregnant.
ONE
One = One drink per hour sets the pace for moderate drinking.
AND
THREE
Three = No more than three drinks per day, and never daily.
WEEKENDS

figure 5.5

The "Zero-One-Three" strategy for lower-risk drinking.

From the Enjoy Michigan Safely Coalition, Michigan Substance Abuse and Traffic Safety Information Center, Lansing, Mich. Reprinted by permission of the Michigan Resource Center.

Chapter Summary

1. Problem drinking is the use of alcoholic beverages resulting in some type of damage or harm to the drinker, the drinker's family, or the drinker's community.
2. Alcohol abuse is a form of problem drinking that involves a repeated maladaptive pattern of drinking leading to significant impairment or distress.
3. Significant expenses associated with alcohol abuse and work performance are due to reduced productivity, off-the-job absenteeism, and on-the-job absenteeism. Work-related risk factors that tend to encourage problem drinking include pro-alcohol cultural factors, lack of social controls, alienation of employees from their jobs, and the degree of work stress in the workplace.
4. Frequent alcohol-related law violations include public intoxication and driving under the influence of alcohol. Alcohol is involved in a high percentage of alcohol-related criminal offenses including homicide, assaults, and rape, as well as property offenses and public order offenses. In such cases, alcohol may act as a disinhibitor of aggressive behavior, an intensifier of anger, a trigger for aggressive behavior, or as a relaxer of social norms.
5. In addition to alcohol-related auto crashes and deaths, alcohol use and abuse have been linked to other types of accidental injuries and fatalities, including falls, drownings, and fires and burns.
6. More than 40 percent of fatal motor vehicle crashes are alcohol-related. Nearly two out of five Americans will likely be involved in an alcohol-caused crash in their lifetime.
7. An elevated blood-alcohol concentration (BAC) is the first and most important factor influencing the risk of involvement in an alcohol-related car crash. Most states have set a BAC limit of 0.10 percent for drivers age twenty-one and older, although some states have already adopted a lower level, namely 0.08 percent BAC. For drivers under twenty-one years of age, most states have established zero tolerance limits of 0.02 percent BAC or lower, that is, none at all.
8. Many other alcohol countermeasures, including "dram shop acts," open container bans, adoption of sobriety checkpoints, administrative license revocation, and mandatory jail sentences for driving on a suspended license are available to reduce the toll of alcohol-related auto crashes and fatalities.
9. Fetal Alcohol Syndrome is a potentially preventable major birth defect among children whose mothers were alcoholics or heavy drinkers during pregnancy. Principal features include growth deficiency, central nervous systems damage, and head and facial abnormalities.
10. Alcohol abuse and alcoholism often result in a serious psychological, social, and physical disorder within the family unit, leading to a family not-at-ease, a family disease. Children of alcoholics (COAs) are at an extremely high risk of developing alcohol and other drug problems, and often assume coping roles of the "hero," "scapegoat," "lost child," and "family mascot." As adults, these COAs also have a strong predisposition toward psychiatric symptoms and increased risk for marital difficulties. Co-dependence describes the unusual coping mechanisms, attitudes, and behavior that family members sometimes develop in response to a problem-drinking parent, spouse, child, or sibling.
11. Alcoholism may be defined as a complex illness or disability involving the recurring use of alcoholic beverages that contribute to various personal or social problems. Alcoholism may also be described as the disease of alcohol dependence characterized by tolerance,

withdrawal, impaired or loss of control over the use of alcohol, and craving. Jellinek's original research revealed at least four major types of alcoholism, while the American Psychiatric Association now views alcoholism as a substance dependence disorder with several distinct criteria for diagnosis.

12. Among the possible causes of alcoholism are factors relating to alcohol (the agent); the drinker (host) with unique genetic, biochemical, and psychological forces; and the psychosocial and cultural setting (environment) in which drinking occurs.
13. Signs and symptoms of alcoholism are often viewed in a series of developmental phases or stages of progression: prealcoholic, prodromal, crucial, and chronic.
14. Treatment for alcoholismic individuals begins with detoxification, includes medical care for specific health problems, and progresses to changing long-term behaviors that have contributed to destructive drinking patterns. Specific treatments include drug therapy, (e.g., Antabuse, Naltrexone), psychotherapy, family therapy, behavioral therapy, transactional analysis, and the self-help techniques of groups like Alcoholics Anonymous and secular alternatives to AA.
15. Reduction of problem drinking begins with "immunizing" strategies employed by parents with their children, relies upon responsible actions taken by hosts and hostesses at drinking parties, and ultimately depends upon the prudent actions of drinkers who wish to preserve alcohol use as a nondestructive part of social functions.

World Wide Web Sites

Al-Anon Family Group Headquarters

www.al-anon.alateen.org

Alcoholics Anonymous (AA) World Services

www.alcoholics-anonymous.org

National Council on Alcoholism and Drug Dependence

swww.ncadd.org

Review Questions and Activities

1. Why is the identification of an alcohol-related problem sometimes complicated? Give two examples of alcohol-related problems and indicate what criteria you used in defining these conditions or practices as problematic.
2. How does the American Psychiatric Association describe alcohol abuse? What criteria does this organization apply to the designation of drinking as alcohol abuse?
3. How can various workplace situations or environments encourage excessive use of alcoholic beverages? Have you ever "worked" in such a situation?
4. What is the difference between off-the-job absenteeism and on-the-job absenteeism in the workplace? Can such conditions apply to classroom situations, family living, church attendance, and so forth?
5. Contact local law enforcement officials and determine how your community handles or processes those who become intoxicated in public. Does the response suggest that public intoxication is still a criminal offense or a public health problem?
6. What are the legal penalties for various alcohol-related criminal offenses, such as homicide, killing a person in an alcohol-caused auto crash, assault, rape, child abuse? Does the involvement of alcohol serve to mitigate or lessen the severity of the penalty or sentence?
7. Undertake a college/university study in conjunction with campus health officials, student personnel services, campus police, student government leaders, counseling services, office of the dean of students, and the campus newspaper to identify serious alcohol-related problems affecting the college/university community.
8. What blood-alcohol concentration limits are enforced in your state for operating a motor vehicle while intoxicated or under the influence of alcohol?
9. Distinguish among the following terms: *prima facie* evidence of driving under the influence of alcohol, "per se" laws regarding drinking and driving, and zero tolerance limits.
10. Identify several additional alcohol countermeasures that can be used to help reduce the epidemic of alcohol-impaired driving skills and related crashes, injuries, and fatalities.
11. Distinguish between the following conditions possibly resulting from prenatal alcohol exposure: Fetal Alcohol Syndrome and Fetal Alcohol Effects.
12. What are the principal features associated with Fetal Alcohol Syndrome?
13. Briefly describe the following possible mechanisms of damage in FAS: maternal nutrients, hormonal deficiencies, local growth factors, prostaglandins, and reduced oxygen levels.
14. Explain why alcohol abuse or alcoholism is often referred to as a "family disease."
15. Why do you think co-dependence sometimes develops in a family setting? In what way is "external referenting" related to co-dependence?
16. Identify several of the characteristics often observed in children of alcoholics.
17. Define alcoholism in terms of fundamental characteristics of alcohol dependence, Jellinek's species, and the proposals offered by the American

Society of Addiction Medicine and the American Psychiatric Association (APA). What criteria are used by the APA to identify alcoholism as a substance dependence disorder?

18. Identify at least three agent-related, three host-related, and three environment-related factors that might cause or contribute to alcoholism.

19. Describe the progressive nature of alcoholism by citing specific signs and symptoms typical of the four phases of this disease.

20. What therapies are used in treating alcoholics? You may want to attend an open meeting of Alcoholics Anonymous and report on your findings.

21. To what extent do you agree or disagree with the recommendations in the text to reduce problem drinking?

References

1. Harry Levine, "The Promise and Problems of Alcohol Sociology," chap. 3 in *Alcohol: The Development of Sociological Perspectives on Use and Abuse,* edited by Paul Roman (New Brunswick, N.J.: Rutgers Center of Alcohol Studies, 1991), 87–112.
2. Gail Milgram and the editors of Consumer Reports Books, *The Facts About Drinking* (Mount Vernon, N.Y.: Consumers Union, 1990), 50–51.
3. American Psychiatric Association, *Diagnostic and Statistical Manual of Mental Disorders,* 4th ed. (Washington, D.C.: American Psychiatric Association, 1994), 182–83, 196.
4. National Institute on Drug Abuse, *National Household Survey on Drug Abuse: Main Findings* (Washington, D.C.: GPO, 1993).
5. National Council on Alcoholism and Drug Dependence, *NCADD Fact Sheet: Alcohol and Other Drugs in the Workplace* (New York: National Council on Alcoholism and Drug Dependence, 1992), 1.
6. Harrison Trice and William Sonnenstuhl, "Job Behaviors and the Denial Syndrome," chap. 32 in *Society, Culture, and Drinking Patterns Reexamined,* edited by David Pittman and Helene Raskin White (New Brunswick, N.J.: Rutgers Center of Alcohol Studies, 1991), 631–49.
7. Terry Blum, Paul Roman, and Jack Martin, "Alcohol Consumption and Work Performance," *The Journal of Studies on Alcohol* 54, no. 1 (January 1993): 61–70.
8. Harrison Trice and William Sonnenstuhl, "Job Behaviors and the Denial Syndrome," 635.
9. William Sonnenstuhl and Harrison Trice, "The Workplace as Locale for Risks and Interventions in Alcohol Abuse," chap. 12 in *Alcohol: The Development of Sociological Perspectives on Use and Abuse,* edited by Paul Roman (New Brunswick, N.J.: Rutgers Center of Alcohol Studies, 1991): 255–88, and Harrison Trice, "Work-Related Risk Factors Associated with Alcohol Abuse," *Alcohol Health & Research World* 16, no. 2 (1992): 106–11.
10. National Institute on Alcohol Abuse and Alcoholism, *Alcohol Alert: Drinking and Driving,* no. 31, PH 362 (January 1996), 2
11. Susan Martin, "The Epidemiology of Alcohol-Related Interpersonal Violence," *Alcohol Health & Research World* 16, no. 3 (1992): 230–37.
12. James Collins, "Drinking and Violations of the Criminal Law," chap. 33 in *Society, Culture, and Drinking Patterns Reexamined,* edited by David Pittman and Helene Raskin White (New Brunswick, N.J.: Rutgers Center of Alcohol Studies, 1991), 650–60.
13. Ibid.
14. U.S. Publication Health Service, *Healthy People 2000: National Health Promotion and Disease Prevention Objectives* (Boston: Jones and Bartlett Publishers, 1991), 64. Reprinted from the DHHS Publication no. (PHS) 91-50213.
15. National Institute on Alcohol Abuse and Alcoholism, *Alcohol and Health: The Seventh Special Report to the U.S. Congress* (Washington, D.C.: GPO, 1990) 163.
16. "Alcohol and Injuries: Problems and Responses," *The Bottom Line on Alcohol in Society* 14, no. 1 (spring 1993): 69–73; and "Alcohol Involvement in Pedestrian Fatalities—United States, 1982–1992," *Morbidity and Mortality Weekly Report* 42, no. 37 (24 September 1993): 716–19.
17. National 3D Prevention Month Coalition, *National Drunk and Drugged Driving (3D) Prevention Month Background and Resource Guide* (Washington, D.C.: U.S. Department of Transportation, 1993), 3.
18. Kevin Johnson and Carrie Dowling, "After Decade of Decline, a Deadly Statistic Rises," *USA Today* (2 July 1996): 2A.
19. "Multiple Offenders," *Prevention Pipeline* 8, no. 1 (January/February 1995): 36.
20. National Institute on Alcohol Abuse and Alcoholism, *Alcohol Alert: Drinking and Driving,* no. 31, PH 362 (January 1996) 1–4.
21. Ibid.
22. "Alcohol-Related Traffic Deaths in Young Drivers," *Journal Watch* 16, no. 1 (1 January 1996): 5. (Summarized from "Alcohol-Related Traffic Crashes and Fatalities Among Youth and Young Adults—United States, 1982–1994," *Morbidity and Mortality Weekly Report* 44 (1 December 1995): 869–74.)
23. David A. Sleet, Alexander C. Wagenaar, and Patricia F. Waller, "Introduction: Drinking, Driving, and Health Promotion," *Health Education Quarterly* 16, no. 3 (fall 1989): 319–33.
24. Herbert Moskowitz and Marcelline Burns, "Effects of Alcohol on Driving Performance," *Alcohol Health and Research World* 14, no. 1 (1990): 12–14.
25. Ralph Hingson, Timothy Heeren, and Michael Winter, "Lowering State Legal Blood Alcohol Limits to 0.08%: The Effect on Fatal Motor Vehicle Crashes," *American Journal of Public Health* 86, no. 9 (September 1996): 1297–99.
26. "How Much Is Too Much?" *The Bottom Line on Alcohol in Society,* 10 (1990): 18–23.
27. Center for Substance Abuse Prevention, *Making the Link: Alcohol, Tobacco, and Other Drugs & Pregnancy and Parenthood,* ML 010 (Rockville, Md.: Substance Abuse and Mental Health Services Administration, 1995), 1–2.
28. Nancy Day, "The Effects of Prenatal Exposure to Alcohol," *Alcohol Health and Research World* 16, no. 3 (1992): 238–44; and National Institute on Alcohol Abuse and Alcoholism, *Alcohol and Health,* 203.
29. Beatrice Larroque and others, "Moderate Prenatal Alcohol Exposure and Psychomotor Development at Preschool Age," *American Journal of Public Health* 85, no. 12 (December 1995): 1654–61.
30. George Steinmetz, "The Preventable Tragedy: Fetal Alcohol Syndrome," *National Geographic,* February 1992, 36.
31. Elias Michaelis and Mary Michaelis, "Cellular and Molecular Bases of Alcohol's Teratogenic Effects," *Alcohol Health & Research World* 18, no. 1 (1994): 17–21.
32. Paddy Cook, Robert Peterson, and Dorothy Moore, *Alcohol, Tobacco, and Other Drugs May Harm the Unborn* (Washington, D.C.: GPO, 1990), 18.
33. Enoch Gordis, "Fetal Alcohol Syndrome: A Commentary," *Alcohol Alert* no. 13, PH 297 (July 1991): 3.
National Institute on Alcohol Abuse and Alcoholism, *Alcohol Alert: Fetal Alcohol Syndrome: A Commentary,* no. 13, PH 297 (July 1991), 2.
34. James J. Collins, "Epidemiology of Alcohol-Related Violence." *Alcohol Health and Research World* 17, no. 2 (1993): 93–100.
35. National Institute on Alcohol Abuse and Alcoholism, *Alcohol and Health: The Eighth Special Report to the U.S. Congress* (Rockville, Md: National Institutes of Health, 1993): 247.
36. Ibid.
37. Robert N. Parker, "The Effects of Context on Alcohol and Violence," *Alcohol Health and Research World* 17, no. 2 (1993): 117–32.
38. Office for Substance Abuse Prevention, *Some Questions and Answers about Children of Alcoholics,* DHHS Pub. no. (ADM) 92-1914 (Rockville, Md.: National Clearinghouse for Alcohol and Drug Information, 1992).
39. Donald Jorgensen and June Jorgensen, *Secrets Told by Children of Alcoholics* (Blue Ridge Summit, Pa.: Tab Books, 1990), 21–44.

40. National Institute on Alcohol Abuse and Alcoholism, *Alcohol Alert: Children of Alcoholics: Are They Different?* (1990), 1–2.
41. Judith Seixas and Geraldine Youcha, *Children of Alcoholism: A Survivor's Manual* (New York: Perennial Library/Harper & Row, 1985); and Sharon Wegscheider, *Another Chance: Hope and Health for the Alcoholic Family* (Palo Alto, Calif.: Science and Behavior Books, 1981).
42. William H. Crisman, *The Opposite of Everything Is True: Reflections on Denial in Alcoholic Families* (New York: William Morrow, 1991), 72–78.
43. Tom Dunkel, "Dealing with Demons of a New Generation," in *Annual Editions: Drugs, Society, and Human Behavior 94/95* (Guilford, Conn.: Dushkin, 1994), 128–30. (Originally published in *Insight,* 1993.)
44. Sharon Wegscheider-Cruse, *The Miracle of Recovery* (Deerfield Beach, Fl.: Health Communications, 1989), 35.
45. Anne Wilson Schaef, *When Society Becomes an Addict* (San Francisco: Harper & Row, 1988), 30.
46. National Institute on Alcohol Abuse and Alcoholism, *Alcohol Alert: Neuroscience Research and Medications Development—A Commentary,* no. 33, PH 366 (July 1996), 3.
47. E. M. Jellinek, *The Disease Concept of Alcoholism* (New Brunswick, N.J.: Hillhouse Press, 1960), 35–38.
48. American Medical Association, *Manual on Alcoholism,* 3d ed. (Chicago: American Medical Association, 1977), 4.
49. Robert Morse and Daniel Flavin, "Report for the Joint Committee of the National Council on Alcoholism and Drug Dependence and the American Society of Addiction Medicine to Study the Definition and Criteria for the Diagnosis of Alcoholism," *Journal of the American Medical Association* 268, no. 8 (26 August 1992): 1012–14.
50. American Psychiatric Association, *Diagnostic and Statistical Manual of Mental Disorders,* 4th ed. (Washington, D.C.: American Psychiatric Association, 1994), 181 195; and National Institute on Alcohol Abuse and Alcoholism, *Alcohol Alert: Diagnostic Criteria for Alcohol Abuse and Dependence,* no. 30, PH 359 (October 1995), 4–5.
51. Lester Grinspoon, and others, "Alcohol Abuse and Dependence," *Harvard Medical School Mental Health Review* (1990): 5.
52. Donald Goodwin, *Is Alcoholism Hereditary?* 2d ed. (New York: Ballantine, 1988), 83–156.
53. Andrew Heath, "Genetic Influences on Alcoholism Risk," *Alcohol Health & Research World* 19, no. 3 (1995): 166–71; and Marc Schuckit, "A Long-Term Study of Sons of Alcoholics," *Alcohol Health & Research World* 19, no. 3 (1995): 172–75.
54. Shirley Hill, "Neurobiological and Clinical Markers for a Severe Form of Alcoholism in Women," *Alcohol Health & Research World* 19, no. 3 (1995): 249–56.
55. C. Robert Cloninger, Soren Sigvardsson, and Michael Bohman, "Type I and Type II Alcoholism: An Update," *Alcohol Health & Research World* 20, no. 1 (1996): 18–23; and Samuel Ball, "Type A and Type B Alcoholism," *Alcohol Health & Research World* 20, no. 1 (1996): 30–35.
56. Mark Schuckit, "A Clinical Model of Genetic Influences in Alcohol Dependence," *Journal of Studies on Alcohol* 55 (1994): 5–17.
57. Grinspoon, Bakalar, and others, "Alcohol Abuse and Dependence," 5.
58. Marc Schuckit and Tom Smith, "An 8-Year Follow-up of 450 Sons of Alcoholic and Control Subjects," *Archives of General Psychiatry* 53, no. 3 (March 1996): 202–10.
59. R. J. Solberg, *The Dry-Drunk Syndrome* (Center City, Minn.: Hazelden Educational Services, 1980), 3–4.
60. Mary McCaul and Janice Furst, "Alcoholism Treatment in the United States," *Alcohol Health & Research World* 18, no. 4 (1994): 253–60; and Paula Kurtzweil, "Medications Can Aid Recovery from Alcoholism," *FDA Consumer* 30, no. 4 (May 1996): 23–25.
61. William Hobbs, Theodore Rall, and Todd Verdoorn, "Hypnotics and Sedatives; Ethanol," chap. 17 in *Goodman & Gilman's The Pharmacological Basis of Therapeutics,* 9th ed. (New York: McGraw-Hill Health Professions Division, 1996), 391.
62. National Institute on Alcohol Abuse and Alcoholism, *Alcohol Alert: Neuroscience Research and Medications Development,* no. 33, PH 366 (July 1996), 3.
63. H. Thomas Milhorn, *Drug and Alcohol Abuse: The Authoritative Guide for Parents, Teachers, and Counselors* (New York: Plenum Press, 1994), 176.
64. George Vaillant, "A Long-term Follow-up of Male Alcohol Abuse," *Archives of General Psychiatry* 53, no. 3 (March 1996): 243–49.

Chapter 6

Narcotics: Opioid analgesics

KEY TERMS

Analgesia
Antitussive
Codeine
Comprehensive Drug Abuse Prevention and Control Act
Darvon
Endogenous Opioid
Endorphins
Enkephalins
Exempt Narcotic
Fentanyl
Harrison Narcotics Act
Heroin
LAAM
Mainlining
Methadone
Methadone Maintenance
Morphine
MPTP
Multimodality Therapeutic Approach
Narcotic Antagonist
Narcotics Anonymous
Natural "High"
Opioid
Opium
Papaver somniferum
Psychotherapy
Pure Food and Drug Act
Receptors
"Rush"
Skin-Popping
Snorting
Therapeutic Community

chapter objectives

After you have studied this chapter, you should be able to do the following:

1. Define the key terms.
2. Classify common opioids as natural, semisynthetic, synthetic, or endogenous.
3. Identify several common side effects and adverse drug reactions associated with using narcotics.
4. Explain how the following narcotics are related in their derivation or origin: opium, morphine, China White heroin, and codeine.
5. Distinguish the unique status of an "exempt narcotic" from opioids such as morphine and methadone.
6. Explain how lifestyle could influence the health of a person abusing heroin.
7. Compare the effects of methadone and LAAM with those of morphine-based drugs.
8. Compare and contrast "designer narcotics" with "new-wave narcotics" in terms of origin, effects, and street names.
9. Describe drug dependence as an endorphin deficiency.
10. Discuss the historical influences in the early part of the twentieth century that led to the enactment of the first Federal Food and Drug Act of 1906 and the Harrison Narcotics Act of 1914.
11. Identify the major provisions of the Comprehensive Drug Abuse Prevention and Control Act of 1970 that affected the availability, distribution, and possession of narcotics.
12. Distinguish from one another each of the following, pertaining to the treatment of narcotic-dependent individuals: psychotherapy, detoxification, therapeutic communities, methadone maintenance, Narcotics Anonymous, and narcotic antagonists.
13. Explain the meaning of the term *cold turkey* as it relates to the condition of narcotic drug dependency.
14. Discuss the pros and cons of methadone or LAAM maintenance as a technique for reducing problems of heroin dependency.
15. Describe the major elements of the "multimodality approach" to the treatment of narcotics dependency.

General Characteristics of Narcotics

Although the term *narcotic* has several meanings—one of which refers to all illegal drugs of abuse—it will be used exclusively in this text to describe a family of drugs having a stupor- or sleep-inducing action and an analgesic (pain-relieving) action.

Classification of Opioids

Sometimes the narcotic drugs are called **opioids** or *opiates* because they are derived from the opium poppy plant or made synthetically to have the same drug actions of morphine, a major ingredient of opium.

As shown in figure 6.1, the opioids may be classified as

1. *natural substances,* such as opium, morphine, codeine, and thebaine;

2. *semisynthetic narcotics,* such as heroin, hydromorphone (dihydromorphinone), thebaine derivatives, and etorphine, all produced by modifying the chemicals contained in opium;
3. *synthetic products* made entirely in the laboratory, such as meperidine (Demerol), methadone, and propoxyphene (Darvon); or
4. *endogenous opioids,* natural, internal bodily substances identified as enkephalins, endorphins, and dynorphins that originate within the body and have opioidlike effects within the body.

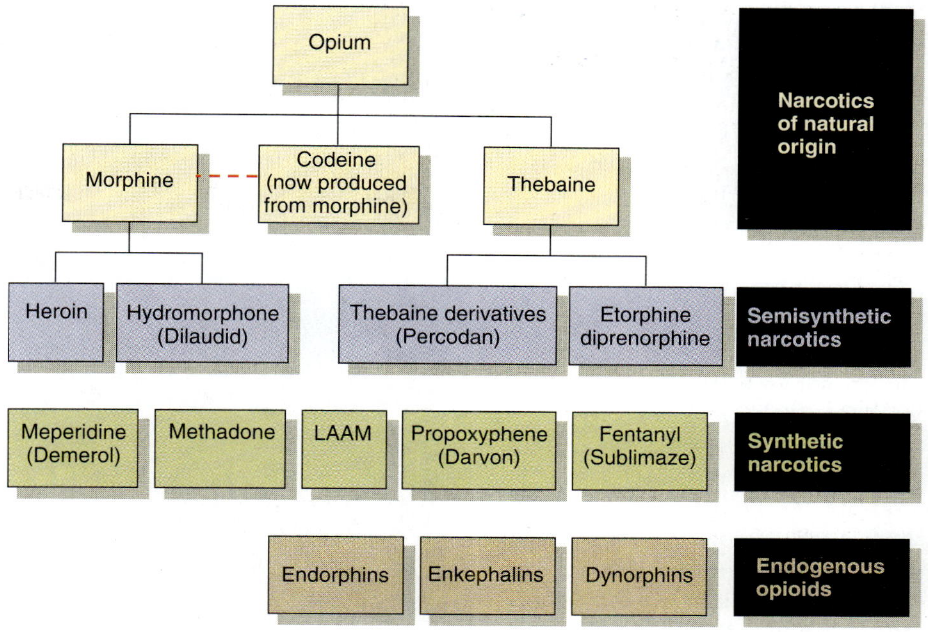

figure 6.1

The narcotics: Opioid analgesics.

Medical Use and Addiction

Although the opioids have been used medically for **analgesia** (pain relief), treatment of diarrhea, and the relief of coughing, they are also addictive. Their heavy use or even occasional use over a long period will likely result in opioid abuse and dependence, characterized by daily use, inability to stop usage, constant or repeated intoxication with a narcotic drug, overdoses, tolerance, and withdrawal.[1]

Words such as *addictive, addiction,* and *addict* have been replaced by the more modern, precise, and accurately descriptive terms *dependency producing, drug dependence,* and *drug* or *chemically dependent person,* respectively.

For some, addiction refers to a lifestyle focused on getting and using dependency-producing drugs, despite severe adverse consequences. Others use the term drug dependence with reference to using a particular drug to block or delay the withdrawal syndrome. Nevertheless, the *addiction* terminology still appears frequently as an equivalent to drug dependency in current professional literature and in mass media reports dealing with narcotics and compulsive drug use.

Many artificial morphine-like drugs have been produced in the laboratory to duplicate the medical usefulness of, yet avoid the chemical dependence often associated with, the opioids. Some of these newer nonnarcotic drugs are used for the relief of coughing. However, morphine, codeine, and the synthetic narcotics still play vital roles in the medical relief of pain.[2] Morphine remains the standard against which new analgesics are measured, because no other drug has been proven to be clinically superior in relieving severe pain.[3]

Narcotics are rarely used alone to induce sleep because of their euphoria-producing effects and the likelihood of their misuse and abuse. In addition to pain relief and a general feeling of well-being, opioids also produce drowsiness that leads to sleep. With high doses, these drugs cause a clouding of mental function due to central nervous system (CNS) depression. Unlike other CNS depressants, there is usually no loss of motor coordination or consciousness, and no slurring of speech, unless a large dose is administered or the person is already ill or fatigued.

Other Opioid Effects

Behavioral effects of the narcotics usually depend upon whether the individual is experiencing pain or is pain-free. When given a therapeutic dose of morphine, for instance, a patient in pain and suffering from anxiety tends to experience relief from the pain and from the anxiety. However, when pain is not present, a person taking the same dose may develop mental distress, such as fear, nervousness, and nausea.

Common side effects include constipation, constriction of the eye's pupil, and respiratory depression that leads to irregular breathing. Less commonly experienced are nausea, vomiting, dizziness, and shortness of breath. There is little doubt, however, that the most attractive nonmedical effect of the opioids is the experience of well-being, ranging from a mild euphoria to a tingling sensation often interpreted as a sexual orgasm.

When used medically, narcotics are given orally or by intramuscular injection. When abused, they may be smoked, sniffed (**"snorting"**), or self-administered by either subcutaneous (**"skin-popping"**) or intravenous (**"mainlining"**) injection.

Unlike ethyl alcohol and the barbiturates, the opioids, even when they are abused, usually do not cause physical damage to the brain, liver, or heart. Unlike the stimulant drugs—cocaine and amphetamine—the opioids do not induce psychotic experiences or increase susceptibility to seizures.[4] The health problems so often associated with the abuse of narcotics are typically related to the neglect of personal health and safety, as detailed later in this chapter.

Narcotics of Natural Origin

Included in this section are those opioids that are present in or produced by nature, that is, not artificial or synthetic in their origin.[5]

Opium

Known as the "mother drug" because it is the main source of nonsynthetic narcotics, **opium** is produced from the opium poppy, ***Papaver somniferum.*** Cultivated in many countries around the world, the poppy flower is grown in large quantities in Burma, Turkey, Thailand, Afghanistan, Laos, Pakistan, Mexico, and Colombia.

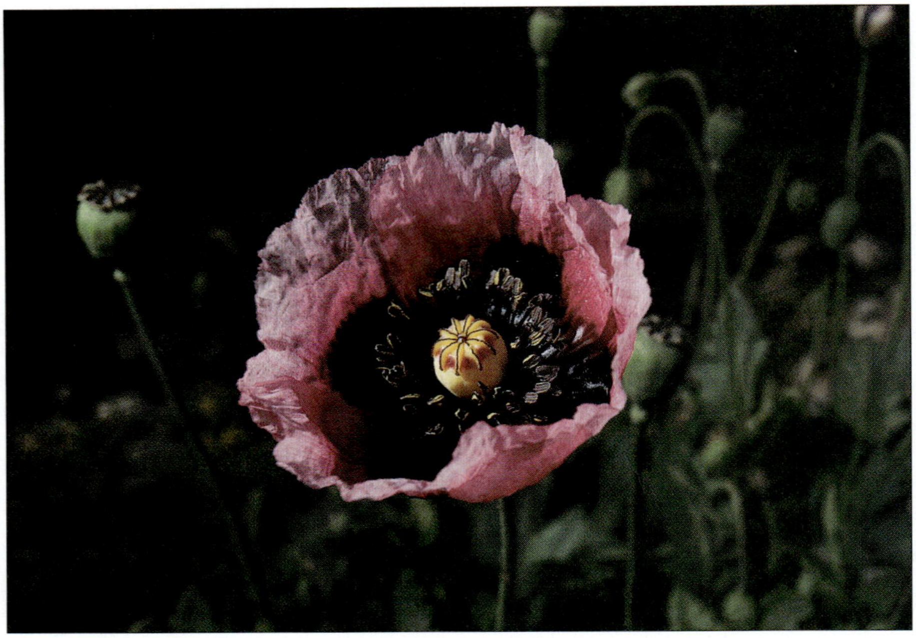

A close-up view of the poppy, Papaver somniferum, from which opium is produced. This particular poppy is the main source of nonsynthetic narcotics.

Opium is derived from the unripe poppy pod, which is slit with a knife. Milky fluid oozes from the seedpod, which is allowed to "bleed" overnight. Early the next day, the dried exudate is scraped off the leaves and air-dried to yield a brownish gum known as "crude" or "raw" opium. An alternate method of harvesting opium is the industrial poppy straw process, in which chemical substances known as alkaloids are extracted from the mature dried plant. This extract may be either a liquid, a solid, or a fine brown powder.

The dried raw opium or extract usually is smoked, with inhalation of its vapors. Sometimes, though, the crude opium is swallowed. Widely used throughout the world until the beginning of the twentieth century, opium is not often abused in America because of its strength of action and massive bulk, which interferes with trafficking. With current drugs of abuse that produce an even greater euphoria, opium seems to have lost its cultural popularity.

Only a small amount of opium is imported for making antidiarrheal preparations. Most of the legally imported opium gum and almost all of the illegal substances destined to enter America are chemically treated for the constituent alkaloids (basic nitrogenous compounds) of the "mother drug." Legal derivatives of opium include morphine, codeine, Dilaudid, and metopon, all of which have valid medical uses. The major illegal narcotic derived from opium is heroin.

Morphine

The chief alkaloid ingredient of opium, ranging from 4 percent to 21 percent concentration, is **morphine.** It is used medically as a sedative and an analgesic, being one of the most effective drugs known for relief of pain. Large doses have been used to provide anesthesia during heart surgery because morphine, unlike most anesthetics, has no depressant effect on the cardiovascular system. Sometimes morphine is also used to control post-operative pain and pain associated with cancerous conditions.

Manufactured in several different forms, morphine is usually available in tablets and injectable preparations. The white crystal form is illegal. When taken orally, morphine has a bitter taste. It is more frequently administered by subcutaneous, intramuscular, or intravenous injection; the latter method is most frequently used by morphine-dependent individuals.

Known on the street by names like "Big M," "Miss Emma," "white stuff," "M," "encel," "hocus," "unkie," "hard stuff," and "morpho," morphine is often obtained for illegal use through theft, diverted shipments, and counterfeit prescriptions. Used nonmedically, morphine produces a typical "high," a feeling of extreme well-being, and then drowsiness. Tolerance and physical dependence develop rapidly among users, depending upon the frequency of use and potency or dosage of the drug consumed.

A small portion of the morphine obtained from opium is used for medical purposes. Most of this opioid is converted to several other medically useful drugs, particularly codeine and hydromorphone (Dilaudid), both described in this chapter.

Codeine

Occurring naturally as a minor alkaloid ingredient in raw opium, **codeine** is more often produced from morphine. In terms of chemical structure, codeine is closely related to morphine, although it is less potent and thus produces less pain relief, sedation, and respiratory depression.

Codeine is marketed in tablets for oral administration, in combination with aspirin or acetaminophen (Tylenol), in liquid preparations (Actifed with codeine) for relief of coughs (**antitussives**), and in injectable forms. Potentially addictive, codeine infrequently causes physical dependence when taken under medical supervision for only a short time. As such, it is the most widely used naturally occurring narcotic in medical practice.

Particularly effective as an antitussive, codeine is sold in over-the-counter, nonprescription combination cough products in some states.[6] Such availability without a prescription demonstrates the **exempt narcotic** status of codeine. An exempt narcotic is a drug preparation that contains a narcotic substance but can be purchased without a physician's written prescription. Most states require that the purchaser be an adult, have personal identification, and sign a special record book at the pharmacy when buying such a drug. An exempt narcotic preparation usually contains less than one grain of narcotic per fluid ounce of the liquid product.

As an exempt narcotic, codeine has been somewhat appealing to certain drug abusers. The syrup form of codeine, as found in cough syrup and Tylenol #4 medicine, is frequently used in combination with gluthethimide (Doriden), a nonbarbiturate sedative-hypnotic. Known as "hits," this mixture is used by those who want the effects of heroin but are reluctant to use drugs intravenously.

Some people who are dependent on "harder" drugs make the rounds of drugstores to purchase large quantities of codeine-containing cough suppressants when other opioids are temporarily not available on the street. The liquid is then boiled down until only a white, powdery residue remains that is eventually prepared for injection into a vein. Others drink the codeine cough syrup to experience a "drunken glow," the result of a slight narcotic experience in combination with alcohol—nearly 40 percent of the total mixture. Such drug abuse has declined somewhat, due largely to codeine's removal from its exempt status in several states.

Thebaine

One of the minor components of opium, *thebaine* is chemically similar to morphine and codeine. However, thebaine has stimulant effects rather than depressant ones, and it is not used in this country for medical purposes. It is converted into various other medically important compounds, including codeine, naloxone, and etorphine. Thebaine is controlled in Schedule II of the Controlled Substances Act.

Semisynthetic Narcotics

This section describes some of the more significant semisynthetic or half-synthetic opioids, substances that have been derived indirectly from a natural narcotic by modifying the chemicals contained in opium.

Hydromorphone

Commonly known as Dilaudid, *hydromorphone* is a semisynthetic narcotic analgesic derived from morphine. Marketed in tablet and injectable form, it is shorter-acting and more sedative than morphine. Its potency is two to eight times as great as that of morphine. Therefore, it is a highly abusable drug, often illegally procured through fraudulent prescription or theft.

Oxycodone

Synthesized from thebaine, *oxycodone* is similar to codeine but more potent. It also has a higher dependence potential. Taken orally, it is marketed in combination with other drugs, especially Percodan, for the relief of pain. Drug abusers often take Percodan by mouth or dissolve Percodan tablets in water, filter out insoluble material, and then "mainline" the active drug.

Etorphine

Derived from thebaine, *etorphine* is more than a thousand times as potent as morphine in its analgesic, sedative, and respiratory depressant effects. As such, its potential for human use is distinctly limited by the danger of overdose. One form of this semisynthetic narcotic is used by veterinarians to immobilize large, wild animals. Another thebaine derivative, diprenorphine, counteracts the effects of etorphine. The production and distribution of both drugs are strictly regulated by the Controlled Substances Act.

Heroin

Of all the narcotics, heroin accounts for nearly 90 percent of the opioid abuse in the United States. With consumption having doubled since the mid-1980s, it is now estimated that there are over 300,000 occasional users and over 800,000 chronic users reflecting the big comeback heroin is making.[7]

Glamorized by the entertainment and fashion industries, "heroin chic" is frequently portrayed as safe, "cool," and trendy.[8] Though most users are still long-time addicts who inject, new heroin users are increasingly young and usually snort the drug.[9]

One of the more powerful dependency-producing drugs, **heroin** is a semisynthetic drug made by treating morphine with acetic anhydride to yield diacetylmorphine. In 1898 it was introduced into medical practice as a cough suppressant under the name *heroin.* This name is derived from a German word meaning long or powerful. Heroin's impact on individuals and society is described appropriately by this original meaning.

Characteristics of Heroin

Initially, the use of heroin in medical practice met with worldwide acceptance. There were fewer undesirable side effects than with morphine, and most people and physicians were unaware of heroin's potential for causing drug dependency. However, within twenty years, heroin had gained a bad reputation in the United States—a reputation evident in the slang words describing the drug: *junk, smack, scag, H,* and *hard stuff.*

Pure heroin is a white powder with a bitter taste. It may vary in color from white to dark brown due to impurities remaining from the manufacturing process or the presence of additives. Since 1924, its production and importation have been outlawed in the United States, where heroin is no longer used medically. Experiments with cancer patients to determine its possible use as a pain-relieving drug, however, may rehabilitate heroin's therapeutic value in the future.

The possession of heroin is illegal. Bought "on the street" from a "pusher" or dealer, heroin is invariably mixed or "cut" with other substances, including powdered milk, sugar, starch, quinine, and even strychnine and arsenic. Consequently, users seldom know precisely what they are buying.

More Potent Forms of Heroin

During the 1980s, a cheaper and more powerful form of heroin, known as "black tar" or "tootsie roll," became widely available throughout the United States. Resembling roofing tar, black tar is a crudely processed heroin that originates in Mexico. It is still sold on the street in extremely small pieces that can be "cut down" to a powder form. This new form of heroin ranges between 40 to 80 percent pure at the dealer level, a figure nearly forty times higher than regular heroin of an earlier time.

Then by 1995, Colombia, a nation in South America, emerged as the foremost heroin pipeline into the United States. Averaging a purity of about 63 percent, Colombian heroin soon became widely available, cheap enough to buy, and pure enough to snort or smoke. One particular variety named Red Rum—"murder" spelled backwards—had a purity of up to 70 percent. This is the heroin that claimed the famous musician, Jonathan Melvoin of the Smashing Pumpkins, who died of an injected overdose. Experienced addicts tend to snort or smoke this high purity heroin or use much less of the drug when injecting it.[10]

At almost the same time, a potentially even more dangerous form of heroin, known as "China White," was introduced into this country by secret Chinese "triads," or criminal societies.[11] With a purity of nearly 90 percent, China White is widely smoked or snorted. No longer confined to the inner city, use of China White has appeared in trendy metropolitan clubs where middle-class teenagers often snort heroin to counteract the effects of cocaine. Increasing numbers of college students reportedly snort heroin to relax when they are anxious about exams.[12]

Smokers and snorters do not need a syringe to get a fix, and thus they avoid the fear of HIV infection and AIDS often associated with a "dirty" needle.

New heroin users have a rather positive image of this drug, tend to look down on heroin injectors and crack users, and do not identify with the addicts of their parents' generation.[14] They invari-

At Issue

Should intravenous (IV) drug abusers be allowed to exchange dirty needles for new ones to reduce the spread of AIDS?

Point: HIV infection and AIDS are widespread among drug addicts who inject cocaine or heroin. According to the National Commission on AIDS, a majority of female AIDS cases are linked to IV drug use; a third of AIDS cases are related to IV drug use; and a growing number of male AIDS cases are directly associated with IV drug use. The individuals behind these statistics transmit HIV to one another by sharing blood-contaminated needles and syringes. Allowing IV drug abusers to exchange dirty needles for new, clean ones is an enlightened, simple, compassionate, and effective way of reducing the spread of a potentially fatal disease. Such exchange programs enable the needle distributors to gain the confidence of drug users, who might then respond to invitations or encouragement to get treatment.

The continuing uncertainty about laws restricting the possession or delivery of drug paraphernalia, including syringes, serves as a barrier to preventing HIV infection; and increases the likelihood of needle sharing and the further transmission of the AIDS-causing virus.*

*Scott Burris, David Finucane, Heather Gallagher, and Joseph Grace, "The Legal Strategies Used in Operating Syringe Exchange Programs in the United States," *American Journal of Public Health,* Vol. 86, No. 8 (August, 1996): 1161–1166.

Counterpoint: Wake up, you dreamers! Needle-exchange programs should be forbidden, because they are equivalent to government's endorsement of illegal drug use. There is only limited evidence that such programs are effective; even if they could prevent needle sharing, this so-called prevention approach will not reduce the spread of HIV virus from IV drug users to people who do not use drugs. Today, AIDS is being spread increasingly in the United States by heterosexual intercourse, primarily through transmission of the HIV virus from IV drug users to their sexual partners. To be blunt, clean needles will never alter irresponsible sexual behavior. Force these IV drug abusers into treatment. Giving them clean needles only interferes with their movement into treatment programs. Providing clean needles to intravenous drug users sends the wrong message and might even encourage current nonusers to become IV drug users.*

*The federal government's National Drug Control Policy has taken the position that federal funds should be spent on treating addicts for long term benefits rather than focusing on short term, harm reduction methods like needle exchange programs. The government is also concerned that needle exchange programs are usually located in disadvantaged minority neighborhoods where these programs tend to increase violence, crime, and gang activity.[13]

Box 6.1 New-Wave Narcotics

Heroin appears to be making a big comeback among Americans. Some young people are scared by the devastating effects of crack cocaine and choose heroin instead. Others prefer the mellower high and cheaper cost of heroin in comparison with crack. With high-purity heroin available at "bargain basement" prices, snorting or sniffing is "in," while injecting heroin is on the decline. The needle is "out," due to the threat of contracting HIV and AIDS.

But an alarming number of drug abusers also dabble in "new-wave" narcotics—esoteric combinations of two or more psychoactive drugs, one of which is an opioid. Some of these new-wave narcotics are identified here.

Narcotic	Used in Combination With	Anticipated Effects	Common or Street Name
Codeine (from Empirin #4 and Tylenol #4)	Doriden (a CNS depressant)	• Euphoria • Sedation	Loads, Four Doors, Hits
Talwin (partial narcotic antagonist with analgesic effect)	Pyribenzamine (an antihistamine)	• Heroin-like rush with prolonged euphoria	T's and Blues
Heroin	Cocaine (a CNS stimulant)	• Smoother stimulating effect • Reduced excitability after crashing	Speedball, Goofball, Dynamite, Hot Rocks
Heroin	Marijuana (a sedative/ psychedelic)	• Euphoria • Relaxation • Pain reduction	Atom Bomb, Dusting
Morphine	Cocaine (a CNS stimulant)	• Smoother stimulating effect • Reduced excitability after crashing	C & M
Heroin	Morphine (a narcotic) and cocaine (a CNS stimulant)	• Smoother stimulating effect • Reduced excitability after crashing	Cottonbrothers

ably begin with snorting, but often progress to the more efficient method of injection, especially when tolerance begins to progress.

There is little doubt that the increased purity and low cost of white heroin have led to a general increase in usage and to a sudden rise in heroin-related emergencies at the nation's hospitals. Due to this drug's extremely high purity, it is fairly certain that overdoses are likely to be fatal. Users are also mixing heroin with other drugs, such as crack; marijuana; alcohol; methamphetamine; and even the so-called "club drugs," including MDMA, ketamine, 2 C-B, and GHB (see box 6.1). Whether it is a lethal combination of heroin and other drugs or merely the wild fluctuations of the narcotic's purity, between 3,000 and 4,000 people die of heroin overdoses each year.

The Heroin "Rush"

Whether by "skin-popping" or "mainlining," or by snorting or smoking, once heroin reaches the brain, it quickly binds to the special opioid receptors found in many brain regions and in other parts of the body. Activation of these receptors in the pleasure circuit—nerve cells in the limbic system's nucleus accumbens, the frontal region of the cerebral cortex, and the brain stem—causes an intense, brief period of euphoria, known as the **"rush."**[15]

As it binds to opioid receptors in other parts of the brain and body, heroin can also stop diarrhea, slow breathing, and cause nausea and vomiting. Activation of the opioid receptors found in neurons controlling breathing may cause these nerve cells to slow down or even stop working, resulting in death.

In addition to the euphoria of the rush, common reactions may include reddening of the face and constriction of the pupils of the eyes. Emotionally, there is a feeling that everything is fine. Some people also report a reduction of aggressive tendencies, depressed appetite and sex drive, and a generalized decline in the level of physical activity. Tensions are reduced; worries disappear; the sharp edges of reality are dulled. Eventually, a period of stuporous inactivity follows. This calm, tranquil, carefree, forgetful state of mind, the so-called "high," lasts from three to six hours. It is the allure of heroin and the undoing of the heroin user who takes the drug with any regularity.

Heroin Dependency

Within several weeks of continued use, the drug taker often needs to increase the dose to achieve the desired "high." This change, which develops rapidly, indicates that tolerance has been established. Often the individual no longer experiences euphoria but is compelled to continue taking the drug to prevent withdrawal. Now the user has become physically dependent on the drug.

Eight to twelve hours after the last dose is taken, withdrawal symptoms appear. Perspiration, tearing, tremors, chills, diarrhea, nausea, and sharp abdominal and leg cramps occur and become progressively worse for two or three days. After a week, the heroin abuser is free of withdrawal symptoms, but minor depression and insomnia may last for several months.

Although the withdrawal process is painful, death from withdrawal occurs only in extreme cases. If a fetus has been drugged sufficiently while still in its heroin-using mother's uterus, the newborn infant will likely experience the heroin withdrawal process. Such withdrawal symptoms may last several weeks or months. Many babies so afflicted eventually die.

Potential hazards associated with abusing narcotics are related to the specific opioid used, its source, potency, dose, and the way it is used. The physical dangers so often reported with heroin and other opioid abuse are more closely related to the unhealthy lifestyle many addicts lead. Diseases, injuries, and deaths commonly observed are caused by uncertain dosage levels, use of unsterile needles and other paraphernalia or contaminants in the drug (see box 6.2).

There is no doubt that heroin in particular and opioids in general are drugs capable of inducing a powerful drug dependency. Therefore, the assumption is widely held that anyone who uses heroin with any frequency will inevitably develop tolerance to and physical dependence on the drug.

This assumption has been challenged by the discovery of people who have used heroin with some regularity and have avoided drug dependency. Apparently these occasional users (referred to as "chippers") space out their drug intake and limit their doses to extremely small amounts of low-potency heroin.

Studies of Vietnam War veterans indicate that nearly three-quarters of those who used heroin at least five times while in Vietnam became addicted, but among veterans who used heroin in the United States after their return from Vietnam, only 28 percent became drug dependent. Some analysts believe the difference in the percentage of addiction was due to the high purity of heroin in Vietnam (nearly 90 percent). At the time of these studies, heroin in the United States had a purity of only about 5 percent. However, others contend that the "peacetime drug setting" of America versus the "wartime setting" of Vietnam was the important factor.

It is apparent that the development of narcotics dependency is related to a number of factors: frequency of drug use, potency of the drug, dosage consumed, the setting of use, and the mind-set of the user. In some cases, physical dependency to heroin develops several months, or as long as a year and a half, after "experimental" use begins.

Unlike the physical trauma frequently associated with the abuse of alcohol and barbiturates, continuing use of heroin and the other opioids does not damage the brain, liver, or heart.[16] However, heroin abusers are subject to numerous life-endangering conditions, because they tend to neglect their health, fail to detect common signs of illness, and frequently resort to intravenous injecting of opioids with shared needles. Commonly observed problems include the transmission of HIV, AIDS, viral hepatitis (hepatitis B virus), inflammation of the heart's lining, blood poisoning, tetanus, malaria, syphilis, blood vessel inflammation, heart valve infection, malnutrition, festering sores on the arms and legs, the toxic effects of overdose, withdrawal syndrome, and the rare possibility of degenerative nerve damage.

Despite these problems, the heroin-dependent individual eventually has but two concerns: fear of running out of the drug and fear of running out of accessible veins for injection.

Box 6.2 Opioid Overdose and First-Aid Treatment

Overdose of an opioid is usually the result of an addict's accidental injection of impure "street heroin," for instance, rather than any inherent properties of the drug itself. Accustomed to specific doses of impure "street heroin," opioid-dependent individuals sometimes unknowingly buy drug packets that have not been "cut" as much as usual. Injection of the so-called right dose becomes an overdose. Such accidental overdosing with high-potency heroin occasionally leads to death.

Symptoms of Opioid Overdose

Stuporous condition, or deep sleep, cannot be aroused easily

Low respiration (slow or shallow breathing)

Blueness of lips and skin

Pinpoint pupils of the eyes

Needle marks on the body

First-Aid Treatment of Opioid Overdose

Try to keep the overdose victim awake by talking

Maintain an open airway

Give mouth-to-mouth resuscitation if needed

Place the unconscious person on his or her side

Monitor the unconscious person's vital signs—breathing, pulse, temperature

Call paramedic/ambulance service for transportation to a medical facility

Synthetic Narcotics

In contrast with opioids derived directly or indirectly from sources of natural origin, synthetic narcotics are produced entirely within the laboratory. Some of these are described in the next sections. Research has been accelerated to find a drug that retains the analgesic properties of morphine but avoids the dangers of tolerance and physical dependence. To date, no such drug has been synthesized that is not susceptible to abuse.

Meperidine

The first synthetic narcotic produced was *meperidine*. Chemically unlike morphine, it does resemble the opium extract in its analgesic potency. It is used widely under the brand name Demerol for the relief of moderate to severe pain. Available in pure form and in products containing other medications, it is administered orally or by injection. Tolerance and dependence occur with long-term use, and large doses can result in convulsions.

A designer analogue of meperidine, known for several years as MPPP, was formulated again in 1982 by an "underground" chemist. However, during its production, the derivative of Demerol was accidentally contaminated with a toxic by-product, named **MPTP** (1-methyl-4-phenyl-4-propionoxypiperidine). This Demoral look-alike, sold in the "street market" as China White, new heroin, or synthetic Demoral, is not easily distinguished from authentic heroin or cocaine.

MPTP is extremely neurotoxic (nerve damaging) and attacks the part of the brain that regulates movement, resulting in permanent symptoms like those of Parkinson's disease. Use of this "designer heroin" causes arthritis-like symptoms at first, such as stiffness, tremors, body seizures, and difficulty in speaking, and eventually results in a stiffening body paralysis.

MPTP and other meperidine derivatives have been sold not only as designer heroin, but also as methamphetamine, PCP, and cocaine (see box 6.3). Two other synthetic narcotics, **methadone** and **LAAM,** will be described later in the chapter under "Maintenance Therapy."

Box 6.3 Designer Drugs *Narcotics*

For many years, illegal drugs have been defined in terms of their chemical formulas. To avoid such legal restrictions and outwit officials of the Drug Enforcement Administration, so-called underground chemists have modified slightly the molecular structure of certain illegal drugs to produce chemical variants or analogues known as "designer drugs." (An analogue is a substance derived from a chemically similar compound.) These chemically engineered analogues can be several hundred times stronger than the drugs they are designed to imitate.

The narcotic analogues—now outlawed—can cause symptoms such as those seen in Parkinson's disease: uncontrollable tremors, drooling, impaired speech, paralysis, and irreversible brain damage.

Type	Street Name	Appearance	Methods of Use
Analogues of of fentanyl (narcotic)	Synthetic heroin "China White"	White powder resembling heroin	Inhaled through nasal passages Injected
Analogues of of meperidine (narcotic)	Synthetic heroin MPTP (new heroin) MPPP PEPAP	White powder	Inhaled through nasal passages Injected

Propoxyphene

Another close relative of methadone, *propoxyphene* was first marketed in 1959 under the trade name **Darvon.** It has been used for the relief of mild to moderate pain, with millions of prescriptions written each year. Darvon is somewhat less dependence-producing than other opioids and also less effective as an analgesic. This prescription drug is available in propoxyphene-only preparations and in combination with acetaminophen (Darvocet, Wygesic), and with aspirin and caffeine (Darvon Compound-65).

An early controversy has continued about Darvon's effectiveness as an analgesic. When it was first manufactured in 1957, Darvon was widely promoted as a safe, nonaddicting substitute for codeine.[17] Since then, research indicates that propoxyphene is no more effective than aspirin or codeine and is much more dangerous than aspirin. Darvon has the potential for addiction and overdose and poses a special threat for the elderly.[18]

Because propoxyphene can be misused and abused, and due to its dependency-producing qualities and potential for accidents and overdoses, Darvon has been placed in Schedule IV of the Controlled Substances Act.

Fentanyl

In 1968 another synthetic narcotic, **fentanyl,** was introduced as an intravenous analgesic-anesthetic. It is used in surgical procedures for the control of pain because of its almost immediate and short duration of action—about one to two hours.[19]

Marketed under the trade name Sublimaze, fentanyl is an extremely potent drug. A dose of just 0.1 milligram is approximately equivalent in pain-killing activity to 10 milligrams of morphine.[20] In a medical setting, fentanyl is used only by injection. Although there are no legally produced oral forms of this drug, there is evidence that some individuals abuse fentanyl by smoking or snorting special preparations of this substance.

Due to fentanyl's extreme potency, there is considerable risk of respiratory depression and a significant decrease in blood pressure and heart rate resulting in death. It has been reported that some addicts have died so rapidly after using this drug that when they are found, the needle was still in their arms.[21]

By manipulating the chemical structure of fentanyl, so-called street chemists have created numerous designer heroins or fentanyl analogues, including alpha-methyl fentanyl and 3-methyl fentanyl. Each new "designer" analogue differs in potency, toxicity, and length of action. While each fentanyl derivative mimics heroin's rush and tends to delay or forestall withdrawal symptoms, certain potent analogues have caused sporadic outbreaks of death from overdosage.[22]

Fentanyl derivatives have been sold to unsuspecting drug users under the names "China White," "synthetic heroin," "Mexican Brown," and "Persian White." Available in powder form, these designer drugs are often diluted with lactose, powdered sugar, or mannitol. Sometimes the fentanyl analogues are mixed with heroin to improve somewhat poor quality or with cocaine. The analgesic potency of designer heroin ranges from 200 to 3,000 times stronger than morphine in the human body (see box 6.3).

Endogenous Opioids

Investigations into the chemistry of brain function revealed that many natural body chemicals—identified as neurotransmitters in chapter 3—serve as communicators by which certain nerve cells send and receive messages. Some of these endogenous ("made-within the body") chemicals were found to act in much the same way as opioid drugs.

During the 1970s, researchers discovered that morphine appeared to bind or attach to natural receptors (specific sites) in the brain.[23] If such receptors exist, it was reasoned, the body must be producing some type of morphinelike chemicals. After intense investigation, scientists discovered natural bodily substances resembling morphine that produce morphinelike effects—euphoria and pain reduction—and also use the same brain receptors as morphine.[24] This linkage of naturally occurring neurochemicals with opioidlike effects provided a new, physical basis for understanding how psychoactive drugs can cause addiction or dependence.

Pertinent research findings related to the **endogenous opioids** (the "morphine within") are:

1. The human brain and gastrointestinal tract were found to contain specific **receptors** or sites where opioid molecules attach to produce the characteristic effects of narcotics. These receptors appear to be concentrated in the limbic system and the thalamus with its associated structures—areas of the brain involved with pain perception, emotions, and behavior control.
2. Opioid receptors were originally thought to be attachment sites for some naturally occurring, internal bodily substance resembling a narcotic. Eventually, such substances were extracted from the brain and the pituitary gland and were named **enkephalins** (from the Greek word meaning "in the head").
3. Shortly after enkephalins were identified, another pituitary extract was also found to have opioid activity. This chemical was named **endorphin** (the "morphine within"). It was found to be forty times more powerful than the enkephalins and 100 times more potent than morphine.

   The term *endorphin* is used to describe any natural, internal bodily substance that has opioid-like activity, including the enkephalins and dynorphins, another form of endogenous opioids. These particular endorphins are compounds consisting of amino acids, the building blocks of proteins.[25]
4. These opioid neurotransmitters are thought to be used by the brain to control and moderate emotions.
5. The endorphins (endogenous opioid peptides) can be displaced from the brain by opioid drugs (heroin and morphine) that use the same receptor sites in the brain to reduce an individual's awareness of pain.

With the identification of many endorphins, scientific inquiry has been accelerated in an attempt to explore the likely relationship between these internal morphinelike substances and several scientifically puzzling conditions, as indicated:

Drug dependence might be an endorphin deficiency. Within a theoretical framework, endorphins act somewhat like hormones (body-regulating chemicals in the blood) in a negative feedback relationship with the pituitary gland. When the concentration of a particular circulating hormone is high, the pituitary gland that triggers the release of the hormone stops production. But when the concentration of that same hormone falls below necessary levels, the pituitary speeds up production again to supply the need.

Applied to drug dependence, this theory suggests that the use of morphine or heroin effectively ties up the receptor sites and fools the natural feedback system. Natural endorphin production is halted. When the external narcotic is also withdrawn, the system experiences an acute shortage of endorphins that cannot be quickly supplied by the manufacturing centers. Thus narcotic withdrawal symptoms appear. It seems likely, then, that long-term use of any narcotic would produce an endorphin shortage. If so, this deficiency could explain the craving for a particular narcotic that exists even after a drug-dependent person goes through withdrawal.

Pain is typically relieved; that is, an individual is enabled to tolerate pain better by the use of some narcotic drug. Endorphins also have potent analgesic effects. Perhaps the endorphins are one's private, internal supply of morphine that is released to alleviate severe pain associated with shock or trauma, including emotional stress.

Placebo relief of pain may be produced by the release of endorphins that act as neurotransmitters on nerve cells to deaden pain. This effect occurs when a pharmacologically inert substance is given to a person instead of an active drug.

Acupuncture, an ancient Chinese procedure for reducing pain and treating various diseases by the insertion of extremely fine needles into the body, might produce its analgesic effect when the inserted needles trigger the brain's production of endorphins.

Schizophrenia, other mental illnesses, and even specific behavioral roles, may be the result of altered endorphin production and function. Though this view is still controversial, some researchers believe that certain symptoms of schizophrenia may be due to either an excess or a deficiency of endorphin activity. Some endorphins have caused hallucinations and are possibly an important factor contributing to a variety of mental illnesses and abnormal mental functioning.

Sexual activity might be related to endorphins that function as regulators of

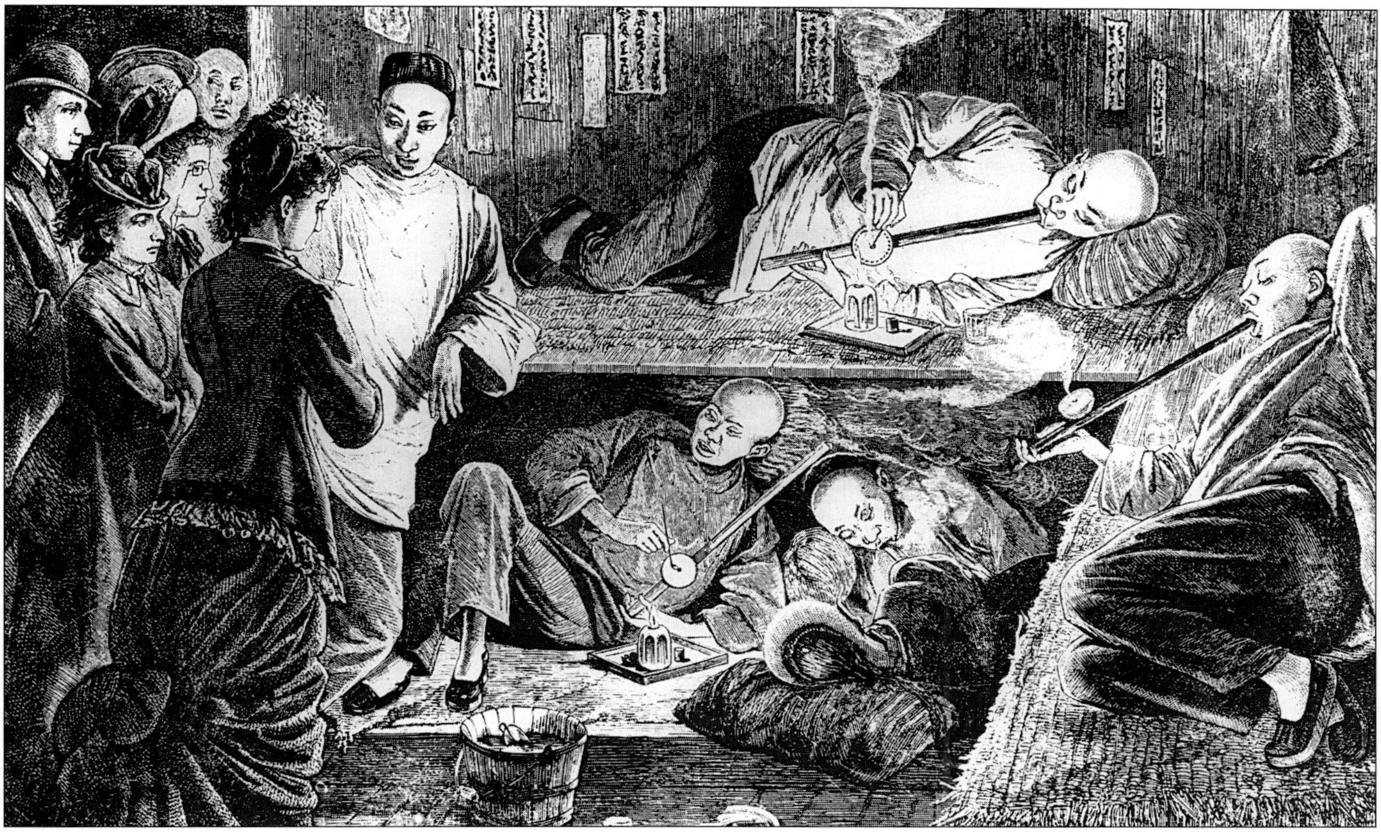

The pursuit of the poppy for recreational purposes is not of recent origin. Shown here are some citizens of San Francisco as they observe newly arrived Chinese immigrants in a popular opium den on Kearney Street in 1878.

The Bettmann Archive

sexual behaviors. People who possess high levels of endogenous (internal) opioids will probably be sexually inactive, but those with low levels should, according to this view, be highly sexual.

The **natural "high"** of exercise is likely the result of increased production of endorphins. People who exercise vigorously often experience a feeling of elation similar to a druglike high. This perceived condition of euphoria is known among joggers as "runner's high" and occurs with regular, sustained exercise.

Researchers relate physical conditioning with increased blood levels of endorphins. Although still somewhat controversial, these findings suggest that daily exercise (e.g., jogging and running) can be addictive. Joggers frequently complain of unsettled feelings and being out-of-sorts when they miss their daily "fix" of exercise. Without their sustaining endorphins, they experience withdrawal symptoms from the "morphine within." Upon resuming their regular exercise, the joggers' moods and emotions seem to improve with elevation of their endorphin levels.

Continuing scientific investigations suggest that endorphins are fundamental to normal physiological functioning. Endorphins are thought to influence our "appetite clocks"; reproductive hormone cycles; the onset of puberty; pregnancy and labor; and even esthetic and emotional experiences of thrills, laughter, and tears.[26]

Historical and Legal Perspectives

The pursuit of the poppy for recreational and medical purposes is not of recent origin. Opium use dates back to at least 3000 B.C., when ancient Egyptians derived significant benefits from their "joy plant." It is likely that early Greeks, Romans, and Arabians were aware of the healing power and the addicting quality of opium.

Over the centuries, the smoking of opium became widespread in much of the Middle East and Far East. By the seventeenth century, opium was firmly established in Europe. A profitable trade between the Orient and Great Britain developed around the exportation and importation of opium. This international arrangement was jeopardized temporarily by the Chinese emperors who attempted to prohibit the cultivation and use of opium through strict antiopium laws, and eventually by the Opium Wars of the nineteenth century.

Until the beginning of the nineteenth century, opium was the sole narcotic. Then in 1806 a German pharmacist, Friedrich Serturner, isolated the principal active ingredient of opium. After using this opium extract, he and his associates named the new drug morphine, after Morpheus, the Greek god of sleep. Although the dangers of opium dependence were well known, the hazards of morphine abuse were not recognized for many years. The new opium extract was hailed as a "wonder drug" in the treatment of pain and relief of diarrhea. Less than fifty years after its initial introduction, the abuse of morphine—and many other drugs—was enhanced by the perfection of the hypodermic syringe.

By the dawn of the twentieth century, the addictiveness of morphine was finally acknowledged. The "cure" had become worse than the diseases for which morphine had been taken. Then in 1898 the Bayer Company of Germany introduced a new "wonder drug." It was derived from morphine, supposedly nonaddicting, and yet more powerful than morphine as an analgesic. Heroin, as the new drug was named, was promoted as a treatment for morphine dependency and withdrawal. The medical profession was slow in recognizing the addictive nature of heroin, while opium and morphine addicts were switching rapidly to heroin as the "drug of choice." Heroin soon reigned supreme and unrestricted.

Box 6.4 The Narcotic Paradise

During much of the nineteenth century, the United States could properly be called the narcotic's paradise. Millions of people pursued the poppy and its natural and semisynthetic derivatives. The following examples demonstrate the prevalence of narcotic use and abuse during one phase of American history.

Opium was legal and a major ingredient in numerous patent medicines, such as "snake oil," teething syrups for infants, cough medicines, and painkillers.

Physicians legally prescribed opium, then morphine, and—by the end of the century—heroin.

Medications containing opium and morphine could be ordered by mail, if such preparations were not available at groceries and drugstores.

Children were routinely given opium-containing drugs to quiet them down and to treat colic (abdominal pain).

In an age when drinking alcohol was often considered unladylike or too embarrassing, women took narcotic medications in the form of elixirs for "female troubles" (menstrual cramping and menopausal discomfort).

Alcoholics desiring to give up liquor often took opium or morphine for a fast cure. They were quickly converted from being alcoholics to being "opioidolics."

Opium was legally imported, and later morphine was legally manufactured from opium.

Despite its dependency-producing potential, opium's reputation was favorable, as reflected in its nickname—God's Own Medicine, or "G.O.M."

In the United States, morphine was first used extensively during the Civil War (1861–65) as an analgesic for battle wounds. Morphine addiction was soon known as the "soldier's disease" because tens of thousands of soldiers eventually became drug dependent.

When first introduced on the American drug scene, heroin was thought to be a cure for morphine dependence.

Historical Sources: Edward M. Brecher and the editors of *Consumer Reports, Licit and Illicit Drugs,* pages 3–7, Consumers Union, Mt. Vernon, N.Y., 1972; and Michael Burkett, *The History and Use of Opiates: Facts, Myths, Realities.* Do It Now Foundation, Phoenix, Ariz., 1975.

Pure Food and Drug Act

The first nationwide response to the growing epidemic of narcotic abuse in America was the passage of the original **Pure Food and Drug Act** of 1906. This law prohibited interstate commerce in misbranded and adulterated drugs. A particular target of the law was the secretly formulated "cure-all" patent medicines. Many of these nonprescription drugs contained either opium or morphine in combination with alcohol (see box 6.4). Now the drug makers would have to reveal the narcotic contents on the labels of their products and assure the purity of their medicines.

Harrison Narcotics Act

In 1914, the federal government officially entered the area of narcotics control with the enactment of the **Harrison Narcotics Act.**[27] This law established a mechanism of recordkeeping for the importation, manufacture, distribution, sale, and prescription of narcotic drugs. While this effectively outlawed the nonmedical use of heroin, physicians were still allowed to prescribe narcotics; and numerous over-the-counter medications containing small amounts of opium, morphine, heroin, and cocaine were permitted to be sold. Cocaine was considered to be a "stepping-stone" to heroin abuse, so it was mistakenly classified as a narcotic.

With the enactment of the Harrison Narcotics Act, dispensing narcotics to known addicts was forbidden. Clinics that had been established to provide opioid drugs to "registered addicts" on a maintenance or continuing dose level were closed within a few years. These policies effectively ended the medical profession's involvement in the treatment of drug dependency for nearly forty years.

Then, in 1924, the importation of heroin was outlawed. Deprived of medical sources for their supply of narcotics, addicts eventually turned to the black market and to crime to finance their drug dependency. Amazingly, the cultivation of the opium poppy in the United States was not banned by Congress until 1942.

During the decade of the national economic depression, the federal government constructed two narcotics "farms" for the compulsory treatment of criminals convicted of drug addiction. Both facilities also admitted patients on a voluntary basis. Under the direction of the Public Health Service, the hospital "farms" were established in Lexington, Kentucky (1935) and Fort Worth, Texas (1938). Treatment at these hospitals usually consisted of withdrawing the drug-dependent individual by giving progressively smaller doses of morphine. Such treatment was not usually successful, and many patients returned to addictive behavior soon after discharge.

Until new methods of treating drug dependency were developed in the 1960s, the federal government's policy toward drug abuse was to encourage public compliance with restrictive drug laws. This was to be accomplished by imposing high fines and severe prison sentences for first conviction. Increasingly, the United States relied on its criminal justice system to control and punish the narcotics user. Treatment and prevention concerns were largely ignored.

Comprehensive Drug Abuse Prevention and Control Act

The present era of drug law enforcement was spearheaded by a federal government "war on drug abuse" begun in the late 1960s. The **Comprehensive Drug Abuse Prevention and Control Act** of 1970 replaced the crazy-quilt pattern of criminal drug laws and became the legal foundation for reducing the consumption of illicit narcotic and nonnarcotic drugs. Under the provisions of the Controlled Substances Act portion of the legislation, psychoactive drugs were categorized into five schedules according to their presumed potential for abuse and their current acceptability in medical practice.[28]

Additionally, this legislation established mechanisms for reducing the availability of controlled drugs, procedures for bringing substances under control, penalties for the manufacture, distribution, and possession of controlled drugs, criteria for determining control requirements and prescription status, and international obligations for the control of specific drugs. Under the provisions of the Controlled Substances Act, the federal drug bureaucracy was restructured and expanded. The drug law-enforcement functions of the federal government have evolved through a series of bureaus, special offices, agencies, and administrations, and are under the Department of Justice.

Treatment of Narcotic-Dependent Individuals

Before 1900, the treatment for opium and morphine dependence consisted of managing the withdrawal syndrome through *detoxification.* In this process, the blood level of the opioid was gradually lowered by decreasing dosages of some opium-based patent medicine to wean addicted patients from the more potent opioid drug. Eventually both drugs were completely withdrawn from the body. Occasionally, patients were deprived of their drugs and then observed and restrained during the withdrawal process. This sudden withdrawal of a narcotic without medical treatment is often called the "cold turkey" method. The gooseflesh effect—one of the common withdrawal symptoms—resembles that of a plucked turkey.

Even during those "primitive days" of drug-abuse treatment, it was recognized by many that a permanent cure depended upon the reeducation of the patient's attitude after detoxification had been achieved. However, little attention was paid to the psychological and sociological aspects of the drug-dependence and drug-treatment processes. Until the full effects of the Harrison Narcotics Act were felt, many physicians and even some "walk-in" clinics supplied addicted patients with small "maintenance" doses of narcotics. Such treatment was eventually stopped as provisions of the new federal legislation were implemented.

When the federal government opened the two Public Health Service Hospitals for narcotic-dependent individuals in the 1930s, the major therapeutic effort was the "institutional-aftercare model of treatment." This therapy mandated inpatient hospitalization in a drug-free environment and detoxification. Emphasis was then placed on rebuilding physical health status and providing vocational rehabilitation services, counseling, and various social services. After completing a prescribed time of institutional care in the hospital, the patient returned to the non-medical community but was closely supervised to ensure abstinence from narcotics. This supervision was conducted through a parole system in which former patients reported at regular intervals to designated officials.

Several therapies are available for the modern treatment of opioid dependence. These include detoxification; pharmacological treatments, involving maintenance therapy and the use of narcotic antagonists; therapeutic communities; psychotherapy; self-help groups; and acupuncture. Each of these major treatments is described in the following sections.[29]

Detoxification

Unless an addict is to be placed on a so-called maintenance program, the first and basic treatment is still *detoxification.* Defined as controlled withdrawal from an opioid under medical supervision, detoxification is only the first step in recovery from narcotics dependence.

Several drugs may be used in the detoxification process to help the addict become drug-free. Oral methadone, better known for its major role in maintenance therapy, is given in progressively smaller doses each day for one to two weeks. This procedure gradually lowers the blood level of the opioid drug and the tolerance threshold to prevent withdrawal from occurring. Another medication, levo-alpha-acetyl-methadol (LAAM), may also be employed for acute detoxification. Within a medical setting, clonidine is sometimes used for rapid detoxification, because this drug suppresses withdrawal symptoms. Although still controversial, buprenorphine shows promise as another drug that may be used in the detoxification of opioid-dependent individuals, and in maintenance therapy.

Maintenance Therapy

A somewhat controversial form of treating opioid dependence, maintenance therapy involves the continuing use of a drug similar in action to the drug for which it substitutes. In this section, two synthetic narcotics—methadone and LAAM—and narcotic antagonists are described in relation to maintenance therapy for heroin addiction and other opioid dependencies.

Methadone

A synthetic opioid, methadone was developed by German scientists during World War II as a substitute for morphine. In America, methadone was used initially in the detoxification of opioid-dependent patients.

However, methadone was first used on a large-scale basis in the mid-1960s when two physicians, Vincent Dole and Marie Nyswander, pioneered their **methadone maintenance** (continuing use of methadone) program. They recommended that minimal dosages of methadone be used on a regular basis to stabilize heroin patients. This would enable narcotic-dependent individuals to live as functioning members of society, in contrast to the alternating euphoria and desperation associated with illegal heroin use.

Unlike heroin, whose effects last about four hours, methadone's effects last approximately twenty-four hours. Methadone can be administered orally, while heroin is injected intravenously. In effect, methadone use reduces the addict's craving for a drug; eliminates the "rush" of sensation following injection of heroin, and the dangers associated with needles; and permits the patient to move toward conventional patterns of living and improved social functioning. Agencies providing such maintenance services also offer extensive counseling and life reeducation programs for the recovering addict.

During the first several weeks of maintenance treatment, patients visit a licensed or registered practitioner six days each week and take liquid oral doses of methadone under supervision. Gradual reduction of the methadone dose is encouraged, although abstinence from methadone is not always a primary goal.

Critics of maintenance programs view methadone as little more than a substitute of one addictive drug for another. Proponents of such therapy consider methadone maintenance as a lesser evil than heroin dependence. At the least, methadone permits the heroin addict to lead a fairly normal life without involvement in criminal activity. A number of studies have also shown that methadone maintenance programs indirectly help reduce the use of other drugs, such as alcohol and cocaine.[30]

LAAM

Levo-alpha-acetyl-methadol (LAAM) is only the second synthetic narcotic drug approved by the Food and Drug Administration to treat heroin and other opioid addictions through outpatient clinic maintenance programs. Like methadone, LAAM blocks the "highs" of other opioids and suppresses the symptoms of withdrawal, such as increased blood pressure and temperature, rapid heartbeat, gooseflesh, runny nose, tremors, insomnia, vomiting, abdominal cramping, restlessness, headaches, and drug craving.

The major advantage of LAAM is that its effects last for 48 to 72 hours after a dose is taken, compared to only 24 hours for methadone. Methadone must be given daily; LAAM use allows patients to reduce their clinic visits to only three per week. Consequently, with fewer required visits to a clinic, patients can lead a more normal life, and clinics have the option to treat more patients than with methadone.

In addition to methadone or LAAM maintenance therapy, licensed clinics and hospitals must also provide comprehensive medical services, counseling, vocational rehabilitation, and general treatment plans for narcotics-dependent patients.

Narcotic Antagonists

Research for an effective analgesic that is not dependency-producing led to the development of a class of chemical compounds known as **narcotic antagonists.** These drugs tend to block and even reverse the effects of narcotics and are therefore useful in treating opioid dependence. Some of these antagonists have analgesic activities, while others lack any narcotic action.

Naltrexone and *cyclazocine* chemically prevent heroin from having any effect on the opioid-dependent person, except the shortening of the withdrawal syndrome. Another antagonist, naloxone (Narcan) is used frequently for the treatment of narcotic poisoning, that is, as an antidote for opioid overdose.

A "partial antagonist," *pentazocine* (Talwin) provides effective analgesia but also possesses narcotic antagonistic activity. When taken orally, pentazocine has little potential for abuse. Intravenous self-administration, however, has led to instances of drug dependence. Nevertheless, the narcotic antagonists seem to be ideally suited for individuals who wish to leave therapies such as methadone maintenance and therapeutic communities.

Therapeutic Communities

The concept of drug-free **therapeutic communities,** directed by ex-addicts, was first established in 1958 as a basic treatment for narcotic and other drug dependencies. This approach to therapy was based on the belief that only former addicts could break through the shell of projection, denial, and lying common to the narcotics addict. The ultimate goal of such residential communities is to enable an addicted individual to develop a socially productive, drug-free lifestyle.

Synanon, the original such community, was founded in Los Angeles, California, by Chuck Dederich in 1958. Former addicts were used as role models for patients, who also participated in the process of group therapy.

In addition to encounter group therapy, these communities used tutorial learning sessions, remedial and formal education classes, assignment of jobs within the residence, and eventually "living-out" situations within the local community.

Before long, other residential therapeutic communities developed, such as Daytop Village, Phoenix House, and Gateway House. Some of the communities added degreed professionals to their staffs to complement the nondegreed former addicts and alcohol abusers.

However, these groups have maintained their hostility to the use of drugs for either "withdrawal" or "maintenance." Additionally, all have programs of varying lengths aimed at changing personal lifestyle patterns of self-destructive behavior. The basic goal of therapeutic

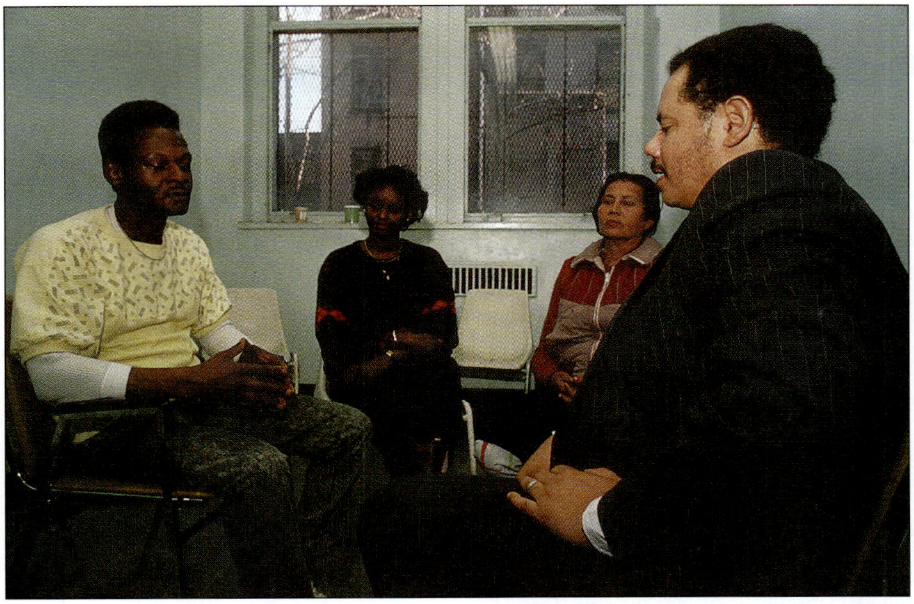

Group counseling and family therapy are important of the multimodality approach to the treatment of narcotics dependency. Pictured here are former heroin addicts who are now alcoholics in a counseling session at a methadone clinic.

© J. Griffin/The Image Works

communities is to bring about a change in living—specifically, abstinence from drugs; elimination of criminal behavior; and development of employable skills, self-reliance, and personal honesty.

Therapeutic communities have begun to serve criminal offenders and socially disadvantaged people, including the unemployed and newly arrived immigrants, in addition to drug abusers.

Psychotherapeutic Approaches

In general, **psychotherapy** is any form of treatment that uses psychological, rather than physical, means or medications in helping patients cope with various mental problems and mental disorders. Psychotherapeutic procedures feature verbal and nonverbal communication between a patient (or client) and a trained therapist. Goals of verbal therapy attempt to promote deeper self-understanding, provide insights into oneself and one's personal meaning, and bring disturbed and dysfunctional people into closer contact with the split elements of their mental lives. Such therapy tends to analyze and then resynthesize the self and also permits the individual to vent rage, frustration, and hate without fear of condemnation.

Psychotherapy has expanded beyond inner conflicts and unconscious drives and deals with interpersonal relationships and events outside the self. Several forms of group therapy and family therapy evolved from this new approach. For instance, an individual's problems are frequently viewed as being rooted in relationships with others, especially family members. Thus the entire family becomes involved in treatment. Role-playing, in which individuals assume different characters within the family for purposes of expression and interpretation of behavior, is one technique sometimes used in family therapy.

Narcotics Anonymous

Many self-help groups have been formed in which recovering addicts offer help to others seeking recovery from opioid dependence. In Narcotics Anonymous (NA), members employ a twelve-step program similar to that of Alcoholics Anonymous. On a voluntary basis, NA members meet regularly to promote and stabilize their own recovery. Founded in 1953, Narcotics Anonymous has close to four thousand groups in the United States and throughout the world (see box 6.5). For more information on Narcotics Anonymous, contact:

Narcotics Anonymous
World Service Office
P.O. Box 9999
Van Nuys, CA 91409

Acupuncture

A form of alternative medicine has emerged on the health care scene. The ancient art of acupuncture, as practiced in Asia for thousands of years, has generated considerable interest among physicians and dentists, and it might have some beneficial application in the treatment of heroin addiction.

According to the traditional Chinese definition, acupuncture is a procedure of treating certain diseases and alleviating pain by the insertion of extremely fine needles into the human body at specific points called loci. After initial insertion, which causes only a slight feeling of soreness and swelling, the stainless steel or copper needles are twisted for varying lengths of time by manual twirling or by electrical stimulation.

Since the introduction of acupuncture into the United States in the 1970s, scientific investigations have been undertaken to learn more about its therapeutic applications. Specifically, its use in reducing the pain of withdrawal from heroin has been researched, as has the procedure's seeming ability to relieve chronic pain and to produce surgical anesthesia. However, the precise mechanism of acupuncture's effectiveness has not been established.

A Multimodality Approach to Treatment

There is no single therapy for all opioid dependents. Also, the most important predictor of therapeutic success is time spent in treatment. Consequently, the individual addict must be matched with an individualized comprehensive therapeutic program to assure maximum effect. A

Box 6.5 Narcotics Anonymous

Narcotics Anonymous (NA) is a fellowship of men and women learning to live without drugs. The NA program is one of abstinence from all drugs, and its primary purpose is to bring the message of recovery to other addicts. Although NA is not a religious organization, its programs consists of a set of spiritual principles through which members recover from an apparently hopeless state of mind and body.

There is only one requirement for membership—the desire to stop using drugs. However, the members are guided along their way to recovery by the Twelve Steps of Narcotics Anonymous and the fellowship meetings where interacting with, talking with, and helping other addicts become the means of staying clean from drugs. Members believe that their addiction provides a common ground for understanding one another and for handling their painful past.

According to the Twelve Step program of NA, members admit their powerlessness over their addiction and come to believe that a power greater than themselves could restore them to sanity. Basic to recovery from addiction are two healing forces—forgiveness and gratitude—learned by practicing the Twelve Steps of Narcotics Anonymous. Forgiveness releases the grip others have on recovering addicts for real or imagined wrongs. Gratitude for being clean helps recovering addicts break old habits that promoted the continuing use of drugs.

Source: Modified from *Treatment to N.A.* **Hazelden Foundation,** Center City, Minn., 1988.

multimodality therapeutic approach, one with several components or aspects, would properly identify a full range of treatment services to meet the physical, mental, social, and spiritual needs of each patient. Such a comprehensive program might include the following:

Rapid admission to a health care facility on a voluntary or compulsory basis for necessary medical care, including emergency procedures.

Detoxification under supervision, with or without the use of other drugs to ease the discomfort of withdrawal.

Medical services, including tuberculosis skin testing, HIV counseling, and random urine testing for drugs of abuse. In maintenance programs, individualized dosage will be determined to control withdrawal symptoms without causing sedation or other effects of intoxication.

Extensive *vocational rehabilitation* leading to the acquisition of job skills that, in turn, will improve the self-image of the individual and provide the basis for independent living.

Transitional care in a "halfway house" or a residential center until the patient is ready for complete, full-time reentry into the community.

Long-term outpatient care provided in a hospital, public clinic, or day center, offering counseling, casework, psychotherapy, spiritual renewal, and the optional use of methadone maintenance or narcotic antagonists.

Provision of *emergency services* through "crash pads," information and referral centers, free clinics, telephone hot lines, and in hospital emergency rooms.

Chapter Summary

1. Narcotics are psychoactive drugs that induce sleep and relieve pain. Derived from the opium poppy plant or made synthetically to have narcotic drug actions, these drugs are also known as opioids or opiates.
2. Opioids are classified as natural substances, semisynthetic narcotics, synthetic products, and internal bodily substances (endogenous opioids) that have opioidlike effects within the human body.
3. Continuing use of opioids frequently leads to opioid dependence—inability to stop usage, constant or repeated intoxication, overdoses, tolerance, and withdrawal symptoms—often described as addiction.
4. Certain narcotics have legitimate medical uses. Morphine sedates and relieves pain; codeine acts as an antitussive; dihydromorphinone (Dilaudid) is a powerful analgesic; and methadone and LAAM are used in treating heroin-dependent individuals.
5. Heroin, a powerful, dependency-producing derivative of morphine, is considered the most frequently abused narcotic in America.
6. Many physical dangers associated with heroin abuse are related to uncertain dosage levels, use of unsterile needles for injection, contaminants in the heroin sample used, and the combination use of heroin with barbiturates and/or alcohol.
7. Heroin withdrawal, though not usually fatal, can be very painful and includes sweating, tearing, tremors, chills, diarrhea, nausea, sharp abdominal and leg cramps, mental depression, and insomnia.
8. Research has revealed the existence of natural, internal bodily chemicals (endogenous opioids) that have opioidlike effects. Known as endorphins, or "the morphine within" the head or body, these substances are thought to possibly be related to drug dependence (a deficiency of endorphins), toleration of pain, acupuncture, mental illness, and the natural "high" of vigorous exercise.
9. The widespread and indiscriminate therapeutic use of opium, morphine, and heroin (especially in "patent medicines"), in the nineteenth and early twentieth centuries in America, led to enactment of the Federal Pure

Food and Drug Act of 1906 and the Harrison Narcotics Act of 1914.

10. The legal foundation for reducing the illicit use of narcotic and nonnarcotic drugs is the Comprehensive Drug Abuse Prevention and Control Act of 1970. This drug law categorizes most psychoactive drugs into five schedules of decreasing restrictiveness according to their presumed potential for abuse and current acceptability in medical practice.
11. Treatment of opioid dependency might involve detoxification and psychotherapy, participation in therapeutic communities, admission to methadone or LAAM maintenance programs, and use of narcotic antagonists.
12. A multimodality approach to treating opioid dependency meets various physical, mental, social, and spiritual needs of addicts through rapid admission for medical care, supervised detoxification, placement in a halfway house or long-term outpatient clinic program, extensive counseling and psychotherapy, and a spiritual reawakening often achieved through participation in Narcotics Anonymous. Sometimes methadone or LAAM maintenance or narcotic antagonists are also employed.

World Wide Web Sites

Narcotics Anonymous World Services

www.wsoinc.com

National Institute on Drug Abuse Research Reports

www.nida.nih.gov/ResearchReports/Heroin/heroin.html

Review Questions and Activities

1. In what ways are the various narcotic drugs classified?
2. What are the major drug actions or effects of opioids?
3. Describe some of the legitimate therapeutic uses of the opioids—specifically, morphine, codeine, and methadone.
4. Distinguish between the heroin "rush" and the heroin "high."
5. Explain why there are so many physical dangers associated with heroin abuse, because heroin does not usually cause long-term physical damage or illness.
6. Interview a local police officer who specializes in narcotics investigations and related criminal offenses. Do narcotics violations involve illegal drugs other than the opioids? Are narcotics a significant part of the "drug scene" in your community or not? Explain.
7. Investigate the lives and works of poet Samuel Taylor Coleridge and author Thomas De Quincey and their involvement with laudanum (tincture of opium).
8. Report on one or more of the following literary works dealing with opioids: Dean Latimer and Jeff Goldberg's *Flowers in the Blood: The Story of Opium* (New York: Franklin Watts, 1981); Richard Ashley's *Heroin: The Myths and the Facts* (New York: St. Martin's Press, 1972); Arnold Trebach's *The Heroin Solution* (New Haven: Yale University Press, 1982); Jean Cocteau's *Opium: The Diary of a Cure* (New York: Grove Press, 1980); Nelson Algren's *The Man with the Golden Arm* (New York: Penguin, 1977); Peter Maas's *China White* (New York: Simon & Schuster, 1994); Jim Carroll's *The Basketball Diaries*, and *Forced Entries* (New York: Penguin Books, 1978 and 1987).
9. Explain how opioids such as methadone and LAAM can be used in the treatment of heroin dependency.
10. Discuss the probable relationship between the endorphins and drug dependence as well as general physiological functioning.
11. Describe the use of opium, morphine, and heroin as therapeutic drugs during the part of American history before the enactment of the Harrison Narcotics Act and the Comprehensive Drug Abuse Prevention and Control Act.
12. What factors are thought to play a part in the development of opioid dependency?
13. What are the unique features of a "therapeutic community" as a treatment approach to drug dependency?
14. How does a methadone maintenance program work as a treatment for heroin dependency?
15. What would likely happen if an individual no longer dependent on an opioid were to take a narcotic antagonist?
16. How does an opioid detoxification program differ from the "cold turkey" treatment?
17. Do you believe that psychotherapy and Narcotics Anonymous are effective means of reducing opioid abuse? Explain.
18. What opioidlike drugs have been identified as "China White" on the illegal street market?

References

1. Lester Grinspoon and James Bakalar, *The Harvard Medical School Mental Health Review: Drug Abuse and Addiction* (Boston: Harvard Mental Health Letter, 1993), 25.
2. Robert Julien, *A Primer of Drug Action*, 7th ed. (New York: W. H. Freeman and Company, 1995), 242, 252–53.
3. Terry Reisine and Garril Pasternak, "Opioid Analgesics and Antagonists," chap. 23 in *Goodman & Gilman's The Pharmacological Basis of Therapeutics*, 9th ed. (New York: McGraw-Hill Health Professions Division, 1996), 527.
4. Grinspoon and Bakalar, *The Harvard Medical School Mental Health Review*, 25.
5. Unless otherwise indicated, the basic description of the opioid drugs is derived from Drug Enforcement Administration, U.S. Department of Justice, *Drugs of Abuse* (Washington, D.C.: GPO, 1989), 12–23.
6. Editors of Consumer Reports Books, *The New Medicine Show* (Mount Vernon, N.Y.: Consumers Union, 1989), 27; and *Physicians' Desk Reference*, 50th ed. (Montvale, N.J.:

Medical Economics Company, 1996), 1067, 2888.

7. Office of National Drug Control Policy, *What American Users Spend on Illegal Drugs: 1988–1995* (Washington, D.C.: Office of National Drug Control Policy, 1997), 8.
8. Elizabeth Snead, "Its Dark, Nihilistic Chic Snakes into Pop Culture," *USA Today* (19 July 1996): 1D–2D.
9. John Leland, "The Fear of Heroin Is Shooting Up," *Newsweek* CXXVIII, no. 9 (26 August 1996): 55–56.
10. "Substance Abuse News Briefs: Musician's Overdose Increases Popularity of Killer Heroin," *Substance Abuse Report* XXVII, no. 15 (1 August 1996): 7.
11. Peter Maas, "The Menace of China White," *Parade,* (18 September 1994), 46.
12. Peter Maas, *China White* (New York: Simon & Schuster, 1994); and "Heroin's New Purity Creates New Customers: Snorters," *Substance Abuse Report* 24, no. 24 (15 December 1993), 1–3.
13. Drug Czar's Statement on Needle Exchange and Minority Communities (Wash., D.C., April 24, 1998); and Office of National Drug Control Policy, Comments on Needle Exchange Research (Aug. 20, 1997), Released by the Family Research Council.
14. U.S. Department of Health and Human Services, National Institute on Drug Abuse, *Epidemiologic Trends in Drug Abuse,* vol. 1: Highlights and Executive Summary, June, 1995.
15. Clinical Center Communications, National Institutes of Health, *Medicine for the Public: Drugs and the Brain* (Bethesda, Md.: National Institutes of Health, 1991), 9–11.
16. Reisine and Pasternak, "Opioid Analgesics and Antagonists," 545.
17. Jim Parker, *Darvon, Darvocet, and Other Prescription Narcotics* (Tempe, Ariz.: Do It Now, 1990), 2–3.
18. Sidney Wolfe, Rose-Ellen Hope, and Public Citizen Health Research Group, *Worst Pills Best Pills II* (Washington, D.C.: Public Citizen Health Research Group, 1993), 279–80.
19. Harold Doweiko, *Concepts of Chemical Dependency,* 2d ed. (Pacific Grove, Calif.: Brooks/Cole, 1993), 118–19.
20. *Physicians' Desk Reference,* 1307.
21. Doweiko, *Concepts of Chemical Dependency,* 119.
22. Julien, *A Primer of Drug Action,* 253.
23. Tibor Palfai and Henry Jankiewicz, *Drugs and Human Behavior* (Dubuque, Iowa: Brown & Benchmark, 1991), 153.
24. Andrew Weil and Winifred Rosen, *From Chocolate to Morphine,* rev. ed. (Boston: Houghton Mifflin, 1993), 28–29.
25. Grinspoon and Bakalar, *The Harvard Medical School Mental Health Review,* 24.
26. Janet Hopson, "A Pleasurable Chemistry," *Annual Editions: Drugs, Society, and Behavior 94/95* (Guilford, Conn.: Dushkin, 1994), 59–62. (Reprinted from *Psychology Today* July–August 1988, 29–30, 32–33.)
27. Bureau of Justice Statistics, U.S. Department of Justice, *Drugs, Crime, and the Justice System: A National Report* (Washington, D.C.: GPO, 1992), 80.
28. Ibid., 82, 84.
29. Barry Stimmel and the Editors of Consumer Reports Books, *The Facts about Drug Use: Coping with Drugs and Alcohol in Your Family, at Work, in Your Community* (New York: Haworth Medical Press, 1993), 155–70; "Pharmacological Treatments for Opiate Dependence: Methadone and More," *Substance Abuse Report* 25, no. 1 (1 January 1994): 1–2; "Maintenance Pharmacotherapy: Turning Addicts into Taxpayers," *Substance Abuse Report* 25, no. 12 (15 June 1994): 3; "How Pharmacotherapies Work: Agonists and Antagonists," *Substance Abuse Report* 25, no. 1 (15 June 1994): 4–5; and Dixie Farley, "New Drug Approval Approach Boosts Fight against Heroin Addiction," *FDA Consumer* 28, no. 9 (November 1994): 11–15.
30. J. S. Ball, and A. Ross, *The Effectiveness of Methadone Maintenance Treatment.* (New York: Springer-Verlag, 1991).

Chapter 7

Sedative-hypnotics and inhalants

KEY TERMS

Antianxiety Agent
Appetitive Drug Use
Barbiturate
Benzodiazepine
Bromide
BuSpar
Cross-Dependence
Cross-Tolerance
Dalmane
Escape-Avoidance Drug Use
Halcion
Hypnotic
Major Tranquilizer
Minor Tranquilizer
Potentiating Drug Interaction
Rauwolfia serpentina
Reserpine
Rohypnol
Sedative
Sedativism
Synergistic Drug Interaction
Valium
Xanax

chapter objectives

After you have studied this chapter, you should be able to do the following:

1. Define the key terms.
2. Describe the general pharmacological effects of the sedative-hypnotic drugs.
3. Identify the major types or families of psychoactive drugs that are central nervous system depressants and also produce a calming effect, induce euphoric intoxication, and promote sleep.
4. Explain why sedative-hypnotics are frequently misused and abused.
5. Differentiate between appetitive motivations and escape-avoidance motivations in relation to the use of sedative-hypnotics.
6. Describe the general characteristics shared by nearly all of the sedative-hypnotics.
7. Distinguish between potentiating and synergistic drug interactions.
8. Explain how automatism and maximum tolerance level may be contributing factors to barbiturate overdose.
9. Describe the process of barbiturate withdrawal.
10. Identify three nonbarbiturate sedative-hypnotics.
11. Discuss the brief history of the popularity of methaqualone (Quaalude) as a recreational drug.
12. Distinguish major tranquilizers from minor tranquilizers in terms of their drug actions.
13. Discuss the alleged controversies surrounding the use of antianxiety drugs in the general population.
14. Relate the use of Rohypnol to the increasing problem of "roofie rape."
15. Explain why many young people may become involved in the abuse of inhalants.
16. Identify three inhalants that have become popular among some adults.

Introduction

This chapter examines those psychoactive drugs that have been used to restore sleep to the sleepless and to calm the anxious patient—persistent goals of medical practice. When chemical alternatives to the opioids were developed, there was international praise for the new drugs that would help people achieve what the narcotics could not bring—tranquilization by day and relaxing sleep by night. It was not long, however, before the new sleep inducers and antianxiety agents were found to have serious and sometimes health-threatening characteristics.

When taking less than sleep-inducing doses of these new drugs, many people experienced a pleasant, euphoric state of intoxication, known as a "high." This calm "high," achieved through the "downer" drugs, soon became the focal point for millions of recreational drug abusers. At last, one could get drunk without booze!

These depressant, nonalcoholic, nonopioid drugs—barbiturates and nonbarbiturate sedative-hypnotics, the antianxiety minor tranquilizers, and the inhalants—are the major focus of this chapter, along with the people who use them and abuse them.

Drugs That Calm and Promote Sleep

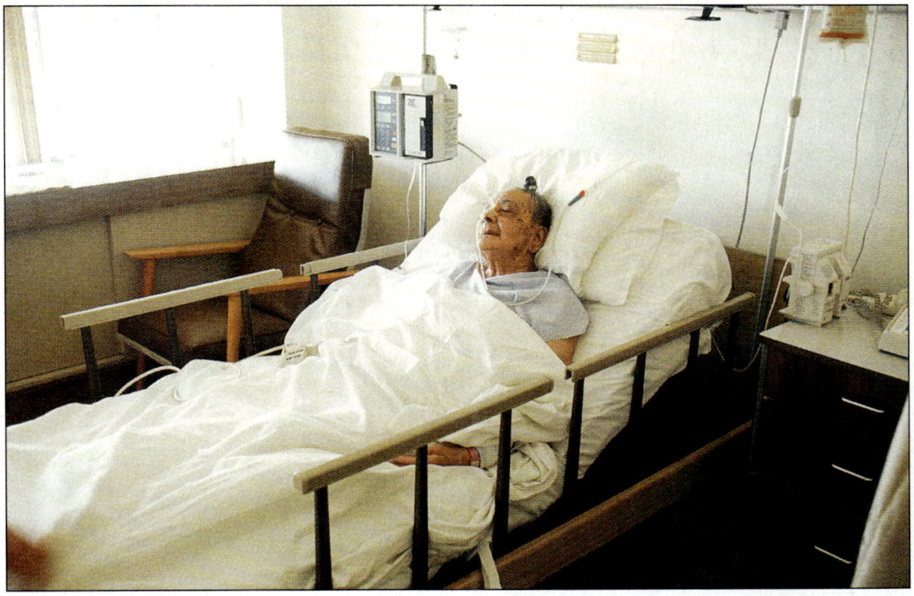

Many elderly people have used sedative-hypnotic drugs for years to relieve minor anxieties and to secure proper sleep—an unrelenting human desire. Such persistent dependence on these drugs is broken only upon hospitalization.

© Tony Freeman/Photo Edit

Drugs that slow down mental and physical functions of the body are known generally as central nervous system (CNS) *depressants*. Because these chemical agents tend to produce a calming effect, relax muscles, and relieve feelings of tension, anxiety, and irritability, they are also described as having a sedative or sedating effect. Such drugs are referred to as **sedatives.**

At higher dose levels, sedatives also produce drowsiness and eventually a state resembling natural sleep. Drugs that have such a sleep-inducing effect are called **hypnotics.** This hypnotic effect has nothing to do with the artificially induced state of suggestibility often associated with the word *hypnosis.* Nevertheless, the combination term *sedative-hypnotic* appropriately identifies the major pharmacological effects of these drugs. In reality, almost any drug that calms, soothes, and reduces anxiety is also capable of relieving insomnia (sleeplessness).[1]

Ethyl alcohol and the narcotic analgesics, such as morphine and heroin, are also classified as CNS depressants but are discussed in separate chapters. Along with the sedative-hypnotics, they are considered "downers," as they too decrease activity and reduce excitement. Although the narcotics and the sedative-hypnotics share many of the same actions, the latter drugs have no practical pain-relieving properties. Unlike the narcotics, intoxicating doses of the sedative-hypnotics almost always result in impaired judgment, slurred speech, and loss of motor coordination.

Due to chemical differences, the sedative-hypnotics include several related families of drugs having common characteristics but somewhat diverse effects and therapeutic uses. The family members of the sedative-hypnotic classification are (1) barbiturates, (2) nonbarbiturate sedative-hypnotics, (3) minor tranquilizers, and (4) abused inhalants that have mind-changing actions similar to those of alcohol, barbiturates, and benzodiazepines.[2] Their abuse potential is so high, therefore, all but the inhalants are strictly regulated under the provisions of the Controlled Substances Act. The prescribed sedative-hypnotics and commonly abused volatile solvents and chemicals are listed in table 7.1, along with examples of common trade-name drugs.

A fifth family member, the **major tranquilizers** or antipsychotics, are also sedative-hypnotics. Unlike the minor tranquilizers, these major antipsychotics are not controlled drug substances. Moreover, these major tranquilizers produce their desired effect almost exclusively among psychotic patients, have almost no addictive potential, and are not typically abused substances.

Sedative-hypnotics are among the most widely prescribed psychoactives in the United States. Taken under medical supervision, they have improved the quality of life for millions of people. Beneficially employed for the specific treatment of insomnia and the relief of anxiety and tension, the sedative-hypnotics have also become important additions to surgical anesthesia because of their sleep-inducing actions. One drug, phenobarbital, is often the drug of choice in controlling grand mal epileptic seizures and all types of partial seizures.[3]

Although their use in medical practice has declined steadily and rather significantly, barbiturates are still used as surgical anesthetics and only occasionally as sleeping pills. Specific barbiturates designated as "short-acting" and "intermediate-acting" were once the favorites of drug abusers. However, with a reduction in their prescription and manufacture, barbiturates are not as likely to be diverted from approved medical use.

Among the most frequently abused nonbarbiturates are glutethimide (Doriden); ethchlorvynol (Placidyl); and, until its United States production ceased in 1983, methaqualone (Quaalude, Sopor)—all prescribed to induce sleep. Benzodiazepines (frequently used minor tranquilizers) are often prescribed as antianxiety medicines and sleep-promoting medications. These tranquilizers are also commonly abused.

table 7.1 Depressants: Sedative-Hypnotic Drugs and Inhalants

Barbiturates	Inhalants
Amobarbital (Amytal)*	Benzene
Butabarbital (Butisol)	Butane
Hexobarbital (Sombucaps)	Gasoline
Phenobarbital (Luminal)	Toluene
Secobarbital (Seconal)	Naphtha
Pentobarbital (Nembutal)	Carbon tetrachloride
Amobarbital/Secobarbital (Tuinal)	Acetone
Minor Tranquilizers	Methyl ethyl ketone
	Freons
Meprobamate (Miltown, Equanil)	Propane
Benzodiazepines	Nitrous oxide
Alprazolam (Xanax)	Amyl nitrite, butyl nitrite
Chloridazepoxide (Librium)	Organic nitrogen room odorizers
Clonazepam (Clonopin)	**Major Tranquilizers**
Clorazepate (Tranxene)	
Diazepam (Valium)	Reserpine (Serpasil)
Flurazepam (Dalmane)†	Phenothiazines
Lorazepam (Ativan)	Chlorpromazine (Thorazine)
Oxazepam (Serex)	Prochlorperazine (Compazine)
Prazepam (Centrax)	Mesoridazine (Serentil)
Temazepam (Restoril)†	Butaperazine (Repoise)
Triazolam (Halcion)†	Thioridazine (Mellaril)
	Haloperidol (Haldol)
Nonbarbiturate Sedative-Hypnotics	
Chloral hydrate (Noctec)	
Glutethimide (Doriden)	
Ethchlorvynol (Placidyl)	
Buspirone (BuSpar)	

* Common trade names occur within parentheses. Many of these drugs are sold under a variety of trade names.
† These drugs are used almost exclusively as a bedtime sedative to induce sleep.

Motivational Factors in Misuse and Abuse

The unrelenting human quest for sleep, along with physicians' over prescription of "sleeping pills," is the basis for much misuse and abuse of the sedative-hypnotics. People who have difficulty sleeping or who have trouble coping with stress, the pressures of modern living or anxiety, sometimes overuse or become dependent on sedatives. Patients on prescribed barbiturates soon discover that taking smaller doses produces a feeling of drowsy well-being while still awake. Similar to the pleasant feelings of alcohol intoxication, the response attracts those who do not really need these drugs and promotes overuse by those who do.

Misuse of the sedative-hypnotics is thought to be extensive. Many people, especially the elderly, have used these drugs for years—out of habit or by tradition—to relieve minor anxieties and to secure "proper" sleep.

Recreational drug use often includes a desire for some pleasure or an escape from worry. Certain individuals value the feelings of relaxation and tranquility, the sensation of decreased tension, and the tingling euphoria resulting from use of the sedative-hypnotics. The enjoyment of such effects describes **appetitive drug use,** or drug-taking behavior motivated by the hunger or desire for pleasurable responses and sensations.

While others may also enjoy the various pleasures of intoxication, their primary concern in drug taking is, by contrast, to get relief from unpleasant sensations, tension, disturbed interpersonal relationships, fears, and anxieties. Such motivation for taking drugs is called **escape-avoidance drug use.** These two basic motivations—desire for pleasure (appetite use) and relief from tension (escape-avoidance use)—represent the extremes on a spectrum of psychological factors that give rise to drug-taking behavior.

As with alcohol, sedative-hypnotic intoxication can also bring about a temporary period of disinhibition. Desirable social behaviors may vanish, and internal feelings of anger, rage, and even depression may be released. Contrary to common belief, this emotional upheaval is sometimes enjoyed by drug takers.

On occasion, heroin abusers take sedative-hypnotics to increase the effects of narcotics. Stimulant users often take sedatives to moderate or offset the undesirable, jittery feelings that stimulants produce. Alcoholic beverages are also used with various sedative-hypnotics, especially the minor tranquilizers.

Whether they are used for recreation, self-medication, or merely to prevent withdrawal symptoms, the depressant drugs are frequently taken with little consideration of possible adverse consequences. Moreover, they are often acquired not only within a legitimate and supervised patient-physician relationship, but also as a result of illicit prescribing, inadequate medical supervision of a patient's medical condition, and patient manipulation of the prescriber. Nonprescription channels of acquiring these drugs include thefts at the retail or wholesale levels, prescription forgeries, smuggling, illegal manufacture, and "street sales."

General Characteristics

Several effects of the sedative-hypnotics are shared by nearly all drugs in this classification because of their pharmacologic similarity.[4]

1. These sedative-hypnotics tend to produce a *widespread depression,* or slowing down of the brain and central nervous system, including a reduction in the state of wakefulness.

   Barbiturates and benzodiazepines activate the brain's pleasure center resulting in an increase of dopamine neurotransmitter. One of the brain's chemical signals, dopamine is associated with the initial feeling of euphoria, which is sufficient to reinforce the continuing consumption of these drugs.

   However, both of these major types of sedative-hypnotics also produce a more evident depressant effect on the central nervous system. This comes about by inhibiting or preventing the transmission of nerve impulses at the synapses between nerve cells. Barbiturates and benzodiazepines mimic the effects of the inhibitory neurotransmitter identified as GABA. When these drugs are bound near the receptor sites on the presynaptic neurons, such an action enhances the inhibitory neurotransmitter and reduces the excitability of neurons. Consequently, the transmission of nerve impulses across the synapses is inhibited, and sedation occurs.

   Valued primarily for their calming and sleep-inducing effects, the sedative-hypnotics are prescribed variously as antiepileptic agents, muscle relaxants, and antianxiety drugs. Some of the sedative-hypnotics are used to produce general anesthesia, that is, drug-induced absence of all sensation.
2. With increasing dosage, nearly all of these drugs produce a variety of behavioral alterations in a continuum of sedation. Beginning with relief from anxiety at low doses, the behavior progresses to disinhibition (a state of euphoria); sedation; hypnosis; general anesthesia; coma; and then, at high doses, death, resulting from depression of the brain's respiratory center. However, the benzodiazepines do not induce general anesthesia.
3. The combined effects of sedative-hypnotics are often described as *potentiating* or *synergistic* with respect to depressant characteristics, as described in box 3.3 on drug interactions. **Potentiating** and **synergistic drug interactions** result in an exaggerated depressant effect on the central nervous system when sedative-hypnotics, narcotics, or ethyl alcohol are taken in combination. As such, these two descriptive terms are often used interchangeably.

   More precisely, *potentiation* involves one drug's intensifying the action of another that originally had no clinical effect or only a minor drug effect, while *synergism* describes the cooperative, facilitative, and supraadditive effect of two or more drugs that have the same drug action. Therefore, the joint use of barbiturates and alcohol or two or more other sedative-hypnotics (all central nervous system depressants) would be a synergistic interaction that contributes to the serious problems of drug overdose and even death.
4. With repeated use over a prolonged period these drugs are capable of inducing *psychological dependence, tolerance,* and *physiological dependence.* Such dependency on sedative-type psychoactive drugs has become known as **sedativism,** an all-too-common American affliction.
5. To a remarkable degree, **cross-tolerance** and **cross-dependence** are exhibited by the sedative-hypnotics. In cross-tolerance, the tolerance to one drug, *A,* results in a lessened or reduced pharmacological response to another, *B* of the same drug class, even though the person never used drug *B* before.

   By contrast, cross-dependence is a condition in which one drug can prevent withdrawal symptoms associated with physiological dependence on a different drug. Significantly, in cross-dependence, any sedative-hypnotic can be substituted for any other drug in the same drug class.

Historical Perspectives

The use of depressant drugs has its origin in antiquity. Secret potions of herbs, opium, alcohol, or cannabis were employed to induce stupor and sleep. Although the legendary oracle of Delphi—an ancient Greek priestess—did not know the precise scientific reasons for carbon dioxide's effects, the inhaled gas permitted her to make her predictions in a trancelike state. During the nineteenth century, "ether frolics," "chloroform jags," and nitrous oxide ("laughing gas") demonstrations popularized the inhalation of vapors to produce an altered state of consciousness.

Rauwolfia serpentina, the Indian snakeroot shrub common to India and Southeast Asia, had been used for centuries to treat many diseases, including high blood pressure and even mental disorders. It was not until the 1950s that *Rauwolfia's* active ingredient, **reserpine,** was used clinically as an antipsychotic agent. Reserpine ushered in the age of the "major tranquilizers," which revolutionized treatment of the mentally ill. Because of reserpine's adverse side effects, the derivative of the Indian snakeroot was soon replaced by the phenothiazine family of antipsychotic agents.

The first drug introduced as a sedative-hypnotic was **bromide.** In the 1860s, potassium bromide entered the practice of medicine as a treatment for epileptic convulsions. Due to its irritating effects on the gastrointestinal tract and its tendency to accumulate in the body, leading to chronic bromide intoxication (bromism), bromide was replaced by the barbiturates upon their introduction in the early 1900s.

Synthesized first in 1862, **barbiturates** were initially used in medical practice under the name *barbital.* Unlike the acid, from which it was derived, barbital not only sedated but also induced sleep. Since the introduction of barbital, more than 2,500 barbiturates have been synthesized. Only about fifty of these drugs have ever been distributed as prescribed medications.

Although *chloral hydrate* and *paraldehyde* were synthesized and marketed before 1900, the barbiturates proved so successful as sedative-hypnotics that they remained the number one depressant-type medication until 1960. Still prescribed barbiturates have been replaced in large measure by the newer minor tranquilizers—benzodiazepines. These relatively new antianxiety drugs, also referred to as *anxiolytics* (dispellers or dissolvers of anxiety), are usually less sedating, much safer, and slower to induce tolerance, and they demonstrate greater antianxiety effects with less sedation than the barbiturates.[5] However, they are also dependency-producing drugs.

Barbiturates

Among those drugs employed as hypnotics, sedatives, anesthetics, and anticonvulsants are the barbiturates. Of the nearly fifty derivatives of barbituric acid ever marketed for medical use, fewer than fifteen are in common use today. Easy to use, barbiturates almost always come prepared in capsule or tablet form. A few of them are injectable.

Still prescribed for conditions requiring central nervous system depression, small doses of barbiturates tend to calm nervous individuals, while large doses cause drowsiness and sleep. Short-term effects are similar to those of alcohol intoxication, with a reduction of tension and anxiety, a calming relaxation, slower reaction time, and varying degrees of motor incoordination. However, these drugs are not effective as painkillers.

Since the early 1970s, safer, less toxic, and less sleep-producing benzodiazepines have been replacing the medical use of barbiturates, especially for treatment of insomnia and daytime nervousness or tension.[6] As physicians reduced their prescribing of the barbiturates, a corresponding decline in barbiturate-related overdoses and suicides has also occurred.

Though not strongly supported by clinical studies, the several barbiturates are classified according to their onset and duration of action, as well as their therapeutic uses, as follows.[7]

1. *Ultrashort-acting barbiturates* with rapid onset of effects are used as surgical anesthetics. These drugs produce anesthesia within one minute after intravenous administration. Their rapid onset and brief duration of action (from 15 minutes to 3 hours) make them undesirable for purposes of abuse. Examples of ultrashort-acting barbiturates include thiopental (Pentothal), hexobarbital (Evipal), and thiamyl (Surital).
2. *Short-intermediate-acting barbiturates*, used mostly as sedative-hypnotics, have an onset time of action between 15 to 40 minutes after administration by mouth. The duration of action lasts up to six hours, a characteristic that makes these drugs the preferred barbiturates of most abusers. These drugs are sold in capsules and tablets, as well as in a liquid form or suppositories. Representing this classification are the following barbiturates: secobarbital (Seconal), amobarbital (Amytal), pentobarbital (Nembutal), butabarbital (Butisol), talbutal (Lotusate), and aprobarbital (Alurate). Two of these barbiturates, amobarbital and secobarbital, are combined and sold under the trade name Tuinal.
3. *Long-acting barbiturates* have onset times of up to one hour after use, but their durations of action approach sixteen hours. Their relatively slow onsets of action discourage these barbiturates from being used for episodic intoxication. Consequently, they are not usually distributed on the illicit market. In medical practice, these barbiturates are used as sedatives, hypnotics, and anticonvulsants in the control of epilepsy. Frequently prescribed barbiturates include phenobarbital (Luminal), mephobarbital (Mebaral), and metharbital (Gemonil). Unlike other barbiturates, phenobarbital does not usually produce the "high" typical of depressants.

The many years of barbiturate use in medical practice and barbiturate abuse have revealed both the benefits and problems of these sedative-hypnotics. For instance, prescribed for only short periods, barbiturates are relatively safe when taken under medical supervision. However, the aftereffects of such legitimate use can include a residual depression of the central nervous system (a "hangover") on the day following use.[8] This hangover is characterized by motor incoordination, listlessness, nausea, and emotional disturbances—all related to barbiturates' disruption of normal rapid eye movement (REM) or dream, sleep.

Nonmedically approved uses of the sedative-hypnotics include the simultaneous consumption of barbiturates and amphetamines, CNS stimulants. Such a combination is alleged to produce super-mood elevation. The same combination involves an alternating cycle of sedation and stimulation, that is, taking amphetamines during the day to overcome a drowsy hangover, and then taking barbiturates at night to overcome insomnia. "Speed freaks" also use barbiturates to produce sleep after several days of almost continuous amphetamine injection.

Illegally sold barbiturates pose special hazards for drug abusers. In addition to their high price, barbiturates manufactured and packaged as "street drugs" lack quality control. Street-obtained downers, for example, often contain toxic contaminants and little of the hoped-for sedative-hypnotic. For instance, barbiturates, especially those in capsule form, are often cut with weaker drugs or with traces of tranquilizer; strychnine; arsenic; laxative; heart medication; or inactive substances, such as milk sugars. Homemade capsules may appear genuine, but any red capsule is sometimes offered as Seconal and any yellow capsule may masquerade as Nembutal.

The main reasons for the declining medical uses of barbiturates relate to the risks of fatal overdose, the rapid increase of tolerance, the disruption of normal REM sleep, and the sheer addictiveness of these drugs.[9]

There is also concern about the use of one particular barbiturate, namely, phenobarbital. Although prescribed less than during the 1960s, 1970s, and early 1980s, phenobarbital is still an important treatment for seizure disorders among pregnant women. Research suggests that

Box 7.1 Overdose with Depressants and First-Aid Treatment

Among the frequently abused depressants are both the barbiturate and the nonbarbiturate sedative-hypnotics, the minor tranquilizers, and ethyl alcohol. Although these drugs tend to slow down body function, the physical symptoms of overdose may vary considerably, depending on the specific drug used, the method of administering the drug, and the particular stages of intoxication reached by the drug user.

Symptoms of Depressant Overdose

Confused behavior, often with slow and slurred speech.

Aggressive behavior is possible.

Slow, shallow, or irregular breathing.

Glazed eyes with slow reaction to light.

Person may be either semiconscious or unconscious.

Coma is a possibility.

If individual falls asleep, he or she is difficult to awake.

Muscles may be either flaccid or rigid.

First-Aid Treatment of Depressant Overdose

Try to keep overdose victim awake by talking.

If individual falls asleep or becomes unconscious, watch for sudden cessation of breathing.

Give mouth-to-mouth resuscitation, if possible.

Maintain an open airway to promote unobstructed breathing.

Place unconscious person on his/her side.

If person is conscious, consider diluting the drug taken, inducing vomiting, and then transporting the individual to the nearest medical center as soon as possible.

Be watchful of possible emotional depression and suicidal tendencies.

men whose mothers took this barbiturate during pregnancy were twice as likely to have lower intelligence scores than other men in the study.[10] While factors other than phenobarbital may have affected the men's intelligence scores, this study emphasizes once again the serious effects of parental drug use on the health and development of children. According to the National Institute on Drug Abuse, an estimated 22 million children were born in the United States during the 1960s and 1970s who were exposed in utero to prescribed barbiturates.

Barbiturate Overdose

The long-term use of barbiturates has the potential for serious, even lethal, effects, especially among those who increase their prescribed dosage without medical advice or abuse nonprescribed forms of these drugs (see box 7.1). Even occasional recreational use or self-medication may lead to an overdose condition resulting in respiratory depression, collapse of the blood-circulatory system, kidney failure, and coma. Taking only ten times the hypnotic dose is highly toxic and sometimes fatal, while 15 to 20 times the hypnotic dose is usually fatal.

Among those who develop a tolerance, a "maximum tolerance" level is eventually established for each kind of barbiturate. Unfortunately, this maximum tolerance, or uppermost dosage limit or cutoff point, is never precisely known to the barbiturate abuser until it is too late for preventive action. The usual dose becomes dangerously close to the lethal dose. For instance, if a person having a maximum tolerance of twenty-five barbiturate capsules per day were to take in twenty-three or twenty-four capsules to achieve a desired "high," then consuming only a few extra capsules could easily result in an overdose condition. This is assumed to be what happened to Judy Garland, the famous singer-actress who died allegedly of barbiturate overdose.

Overdosing can occur well under the maximum-tolerance level if barbiturates are combined with alcohol or some other depressant drug. Alcohol enhances the toxic effect of the barbiturate.

Barbiturate Dependence

As indicated earlier, tolerance, psychological dependence, and physiological dependence occur rather easily with the barbiturates. Tolerance to the euphoric effects builds quickly after a few weeks.

Many people find that taking just one barbiturate the first day produces a desired high. By the second or third day, the same dose only makes them sleepy. To get high, they must increase the daily dosage. This pattern is repeated until the dose required for the euphoric effect builds to a high of twenty-five or more capsules per day. But as tolerance increases, the overdose threshold remains relatively unchanged; it does not increase proportionately. Too often the outcome of barbiturate abuse is overdose and death.

While differing from person to person, physical dependence occurs when large quantities of barbiturates (4 to 6 times the average hypnotic dose) are taken for a prolonged period of time, often within 2 to 6 months after the initial excessive dose.

Barbiturate Withdrawal

Most people do not understand how serious and extremely dangerous withdrawal from barbiturates can be. Unlike heroin-dependent individuals, those who experience barbiturate withdrawal symptoms cannot "kick" their drug alone. They must receive medical assistance in a hospital because the abstinence syndrome for barbiturates *is* a medical emergency.

Within only twelve hours after the last dose, the dependent person without medical care begins returning slowly to a nonintoxicated state. Several hours later, this individual usually begins to experience nervousness, weakness, insomnia, nausea, and tremors of the arms and legs.

Then, 48 to 72 hours later, the withdrawal symptoms intensify. The person begins to vomit; has a drop in blood pressure; and develops extreme weakness, delirium, hyperexcitability, fever, and severe body convulsions or seizures. Death can occur from physical exhaustion and collapse of the cardiovascular (heart-blood vessel) system.

Nonbarbiturate Sedative-Hypnotics

In this section, three nonbarbiturate sedative-hypnotics—chloral hydrate, glutethimide, and methaqualone—and other similar hypnotics are discussed.

Chloral Hydrate

One of the oldest sedative-hypnotics still in use, chloral hydrate was first synthesized in 1862. Advantages originally associated with use of this drug included its lack of side effects in therapeutic doses, such as hangover and respiratory depression. However, the popularity of chloral hydrate declined substantially after barbiturates were introduced in 1903.

A liquid marketed in syrups and soft gelatin capsules, chloral hydrate induces sleep shortly after a normal therapeutic dose. The sleep typically lasts about five hours. At one time, the hypnotic drug was added to an alcoholic beverage to concoct the infamous "Mickey Finn" or "knockout drops"—a potent, quick-acting, and sometimes lethal sleep-inducing preparation.

In addition to its continued use as a daytime sedative and a short-term hypnotic, chloral hydrate is sometimes given before surgery or certain medical procedures to relieve anxiety or tension. On occasion, this drug is also used to keep children calm during dental surgery and during various medical imaging processes.

Easily capable of producing a drug dependency with symptoms of withdrawal resembling those of alcohol dependence, chloral hydrate is rarely used as a "recreational" drug. The hypnotic is primarily misused by older adults who take the prescribed drug as a sedative despite its tendency to cause gastric disturbances. Studies conducted by the Environmental Protection Agency suggest the possibility that chloral hydrate might cause cancer and genetic damage. If this drug proves to be a carcinogen, its limited use, especially among the elderly, will further decline.

Glutethimide

First introduced in 1954 as a substitute for the barbiturates, glutethimide was distributed under the trade names Doriden and Dormtabs. This drug treatment for sleeplessness was supposedly less toxic and less dependency-producing than barbiturates. Neither of these hoped-for characteristics was demonstrated in medical practice. Doriden is prescribed only occasionally because it is considered as somewhat obsolete by many physicians.

Within thirty minutes of oral intake, glutethimide produces a sedative-hypnotic effect that lasts approximately six hours. However, if glutethimide is used daily to help produce sleep, it is usually not effective for more than seven days.

At ten times the hypnotic dose, the drug is likely to induce severe intoxication. The lethal dose is estimated at 20 to 40 times the usual hypnotic dose. Doriden has a relatively long duration of action, therefore, it is difficult to reverse overdoses, which often result in death. In terms of lethality, glutethimide is considered several times more hazardous than barbiturates.

Methaqualone

A synthetic drug originally marketed under the trade name Quaalude, *methaqualone* was first introduced in the United States in 1965 as a safe, effective, and nondependency-producing medicine to replace the dangerous barbiturates.

By the late 1970s, it became one of the most frequently prescribed sedative-hypnotics. Additionally marketed under the brand names Sopor, Mequin, Somnafac, Parest, and others, methaqualone—like many other sedative-hypnotics—was not usually effective for more than two weeks when taken regularly for insomnia.

Methaqualone soon became a popular recreational drug because of its alleged safety and widespread availability. It was known variously as "ludes," "sopors," "sopes," "lemmons," and "714s." The chief nonmedical attractions were that the drug produced a euphoric; alcohol-like high; a general feeling of relaxation; and the anticipated enhancement of sexual performance, because methaqualone was thought to have aphrodisiac properties.

Quaalude became one of the leading drugs of abuse in the 1970s and early 1980s.

Relatively safe when used wisely under medical supervision, methaqualone could cause loss of inhibitions and motor coordination, dizziness, sleep, and hangover the next day. Prolonged use sometimes led to tolerance and psychological and physical dependence. Overdose was common and occasionally fatal, especially when combined with an alcoholic beverage. Without medical supervision, withdrawal from methaqualone often proved deadly.

Such a reputation of toxicity and fatal consequences was responsible for the reclassification of methaqualone from its uncontrolled prescribed drug status first to a Schedule II drug and eventually to a Schedule I drug, under provisions of the Controlled Substances Act. Continuing widespread abuse soon led the sole manufacturer to stop production of Quaalude in 1983. Since then, methaqualone has practically disappeared as a drug problem due to international controls on production.

However, several varieties of "street" or "bootleg" methaqualone have become available after being smuggled into the United States. These fake Quaaludes have contained methaqualone substitutes, such as diazepam (Valium), phenobarbital, antihistamines, and even PCP (angel dust).

Other Nonbarbiturate Hypnotics

Other nonbarbiturates are also available for use as sleep-inducing medications. One of these, *ethchlorvynol* is still prescribed, but much less now than in the past. Three others—*flurazepam*, *temazepam*, and *triazolam*—belong to the

benzodiazepine drug group of antianxiety medications but are promoted almost exclusively as hypnotics. These latter three benzodiazepines are among the most frequently prescribed sleeping pills.

Ethchlorvynol (Placidyl) is marketed as a hypnotic agent with a rapid onset and short duration of action. With regular use, however, its effectiveness rarely lasts for more than one or two weeks. This drug can cause death at as low as fourteen times the hypnotic dose, although there is considerable individual variation. With overdose there may be low blood pressure, decreased breathing and heart rate, and coma.

Marketed under the brand name **Dalmane,** *flurazepam* is one of the most widely prescribed hypnotics. Due to its relatively long duration of sedative action, flurazepam is used primarily to treat insomnia characterized by difficulty in falling asleep and frequent nighttime and early awakenings.[11] Dalmane is not used for daytime sedation because its metabolites (breakdown by-products) have sedative effects and tend to accumulate in the body. When used on consecutive nights, the drug increases gradually in the patient's body and is thought to result in reduced alertness and impaired visual motor coordination during the waking hours. There has been a high incidence of adverse effects, therefore, older adults have been cautioned to avoid using this drug.

Nevertheless, flurazepam possesses certain desirable properties not shared by other hypnotic agents. It is often effective as long as twenty-eight nights; it promotes more sleep time on the first three nights of therapy; it avoids the problem of rebound insomnia when therapy is discontinued. Tolerance to the effects of flurazepam develops more slowly than to the barbiturates. Furthermore, medically supervised use of this drug does not typically result in physical dependence unless it is taken for more than three months. Even after massive doses, most people do not experience a toxic reaction unless flurazepam is taken along with alcohol or some other CNS depressant.

Since its introduction in the early 1980s, *triazolam* **(Halcion)** has become one of the most widely used sleeping medications in the United States. A benzodiazepine hypnotic, Halcion has a rapid onset and a short duration of action. Consequently, it is less likely than some of the other benzodiazepines to cause drowsiness the following day. Its primary use as a hypnotic is for the short-term treatment of insomnia.

Despite Halcion's popularity and apparent effectiveness, special concerns have arisen about its widespread use, especially regarding its causing memory loss, increased wakefulness during the last third of the night, and increased signs of daytime anxiety or nervousness. In addition, numerous reports of serious adverse reactions to taking this medicine have been reported to the U.S. Food and Drug Administration. Harmful reactions have included amnesia to events occurring after taking the drug, anxiety, anorexia (loss of appetite for food), agitation, bizarre and aggressive behavior, confusion, delirium, depression, hallucinations, paranoia, seizures, suicidal thinking, and a feeling of detachment from reality.[12]

Some patients have experienced serious psychiatric side effects when using Halcion, therefore, this medication was taken off the market in the United Kingdom and severely restricted in Canada.[13] In the United States, the Food and Drug Administration has required the manufacturer of Halcion to provide consumers with more detailed information about the risks and benefits of this drug.

Temazepam (Restoril) is another benzodiazepine hypnotic that has a relatively long duration of sedative action. This characteristic makes the drug especially useful for people who tend to wake early. Although Restoril has had many fewer reported dangerous side effects (adverse reactions) than other benzodiazepines, the main disadvantage of this hypnotic is its tendency to cause a hangover—a drowsy, light-headed feeling—the following day. Like all the benzodiazepines, the continued use of Restoril can result in drug dependence. In addition, the sleep-inducing effects of this medication may decline with time.

Several drugs intended for other medical purposes also possess sleep-inducing characteristics. Some of these are prescribed as such by physicians. Examples include prescription-only sedating antihistamines (Atarax, Vistaril, and Benadryl); an antipsychotic drug, such as thioridazine (Mellaril) used in treating severe mental disorders; and an antidepressant, such as amitriptyline (Elavil). Over-the-counter hypnotics are discussed in chapter 12.

Self-Care for Inducing Sleep

While various drug and nondrug therapies have been developed for the condition of insomnia, many people have found relief from sleeplessness by engaging in one or more forms of self-care or self-medication.[14] Some of these acceptable alternatives are:

1. Do not take naps during the day or go to bed earlier than usual.
2. Change the bedroom environment so that it is as quiet and dark as possible. Use special window shades that eliminate most external light. Use electronic devices that emit rest-promoting sounds that mask many noises from within and outside one's home. Maintain a comfortable room temperature for sleeping and keep it consistent from night-to-night.
3. Do not consume caffeine-containing beverages (coffee, tea, and cola drinks) or chocolate within eight hours of your anticipated bedtime.
4. Do not eat a heavy meal in the evening, especially just before retiring. Drink a mixture of warm milk and "instant breakfast" to which a spoonful of malt has been added. Milk and malt are high in the chemical tryptophan (an essential amino acid found in food), which can have a natural sedative effect.
5. Engage in exercise on a daily basis. Regular physical activity tends to promote a good night's sleep.
6. Take an unhurried warm bath about three hours before bedtime. This procedure tends to be relaxing. Other bedtime routines, such as reading a pleasant book, listening to music, or

watching TV just before retiring, can also help promote sleep.

7. Do not use any drugs that might affect the central nervous system. Chief offenders tend to be alcohol, tobacco, nose drops, and nasal decongestants, in addition to caffeine. Under a physician's care, change the intake of any prescribed medicine that might also affect the central nervous system.
8. Each day, get up early at the same time, even when you have slept poorly and especially on nonworking days. This consistent behavior will help you avoid the "late-sleeping syndrome"—the feeling of being "out-of-sorts" after sleeping late in the morning.
9. If sleeplessness is the result of worry or grief, try to resolve your basic problem by confiding in a friend, joining a support group, or consulting a counselor.
10. Resist the urge to be a clock watcher at night. Turn the clock to the wall or reposition your bed to avoid looking at the clock.

Another nondrug approach to insomnia is the use of a behavior therapy technique called "systematic desensitization." In this process, an individual engages in various relaxation exercises. Then the person visualizes scenes related to going to bed while in a relaxed state. The ultimate goal is to associate bedtime with a sense of relaxation incompatible with anxiety.

Minor Tranquilizers

The term **minor tranquilizer** is somewhat misleading because it implies that such a drug acts like a "major tranquilizer," but to a lesser degree. Nothing could be more incorrect! The major tranquilizers, such as chlorpromazine (Thorazine) and reserpine (Serpasil), relieve symptoms of severe mental disorders, such as schizophrenia and paranoia; they are therefore more appropriately called "antipsychotics."

The minor tranquilizers, though, function more like sedative-hypnotics. The preferred descriptive term for the minor tranquilizer is **antianxiety agent** because these minor tranquilizers are useful in treating anxiety and neurotic conditions. While the antianxiety drugs do tranquilize a person, the antipsychotics seldom produce such a state in a nonpsychotic individual. Consequently, the major antipsychotics are rarely abused drugs, and, unlike the minor tranquilizers, they are not even controlled substances.

Meprobamate

Ushering in the era of antianxiety drugs, meprobamate was first marketed in the mid-1950s under the trade names Miltown and Equanil. This drug not only possessed a muscle-relaxant effect but was also found to be an antianxiety agent. It was soon prescribed widely for relief of anxiety, tension, and muscle spasms.

The success of this new "minor tranquilizer" was related to its calming effects without producing sleep when taken at low therapeutic doses. Meprobamate was able to provide relief from anxiety and free-floating fears without heavy sedation. After several years of clinical use, meprobamate was found to be somewhat less toxic than barbiturates. With excessive use, however, psychological and physical dependence developed.

Benzodiazepines

Meprobamate's initial success was soon followed by the discovery of a new family of antianxiety drugs, the benzodiazepines. In 1960, *chlordiazepoxide* (Librium) was marketed and widely prescribed as a wonder drug in the "age of coping." Three years later, *diazepam* **(Valium),** another tranquilizing agent chemically similar to chlordiazepoxide, entered medical practice. Valium proved to be 5 to 10 times more potent than Librium.

Since its introduction in 1963, Valium soon became the most frequently prescribed psychoactive drug in American medical history. For more than twenty years, it was one of the most widely prescribed medications in the world. By the early 1990s, Valium's therapeutic popularity had been surpassed first by **Xanax** and then by *Ativan,* two other members of the benzodiazepine family and chemical relatives of diazepam.

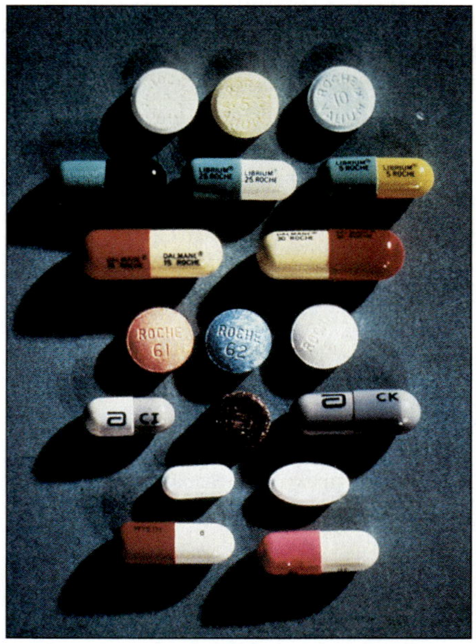

Benzodiazepines pictured here are often prescribed as antianxiety medications, but certain ones are promoted as hypnotics or as anticonvulsant drugs.

Courtesy of the Drug Enforcement Agency

Alprazolam (Xanax) is still the number one antianxiety drug in terms of new and refill prescriptions.[15] This benzodiazepine is promoted as not having the "buzz" effect of Valium, and it is particularly useful in treating panic disorders; anxiety accompanied by agitated depression; and various phobias, including the fear of open spaces (agoraphobia). In addition, Xanax has a somewhat shorter duration of action than Valium.

Characteristics of the Benzodiazepines

In general, the various benzodiazepines currently in use differ mainly in the duration of their effects, and are grouped as follows:[16]

Long-acting benzodiazepines—drugs that stay in the body longer and need to be taken only once or twice per day or every other day:

diazepam (Valium)
clonazepam (Klonopin)
chlordiazepoxide (Librium)
flurazepam (Dalmane)
prazepam (Centrax)
clorazepate (Tranxene)

Intermediate-acting benzodiazepines—shorter-acting drugs that are eliminated more quickly from the body; can be taken three or four times per day or at night:

temazepam (Restoril)
alprazolam (Xanax)

Short-acting benzodiazepines—shortest-acting in this drug group; are eliminated most rapidly from the body and can be taken three or four times per day or at night:

oxazepam (Serax)
lorazepam (Ativan)
triazolam (Halcion)

With the exception of Dalmane, Restoril, and the controversial Halcion (all promoted as hypnotics) and Klonopin (used as an anticonvulsant), the benzodiazepines have been widely prescribed as antianxiety drugs for nearly a quarter of psychiatric patients and for people with arthritis and chronic heart disease.

The primary purpose of these "minor tranquilizers" is to reduce psychic tension and anxiety disorders (the intense fear of impending doom without obvious threat) or for the temporary relief of the symptoms of anxiety. However, most medical authorities do not believe that these drugs should be prescribed to relieve anxieties that are part of the ordinary stresses of everyday life.

Box 7.2 Tranquilizers, Other Sedative-Hypnotics, and Driving: *Why Take the Risk?*

Tranquilizers are central nervous system depressants (drugs that slow down the body) and help relieve tension and anxiety. Major and minor tranquilizers, such as chlorpromazine (Thorazine) and diazepam (Valium), can have pronounced effects on driving skills.

Studies show that prescribed doses of tranquilizers can affect driving skills by slowing reaction time and interfering with eye-hand coordination and judgment. Warnings that caution against taking these medications while driving are often ignored. Research suggests that driving skills are most impaired in the first hour after a tranquilizer is taken.

Flurazepam (Dalmane) is a widely prescribed sleeping pill. Studies show that this drug accumulates in the body, and the buildup can impair driving skills, even the morning after. Elderly people must be especially careful when driving the day after taking this drug, because the drug remains in their bodies longer than it does in younger persons.

Other sedative-hypnotic drugs, including barbiturates, are chemical sedatives that calm people or help them sleep. Sleepy drivers are a hazard on the road. Mixing these drugs with alcohol can double the effects of both and is extremely dangerous.

If your doctor prescribes a tranquilizer or sedative, make a point to discuss how the drug will affect your ability to drive safely. Driving requires a combination of thought and motor skills, a great deal of common sense, and a concern for the safety of everyone on the road. Safe driving requires an observant eye, a steady hand, and a clear head. By mixing drugs with driving, you are only asking for trouble. Why take the risk?

Source: Modified from *Drugs & Driving: Why Take the Risk?* National Institute on Drug Abuse.

Possible Adverse Effects

Usually the benzodiazepines are effective sedatives but are less sleep-inducing than other drugs in the sedative-hypnotic classification. In most patients, judgment and motor coordination are not seriously impaired and a lethal overdose is rare, because there is little depression of breathing.

Nevertheless, there are many possible adverse effects, especially among the elderly. Some common undesirable side effects include clumsiness, dizziness, drowsiness, slurred speech, irritability, nervousness, and trouble sleeping.[17] These symptoms are usually reversed by adjusting or discontinuing the dose (see also box 7.2)

There is no doubt that extensive use of antianxiety drugs has led to their misuse and abuse. These drugs are available for quick comfort during a particular "life panic"—job pressures, family problems, marital difficulties, or stressful academic pressures—therefore overdosing is common and is a frequent cause of visits to hospital emergency rooms.

The benzodiazepines seldom induce respiratory depression, so it is extremely difficult to commit suicide by overdosing with these drugs. However, these "minor tranquilizers" in combination with alcohol or other CNS depressants can be deadly.

One of the less publicized potential dangers associated with the use of benzodiazepines is the occurrence of *impaired anterograde memory.* In this condition (a form of amnesia) the person taking the drug has a reduced capacity for learning and retaining new information presented after taking a therapeutic dose.[18] Older people are more susceptible to this phenomenon than younger individuals.

Benzodiazepine Dependence

The danger of *benzodiazepine dependence* is real, though these drugs are not as powerful reinforcers as are the barbiturates and opioids. Even in therapeutic doses, minor tranquilizers can cause psychological dependence with continued use. While there is little tolerance to the antianxiety effects of benzodiazepines, tolerance to the hypnotic effects of these drugs usually develops after one to two weeks.

The withdrawal reaction, evidence of a physical dependence, may occur at both therapeutic and high doses, and may include the following symptoms:[19] anxiety, numbness in the extremities,

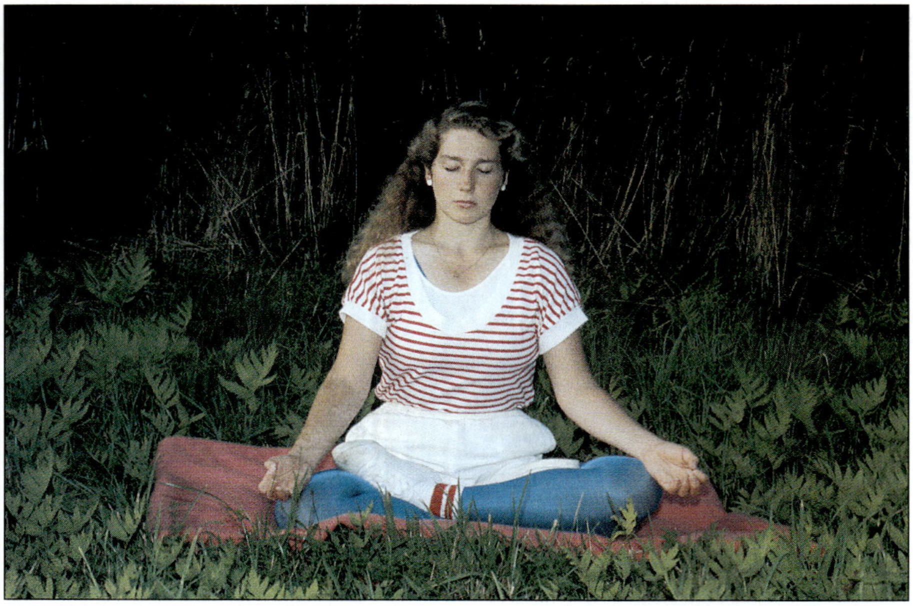

Increasing adoption of nondrug stress reduction techniques, including relaxation exercises, has contributed to the declining use of antianxiety medications, such as Valium.

© Ann Marie Rousseau/The Image Works

unpleasant feelings, intolerance for bright lights and loud noises, nausea, sweating, muscle twitching, and even convulsions. However, withdrawal does not typically involve a craving for the drug.

Recognizing the major problems resulting from the use of minor tranquilizers, physicians prescribe these drugs cautiously. The wider application of nondrug stress reduction techniques, such as biofeedback, self-hypnosis, meditation, and relaxation exercises, has also contributed to the declining use of antianxiety medications.

Rohypnol

Used legally in more than sixty-four nations, **Rohypnol** is one benzodiazepine—flunitrazepam—banned in the United States. Ten times stronger than Valium, Rohypnol is a powerful sleeping pill that also produces disinhibition and short-term amnesia.[20]

Youthful Users and Abusers

While its appeal to drug abusers remains somewhat of a mystery, Rohypnol's illegal use has spread well beyond Florida where it first appeared in 1992 (see fig. 7.1). At present, four different groups of users have been identified: college students and "club" goers; polydrug drug users entering treatment, street and homeless kids; and young Hispanic gang members.

As a sedative-hypnotic, Rohypnol may yet become the Quaalude of the decade. Young people who drive to rave clubs, drink alcohol, take a pill, and then attempt to drive back home are at an increased risk for car crashes, because Rohypnol has an extreme potentiation effect when mixed with alcohol.[21] Among polydrug abusers, Rohypnol is sometimes combined with cocaine to moderate the effect of a binge or to enhance the effects of low-quality heroin.

General Effects and Risks

Rohypnol pills are small white tablets that dissolve easily without a trace in liquids, such as soda pop and beer. The tablets are sealed in bubble packs similar to other legally produced medicines. Such packaging has lead some users to underestimate the drug's potential risks. General effects of Rohypnol include the disinhibition of behavior, feeling of relaxation, short-term memory loss, and extreme sleepiness. Lethal overdoses are unlikely if this drug is taken alone. However, when combined with alcohol or other drugs, it can cause respiratory depression and death.

Like the other benzodiazepines, regular use of this sedative-hypnotic also produces a physical dependency in as little as thirty days. Common withdrawal symptoms include headache, muscle pain, mental confusion, hallucinations, and convulsions. This condition usually requires medical supervision. Serious side effects can also develop from so-called "cold turkey" withdrawal.

"Roofie Rape"

Known on the street as ropies, roofies, R-2's, Mexican valium, roach, rib, rope, the Forget Pill, and the Forget Me Pill, Rohypnol has become notorious. This drug has been used increasingly to incapacitate individuals, almost always females, leaving them with no memory of assault or robbery.

In what has been termed "roofie rape," the odorless, colorless, and tasteless tranquilizer has been added to an alcoholic beverage, which is then consumed by an unsuspecting female. After becoming dizzy and disoriented, the victim often passes out and will have little or no memory of what has happened. As such, the person under the influence of this drug is unable to defend herself from any form of exploitation.

The next morning, after awakening, the person may recall only vaguely that she has been violated and sexually abused, but may not remember precisely what has occurred. This situation makes it difficult for law enforcement officials to prosecute suspected rapists.[22]

Recent Countermeasures

Instances of roofie rape became so numerous that the United States Congress enacted a new law in 1996 to penalize those who use Rohypnol or other date-rape drugs to subdue their victims. An extra twenty-year prison sentence will be added to other penalties for anyone convicted of using an illegal drug as a tool of rape or other violent crime. Simple possession of Rohypnol, with no

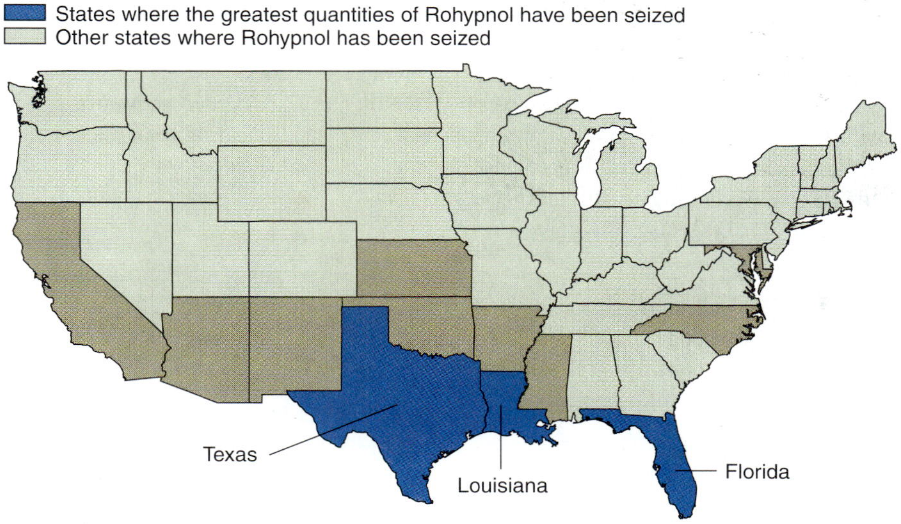

figure 7.1

The abuse of a new sedative-hypnotic. Seizures by law enforcement agencies of the prescription pill, Rohypnol, which is not approved for sale in the United States, have risen sharply in certain states. Since these data were collected, at least thirty-two states have reported one or more criminal cases involving Rohypnol.

Source: Drug Enforcement Administration as published by the Center for Substance Abuse Prevention

proven intent to use as a manipulative drug, carries a penalty of up to three years in prison.

While there is no accepted medical use for Rohypnol in the United States, this sedative-hypnotic has been on Schedule IV of the Controlled Substances Act. The Drug Enforcement Administration is considering moving the drug to the Schedule 1 category, along with heroin. Such action would further increase the penalties for possession, distribution, and trafficking.

Hoffman-La Roche, the United States maker of Rohypnol, is offering free urine tests to law enforcement agencies and rape crisis centers to help determine if rape victims have the drug in their urine. In addition, the company has undertaken an educational campaign warning women to watch their drinks and informing them of the abuses of Rohypnol.[23] Hoffman-La Roche is also cooperating with the federal government on how to stop the illegal diversion of Rohypnol from other countries, including Mexico—where it is legal—into the United States.

Other Antianxiety Medications

In addition to the benzodiazepines, there are three other classes of drugs sometimes used to relieve anxiety—the so-called beta-blockers, the antidepressants, and buspirone.

Beta-blockers (Oxprenolon and Propranolol) are often used in the treatment of angina, hypertension, and irregular heart rhythms. Occasionally, these drugs are also given to reduce anxiety and the shaking and palpitations (extremely rapid actions of the heart) related to anxiety. By blockading the stimulating action of the norepinephrine neurotransmitter, beta-blockers produce a wide variety of effects, including a slowing of heart rate, lowering of blood pressure, and reduction in muscle tremor as seen in anxiety states.

Certain antidepressant drugs, described in more detail in chapter 9, may also be prescribed for anxiety arising out of depressive illness. Although the *tricyclics* and *fluoxetine* (Prozac) are marketed as treatments for serious depression, some physicians might use them to relieve anxiety conditions. Antidepressants work by increasing the level of one or more excitatory neurotransmitters.

Another antianxiety medication, *buspirone* (**BuSpar**), has been introduced recently for medical use. This drug is not a member of the benzodiazepines and is chemically unrelated to other antianxiety compounds. Although the precise mechanism of its action is unknown, buspirone likely affects neurotransmitter functions.

A prescription drug not scheduled as a controlled substance, BuSpar relieves anxiety and nervous tension without causing significant sedation. Moreover, buspirone does not exert anticonvulsant or muscle relaxant effects typically associated with use of benzodiazepines.[24]

In human and animal studies, this antianxiety drug has shown no potential for abuse or diversion from legitimate sources, and there is no evidence that its use results in tolerance or either physical or psychological dependence. These qualities make BuSpar an attractive alternative to the benzodiazepines. Moreover, buspirone has proved particularly useful in the elderly and among alcoholics and addiction-prone people because of its lack of significant sedative effects and abuse potential.[25]

Inhalants

According to the National Institute on Drug Abuse, inhalants are a wide-ranging group of breathable chemicals that produce mind-altering vapors. Representative inhalants include various commercial products used as cleaners, cosmetics, paint solvents, glues, motor fuels, and aerosol sprays. More than 1,400 such items—present in the home and available in the marketplace—cause giddiness or intoxication when they are sniffed or "huffed" by users.[26] They were never meant to be inhaled for either medical or recreational use, so many people do not even think of these products as drugs.

Although inhaling volatile substances (chemicals that evaporate easily and are breathable) is an ancient method of achieving intoxication, this behavior has seldom generated the public interest and professional concern surrounding other abused substances.

Such general reluctance to approach inhalant abuse in a systematic way has persisted despite the numerous abused medicinals inhaled or sniffed for centuries. Often considered a minor problem, the abuse of certain solvents might be more prevalent than the "common" drugs of abuse. It is certain that the toxicity of some inhalants exceeds that of other abused substances.

Commercial solvents, including toluene, and gasoline tend to be the intoxicants of the very young and young adolescents, and more often of males than females.[27] With about 6 percent of United States children having tried one of these breathable chemicals by the fourth grade of school, inhalants have become the gateway drug for a significant segment of youth. Inhalants are often the first psychoactive substance used nonmedically, before either tobacco or alcohol.

Increasingly, though, numbers of male and female adults looking for a quick and inexpensive high have been engaging in sniffing certain aerosols and anesthetics. Although not aphrodisiacs, amyl nitrite and butyl nitrite seem to intensify sexual orgasm when inhaled close to the peak of passion. These chemicals rapidly gained favor as "love drugs," particularly among homosexual males who discovered that amyl and butyl nitrite help relax the anal sphincter, making penetration easier.[28] For the past several years, nitrogen oxide, or "laughing gas," has become a popular intoxicant among high school and college-age persons, and among some young urban professionals.

Reasons for Use

Most people find it difficult to comprehend why anyone would deliberately breathe in strange compounds whose toxic potential has either remained uncertain or been considered a major threat to health and life. Nevertheless, evidence indicates that the use of inhalants continues to increase, especially among youth exposed to poor socioeconomic conditions within a given community. In addition, increased inhalant use seems to be related with lack of success in school.

Surveys of juveniles who had developed a dependence on solvents suggested several categories of justification for use of inhalants. According to the National Institute on Drug Abuse, the categories are:

> **Peer-group influence**—This is perhaps the strongest factor in beginning and continuing the use of a particular inhalant.
>
> **Cost effectiveness**—This is a prime factor in determining whether to use one of the inhalants, especially if the abuser is from a low-income family. A seventy-five cent can of varnish remover can intoxicate more people than a gallon of cheap wine.
>
> **Easy availability**—Industrial and household substances can be found easily, even in places where alcoholic beverages are not present. Gasoline, paints (especially spray paints), and various aerosols are more prevalent than liquor, and they can be found at service stations, paint stores, auto body shops, convenience stores, supermarkets, hardware stores, and pharmacies. If they cannot be purchased, they can be shoplifted.
>
> **Convenient packaging**—Many inhalants come in small, compact packages that permit concealment and mobility. A bottle of nail polish remover can be hidden more easily than a pint of wine. Such convenient packaging permits the abuser to bring the inhalant to school for between-class sniffs.
>
> **Experience of a "high"**—Similar but not identical to alcohol intoxication, the inhalant-induced high is a major attraction or thrill of the volatile substances. Users describe the high as a floaty euphoria and a blotting out of unpleasant aspects of their lives.
>
> **Course of intoxication**—Inhalation produces a more rapid onset of the high than does drinking alcohol or eating other drug substances. Effects subside after one or two hours, and the hangover is regarded as less unpleasant than that of alcohol. Inhalants are considered more reliably intoxicating than marijuana.
>
> **Legality**—Inhalants are usually legal compounds, at least for adults, and most of the volatile substances are produced, distributed, and sold for legitimate purposes.

Thus, from the consumer's viewpoint the use of inhalants is more understandable. As indicated, the volatile substances have certain advantages over other psychoactive substances.

General Effects

The volatile substances are CNS depressants and tend to slow down the function of the brain and spinal cord. When inhaled, the vapors soon produce a state of intoxication or a dreamlike high closely resembling drunkenness.

At low doses, users might experience a relaxed, somewhat light-headed giddy feeling with reduced inhibitions; at higher doses, they might undergo a numbing of senses, sustain hallucinations, and eventually lose consciousness. Headache, nausea, dizziness, slurred speech, shakiness, uncoordinated actions, double vision, and muscle spasms often accompany the sniffing of these chemicals.

Categories of Abused Inhalants

The inhalants are usually classified into three major groups, all of which are potentially hazardous to users.

1. *Commercial solvents,* such as toluene (a popular and preferred inhalant), xylene, benzene, naphtha, acetone, and carbon tetrachloride are components of commercial products, such as airplane glue, plastic cement, paint thinner, gasoline, cleaning fluids, nail polish remover, cigarette lighter fluid, and typewriter correction fluid.
2. *Aerosols* are suspended particles in a gas. These foglike mixtures are the propellant gases in many household and commercial sprays. Containing

various hydrocarbons, these propellants are abused in products such as cooking sprays, glass chillers, spray paints, and hair sprays. Also in this category are Freon gas, used in refrigerators and air conditioners, and propane gas, a widely used fuel.

Amyl nitrite, an inhalant prepared in cloth-covered glass capsules (ampules), has a legitimate medical use in treating heart patients. This prescribed drug relieves the suffocation effect and associated fear common in angina pectoris. In addition, it produces a dilation (expansion) effect on the brain's arteries and thus induces a flushing sensation with feelings of light-headedness. Upon breaking, the amyl nitrite capsules make a snapping or popping sound that has given rise to their common street names, *snappers* and *poppers*.

Butyl nitrite, a substance legally manufactured and formerly sold as a room odorizer or liquid incense, produces a short high when sniffed. A clear yellow liquid, sometimes packaged in ampules, this frequently abused product was commonly known as "Rush," "Locker Room," "Super Bullet," and "Jacaroma." The odor of butyl nitrite was comparable to the smell of rotting apples or dirty sweatsocks and other athletic gear affected by mildew.

3. *Anesthetics,* such a chloroform, ether, and halothane (all volatile liquids), and nitrous oxide and cyclopropane gases are abused inhalants. When tanks of nitrous oxide (laughing gas) cannot be diverted from medical sources, the intoxicating gas can be obtained from whipped-cream propellants, pressurized pellets, and tracer gas used to detect pipe leaks.

Health Hazards

The shared effect of these volatile chemicals, the euphoria of intoxication, is also the common danger, with the impairment of judgment and motor functioning. Acute intoxication may be relatively short—a matter of several seconds to several minutes—or it may last up to an hour or two, depending on the substance used and the dosage. Similar to that of clinical anesthesia, the high may be characterized by delirium, impulsive behavior, sedation, hallucinations, and delusions. Tolerance can develop with regular use, but physical dependence has not been established.

Though some of the dangers associated with inhalant use have been exaggerated, excessive intake presents definite hazards. Overdoses can result in nausea, vomiting, loss of motor coordination, paralysis, and coma. Even more serious problems should not be underestimated.[29] Fatal accidents do occur, for example, inhaling vapors from a plastic bag held over the head or from a balloon can result in a lack of oxygen or suffocation. Lead poisoning may develop from inhaling vapors of lead-based paints, transmission fluid, and various petroleum products. When inhaled, Freon gas is so cold that it can freeze the throat and larynx and cause suffocation. Oily sprays can coat the inside of the lungs, interfere with proper exchange of oxygen and carbon dioxide, and result in asphyxiation.

Long-term or frequent users of amyl and butyl nitrite run the risk of developing glaucoma (increased pressure within the eyeball), red blood cell damage, and Kaposi's sarcoma—a rare form of cancer associated with impairment of the immune system and often seen in AIDS patients.[30] When users of "laughing gas" tap the pressurized tanks of nitrous oxide, there is an increased risk of sustaining brain injury and suffocation (from lack of oxygen), freezing of the lips and throat (due to the cold temperature of the gas), ruptured blood vessels in the lungs, and collapsed lungs.

Certain volatile substances are extremely poisonous. Carbon tetrachloride has been removed from commercial trade because of its toxicity to the kidneys and liver. Leaded gasoline—rapidly disappearing from the marketplace—can cause serious inflammation of the peripheral nerves.

Toluene, a powerful industrial solvent, has been involved in many instances of kidney, nervous system, and bone marrow disorders. This breathable chemical has become one of the most devastating of the inhalants. Chronic use has resulted in numerous "tol heads"—people who live in a chemically induced stupor so disabling that as young adults they often qualify for Social Security disability checks.[31]

Sudden sniffing death or SSD can occur when a solvent or aerosol propellant is inhaled while the abuser engages in strenuous activity. The reduced oxygen content of the blood results in ventricular fibrillation (uncoordinated heart contractions) or other irregularities of heart action, ending in abrupt death.

Prevention of Inhalant Abuse

Various measures have been undertaken with only minimal success in the prevention of inhalant abuse. Most of these substances have valid nonmedical uses and are legally purchased, at least by adults. However, reducing the availability of supplies of certain volatile substances has decreased the numbers of new users and discouraged certain established users from continuing their practice. For instance, some states and cities have outlawed the sale of airplane glue to minors. Perhaps more effective is the Testor Corporation's practice of adding artificial oil of mustard to model airplane cement. Inhalation of the glue's vapors produces nausea. Legislation has also been used in some states to ban the sale of butyl nitrite. However, federal law forbids the manufacture and retail sale of "Rush" as a dangerous and hazardous substance.

Environmental concerns have resulted in a reduction in the use of Freon gases as these propellants and working fluids in refrigeration and air conditioning are being phased out of production. With the eventual elimination of tetraethyl lead from gasolines, morbidity due to lead poisoning from chronic inhalation of gasoline vapors will likely decline.

Other prevention approaches include changes in product composition to lessen the euphoric effects of inhalation; reformulation of volatile substances to reduce their toxicity; modification of warning labels to better identify potential dangers; and more-effective educational campaigns, including radio, television, and school-based drug-information programs. One of the best educational messages about volatile substances is to caution individuals about the dangers of prolonged inhalation, whether by accident or on purpose. For more information on inhalants, contact:

International Institute for Inhalant Abuse 799 East Hampden Avenue, Suite 500 Englewood, CO 80110

and

Solvent Abuse Foundation for Education (SAFE) 750 17th Street, N.W., Suite 250 Washington, D.C. 20006

Chapter Summary

1. Sedative-hypnotics are psychoactive drugs that have a depressant effect on the central nervous system. They are prescribed to produce a calming effect and to induce sleep.
2. Major sedative-hypnotics include the barbiturates, nonbarbiturate sedative-hypnotics, minor tranquilizers, and abused inhalants. These drugs tend to be widely misused and abused.
3. Recreational use of these drugs is often related to the enjoyment of pleasurable responses (appetitive use) or the relief from worry or unpleasant sensations (escape-avoidance use).
4. In general, the sedative-hypnotics tend to produce a CNS depression, a continuum of sedation, additive and potentiating or synergistic drug interactions, tolerance, psychological and physiological dependence, and even cross-tolerance and cross-dependence.
5. Barbiturates are classified as ultrashort-acting (Pentothal and Surital); short-intermediate acting (Seconal and Nembutal); and long-acting (Luminal and Mebaral).
6. Barbiturate withdrawal is extremely serious and dangerous and can lead to death.
7. Before its production stopped in 1983, methaqualone (Quaalude) was one of the most frequently abused sedative-hypnotics.
8. Technically antianxiety drugs or "minor tranquilizers," flurazepam (Dalmane), triazolam (Halcion), and temazepam (Restoril) are benzodiazepines promoted as hypnotics.
9. Self-care for inducing sleep includes establishing a consistent sleep pattern and a favorable sleeping environment, drinking a mixture of warm milk and malt, exercising daily, taking an unhurried bath about three hours before bedtime, and practicing systematic desensitization.
10. So-called minor tranquilizers act like sedative-hypnotics and are appropriately described as having an antianxiety effect.
11. Minor tranquilizers include meprobamate and the widely prescribed benzodiazepines (Xanax, Valium, and Serax). Extensive use of these antianxiety drugs has led to their misuse and abuse.
12. Dependency-producing with prolonged use, antianxiety medications can be deadly when used in combination with alcohol or another CNS depressant.
13. Although it is not legally available in the United States, Rohypnol, a prescribed benzodiazepine that produces a temporary amnesia, has become a tool of rape and other violent crime.
14. Abused inhalants—chemicals that produce mind-altering vapors—slow down CNS function and produce a dreamlike high resembling drunkenness.
15. There are significant health hazards associated with using inhalants, such as commercial solvents, aerosols, and anesthetics. Physical dependence is not observed.

World Wide Web Sites

National Inhalent Prevention Coalition

www.inhalants.org

National Institute of Mental Health Anxiety Disorders

www.nimh.nih.gov/publicat/anxiety.htm

Review Questions and Activities

1. What is a sedative-hypnotic psychoactive drug?
2. What drug families, or groupings of psychoactive drugs, are considered to be sedative-hypnotics?
3. How do the sedative-hypnotics differ from the narcotic analgesics?
4. What factors account for the medical use and recreational abuse of the sedative-hypnotics?
5. How does the combination use of sedative-hypnotics contribute to drug overdose and death?
6. Do you believe that sedativism is prevalent in America? What psychoactive drugs other than the sedative-hypnotics contribute to sedativism?
7. Trace the major historical factors in the evolving development of sedative-hypnotic drugs and their use.
8. What factors make the recreational use of barbiturates particularly hazardous?
9. What factors contributed to stopping the production of methaqualone?
10. What effects, if any, do the sedative-hypnotics have on the normal sleep pattern?
11. Explain why the major tranquilizers are rarely abused as recreational drugs.

12. Why have the benzodiazepines largely replaced the barbiturates in the practice of medicine?

13. Do you believe that America is a "tranquilized" society? What evidence might you offer to support your response?

14. What countermeasures have been taken to prevent the use of Rohypnol in the commission of rape?

15. Explain why women are alleged to use minor tranquilizers more frequently than men.

16. Which prevention activity is the most effective in reducing the abuse of inhalants? Explain.

References

1. Lester Grinspoon and James Bakalar, *The Harvard Medical School Mental Health Review: Drug Abuse and Addiction* (Boston: Harvard Mental Health Letter, 1993), 22.
2. Avram Goldstein, *Addiction: From Biology to Drug Policy* (New York: W. H. Freeman, 1994), 124.
3. James Rybacki and James Long, *The Essential Guide to Prescription Drugs* (New York: Harper Perennial, 1996), 787–92.
4. Anthony J. Trevor and Walter L. Way, "Sedative-Hypnotics," chap. 21 in *Basic and Clinical Pharmacology,* 4th ed., ed. Bertram Katzung (Norwalk, Conn.: Appleton & Lange, 1989), 264–77.
5. Joe Graedon and Teresa Graedon, *The People's Guide to Deadly Drug Interactions* (New York: St. Martin's Press, 1995), 160–67; and Jim Parker, *Downers: A Guide to Depressant Drugs* (Tempe, Ariz.: Do It Now, 1993), 4–6.
6. United States Pharmacopeia, *Complete Drug Reference* (Yonkers, N.Y.: Consumer Reports, 1995), 357.
7. Drug Enforcement Administration, U.S. Department of Justice, *Drugs of Abuse* (Washington, D.C.: GPO, 1989), 26; and Barry Stimmel and the editors of Consumer Reports Books, *The Facts about Drug Use: Coping with Drugs and Alcohol in Your Family, at Work, in Your Community* (New York: Haworth Medical Press, 1993), 97–99.
8. William Hobbs, Theodore Rall, and Todd Verdoon, "Hypnotics and Sedatives; Ethanol," chap. 17 in *Goodman & Gilman's The Pharmaceutical Basis of Therapeutics,* 9th ed. (New York: McGraw-Hill Health Professions Division, 1996), 378.
9. Parker, *Downers,* 2.
10. June Reinisch and others, "In Utero Exposure to Phenobarbital and Intelligence Deficits in Adult Men," *Journal of the American Medical Association,* 274, no. 19 (15 November 1995): 1518–25.
11. *Physicians' Desk Reference,* 50th ed. (Montvale, N.J.: Medical Economics Company, 1996), 2173.
12. "The Halcion Story: What You Need to Know, but the FDA Won't Tell You," *Public Citizen Health Research Group Health Letter* 6, no. 1 (January 1990): 1–3, 8.
13. "Halcion and Other Sleeping Pills," *University of California at Berkeley Wellness Letter* 8, no. 10 (July 1992): 3.
14. Quentin Regestein, David Ritchie, and the editors of Consumer Reports Books, *Sleep: Problems and Solutions* (Mount Vernon, N.Y.: Consumers Union, 1990), 182–85.
15. "Top 200 Drugs of 1995," *Pharmacy Times* 62, no. 4 (April 1996): 27–36.
16. Grinspoon and Bakalar, *The Harvard Medical School Mental Health Review,* 22.
17. United States Pharmacopeia, *Complete Drug Reference,* 381.
18. Harold Doweiko, *Concepts of Chemical Dependency,* 2d ed. (Pacific Grove, Calif.: Brooks/Cole, 1993), 63.
19. Lester Grinspoon and James Bakalar, "Substance Use Disorders," chap. 19 in *The New Harvard Guide to Psychiatry,* ed. Armand M. Nicholi, Jr. (Cambridge, Mass.: Belknap Press/Harvard University Press, 1988), 425.
20. Center for Substance Abuse Prevention, "Rohypnol Update," *Prevention Pipeline* 9, no. 4 (July/August 1996): 13.
21. Peggy Lytton, "Rohypnol: Looming Problems from a New Drug," *Prevention Pipeline* 9, no. 1 (January/February 1996): 27–29.
22. Ibid.
23. "Date-Rape Pill May Be Banned," *Substance Abuse Report* XXVII, no. 14 (15 July 1996): 4.
24. *Physicians' Desk Reference,* 737.
25. Rybacki and Long, *The Essential Guide to Prescription Drugs,* 144–46.
26. Jim Parker, *All About Sniffing* (Tempe, Ariz.: D.I.N. Publications, 1996), 1–2.
27. Ruth Edwards and E. Oetting, "Inhalant Use in the United States," *Epidemiology of Inhalant Abuse: An International Perspective,* NIDA Research Monograph No. 148 (Rockville, Md.: National Institute on Drug Abuse, 1995), 8–28.
28. H. Thomas Milhorn, *Drug and Alcohol Abuse* (New York: Plenum Press, 1994), 314.
29. Isabel Burk, "Huffing: Invisible Substances Right Under Our Noses," *Student Assistance Journal* 7, no. 3 (November–December 1994): 20–23.
30. Samuel Irwin, *Drugs of Abuse: An Introduction to Their Actions & Potential Hazards,* 11th ed. (Tempe, Ariz.: D.I.N. Publications, 1995), 15.
31. Wendy Hundley and Steve Bennish, "Toluene: Dayton's Nightmare Drug," *Dayton Daily News,* 21 July 1996, sec. E, p. 1.

Part Three

The Stimulants

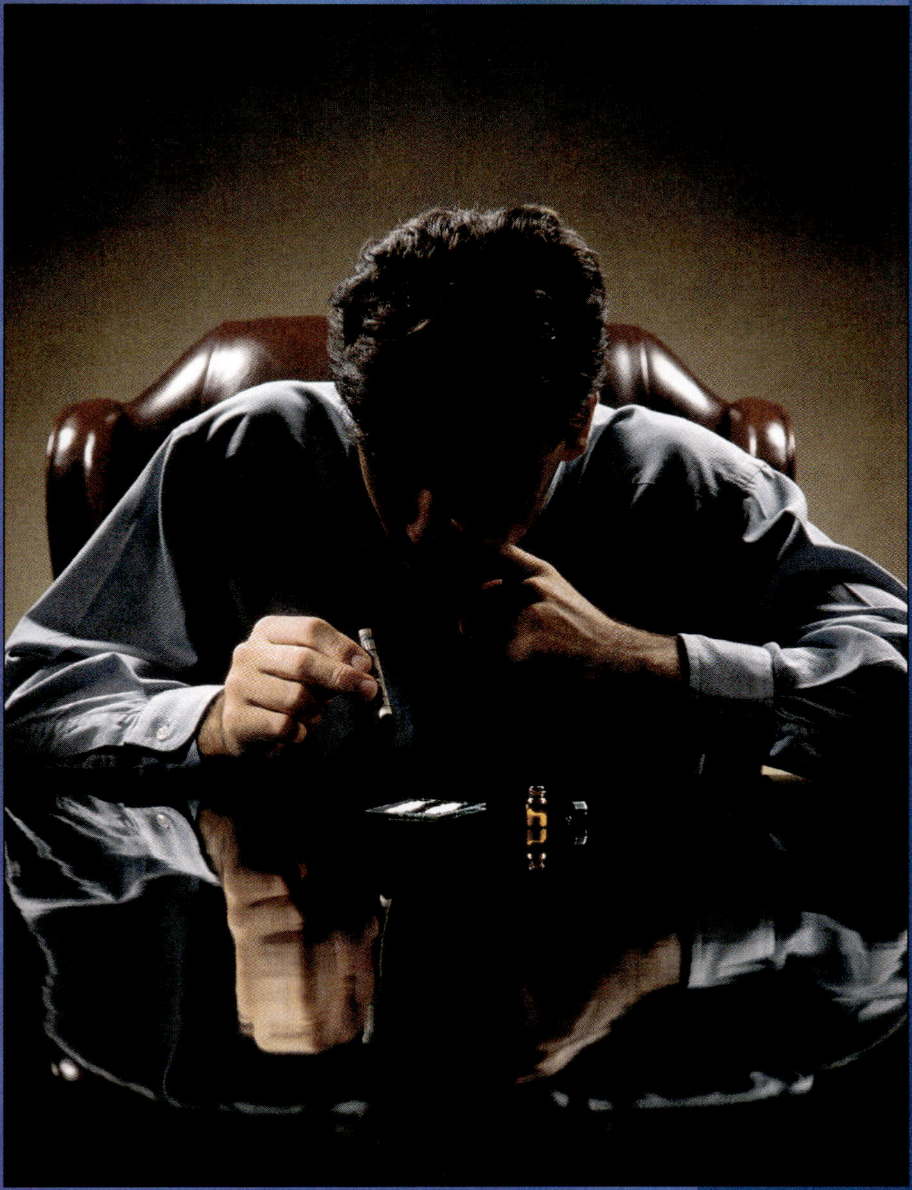

Questions of concern

1. What is the likelihood that America will eventually become a tobacco-free society?
2. While cocaine has assumed the status of a life-threatening drug. why is there still a crack cocaine epidemic?
3. Despite the personal and social problems related to the use of stimulants, wouldn't many Americans benefit from such drugs if they counteract the depressing and monotonous aspects of daily living?

Chapter 8

Tobacco: A persistent health threat

KEY TERMS

Bronchogenic Carcinoma
Carbon Monoxide
Carcinoma *in situ*
Cardiovascular Disease
Chewing Tobacco
Chronic Bronchitis
Chronic Obstructive Lung Disease (COLD)
Cigarette
Ciliary Function
"Cold Turkey"
Coronary Heart Disease
Environmental Tobacco Smoke
Hyperplasia
Involuntary Smoking
Lower-Yield Cigarette
Lung Cancer
Mainstream Smoke
Nicotiana tabacum
Nicotine
Nonsmokers' Liberation Movement
Oral Gratification
Particulates
Passive Smoke
Polycyclic Aromatic Hydrocarbons
Pulmonary Emphysema
Sidestream Smoke
Smokeless Tobacco
Snuff
Snuff Dipping
"Tar"
Tobacco
Tobacco Additives

chapter objectives

After you have studied this chapter, you should be able to do the following:

1. Define the key terms.
2. Estimate the number and percentage of Americans who smoke and use smokeless tobacco.
3. Identify several patterns and trends in the use of tobacco products.
4. Explain why smoking less-hazardous cigarettes can sometimes increase health risks.
5. Explain the meaning of the nonsmokers' liberation movement.
6. Describe smoking as a learned behavior.
7. Identify several psychosocial predictors of smoking among American adolescents.
8. Classify smokers according to: stimulation, handling, pleasurable relaxation, tension reduction, craving, and habit.
9. Name the major phases and constituents of cigarette smoke.
10. Explain smoking behavior as a nicotine addiction.
11. Explain what is meant by the term *dose-related* as it pertains to cigarette smoking and excess mortality.
12. Identify several significant findings of research that relate to the health consequences of smoking.
13. List several complications resulting from maternal smoking during pregnancy.
14. Identify at least five major health consequences associated with passive smoking.
15. Name two specific undesirable smoking-drug interactions that can occur in the human body.
16. Explain the probable actions of nicotine and carbon monoxide in the development of cardiovascular disease associated with cigarette smoking.
17. Distinguish each of the following from the others: hyperplasia, loss of ciliary function, and carcinoma *in situ.*
18. Distinguish between pulmonary emphysema and chronic bronchitis.
19. Compare the health hazards associated with smoking with those related to smokeless forms of tobacco.
20. Explain why people continue to smoke despite scientific evidence that smoking is harmful to health.
21. Describe five techniques for reducing the risks of smoking for those who cannot or will not stop.
22. Name at least five benefits of smoking cessation.

Introduction

Since the U.S. surgeon general's first warning about smoking and cancer, heart disease, and other health problems, the nation's smoking rate has fallen dramatically. In the mid-1960s, an estimated 40 percent of the adult population smoked—53 percent of men and 32 percent of women.

Now the rate of cigarette smoking is one of the lowest ever reported, with only 30% of adults classified as regular smokers. Yet 64 million adult Americans and nearly 5 million adolescents continue to smoke, and another 12 million—mostly adolescent males and young adults—use smokeless tobacco. Of the various forms of tobacco use, cigarette smoking remains the most popular and potentially the most dangerous.

Although the increase in popularity of smokeless tobacco has been related to its perceived harmlessness, the persistent use of any tobacco product carries a major risk of endangering health. Such a risk also applies to the upsurge in cigar smoking, which has become a symbol of achievement.

Continuing such life-threatening behaviors is frequently related to the many psychological rewards associated with using tobacco, the influences of marketing campaigns, the impact of peer pressure and role models, and the addictive nature of nicotine.

This chapter begins by examining the patterns and trends in using tobacco products and provides an analysis of the psychosocial aspects of this behavior. Then the serious health consequences of smoking, including passive smoking, and using smokeless tobacco are detailed, with a focus on cardiovascular diseases, lung cancer, and chronic obstructive lung disease. However, reflecting the health promotion and disease prevention theme of the text, the benefits of smoking cessation are included for those smokers convinced that there is no safe cigarette and no safe level of smoking.

Tobacco: America's Smoke-Drug

Although smoked by native Indians for centuries before the European settlers arrived in America, **tobacco** is often considered a newcomer to the American drug scene. One of the night-shade family of plants native to the Western Hemisphere, tobacco leaves have been smoked, chewed, and sniffed in the Western world for only four hundred years.

Supposedly introduced to Europe by Columbus, tobacco was popularized by Jean Nicot, a French diplomat. At first, tobacco was valued for its assumed sanitary and curative properties. However, it was not long before kings and popes denounced tobacco and the practice of smoking as offensive.

Source of Pleasure and Disease

Although the prepared leaves of ***Nicotiana tabacum*** are a popular source of mild stimulation, **cigarette** smoking has assumed a new status. The practice of smoking is more often described as the major cause of preventable illness and premature deaths in the United States.

Increasingly, the use of cigarettes and other tobacco products is seen as addictive suicide.[1] By contrast, stopping smoking is "the single most important step that smokers can take to enhance the length and quality of their lives."[2]

Smoking tobacco cigarettes and cigars, chewing plugs of tobacco, and sniffing powdered tobacco are potentially dangerous practices. Such behaviors can and do lead to various ailments and severe disorders, from discolored teeth and impaired breathing to debilitating and fatal illnesses, especially heart disease and cancer. These facts are widely known and even accepted by most Americans, including many who smoke. Since the first surgeon general's report on smoking and health was issued in 1964, millions of people have quit smoking.

Nevertheless, millions of people continue to smoke, although nearly 70 percent of them claim they want to quit. More than one thousand Americans die each day from smoking-related diseases. On a yearly basis, the tobacco death toll is at least 400,000. Some estimates of these deaths, however, are as high as 450,000 per year.

In the United States, smoking is responsible for more than one of every six deaths. According to the World Health Organization (WHO), approximately 2.5 million people die worldwide each year as a result of using tobacco. The immediate question one might ask is, Why? Why do so many start to smoke and then continue to smoke?

Personal Decisions with Social Consequences

Countless individuals have made personal decisions about smoking—to start, to change brands, to stop, and to start again after a period of abstinence. Why don't more people stop smoking?

Once a person starts to smoke, his or her future choices about smoking appear less freely made, because smoking tobacco is addictive.[3] The smoker becomes "hooked."

While an estimated 34 percent of smokers have tried to quit, only a small fraction have achieved long-term success. Cigarette smoking has become the most widespread example of drug dependency in this country. It is becoming apparent that the addictive qualities of nicotine are sufficient to overpower a smoker's fear of premature death.[4]

More than individuals become tobacco dependent, however. Our society at large is "hooked"—burdened with a king-sized tobacco industry, a mammoth agricultural enterprise, a considerable source of governmental revenues, a significant customer of the print media, and a potent force in regional and national politics.

While public and private health agencies emphasize the serious health risks of smoking and smokeless tobacco, the federal government continues to subsidize tobacco growers. Again the question is, Why? Why should taxpayers support growing a harmful product and then have to finance disease-prevention activities to discourage the use of the same product?

As a nation, we face a major public health problem and a persistent threat to health that costs an estimated $68 billion per year in lost productivity and the treatment of smoking-related diseases. The American Cancer Society claims this economic expense amounts to nearly $2.59 for each pack of cigarettes sold in the United States.[5]

Yet the major health problems associated with tobacco smoking are created largely by individuals who decide to risk well-being for a puff of smoke, a plug of chewing tobacco, or a pinch of snuff. Why?

The questions and issues raised illustrate the complex problem of understanding a learned behavior that often develops into a dependency, and the difficulty in proposing and applying solutions. More than personal satisfaction is involved in using tobacco—America's "smoke-drug." Sociocultural, economic, political, pharmacological, and even moral factors are identified in the continuation of a legal, mind-stimulating activity that is also a primary health risk.

Box 8.1 Smoking Facts

- More than 3 million adolescents smoke on a daily basis, and 1 million males use smokeless tobacco.
- Teenage cigarette use has jumped over 25 percent since the early 1990s, while the adult smoking rate has declined.
- Now, more than one-third of children in grades 9–12 in American schools smoke cigarettes.
- Smoking has been identified as a "pediatric disease" by medical authorities.
- Teenagers get their cigarettes just as adults do. They walk into stores and buy them and few are checked about their age. They also borrow cigarettes from others, give money to others who then buy them, steal them, or buy them in vending machines.
- Despite laws in all states prohibiting underage smoking, teenagers smoke about 500 million packs of cigarettes yearly and spend over $960 million buying them.
- Eighty-two percent of adults who ever smoked started before they reached age eighteen.
- Of the three thousand American teenagers who start smoking every day, one thousand will eventually die prematurely of smoking-related diseases.

Sources: United States Food and Drug Administration and the Office of the Surgeon General

Patterns and Trends of Tobacco Use

Though cigarette smoking has been a popular and widespread practice in the past, smokers are now in the minority. Although smoking was once perceived as an admired status symbol, current smoking activity is at its lowest level in more than forty years, except among teenagers (see box 8.1).

While overall consumption of cigarettes appears to have stabilized for the past few years, further declines seem unlikely for a rather depressing reason: as adult smokers quit, there is a steady supply of teenagers ready to replace them.[6] Each day, about three thousand American teenagers smoke for the first time. These three thousand teen smokers are nearly equal to the daily number of adults who give up smoking or die from the diseases it causes.

Profile of Tobacco Users

Despite the decline in the adult smoking rate, cigarette use seems to be heavily concentrated in the lower socioeconomic classes.[7] Moreover, the prevalence of smoking remains higher among those living below the poverty level. Less-educated people and minority groups have had smaller reductions in usage rates, and so have females in comparison with males. In addition, the highest proportion of smokers is still found among people between the ages of 25 and 44, while the lowest occurs among those seventy-five years or older.

Smoking prevalence is higher for men than women, highest among Native Americans and Alaskan Natives in comparison with other racial and ethnic groups, and highest among men who have dropped out of high school, according to the American Cancer Society.

With fewer smokers now than in the past and with the per capita consumption falling (see fig. 8.1) to just over two thousand five hundred per adult each year, the United States production of cigarettes has jumped to more than 700 billion each year, an all-time high!

The significant increase in domestic production is the result of foreign demand for U.S. tobacco and American manufacturers' offering discounted cigarettes and lower prices on premium brands to Japan, South Korea, countries of the former Soviet Union, and numerous third-world countries.[8] The United States is the largest cigarette-exporting nation in the world.

Since its introduction into Western civilization by explorers returning from America, smoking until recently was viewed almost exclusively as a masculine activity. Before World War I, a woman who smoked was usually considered unfeminine. Since then, however, women have gradually cast aside the moral and social stigmas surrounding cigarette use, and since World War II they have been smoking more like men—and dying like men! Due to the increase in beginning rates of smoking among less-educated young women, the prevalence of daily smoking has been higher among high school senior females than among males.

The proportions of both women and men smokers have declined. But surveys indicate that the number of men smokers dropped more rapidly and to a much greater degree than the number of women smokers. Although some adult women are beginning to quit at rates comparable to those for adult men, the rate of starting to smoke among younger women has not declined.

Although the prevalence of smoking in the adult population has declined, the average daily number of cigarettes consumed by those who continue to smoke has increased. Those who do smoke appear to be smoking more than ever before—a condition some scientists relate to the introduction of filter-tipped and low-tar/low-nicotine cigarettes. The popularity of cigars has increased slightly, while the use of smoking tobacco for pipes has declined, along with cigarettes.

Resisting the general downward trend is the sudden increase in the use of **"smokeless tobacco"—chewing tobacco** and **snuff.** Associated largely with an aggressive advertising campaign, smokeless tobacco has become a fad among junior high, senior high, and college athletes in particular, and younger males in general.[9] Rather than sniffing powdered tobacco, the individual usually inserts the substance between the gum and cheek, a practice known as **snuff dipping.** Though its popularity has increased significantly, smokeless tobacco should not be considered as a safe alternative to smoking. It isn't!

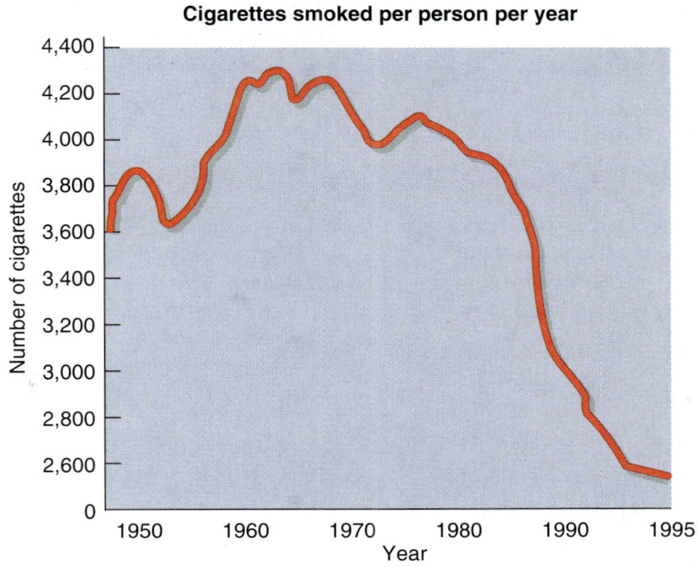

figure 8.1

Per capita consumption of cigarettes, 1950–1995.

Source: Office on Smoking and Health, National Center for Chronic Disease Prevention and Health Promotion, Centers for Disease Control and Prevention, 1996.

The Changing Cigarette

At least 90 percent of U.S. smokers use filter-tip brands, and more than half of the cigarettes consumed are "low-tar" cigarettes, defined as yielding 15 milligrams of "tar" or less per cigarette. (Tar is the particulate matter in cigarette smoke.)

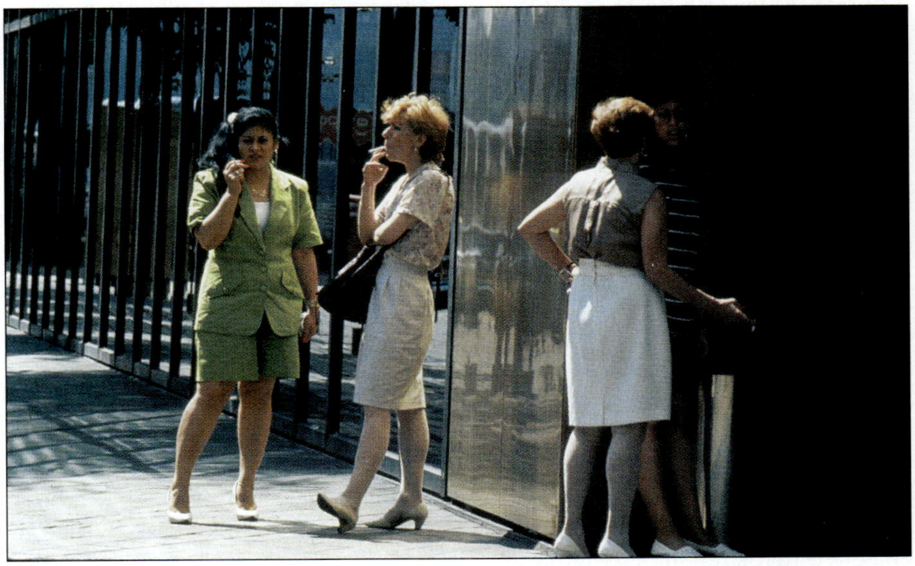

Since the end of World War II, women have been smoking more like men—and dying like men from tobacco-related diseases.

© Lee Snider/The Image Works.

A Switch to Safety?

Preferences for filter-tip, low-tar cigarettes are often related to the public's increased concern about the dangers of smoking. Women smokers are more likely to use these **lower-yield cigarettes** than men are, and smokers of higher income and education also select lower-yield cigarettes in a higher percentage of cases.

In theory, such a change should be protective, because the danger of smoking is believed to be proportional to the dose of inhaled tar, nicotine, and carbon monoxide. Health risk is usually related to the amount of smoke as measured by the number of cigarettes consumed. Smoking these "safer" cigarettes, however, gives only limited reduction of the risks of lung and larynx cancer.

Cancer rates for smokers of such cigarettes are still much higher than

Box 8.2 Tobacco Additives

Tobacco additives are nontobacco substances, including artificial tobacco substitutes and flavoring extracts, typically added to the tobacco mixture of low-tar and low-nicotine cigarettes. These additives are included along with tobacco to speed up or slow down the burn rate of the cigarette, to promote cohesion of the ash, and to improve flavor and aroma.

Among the additives more frequently used in the manufacture of lower-yield cigarettes are:

Artificial tobacco substitutes

Tobacco stems

Flavor extracts of tobacco and other plants

Chemicals specified as "exogenous" enzymes—substances that can promote certain chemical changes

Powdered cocoa flavoring

Licorice

Sugar

Caramel

Freshness-preserving chemicals known as glycols

The precise identity, chemical composition, and potential harmfulness of these additives are not completely known. However, when burned, some are considered to be cocarcinogens—substances that increase the power or activity of cancer-causing chemicals, such as tobacco tars. Until the Food and Drug Administration has the authority to supervise the manufacture of tobacco products, it is likely that many years of research will be required before scientists and smokers learn all of the hazards of the new, "milder" cigarettes.

Another additive, ground cloves, has been responsible for the popularity of "clove cigarettes," or kreteks. Imported from Indonesia, these products contain about 60 to 70 percent tobacco and 30 to 40 percent cloves. However, the smoker is exposed to twice as much tar, nicotine, and carbon monoxide from clove cigarettes as from regular American cigarettes. Typically, clove cigarette smoke is inhaled more deeply and retained in the lungs longer.

The major active ingredient in cloves is the chemical eugenol, which has an anesthetic effect. It is possible that eugenol anesthetizes the backs of smokers' throats and tracheas, thus permitting deeper inhalation and possibly encouraging smoking in some people who would otherwise be discouraged by the harshness of regular cigarettes.

Cloves may improve the fragrance of cigarettes and may produce a mild high, but they certainly do not make tobacco cigarettes less hazardous. Preliminary research indicates that ground cloves can produce serious lung damage and sudden respiratory distress. Accumulation of fluid in the lungs; spasms of the lungs' airways; spitting up or coughing up blood; and increased nausea, vomiting, angina, and respiratory infections have been reported. Other medical problems related to smoking clove cigarettes include severe asthma attacks, difficulty in breathing, chronic coughing, and nosebleeds.

those for nonsmokers. In addition, there is insufficient evidence that the "safer" cigarettes reduce the excess risk of other smoking-related cancers, cardiovascular disease, bronchitis, emphysema, complications of pregnancy, and other disorders linked to smoking. Emphasizing that there is *no safe cigarette* and *no safe level of consumption,* the surgeon general's report on "the changing cigarette" suggested that smoking less-hazardous cigarettes can actually increase one's health risk!

While the foregoing statement appears contradictory, it is based on the common tendency of low-yield smokers to compensate for their decreased intake of nicotine. *Compensation* often takes the form of increasing the number of cigarettes smoked, shortening the interval between puffs, increasing the depth of inhalation, and smoking to a shorter butt. Such compensatory changes may turn a nominally lower-yield cigarette into a higher-yield product. Thus the shift to lower-tar cigarettes may not result in reduced smoke exposure. Any advantage of the lower-yield product is canceled.

Tobacco Additives

An additional concern about low-tar cigarettes deals with health risks related to the design, filtering mechanisms, tobacco ingredients, and additives of the lower-yield products. The chief concern involves the increasing use of **tobacco additives** for processing or flavoring, as described in box 8.2.

Tobacco additives are nontobacco substances that are mixed with the tobacco preparation used in the manufacture of cigarettes. Technically, such items are intended to enhance the flavor and aroma of the tobacco product. However, these additives also affect the burn rate of the cigarette.

Some of these same additives are also known or suspected cancer-causing substances or give rise to carcinogenic substances when burned. The use of these additives may cancel the beneficial effects of reducing the tar yield or might pose increased or new and different disease risks.

A tobacco company has developed a cigarette product that gets nicotine to the smoker without filling the air with sidestream smoke. This new product, known as Eclipse, does not burn tobacco as conventional cigarettes do. Nevertheless, the U.S. Food and Drug Administration is likely to consider Eclipse as nothing more than a nicotine-delivery device. If such a determination is made, then the Food and Drug Administration may be able to regulate this new cigarette, because it is a drug.

To encourage sales of tobacco products and to make them more accessible, smoker-friendly restaurants are opening in otherwise smoke-free airports in major United States cities. Private smoking clubs and retail tobacco shops are also on the rise, sometimes heavily supported by tobacco companies.

The Industry's Response to Falling Sales

To counteract declining numbers of cigarette smokers and domestic cigarette sales, manufacturers have introduced a record number of new brands in an attempt to increase their own market shares. This effort has been achieved largely through a marketing technique known as *targeting.* Through targeting, advertising promotes a "special" product to a limited, narrowly focused population of potential consumers.

For instance, new brand entries have included "designer smokes" for fashion-conscious females; full-flavor (high-tar) cigarettes aimed at Hispanic Americans; premium-priced brands for young upwardly mobile professionals; packaged specialty smokes for Generation X-ers; and even a special cigarette for smokers in the military service, presumably to help new recruits "be all they can be."

At Issue

Should advertising of tobacco products be banned?

Point: Although many "social engineers" favor a prohibition on all advertising of tobacco products, such a ban would be a major infringement on the First Amendment right to free speech. After all, advertising is the voice of free choice in a democratic society. Besides, there is insufficient proof that advertising any tobacco product has ever induced or seduced people to begin using that product. Moreover, in those countries with tobacco advertising bans, such as Canada and Finland, youth smoking rates have not declined. Kids don't begin smoking because of advertising; they smoke because they associate the behavior with being adult. Tobacco advertising is merely an attempt to inform consumers of various brand comparisons and to increase the market share of specific products among the tobacco-using population. As long as tobacco is legal, then advertising tobacco products is just as legal. After all, this is still America!

Counterpoint: Many people would agree with one former Health and Human Services Secretary who said that while tobacco advertising may be legal, it is medically and morally wrong to promote a product that when used as intended, causes death, disease, and addiction. Yes, such ads should be banned! The major concern is not the legality of tobacco advertising, but the health of users and those who come into contact with users' smoke. It is no secret that women, youth, and minority citizens have been targeted with advertising and promotional campaigns aimed at increasing these individuals' consumption of tobacco products. Cigarette advertising typically portrays attractive, healthy people using tobacco in beautiful, pleasant settings that may be interpreted as suggesting a compatibility between smoking and good health. In fact, the two are mutually exclusive and incompatible. The use of young, attractive models conveys the wrong message to our youth who are being actively recruited to replace the 400,000 smokers the industry loses each year due to death.

The Evolution of Tobacco Regulation

Before 1971, there were relatively few laws relating to the sale and promotion of tobacco products in the United States. Taxes had been imposed to raise revenue and were considered as appropriate "vice taxes," along with similar assessments on alcoholic beverages. Licensing of retail businesses selling tobacco products was also a common way of regulating sales and controlling availability of these products. But there was practically no legal concern with "smoke-free indoor air," "youth access to tobacco products," and "advertising of such products."

Then, about thirty years ago, the first federal law was passed banning cigarette ads from radio and television. However, cigarettes, cigars, and smokeless tobacco products have been advertised heavily in newspapers, magazines, direct mail, billboards, posters in trains and buses, bus terminals, subways, and airports, and on small placards in taxis and on the backs of ski-lift chairs. Other tobacco products may still be promoted on radio and television in the United States in an unrestricted manner.

The FDA supports a severe regulation of advertising on billboards, in youth-oriented publications and at sporting events (see "At Issue"). A comprehensive program to prevent children and adolescents from smoking cigarettes or using smokeless tobacco has been finalized (see box 8.3). Provisions of this program are to be enforced by 2000, unless the United States Congress Supreme Court, or the Executive branch of the federal government reverses the antismoking campaign to save children from tobacco, addiction, and smoking-related diseases.

The Nonsmokers' Liberation Movement

For many, regulation or restriction of tobacco use seemed to be another unwanted "big government" intrusion into private life. Smoking had long been considered an individual right. However, little thought or consideration had been given to what right the nonsmoker has to live and work in areas free from air polluted by smoke. It would seem as though the nonsmoker has a right to travel in an airplane, bus, or train; to listen to a lecture or attend a concert in an auditorium; to work; or to eat at a restaurant without

Box 8.3 The Food and Drug Administration's Final Rule Summary on Children and Tobacco

In proposing the final rule summary, the Food and Drug Administration (FDA) has concluded that cigarettes and smokeless tobacco are delivery devices for nicotine, a drug that causes addiction and other significant pharmacological effects. Furthermore, because the United States Supreme Court has upheld restrictions on commercial speech if certain standards are met, the FDA assumes that protecting the health of children under eighteen is a substantial government interest justifying restrictions on tobacco advertising that appeals to children.

The Final Rule on Children and Tobacco calls for:

- Minimum age of 18 to buy tobacco products.
- Ban vending machines and self-service displays, *except* in certain nightclubs and other "adult only" facilities totally inaccessible to persons under 18.
- Ban "kiddie" packs, "loosies," or free samples.
- Mail-order sales permitted.
- Ban billboards within 1,000 feet of schools and playgrounds.
- Other billboards and outdoor and in-store advertising limited to black-and-white text-only, *except* color, imagery permitted in "adult only" facilities if not visible from outside and not removable.
- Advertising in publications with significant youth readership (more than 15 percent or 2 million) limited to black-and-white text only.
- Ban brand-name sponsorship of sporting or other events, including cars and teams: only corporate name sponsorship permitted.
- Ban brand names on hats, t-shirts, gym bags, etc.

In addition to the Rule, the FDA proposes to require tobacco companies to educate children and adolescents about the health risks of tobacco use.

Source: United States Food and Drug Administration, "Saving Our Children From Tobacco," *FDA Consumer*, Vol. 30, No. 8 (October, 1996): 7–8.

being exposed to air filled with the smoke from cigarettes, pipes, or cigars. These concerns have resulted in major changes in public places, first as separate areas for smokers and nonsmokers, then as smoke-free areas, which are increasingly demanded.

Organized groups of nonsmokers, such as Action on Smoking and Health, the Group Against Smokers' Pollution, together with the American Lung Association, the American Cancer Society, the American Heart Association, and professional medical and dental associations, have been successful in restricting or banning smoking in both public and private areas, including work areas, and in establishing the legal right of nonsmokers to be free of others' cigarette smoke, referred to as **"passive smoke."**

The **nonsmokers' liberation movement** has been successful in restricting smoking in hospitals, museums, and elevators, and in lobbying for laws and regulations that require health warnings on cigarette packages (see fig. 8.2) and for separate smoking and nonsmoking sections on commercial interstate buses and national airlines. Federal legislation forbids smoking on most domestic flights, and many airlines are prohibiting smoking on international flights as well.

Specific Efforts at Restriction

Many states and cities have already passed laws requiring either the separation of smokers and nonsmokers or the complete prohibition of smoking in public places, including educational institutions, restaurants, and retail establishments such as grocery and department stores. Some municipalities have attempted to restrict tobacco smoking in private workplaces. A growing number of companies have adopted smoking bans and refuse to hire smokers. Some pay bonuses to employees who quit smoking.

As some companies move to restrict smoking both on and off the job, and thus influence what many consider to be an individual right, smokers have begun to fight back. Several states have passed legislation that forbids the firing of employees who engage in legal off-duty behavior, including smoking. With the full implementation of the federal "Americans with Disabilities Act," employers will be prohibited from asking job applicants if they smoke.

Although roadblocks to a smoke-free American society are constantly being erected by tobacco interests and tobacco-growing states, and possibly by decisions of the United States Supreme Court, tobacco control efforts have been increasing steadily, as indicated:[10]

1. **The FDA Proposal.** The United States Food and Drug Administration has proposed to regulate cigarettes and smokeless tobacco products as drug-delivery devices. This action, if implemented, would involve strict curbs on the promotion of and on minors' access to these items.
2. **Presidential Leadership.** The FDA proposal to regulate tobacco was announced by the president of the United States in 1995. This is the first time any president of this nation has delivered a major statement on tobacco, and then supported a significant proposal to deal with the tobacco problem as a national health concern.
3. **Industry documents.** A tremendous number of internal tobacco industry documents has surfaced revealing the long-standing industry's knowledge of the disease effects of smoking and the drug effects of nicotine.[11]
4. **Litigation.** Several class-action and personal-injury lawsuits have been filed against the industry on behalf of millions of smokers addicted to nicotine or suffering from tobacco-related diseases. By 1997, nearly twenty states seeking reimbursement for Medicaid costs of treating illnesses caused by smoking sued tobacco

SURGEON GENERAL'S WARNING: Smoking Causes Lung Cancer, Heart Disease, Emphysema, and May Complicate Pregnancy.

SURGEON GENERAL'S WARNING: Quitting Smoking Now Greatly Reduces Serious Risks to Your Health.

SURGEON GENERAL'S WARNING: Smoking by Pregnant Women May Result in Fetal Injury, Premature Birth, and Low Birth Weight.

SURGEON GENERAL'S WARNING: Cigarette Smoke Contains Carbon Monoxide.

figure 8.2

Warning labels.

Source: Surgeon General's Public Health Service, Office of the Assistant Secretary for Health.

companies. Tobacco companies agreed to a national antitobacco settlement amounting to over $368 billion. Congress refused to back this settlement and antismoking groups felt the terms, specifically the weak restrictions on marketing to teenagers, were too lenient. However, in 1998, four states reached an out-of-court settlement for over $36 billion. Then, later in that year, the remaining forty-six states also reached a settlement with the major tobacco companies. In return for restrictions on advertising and marketing practices and limited immunity from lawsuits, these states will receive millions of dollars for smoking-related disease costs.

5. **State Programs.** The National Cancer Institute and the Centers for Disease Control and Prevention—agencies of the federal government—have provided grants to states for various tobacco efforts, making possible at least basic tobacco control programs in all fifty states.
6. **OSHA Proposal.** The Occupational Safety and Health Administration (OSHA) has proposed extensive rules that would ban smoking in workplaces except in separately ventilated areas.

The numerous tobacco control measures and proposals described seem to enjoy wide public support. Nevertheless, the tobacco control movement faces powerful pro-tobacco forces. Only time will tell what influences the tobacco industry, politicians, Congress, advertising agencies, tobacco farmers, and restaurant associations, will have on the future of tobacco regulation. For more Information on Smoking, contact:

Action on Smoking and Health (ASH) 2013 H. St., NW Washington, D.C., 20006

Americans for Nonsmokers' Rights (ANR) 2530 San Pablo Ave., Suite J Berkeley, CA 94702

Group Against Smokers' Pollution (GASP) P.O. Box 632 College Park, MD 20741

Stop Teen-Age Addiction to Tobacco (STAT) 511 E. Columbus Ave. Springfield, MA 01105

and the local offices of the American Cancer Society, American Heart Association, and American Lung Association

Psychological Aspects of Smoking

Why do people begin and continue to smoke, when most smokers admit that smoking is harmful to personal health? Many smokers express a desire to quit, undertake a program of cessation, but cannot manage to do so. Perhaps a consideration of the origins and functional aspects of smoking behavior will reveal some of the reasons and motivations involved in the use of cigarettes.

A New Product for Personal Needs

Until the invention of the cigarette manufacturing machine after the Civil War, tobacco was principally consumed in pipes and cigars and in chewing and sniffing. Once mass production of cigarettes was a reality and production costs decreased, cigarettes became readily available. Their preeminence as a tobacco form has been traced to World War I, when they found the favor of the doughboys (soldiers).

Cigarettes became immensely popular because they provided the user with certain personal gratifications unobtainable in other tobacco forms. Cigarettes can be smoked easily and quickly; they can be inhaled; they are readily available and still relatively inexpensive; and they had achieved limited social acceptance or toleration, until the nonsmokers' liberation movement became prominent and active in the 1970s.

Not to be overlooked as a factor in cigarette consumption are the persistent promotional activities of tobacco companies and their advertising agencies. Long ago, motivational research revealed that sales could be increased if products were linked with basic human desires and drives.

Not content with assertions of mildness and good taste, advertisements soon depicted smokers as models of sophistication, eternal youth, handsome ruggedness, enduring beauty, alluring sexuality, and determined individualism, and with athletic prowess sufficient to walk at least a mile for a favorite cigarette.

For many adolescents, smoking a cigarette became symbolic of adulthood and maturity. Or, more simply, as Joe Camel might suggest: smoking is cool! (See the section on advertising in chapter 2.)

A Learned Behavior

Smoking is often viewed as a learned behavior. No one is born a smoker. Curiosity and the desire to imitate adults, especially smoking parents, probably encourage many children to experiment. The initial reaction, however, is likely to be unpleasant.

It is not until adolescence that smoking becomes a real option for most young people. More time is spent away from home with peers; there is increased freedom from authority figures who often discourage or forbid smoking; needs for security and acceptance through group conformity grow; and the demand for immediate need gratification flourishes. The psychological stage for smoking has been set and is powerful enough to produce a million new young smokers each year. Other factors have also been recognized as predictors of tobacco use by young people, as noted in table 8.1.

According to the surgeon general's report *Preventing Tobacco Use among Young People*,[12]

- Nearly all first use of tobacco occurs before high school graduation. If adolescents can be kept tobacco-free, most will remain tobacco-free for the remainder of their lives.
- Male and female adolescents are equally likely to smoke cigarettes, but males are more likely than females to use smokeless tobacco.
- White adolescents are more likely to use tobacco than are African American and Hispanic adolescents, and whites are much more likely to be heavy or frequent smokers.
- Most young people who smoke are addicted to nicotine and report that they want to quit but are unable to do so.
- Tobacco is often the first drug used by young people who later use alcohol and other illegal drugs, especially marijuana.
- Among young people, those with poorer grades and lower self-images are most likely to begin using tobacco.
- Cigarette advertising appears to increase young people's risk of smoking by conveying the message that smoking has important social benefits and that smoking is far more common than it really is.
- Adolescent tobacco use is associated with involvement in fights, carrying weapons, and engaging in risky sexual behavior.

table 8.1 Summary of Factors Appearing to Increase the Risk of Tobacco Use by Young People

Sociodemographic Factors
Young people from families with lower socioeconomic status
Adolescents living in single-parent homes
Environment Factors
Peer influence in beginning experimentation
Peer-group approval of and support of tobacco use by providing experimentation, reinforcement, and cues for continuing use
Social Environment Factors
Adolescents who highly overestimate the number of young people and adults who smoke
Young people who perceive that cigarettes are easily accessible and generally available for use
Behavioral Factors
Perception that tobacco use assists in achieving physical maturity, a coherent sense of self, and emotional independence
Belief that smoking serves positive functions, such as bonding with peers, being independent and mature, and having a positive social image
Lack of confidence to be able to resist peer offers of tobacco
Intention to use tobacco
Experimental smoking

Source: *Preventing Tobacco Use among Young People: A Report of the Surgeon General, Executive Summary*, pages 7–8. Centers for Disease Control and Prevention, 1994.

Psychological Rewards

There are many psychological rewards for the new smoker. Smoking may be the passport to acceptance among one's peers; it may represent freedom or independence from restrictive home life and passive, traditional sex roles, or revolt against parental authority; it may be the result of an unconscious desire to imitate esteemed smokers; it may be nothing more than a soothing and pleasurable way to counteract boredom.

Of course, some people like the taste and smell of cigarettes, and a few enjoy watching the smoke. In essence, the cigarette provides a smoker with a readily available way to deal with a host of personal problems and needs.

Factors in Smoking Behavior

The reasons for beginning cigarette use are not always the same as those for continuing to smoke. Original motives are often replaced by powerful factors, both psychological and biochemical. These factors are most apparent in a classification of experienced smokers according to the major satisfactions people believe they get from using tobacco cigarettes. Six "satisfaction" categories are detailed here to provide an understanding of why people smoke. This brief analysis also offers various alternatives to those who wish to quit.

1. **Stimulation.** Many smokers get a lift from smoking—they feel that it helps them wake up, organize energies, and keep them going. The perking-up effect is due to nicotine's temporary stimulation, which briefly relieves fatigue. If you try to give up smoking, you may want a safe substitute: a brisk walk or moderate exercise whenever you feel the urge to smoke.

2. **Handling—oral gratification.** Having something to handle, manipulate, or fondle can be satisfying. Additionally, having something in your mouth to chew on, such as a toothpick, straw, or pencil can fulfill certain emotional needs. This is called **oral gratification.**

   Why not toy with a pen or pencil? Try doodling or play with a coin, a piece of jewelry, or some other harmless object. If you must put something in your mouth, use candy cigarettes or even a real cigarette if you can trust yourself not to light it.

3. **Pleasurable relaxation.** Other smokers smoke for positive feelings of contentment, achievement, victory, and satisfaction—such as upon completion of a job well done or after a meal.

   Those who do get real pleasure out of smoking may find that an honest consideration of the harmful effects of their habit is enough to help them quit. They could substitute eating, drinking, social activities, and physical activities—within reasonable bounds—and find they do not miss their cigarettes.

4. **Crutch—tension reduction.** Many smokers use the cigarette to manage negative effects, such as stressful situations and feelings of anger, fear, and anxiety. Sometimes the cigarette is used as a tranquilizer or as an escape from cares and worries. Thus smoking represents a tension-reducing activity.

   When it comes to quitting, this kind of smoker may find it easy to stop when everything is going well but may be tempted to start again in a time of crisis. Again, physical exertion, eating, drinking, or social activity—in moderation—may serve as useful substitutes in times of tension.

5. **Craving—psychological and physical addiction.** Quitting smoking is difficult for the person who has developed a "craving." For such an individual, the overpowering desire for the next cigarette begins to build up the moment the old one is put out. A dependent or addicted smoker must have a cigarette after a short time or otherwise experience mild withdrawal symptoms—a "nicotine fit" with its uneasiness; restlessness; nervousness; anxiety; headache; digestive disturbances; and impairment of concentration, judgment, and psychomotor performance.

   Peculiarly, the dependent smoker craves a cigarette, as in chain-smoking, first to increase positive feelings and then to decrease negative feelings of withdrawal. In essence, the smoker satisfies a need to smoke—a physical need for more nicotine.

   The first cigarette each day sends a burst of nicotine to the brain, which produces an immediate feeling of satisfaction and mild euphoria. During the remainder of the day, the smoker tries to maintain this feeling by manipulating the intake of tobacco smoke, inhaling more or less deeply, taking more or fewer puffs, and smoking at different intervals—characteristics of a controlled, compulsive behavior.

   Contrary to popular belief, research suggests that smoking does not reduce anxiety or calm nerves. Under stress, smokers consume cigarettes heavily because stress depletes the body's nicotine. Thus nicotine-deficient smokers smoke more under stress to maintain their usual nicotine level.

   Tapering off is not likely to work for dependent smokers. They must go **"cold turkey,"** that is, quit all at once. It may be helpful for them to smoke more than usual for a day or two, so that the taste of cigarettes is spoiled, and then isolate themselves completely from cigarettes until the craving is gone. Giving up cigarettes may cause so much discomfort that once these people quit, they will find it easy to resist a return to smoking. Otherwise, they know that someday they will have to go through the same agony again.

6. **Habit.** The habit smoker establishes a behavioral pattern almost involuntarily. This individual responds automatically to some cue—a cup of coffee, getting into a car, or nearing the vicinity of an ashtray. Once regarded as psychologically significant, smoking loses its former functions of fulfilling status, relaxation, security, or other emotional needs. Such a smoker no longer gets much satisfaction from cigarettes.

   This smoker may find that it is easy to quit and stay off cigarettes if he or she can break developed habit patterns. Cutting down gradually may be effective if there is a change in the way cigarettes are smoked and the conditions under which they are smoked. The key to success is becoming aware of each cigarette you smoke. Ask yourself, "Do I really want this cigarette?" You may be surprised at how many you do not want.

Health Consequences of Smoking

In the past, many people were willing to accept smoking as long as it did not injure the health of the smoker or cause harm to others. Unfortunately, smoking is a health threat to smoker and nonsmoker alike.[13] Even unborn children can be affected adversely by this multidimensional problem, smoking often leads to self-inflicted disease (morbidity) and premature death (mortality). The smoking problem also results in increased health and welfare costs, added irritating effects of cigarette-induced air pollution, and the persistent threat of home, commercial, and forest fires caused by discarded cigarettes.

Constituents of Tobacco Smoke

The starches, proteins, sugars, and hydrocarbons of the tobacco leaf, when burned, are converted into a complex aerosol mixture of *gases* and *particulate matter* **(particulates)** (see box 8.4). The lighted cigarette generates about two thousand compounds, many of which produce undesirable effects. At the burning zone, the temperature of the smoke is nearly 900° C, although that which reaches the smoker's mouth is in a temperature range from 30° to 50° C.

Box 8.4 Toxic and Carcinogenic Agents in Cigarette Smoke

Compounds *most likely to contribute* to the health hazards of smoking:

Carbon monoxide (gas phase)

Nicotine and "tar" (particulate phase)

Compounds that are *probable contributors* to the health hazards of smoking:

Acrolein, hydrocyanic acid, nitric oxide, nitrogen dioxide (gas phase)

Cresols and phenol (particulate phase)

Compounds that are *suspected contributors* to the health hazards of smoking:

Acetaldehyde, acetone, acetonitrile, acrylonitrile, ammonia, benzene, 2–3 butadione, carbon dioxide, crotononitrile, ethylamine, formaldehyde, hydrogen sulfide, methacrolein, methyl alcohol, and methylamine (gas phase). Butylamine, dimethylamine, DDT, endrin, furfural, hydroquinone, nickel compounds, and pyridine (particulate phase)

Source: Office on Smoking and Health, U.S Department of Health and Human Services.

Common Gases

In the *gas phase* of cigarette smoke are *nitrogen, oxygen,* and *carbon dioxide,* and numerous toxic components, some of which cause cancer, initiate tumors, and damage the hairlike cilia that line the bronchial tubes in the lungs. **Carbon monoxide** is a poisonous component of this smoke and combines with the hemoglobin in red blood cells, thereby reducing the oxygen-carrying capacity of the blood.

Also isolated in this phase of smoke are various *nitrosamines, vinyl chloride, formaldehyde, nitrogen oxides, hydrogen cyanide, ammonia,* and *pyridine.*

Tars and Nicotine

The *particulate phase* of cigarette smoke is composed of tiny particles that irritate the respiratory tract. The major components are *nicotine* and **"tar."** Investigations have shown that more than 90 percent of these particles remain in the lungs of smokers who inhale. When condensed, the particles—regarded as lung-damaging in size—form a yellow-brown sticky mass known as tobacco tar.

The tar contains several *carcinogenic* (cancer-producing) *hydrocarbons,* known as **polycyclic aromatic hydrocarbons** (PAH). Among these PAH are nonvolatile *nitrosamines, aromatic amines, pyrenes, benzo (a) pyrenes,* and *chrysenes.* One of these PAH, benzo (a) pyrene, has been linked with a specific gene that causes lung cancer. Also included in the tar are *phenols, cresols, carboxylic acids, metallic ions, radioactive compounds, agricultural chemicals,* and various *additives* and *flavoring agents.*

Nicotine, the other major component of the particulate, is a colorless, oily compound and an ingredient in certain commercial insecticides. It is usually accepted that nicotine is the principal factor in tobacco responsible for cigarette smokers' pharmacologic responses. In the inexperienced smoker, it is nicotine that sometimes causes nausea and even vomiting until tolerance to these effects develops.

However, nicotine mimics the effects of acetylcholine, an excitatory neurotransmitter, and causes most of its many effects by activating the release of this neurotransmitter in the peripheral and central nervous systems.[14] After contacting lung surfaces in the process of smoking, nicotine enters the bloodstream and is delivered rapidly to the brain. (It takes about 13.5 seconds for an intravenous injection of nicotine in the arm to reach the brain, but by inhalation, the delivery time is only 7.5 seconds.)

Once in the brain, the release of acetylcholine in the peripheral nervous system triggers an increase in blood pressure and heart rate; the production of adrenaline (a hormone from the adrenal glands); blood-vessel narrowing, which lowers skin temperature; increased respiration; release of glycogen from the liver, thus causing the brief stimulating "kick" following smoking; and a reduction of fatigue.

In the central nervous system, nicotine increases the amount of norepinephrine and dopamine neurotransmitters in a complicated process involving nicotine-sensitive acetylcholine receptors in the nerve cells. Norepinephrine's action in the reticular activating system results in arousal; increased alertness; decreased stress reaction; and improved concentration, which may in time help improve task performance.[15]

Within the limbic system, dopamine is released in a small structure, the nucleus accumbens—part of the brain's pleasure circuit and the area that controls the process of addiction. Dopamine neurotransmitter is responsible for the feelings of euphoria that result in repeated drug-taking behavior to experience more pleasure.

According to the director of the National Institute on Drug Abuse, every substance that is addicting leads to an increase in dopamine levels in the brain. This helps explain why people who abuse one substance so often abuse another.[16]

There is no doubt the actions of nicotine soon become reinforcing or rewarding. An individual who smokes only one pack per day can average 70,000 to 80,000 nicotine inhalations per year. As such, the smoking process has many potential conditioned stimuli, ranging from the taste, sight, and feel of the cigarette to the many social settings in which smoking takes place. It is easy to see, therefore, how smokers can also become psychologically dependent on tobacco.

Nicotine Addiction

For many years, people have thought of tobacco use as merely habituating (habit-forming). This attitude prevailed despite that many cigarette smokers, who had repeatedly failed in their attempt to stop smoking, probably realized that their tobacco use was something more than a simple little habit.

Now the scientific community recognizes the addictive or dependency-producing nature of cigarette smoking and tobacco use. This formal acknowledgment, based on the function of dopamine neurotransmitter in the brain, helps explain why so many people continue to use tobacco, despite its known health risks.

After observing smokers' behavior, scientists believe that most cigarette users—perhaps as many as 90 percent—are physically dependent on smoking. Moreover, allegations have been made that cigarette manufacturers have intentionally regulated the nicotine content of their products. Such a practice not only entraps new smokers, but also keeps these smokers addicted. Addicted smokers are, after all, reliable customers who continue to purchase cigarettes despite a strong desire to quit smoking.

The blood plasma half-life of nicotine is about 30 minutes, and the pack-a-day smoker lights up approximately every 30 to 40 minutes of the day. This activity suggests that the smoker is attempting to maintain a constant level of nicotine in the brain.

When deprived of this regular dose, the nicotine-dependent smoker begins to suffer discomfort, jumpiness, irritability, craving for another smoke, nausea, and sometimes headache. Although individuals such as these may desire the pleasant, stimulated feeling provided by a rush of nicotine, they continue to smoke because they want to prevent the unwanted effects of withdrawal.

Upon thorough analysis of available evidence, the surgeon general concluded that cigarettes and other forms of tobacco, too, are addicting.[17] Nicotine is the drug in tobacco that causes this addiction—a fact known for thirty years by the tobacco industry.[18] Nevertheless, top executives of this industry still deny the addictive nature of tobacco smoking.

The core or central element among all forms of drug addiction is that the user's behavior is largely controlled by a substance having a psychoactive effect. There is often compulsive use of the drug despite damage to the individual or to society, and drug-seeking behavior can take precedence over other important life priorities. In addition, the drug is reinforcing, that is, the drug's effect is sufficiently rewarding to maintain self-administration over and over again.

Another aspect of drug addiction is *tolerance,* a condition in which a given dose of a drug produces less effect, or increasing doses are required to achieve a desired response. *Physical dependence* on the drug can also occur and is characterized by a *withdrawal syndrome* (including craving for tobacco, irritability, anxiety, difficulty in concentrating, restlessness, headache, drowsiness, and gastrointestinal disturbances) that usually accompanies drug abstinence. After cessation of drug use, there is a strong tendency to *relapse* or restart using the drug again.

Research demonstrates that tobacco use and nicotine in particular meet these criteria (See box 8.5).

Box 8.5 Criteria for Nicotine Addiction:

One Form of Drug Dependence

Primary Criteria

User's behavior is highly controlled by a drug substance

Drug has a psychoactive (mind-changing) effect

Presence of drug-reinforced behavior

Additional Criteria

Dependence-producing drug use often results in:

- Tolerance
- Physical dependence evidenced by withdrawal syndrome
- Pleasant (euphoric) effects

Addictive behavior often involves:

- Repetitive and stereotypic use patterns
- Quitting episodes followed by resumption of drug use (relapse)
- Compulsive use despite harmful effects
- Recurring cravings or urges to use the drug, especially during drug abstinence

Note: The terms *drug addiction* and *drug dependence* are scientifically equivalent and are often used synonymously.

Source: Modified from *The Health Consequences of Smoking. Nicotine Addiction, A Report of the Surgeon General,* 7, 1988.

Research Findings

Human population studies, health surveys, animal experimentation, and clinical and autopsy studies have been the bases for the present knowledge of the health and disease effects of smoking cigarettes. Following are the significant findings of these research endeavors.

1. **Overall death rates.** Cigarette smokers have overall death rates that are substantially greater than those of nonsmokers. Heart and blood-vessel diseases, including stroke, along with lung cancer, chronic obstructive lung (respiratory) disease, and other cancerous conditions are the major contributors to this excess of smoking-related mortality.
2. **Other cancerous conditions.** In addition to the epidemic of smoking-caused lung cancer, cigarette smoking is also the major cause of cancer of the larynx (voice box), mouth, and

esophagus, and a contributing factor in the development of cancer of the bladder, pancreas, and kidney. Use of tobacco cigarettes is associated with increased risk of cancer of the stomach, uterine cervix, and colon or rectum.[19]

3. **Life expectancy.** Expected life span at any given age is significantly shortened by cigarette smoking. An average drop of seven to nine years in smokers' life expectancy has been reported in comparison with nonsmokers.[20]

4. **Dose-related mortality.** In both men and women smokers, excess mortality is dose related. That is, death rates increase with the *number of cigarettes smoked* and are proportional to the *duration of smoking,* an *earlier age of beginning cigarette smoking, inhalation of cigarette smoke,* and *a higher tar and nicotine content* of the cigarette.

5. **Pipe and cigar smoking.** Pipe and cigar smoking are also associated with elevated mortality for cancers of the upper respiratory tract, including cancer of the oral cavity (mouth and lip), the larynx (throat and vocal cords), and the esophagus. Such smoking results in lower death rates than for cigarette smokers, but higher than for nonsmokers.

6. **Chronic (long-term) health conditions.** In general, male and female cigarette smokers tend to report more chronic health conditions, such as chronic bronchitis and/or emphysema, chronic sinusitis, peptic ulcer disease, and arteriosclerotic heart disease, than people who never smoked. Women who smoke also experience a higher risk of broken bones, because smoking tends to reduce bone density. There is a dose-response relationship between the number of cigarettes smoked per day and the frequency of reporting for most of the chronic conditions cited.

7. **Age-related macular degeneration.** People who smoke more than a pack of cigarettes a day at least double their risk of developing a chronic eye condition, age-related macular degeneration or AMD. This disease is the leading cause of severe visual impairment among the elderly.[21] Treatment is either not available or ineffective for most most patients, therefore, AMD is a major cause of blindness and involves the deterioration of the central portion of the retina—the innermost coat of the rear part of the eyeball. Smoking may slow blood circulation to the retina, speed up the aging of cells, or deplete the body of vital nutrients that protect the eyes from this disease.

8. **Acute (short-term) health conditions.** The occurrence of acute conditions (for example, influenza and the common cold) for males who had ever smoked was 14 percent higher, and for females 21 percent higher, than for those who had never smoked cigarettes.

9. **Lost workdays and disability.** Both male and female current cigarette smokers experienced an excess of workdays lost, days of bed disability, and longer limitation of activity due to chronic diseases than did people who never smoked. Additionally, current and former smokers reported more hospitalization than nonsmokers in the year prior to being interviewed. Significantly, all measures of smoking disability were dose related; that is, the more smoking there was, the greater the likelihood of developing a disability or disablement.

10. **Smoking during pregnancy.** Babies born to women who smoke during pregnancy weigh an average of 200 grams less than babies born to comparable nonsmoking women. The more a woman smokes during pregnancy, the greater the reduction in infant birth weight. The risks of spontaneous abortion, fetal death, neonatal death, placental disorders, bleeding early or late in pregnancy, premature and prolonged rupture of amniotic membranes, and pre-term delivery all increase directly with increasing levels of maternal smoking during pregnancy. Research also suggests that maternal smoking during pregnancy may biologically prime the fetal brain of daughters, predisposing them to smoke years after their birth.[22]

11. **Reproductive problems and male erectile dysfunction.** Studies in women and men suggest that cigarette smoking may impair fertility—the capability of reproducing—by interfering with the production of eggs, sperm, or the conception process. Women who smoked more than a pack of cigarettes a day had two-and-one-half times the chance of developing an ectopic pregnancy—implantation of a fertilized egg outside the lining of the uterus—as women who did not smoke.[23] Those who smoked only a half pack a day were one-and-one-half times as likely to have such a pregnancy. Among men, the more cigarettes smoked over time, the higher the risk of developing male erectile dysfunction. It is thought that nicotine damages the penile arteries, which become narrowed and eventually block the flow of blood, leading to impotence.

12. **Sudden infant death syndrome.** An infant's risk of developing sudden infant death syndrome (SIDS) is increased by maternal smoking during pregnancy. Smoking tends to double the risk in what appears to be a dose-response relationship, that is, the more the mother smokes while pregnant, the greater the likelihood the infant will experience a stoppage of breathing while asleep.[24]

13. **Depression.** Research indicates that mental depression plays an important role in the dynamics of cigarette smoking. Individuals with a history of major depression may be "self-medicating" their psychic pain by smoking tobacco cigarettes. In addition, smokers are more likely than nonsmokers to be depressed, and smokers who are depressed usually find it more difficult to quit

smoking than smokers who are not mentally depressed.[25]

14. **Airway obstruction and slowed lung function.** Cigarette smoking is associated with evidence of mild airway obstruction and slowed growth of lung function in adolescents. Adolescent girls may be more vulnerable than boys to the effects of smoking on the growth of lung function.[26] These effects of relatively small amounts of cigarette smoke on the level and growth of lung function in children and adolescents is another reason to prevent young people from starting to smoke.

15. **Decreased oxygen uptake and exercise tolerance.** Elevated carbon monoxide levels in the blood—a consequence of using tobacco cigarettes—have been shown to decrease maximal oxygen uptake in healthy people and decrease the exercise tolerance of persons with heart disease. Additionally, cigarette smoking tends to impair exercise performance, especially in some types of athletic events and activities involving maximal work capacity.

16. **Smoking and other unhealthy behaviors.** A national research study revealed that smokers tend to display several unhealthy behaviors that may increase the probability, of their developing serious illness and disability and experiencing premature death.[27] Compared with nonsmokers, smokers are more likely to get little sleep (six hours or less per night), skip breakfast, not exercise actively, and drink alcohol heavily (two drinks or more daily). In contrast, smokers were less likely to be overweight and less likely to snack daily than were nonsmokers. The more favorable weight status and snacking behavior tended to be most characteristic of lighter smokers.

17. **Premature facial wrinkling.** Cigarette smoking has been identified as an independent risk factor for the development of premature facial wrinkling.[28] When excessive sun exposure and cigarette smoking occurred together, the risk for developing excessive facial skin wrinkling is multiplied by 12.

18. **Source of drug interactions.** Smoking of tobacco should be considered as one of the primary sources of drug interactions in the human body. For certain drugs, smokers may need a larger dose or may have to take the drug more often than nonsmokers. Smoking may also result in increased risks with drug use, affect an individual's response to certain common diagnostic tests, and interact with certain food constituents.

    One specific smoking-drug problem is the increased risk of heart attack, stroke, and other circulatory diseases among those women who smoke and also use oral contraceptives. This risk is even higher in women older than thirty seven years and among heavy smokers. The official Food and Drug Administration's warning is loud and clear: *"Women who use oral contraceptives should not smoke."*

    Another such smoking-drug interaction is apparent in alcohol use. Beverage alcohol and cigarette smoking show synergistic effects in causing cancer of the upper digestive tract.

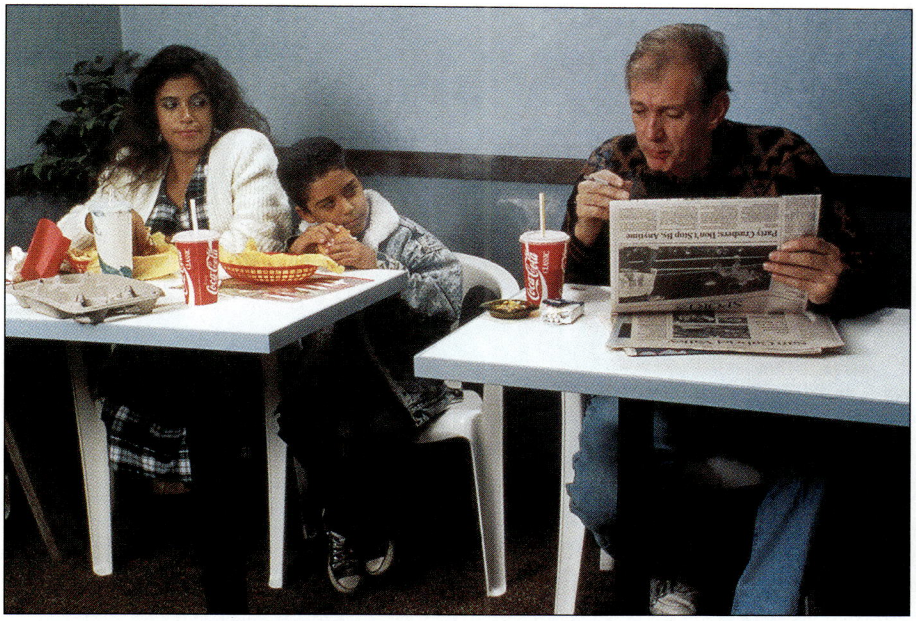

Passive smoking can be more than annoying. In some cases, inhalation of environmental tobacco smoke increases the risk of lung cancer; heart disease; and other cardiac, blood vessel, and blood disorders.

© Stephen McBrady/Photo Edit.

Passive Smoking

Inhaling tobacco smoke from another person's cigarette, cigar, or pipe can be more than annoying. In some cases, it can be deadly.

There is considerable evidence that nonsmokers are exposed to the elements and hazards of tobacco smoke even when they never smoke and do not work or live around people who do. Exposure to nicotine wafted into the air from burning cigarettes finds its way into the lungs of just about everyone, smokers and nonsmokers alike.[29] It is also clear that the tobacco smoke left in the air by smokers can produce some serious diseases in nonsmokers who must breathe the same air.[30]

Secondhand **sidestream smoke** from the burning tobacco products of others, smoke that escapes from the nonburning ends, and **mainstream smoke** that has been inhaled by smokers and then exhaled—mix with air in an enclosed space to form **environmental tobacco smoke,** or ETS. Passive smoking involves the involuntary inhalation of ETS. This environmental tobacco smoke is basically the same, though lower in concentration, as the mixture to which smokers are exposed. It is this ETS that tends to cause a large proportion of healthy nonsmokers to experience irritation of the eyes, nose, and throat.

Sidestream smoke is not filtered (as the smoker's is) and often has higher concentrations of hazardous substances than does mainstream smoke. Concentrations of at least seventeen cancer-causing chemicals are higher in sidestream smoke than in mainstream smoke. For example, the concentration of highly carcinogenic N-nitrosamine is so much higher in sidestream smoke that nonsmokers in smoky rooms for one hour would inhale as much of this chemical as they would by smoking ten to fifteen cigarettes.

Passive cigarette smoke can make a significant and measurable contribution to the amount of indoor air pollution at levels of smoking and ventilation common in the indoor environment. Exposed to an atmosphere of ETS in a confined space, the nonsmoker may also develop varying degrees of stress, discomfort, coughing, wheezing, and allergic reactions. People with certain heart and lung diseases and allergies may also suffer a worsening of their symptoms as a result of exposure to tobacco smoke-filled environments.

The studies summarized here indicate that secondhand tobacco smoke is more than an irritant or a contaminant that merely aggravates the symptoms of those who suffer respiratory diseases (box 8.6).

Box 8.6 Health Consequences of Involuntary (Passive) Smoking

Lung Cancer in Nonsmoking Adults

1. Passive smoking is causally associated with lung cancer in adults.
2. Approximately three thousand lung cancer deaths per year among nonsmokers (never smoked and former smokers) of both sexes are estimated to be linked to environmental tobacco smoke (ETS) in the United States.

Noncancer Respiratory Diseases and Disorders

1. Exposure of children to ETS from parental smoking is causally associated with
   a. increased prevalence of respiratory symptoms of irritation, such as coughing, sputum production, and wheezing;
   b. increased prevalence of middle-ear effusion, a sign of middle-ear disease; and
   c. a small but statistically significant reduction in lung function.
2. ETS exposure of young people and particularly infants from parental (and especially mother's) smoking is causally associated with an increased risk of lower respiratory infections (LRIs), including pneumonia, bronchitis, and bronchiolitis. An estimated 150,000 to 300,000 LRIs occur annually in infants and children less than 18 months of age, resulting in 7,500 to 15,000 hospitalizations annually.
3. Additional episodes and increased severity of asthma in children who already have the disease. It is estimated that ETS exposure worsens symptoms in approximately 20 percent of this nation's 2 million to 5 million asthmatic children and is a major aggravating factor in approximately 10 percent.
4. Evidence is suggestive, but not conclusive, that ETS exposure increases the number of new cases of asthma in children who have not previously exhibited symptoms.
5. Passive smoking has subtle but significant effects on the respiratory health of nonsmoking adults, including coughing, phlegm production, chest discomfort, and reduced lung function.

Source: U.S. Environmental Protection Agency and the U.S. Department of Health and Human Services.

1. The National Academy of Sciences and the surgeon general of the United States have concluded that passive smoke increases the risk of lung cancer among nonsmokers by up to 34 percent, particularly for spouses of smokers. Furthermore, 20 percent of lung cancer deaths among nonsmokers can be attributed to passive smoke—the residue of vapors and particles in the air from burning cigarettes and other tobacco products.
2. The Environmental Protection Agency (EPA) has identified passive smoke as a "class A carcinogen"—a cancer-causing substance that can be as deadly as radon and benzene in humans. As such, environmental tobacco smoke causes nonsmokers to develop an estimated three thousand cases of lung cancer each year.
3. Yale University scientists have found that approximately 17 percent of lung cancers among nonsmokers can be traced to exposure to high levels of cigarette smoke during childhood and adolescence. The apparent risk for getting lung cancer as adults doubled with exposure to twenty-five or more "smoker years"—the number of years a child or adolescent lived in a household multiplied by the number of smokers in the household.[31]
4. For nonsmoking women with spouses who smoke, the risk for developing lung cancer is about 30 percent higher over a lifetime than for those with nonsmoking spouses. This study confirms preliminary data that suggested exposure to ETS during adult life increases risk of lung cancer in lifetime nonsmokers.[32]

5. Other researchers have discovered that passive smoking reduces the blood's ability to deliver oxygen to the heart and lowers the capacity of heart muscles to use oxygen properly. Such effects are seen as reduced exercise capability.[33] Earlier investigations revealed that heart disease is an important consequence of being exposed to environmental tobacco smoke, and that ETS actually causes heart disease.[34] The increase in risk translates into nearly ten times as many deaths from ETS-induced heart disease as from lung cancer. Such deaths contribute greatly to the estimated 53,000 deaths each year from passive smoking.

Still other harmful effects are associated with ETS. Carbon monoxide levels occasionally reached in some **involuntary smoking** situations have resulted in impaired psychomotor function, especially attentiveness and cognitive skills. Data indicate that even fetal growth can be adversely affected when the mother is passively exposed to tobacco smoke during pregnancy.[35]

It has also been recognized that long-term exposure to tobacco smoke in the work environment is dangerous to the nonsmoker and significantly reduces small airway function in the lungs. Based upon tests of the lungs' ability to hold and expel air, research has concluded that passive smoking causes a measurable loss in breathing capacity. Apparently, tiny air tubes and sacs in the airways of the lungs become scarred and permanently damaged.

Smoking and Cardiovascular Diseases

Cigarette smoking is recognized as a major risk factor in the development of specific **cardiovascular** (heart and blood vessel) **diseases,** namely, **coronary heart disease,** *atherosclerosis* (the buildup of blood fats inside the arteries), and *abnormal conditions of the blood vessels in the arms and legs.*

The risk of heart attack due to coronary heart disease is more than twice that of nonsmokers.[36]

Significantly, cigarette smoking is the biggest risk factor for sudden cardiac death—smokers have two to four times the risk of nonsmokers. Exposure to ETS at home increases the risk of death due to heart disease by about 30 percent. ETS exposure in the workplace could increase this risk much higher.

Cigarette use has also been associated with increased mortality from cerebrovascular accidents (strokes) and nonsyphilitic aortic aneurysms (balloonings of the major artery of the body). Though smoking is considered a secondary risk factor in this instance, it affects the risk of stroke indirectly by increasing the risk of heart disease—a primary risk factor for stroke. Compared with nonsmokers, male cigarette smokers have two to three times greater risk of stroke, even when other stroke risk factors are controlled.

The exact mechanisms of cigarette-related cardiovascular diseases are not fully known, but they are thought to involve *nicotine and carbon monoxide as principal malefactors.*

Smoking may initiate a disease process by causing irreversible damage; it may enable or provide positive support to the development of an abnormal condition; it may interfere with and thereby reduce the normal ability of an organism to cope with a disease process; or it may produce temporary conditions that increase the likelihood that some critical event will occur with possibly fatal consequences, such as a heart attack.

One or more of these mechanisms may be operable independently or in conjunction with other factors often associated with cardiovascular diseases: obesity, high serum cholesterol, high blood pressure, and physical inactivity.

Nicotine is responsible for the near-instantaneous increase in heart rate, blood pressure, cardiac output, heart contractions, and consumption of oxygen by heart muscle. Nicotine, because of its blood-vessel narrowing effect, can also decrease peripheral blood flow, thus placing added stress on the smoker's heart.

The smoker's heart is working harder now, therefore, it requires more oxygen to function in its adaptive response to smoking. But carbon monoxide from cigarette smoke tends to displace oxygen from hemoglobin (the substance in red blood cells that carries oxygen and gives blood its red color), thus interfering with the transportation of oxygen and depriving heart muscle of its needed oxygen supply. Such sudden, though temporary, burdens placed on a heart already diseased with clogged coronary (heart) arteries can result in death.

In a compensatory action of adaptation, the body produces more red blood cells, which are associated with increased clotting as the blood becomes viscous or gummy. The body is slowly starved for oxygen, particularly the brain, which is dulled.

It is also possible that carbon monoxide causes damage by injuring the walls of arteries; enhancing the buildup of cholesterol in the development of atherosclerosis, which narrows the arteries; and reducing the supply of oxygen and other nutrients to various body cells. Such actions may explain why young males who smoke or have high blood-cholesterol levels are more likely than others to show signs of heart disease before they reach thirty-five years of age.

Evidence suggests that absorbed nicotine and carbon monoxide jointly contribute to the development of atherosclerosis. Cigarette smoking may also be a factor in increased platelet adhesiveness, which predisposes to blood-clot formation.

Smoking and Lung Cancer

In **lung cancer** victims, cures are rare, and 87 out of 100 people who develop lung cancer will be dead within five years. The survival rate for the first year after diagnosis of lung cancer is only 25 percent.

Studies of the frequency, distribution, causes, and control of cigaette-related diseases have led an overwhelming number of scientists to conclude that *smoking is the major cause of lung cancer* in both men and women (see fig. 8.3). Since 1987, more women have died of lung cancer than of breast cancer, which for over forty years was the major cause of cancer deaths in females.

At present, lung cancer is the leading cause of cancer deaths in the United States, with a yearly toll in excess of 158,000 victims.[37] The incidence or occurrence rate of lung cancer, which had been increasing steadily in both men and women for several decades, has begun to decline in men, but not in women.

This form of cancer, uncontrolled cellular growth, or malignant neoplasm, in the lungs is termed **bronchogenic carcinoma** because it arises in the lining of the bronchial tubes, through which air passes inwardly to various parts of the lungs. The chances of sustaining lung cancer are enhanced with increased numbers of cigarettes smoked per day, with the duration or length of smoking, and with earlier initiation of use. The risks are reduced when smoking ceases.

It is apparent that cigarette smoking triggers a disease process (via the tobacco tars) in which cellular repair and recovery are possible up to some "hazardous point." Beyond this critical point, the process is not reversible in most cases and cancerous growths begin.

Investigations indicate that one particular component of tobacco tars, benzo (a) pyrene, is directly implicated in lung cancer development.[38] When this carcinogenic hydrocarbon enters the lungs, the chemical derivative of benzo (a) pyrene damages a specific gene, P53, in the cells of lung tissue. Typically, the P53 gene keeps the cells dividing normally.

Once damaged sufficiently by benzo (a) pyrene, the gene mutates (changes) and no longer serves its protective function of assuring normal cell division. Now, lung cells begin to divide abnormally. The result is a form of lung cancer known as carcinoma. Nearly 60 percent of lung cancers involve mutations of the P53 gene (see fig. 8.4).

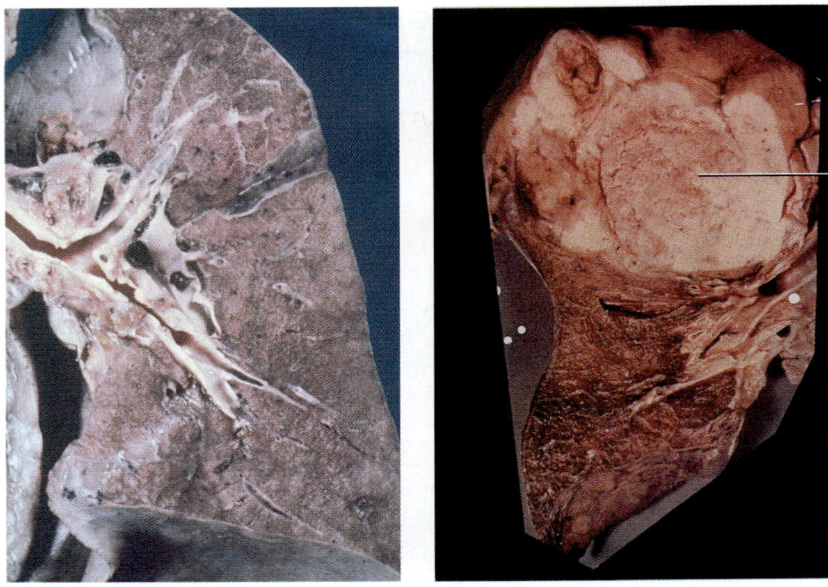

figure 8.3

The lung on the left is healthy. A cancerous tumor has invaded the lung in the right, taking up nearly half of the lung space.

© American Cancer Institute

Laboratory Experiments

In laboratory experiments involving dogs, hamsters, and mice, the cancer-producing (carcinogenic) nature of the tobacco tars, whole cigarette smoke, and filtered smoke has been demonstrated. When applied to test animals by skin painting, tracheal installation or implantation, and inhalation, the components of cigarette smoke were capable of producing cancerous growths similar to those found in the lungs and larynx of smokers.

Autopsy Studies

Even more incriminating evidence against cigarettes has been derived from detailed autopsy studies conducted on patients who died of lung cancer in comparison with noncancer patients. Lung cancer victims were found to have increased presence of bronchial tissue changes considered by investigators to be the precursors (forerunners) of invasive cancer.

Additional studies then compared the frequency of these cancer-related changes in the lungs of smokers and nonsmokers. In nearly every case, there was an increased prevalence of these cellular alterations or adaptations among smokers as compared with nonsmokers. Such changes in the lungs usually occur before cancer cells break through the basement membrane of the bronchial lining and spread throughout the lungs and to other parts of the body. The changes are (1) **hyperplasia,** (2) ***loss of ciliary function*** *in columnar cells,* and (3) **carcinoma *in situ.***

Hyperplasia

Hyperplasia, an increase in the number of layers of basal cells that underlie the inner surface of the bronchial tubes, was the first major effect observed. This condition was prevalent in 95 percent of heavy smokers and in 80 percent of light smokers. It was rarely found in nonsmokers. A typical reaction of surface tissue to irritation, hyperplasia probably results from

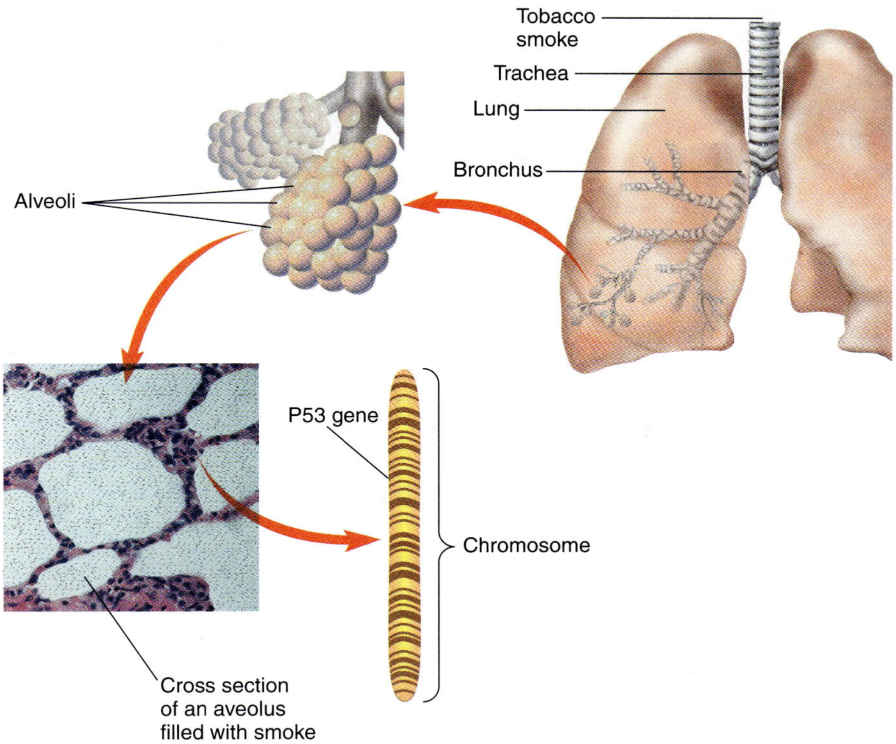

figure 8.4

The smoking-lung cancer link. The link between tobacco smoking and lung cancer involves benzo (a) pyrene, a component of tobacco tar, and the P53 gene, a tiny molecular sphere of influence on a cell's chromosome. One of about 70,000 genes in a human cell, the P53 gene controls normal cell division. As a smoker inhales, tars within the particulate phase of the tobacco smoke pass down the trachea. Entering the bronchus and its branching divisions, the tars are deposited within the alveoli—thin-walled microscopic air sacs lined with simple squamous epithelial cells. Within the tar, the benzo (a) pyrene and its chemical derivative damage the P53 gene which then mutates. No longer serving its protective function, the mutated P53 gene is now responsible for cancerous growth.

the constant bombardment of tobacco smoke products that under certain conditions accumulate on the lining of the bronchial tubes.

Loss of Ciliary Function

Both particulate matter and gaseous components of cigarette smoke have been shown to retard greatly and eventually stop the sweeping movements of cilia, tiny hairlike projections extending from the surface of the columnlike cells of the bronchial tubes (fig. 8.5). Cilia sweep mucus and other debris out of the respiratory tree into the mouth, where it is swallowed or expectorated. Retarded ciliary function interferes with mucus removal and permits the deposit of smoke irritants on the bronchial tube lining, and it gives rise to the smoker's cough. The remaining columnar cells undergo a flattening and enlargement, characteristic of smokers' lung tissue.

Carcinoma in Situ

Characterized by the development of disordered cells with atypical nuclei, carcinoma *in situ*—literally, a cancerous growth remaining at the site of its origin—describes a noninvasive cancer. A major change noted in the lung tissue of smokers, this condition of cancer is confined to the lining (epithelium) layer of the lungs (fig. 8.6). Such a phenomenon usually precedes *metastasis*—the spreading of uncontrolled cell growth throughout an individual's body. Nicotine may promote or enhance the spread of cancer cells.

Significantly, the number of cells with abnormal nuclei decreased noticeably in the bronchial lining of ex-cigarette smokers, depending upon the length of time between cessation of smoking and death.

Chronic Obstructive Lung Disease

Pulmonary emphysema and **chronic bronchitis,** two diseases that were infrequently reported in the population, are reaching epidemic proportions. Often seen together in the same patient, the two diseases are jointly referred to as **chronic obstructive lung disease (COLD),** characterized by slow, progressive interruption of the airflow within the lungs. COLD is one of the leading causes of death in the United States. COLD is also an adaptive response to inhaled irritants and a maladaptation to smoking tobacco.

Cigarette smoking has been identified as the most important cause of COLD, and it greatly increases the risk of dying from pulmonary emphysema and chronic bronchitis. While other factors, including hereditary, predisposition, may contribute to COLD, cigarette smoking is recognized as the major factor in the promotion of "pulmonary cripples." When COLD morbidity is considered, there are more than one million more cases in America than there would be if all people had the same disease rate as those who never smoked.

Pulmonary Emphysema

In pulmonary emphysema, the *alveoli* (tiny air sacs of the lungs) lose the elasticity that ordinarily permits them

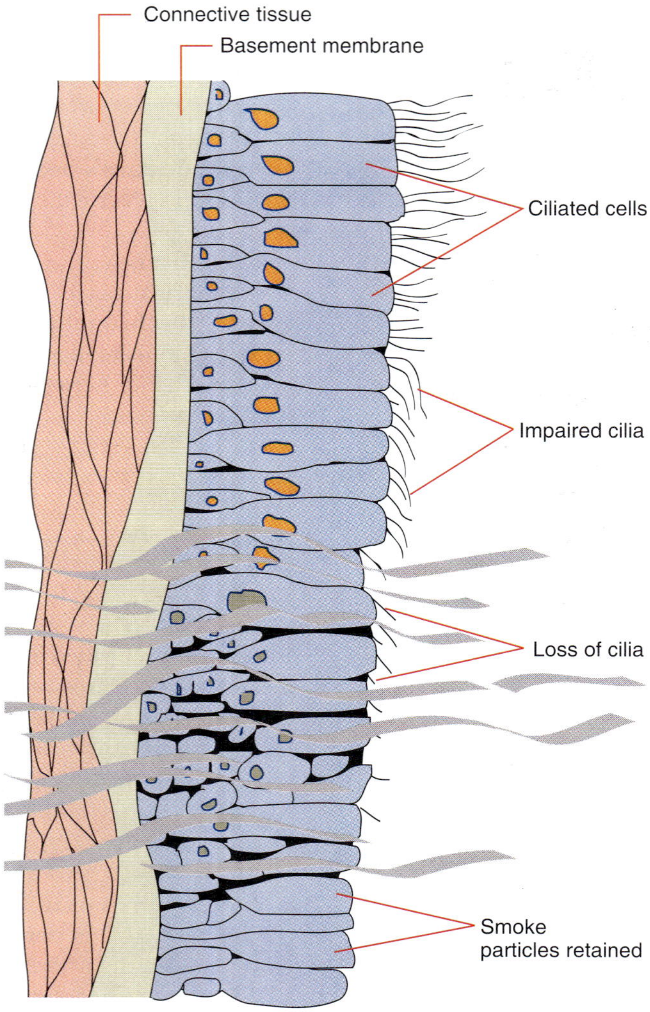

figure 8.5

The effect of tobacco smoke on ciliary function within the bronchial tubes of the lungs.

Source: National Advisory Cancer Council.

to expand and contract. Air becomes trapped in the alveoli. Eventually, many of the air sacs are stretched abnormally, rupture, and are destroyed. In a vain attempt to accommodate the overstretched lungs, the chest cage enlarges, which unfortunately reduces the efficiency of the diaphragm. As this condition progresses, the ability of the lungs to exchange gases is so seriously impaired that the bloodstream becomes low in oxygen and retains carbon dioxide. Typically, the victim develops shortness of breath and an overworked heart, which speeds up to supply body cells with their oxygen requirements.

Chronic Bronchitis

Recurring inflammation of the bronchial tubes with excessive mucus production is common in chronic bronchitis. Invariably, a persistent cough develops in an attempt to dislodge the mucus from the narrowed airways. Deep coughing and thick mucus interfere with normal breathing and reduce normal lung function.

Chemicals in inhaled cigarette smoke irritate the bronchial tubes and alveolar sacs over and over again with each puff. In time, the tissues lining the bronchi thicken; the mucous glands enlarge; and the normal cleansing system of the lungs, especially ciliary function, is impaired. The smoker is now more predisposed to respiratory infections and aggravation of existing ones than is the nonsmoker.

While the relative importance of air pollution in the development of COLD remains controversial, clearly air pollution is a less significant factor under most circumstances than cigarette smoking.

In addition to an increased risk of COLD, cigarette smokers are more frequently subject to, and require longer convalescence from, other respiratory infections than are nonsmokers. Also, if they require surgery, smokers are more likely to develop postoperative respiratory complications.

Smokeless Tobacco

Smokeless tobacco products include chewing tobacco and snuff—mixtures of tobacco leaves and various sweeteners, flavorings, and scents.[39] In chewing tobacco, the leaves are shredded, pressed into bricks or cakes (plugs), or dried and twisted into ropelike strands. A portion of a plug or strand is either chewed or held in place in the cheek or between the lower lip and gum.

Made from powdered or finely cut tobacco leaves, both dry and moist snuff are used in the mouth, or "dipped." A small amount of snuff is usually held in place between the lip or cheek and the gum.

Historically, smokeless tobacco was widely used in the United States before the introduction and social acceptance of cigarettes. During the early part of the twentieth century, the use of smokeless tobacco declined sharply, until the early 1980s. There is ample evidence that chewing tobacco and snuff have regained a degree of popularity.

Typical Users

Original estimates indicated that over 12 million people used some form of smokeless tobacco each year. The National Institute on Drug Abuse estimates that as many as 22 million Americans have used smokeless tobacco products, but only 6.8 million are thought to be regular users. "Dipping" and "chewing" appear to be concentrated among young

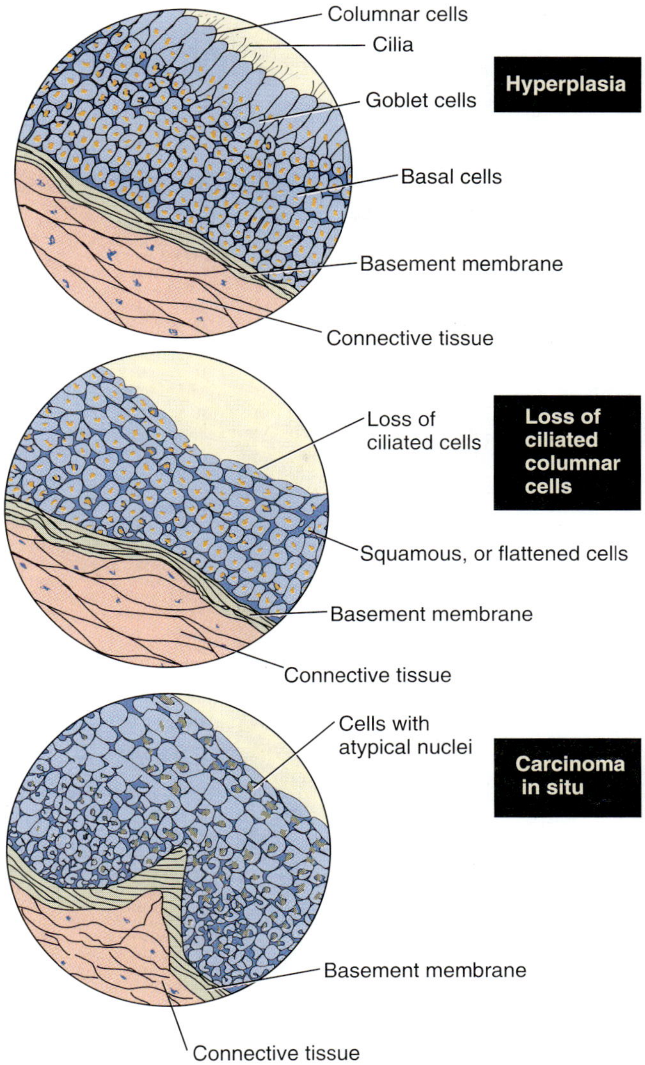

figure 8.6

Cellular changes or alterations in the bronchi of cigarette smokers.

Source: National Advisory Cancer Council.

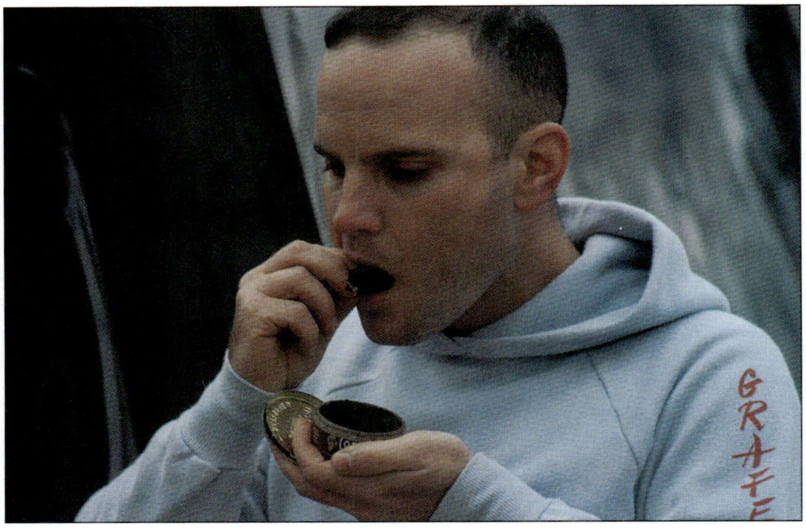

The recent upsurge in use of smokeless tobacco among younger American males has been traced to advertising campaigns featuring athletes and entertainers who engage in chewing, dipping, and spitting as macho art forms.

© M. Edrington/The Image Works

American males—teenagers and college-age youths, especially those who are athletes.

Smokeless tobacco use is prevalent in certain geographic areas as well as within some cultures and populations. For instance, in some Native American tribes, smokeless tobacco use rates among adolescent females approach 45 percent.

Studies of professional baseball players revealed that as many as 39 percent of major and minor league players used smokeless tobacco, mostly snuff, during spring training.[40] Surveys of 2,200 National Collegiate Athletic Association (NCAA) varsity athletes indicated that use of illegal drugs was declining, but smokeless tobacco use increased by 8 percent over a four-year period.[41]

Among males, six of ten baseball players chewed, and 40 percent of football players chewed, while 9 percent of female softball players also chewed tobacco. The overall use of snuff had increased in every racial and ethnic group studied. In reaction to these widespread practices, the NCAA and professional baseball's minor leagues have banned smokeless tobacco.

Origins of Modern Use

Several factors have likely contributed to the renewed acceptance of smokeless tobacco, especially the physical effects of absorbed nicotine. The absorption process results in a gradual release of nicotine over a period of hours, which is felt in a "time-release" action. Particularly appealing are the increase in blood pressure and heart rate, a reduction in one's appetite, a calming action, and a reduced sensitivity to pain and stress for several hours.[42]

Significantly, powerful advertising campaigns that use professional athletes and entertainers to promote smokeless tobacco have established chewing and dipping as art forms and spitters as

Box 8.7 A Common Question; an Uncommon Answer

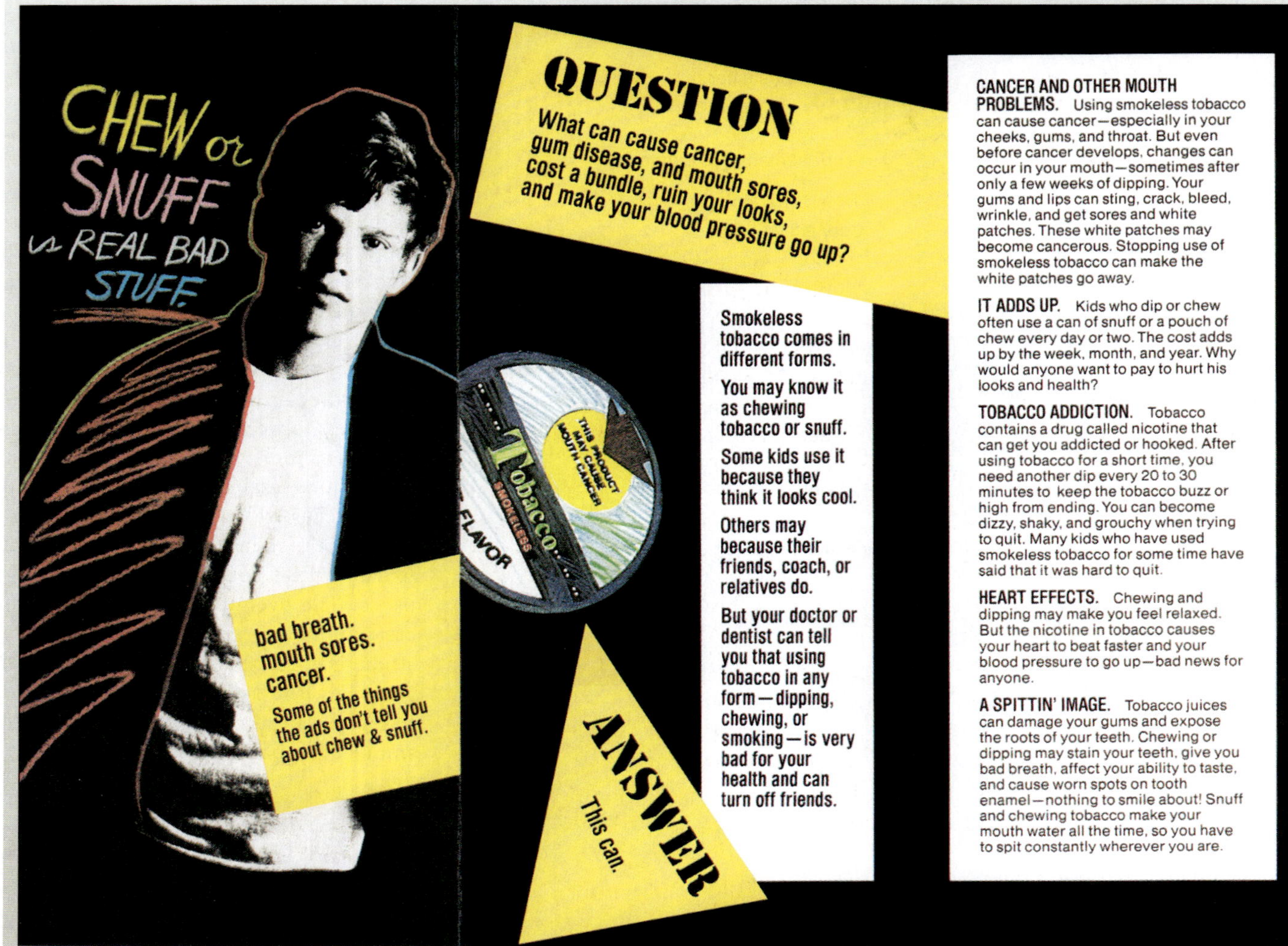

Source: National Cancer Institute, U.S. Department of Health and Human Services.

ultramacho. Not to be overlooked are the clever marketing strategies that display smokeless tobacco products in locations removed from smoking tobacco in grocery and convenience stores, and promotional giveaways on college campuses and at state fairs and sporting events. In addition, the health effects of smokeless tobacco are not so well recognized as is the causal link between cigarette use and harmful health conditions.

Cancer and Smokeless Tobacco

Chemical analysis of various types of smokeless tobacco has revealed the presence of several carcinogenic compounds, including polonium-210, polycyclic aromatic hydrocarbons, and the tobacco-specific nitrosamines. These carcinogens are part of the strong scientific evidence that the use of smokeless tobacco can cause cancers in humans (see box 8.7).

The association between cancer and use of such products is strongest for cancers of the oral cavity (mouth). Oral cancer has been shown to occur several times more frequently among snuff dippers than among nontobacco users, and the excess risk of cancers of the cheek and gum may be nearly fifty times greater among long-term users. Some investigations also suggest that the use of chewing tobacco may increase the risk of oral cancer.

Noncancerous and Precancerous Oral Effects and Smokeless Tobacco Use

Smokeless tobacco use is responsible for the development of a portion of oral *leukoplakias* in teenage and adult users. Leukoplakias are the "white patches" that develop on the mucous membrane surface that lines the inside of the mouth. These white patches occur frequently with smokeless tobacco use. With continued use, the leukoplakias can undergo a transformation to malignant conditions, that is, cancerous tumors.

The degree to which the use of smokeless tobacco affects the tissues of the mouth is variable, depending on the site of action, type of smokeless tobacco product, frequency and duration of use, possible predisposing factors (including smoking), and other factors not yet determined. For example, among snuff users, oral lesions (abnormalities of tissue) were found in 67 percent of baseball players who were year-round users, but in only 32 percent of baseball players who used snuff only during the baseball season.

Although research is not complete, there is some evidence that supports the association of smokeless tobacco use with gingival recession, or receding gums, especially where the tobacco is placed repeatedly. Negative health effects from long-term use of smokeless tobacco also include tooth discoloration, tooth decay and loss, bad breath, and gingivitis (inflammation and destruction of the gums).

Nicotine Exposure and Smokeless Tobacco

The use of smokeless tobacco products can and does lead to nicotine dependence. An examination of nicotine absorption, distribution, and elimination that results from both smoking and smokeless tobacco use indicates that the extent of nicotine exposure is similar for both.

As is the case with most other drugs of abuse, nicotine produces effects in the user that are considered desirable to the user. These effects are caused by the nicotine and not simply by the tobacco leaf or tobacco smoke.

The exposure to nicotine from cigarette smoking and smokeless tobacco is similar, therefore, the health consequences of smoking that are caused by nicotine also would be expected to be hazards of smokeless tobacco use. Areas of particular concern in which nicotine may play a contributing or supporting role in the origin of disease include coronary artery disease, peripheral blood-vessel disease, hypertension, peptic ulcer disease, and fetal mortality and morbidity among pregnant women.

Rewards Versus Risks

The serious health risks just discussed should be sufficient to discourage smokers and users of smokeless tobacco from continuing their life-threatening forms of adaptive behavior and to discourage new tobacco users. However, the mere presentation of facts has little effect upon smokers, tobacco chewers, and snuff dippers, except those who are highly motivated to reduce their exposure to tobacco or to quit using it entirely.

Persistence in smoking might seem contradictory in this enlightened, scientific era, but it is due in part to the effectiveness of early learning that is reinforced thousands of times, puff after puff. In time, tobacco users continue their habits because they have become addicted to nicotine.

Other considerations play a role in maintaining the conflict between smoking behavior and possible health hazards. For instance, not everyone who smokes becomes ill, incapacitated, or dies. Certain cigarette-related diseases may require some genetic, biological, chemical, or physical factor to be operable before smoking takes its toll.

Then, too, rationalization is commonly employed to justify the smoker's action. We often hear these replies to probing inquiries: "Just one cigarette never hurt anybody." "It won't happen to me because I'm lucky." "Why should I quit since I don't feel sick?" "Why worry? They will find a cure for cancer before I die." Do any of these excuses sound familiar? Many of them are based on the remoteness, the delayed action of the possible harmful effects of smoking. If one cigarette caused serious, immediate illness or instant death, smoking would rapidly decline or become extinct.

Recognizing that people have been rewarded with feelings of relaxation, well-being, and stimulation through smoking, the American Lung Association has devised a unique program of helping smokers quit. This plan is based upon establishing a system of personal rewards for quitting smoking.

Although the idea may appear strange, a system of self-rewards greatly improves an individual's chances of becoming a permanent nonsmoker. The rewards should be enjoyable; easy to obtain; occasionally expensive; material and immaterial, in proportion to what has been achieved; and administered as soon as possible after completing some activity in the program.

Suggested self-rewards include reading in bed on a weekend morning, buying and wearing a new piece of clothing, talking with a friend on the telephone, eating a special food, having someone else clear the table, getting a back rub, and going bowling. By devising a system of similar rewards, a person will have an incentive for modifying smoking behavior.

Reducing the Risks

Almost every type of study has led scientists to conclude that increased exposure to cigarette tars, nicotine, carbon monoxide, and other smoke components leads to increased health risks among the smoking and nonsmoking population. Elimination of the exposure to cigarettes is the best and quickest way to reduce dosage and related risks. The benefits of eliminating smoking for the individual smoker are enormous!

People who quit smoking live longer because smoking cessation at all ages reduces the risks of premature death. Quitting smoking carries major and immediate health benefits even to those in older age groups and applies not only to healthy people, but to those already suffering from smoking-related diseases, especially cancer, lung disease, and heart disease.[43]

The longer people refrain from smoking after stopping, the more probable it is their health condition will approach that of their nonsmoking counterparts (see box 8.8). For instance, after fifteen years of nonsmoking, the risk of coronary heart disease is similar to that of

Box 8.8 Benefits of Quitting Smoking

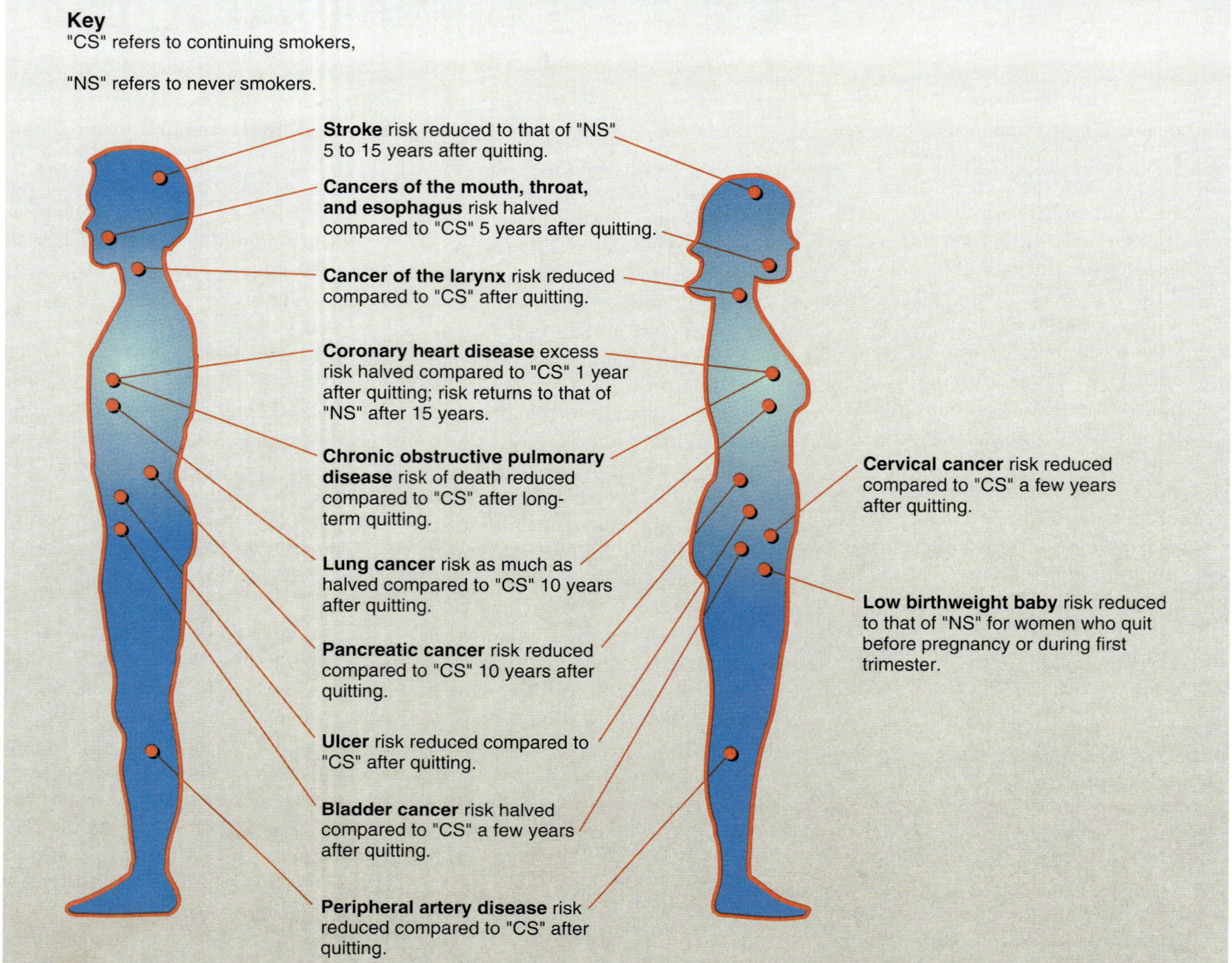

Source: *The Health Benefits of Smoking Cessation: A Report of The Surgeon General, 1990—At a Glance*, U.S. Department of Health and Human Services, publication no. (CDC) 90-8419.

persons who have never smoked (see box 8.9). Smokers who quit smoking will also benefit considerably in terms of stroke risk, regardless of the degree of their previous exposure to smoking. A complete loss of stroke risk, however, is not seen in heavy smokers.[44]

There are some apparent consequences of quitting. Many former smokers report a reduction in smoker's cough, nasal stuffiness and discharge, and sputum production. Shortness of breath usually improves within a few weeks. In time, food tastes better, sleep is sounder, fatigue diminishes, taste in the mouth improves, and yellowish stains on teeth and fingers disappear. The economics of giving up cigarettes should not be discounted. Giving up smoking one $1.90 pack of cigarettes a day over a thirty-year period will result in a savings of more than $20,800!

Although the development of a cigarette that is absolutely safe with respect to all presently associated diseases is not likely, tobacco companies have been successful in reducing the tar and nicotine content of their products. Reconstituted tobaccos and improved filters have met with considerable acceptance by the smoking population. These measures have helped to reduce exposure to potentially harmful substances.

The risk to a filter-cigarette smoker, however, still remains above that of the nonsmoker. Unfortunately, the popular 100-and 120-millimeter cigarettes increase the dosage and risk. Moreover, the addition of menthol may improve the

Box 8.9 What You Should Know About Quitting Smoking

Smokers often try to quit more than once before they succeed. Nearly 70 percent of ex-smokers make one or two quit attempts, while 9 percent quit six or more times before succeeding. So far, more than 38 million Americans have succeeded! About 90 percent of successful quitters eventually do so on their own, but with good cessation programs, 20 percent to 40 percent of participants are able to quit smoking and stay off cigarettes for at least one year.

Some Consequences of Quitting Are . . .

- Nearly 80 percent of those who quit smoking gain weight, compared to 56 percent of continuing smokers.
- Short-term consequences of nicotine withdrawal include anxiety, irritability, frustration, anger, difficulty in concentrating, and restlessness. Possible long-term consequences are urges to smoke and increased appetite.

But at the Same Time. . .

- The average weight gain after quitting is just 5 pounds, and only 3.5 percent of those who quit gain more than 20 pounds after quitting.
- Nicotine withdrawal symptoms peak in the first 1 to 2 days after quitting and subside rapidly during the following weeks. With long-term abstinence, ex-smokers are likely to enjoy favorable psychological changes such as enhanced self-esteem and increased sense of control.
- People who quit smoking are more likely than current smokers to exercise regularly. Exercise may help new quitters to stay off cigarettes and avoid or minimize weight gain.

The Bottom Line . . .

The health benefits of quitting far exceed any risks from the average 5-pound weight gain or any adverse psychological effects that may follow quitting. To help limit any weight gain after quitting, eat a well-balanced diet and avoid the excess calories in sugary and fatty foods; satisfy cravings for sweets by eating small pieces of fruit; have low-calorie foods on hand for nibbling; drink six to eight glasses of water per day; and build exercise into your life by walking 30 minutes a day or doing the physical activity of your choice.

Source: *The Health Benefits of Smoking Cessation: A Report of The Surgeon General, 1990—At A Glance*, U.S. Department of Health and Human Services, publication no. (CDC)90-8419.

taste, but it does not reduce the health hazards.

While *there is no safe way to smoke*, there are some suggestions that smokers can follow if they wish to make their cigarette use less hazardous. The following recommendations are offered by the Public Health Service.

1. *Inhale less.* Cigarette smoke that enters the lungs is the disease-causing agent in pulmonary and cardiovascular disorders. Death rates and morbidity rates increase with the degree and frequency of inhalation. Some smokers may wish to switch to pipes or cigars, in which smoke usually is not inhaled. Having switched, they may reduce their risks of having lung cancer, COLD, and cardiovascular diseases, but they may increase their risks of developing cancer of the larynx, lip, and esophagus.
2. *Smoke fewer cigarettes.* The exposure to health risks is in direct proportion to the number of cigarettes smoked. The fewer smoked, the lower the risks. This procedure can be promoted by making a conscious effort to stretch the existing supply, by postponing smoking, by placing cigarettes in an out-of-the-way location, and by promising oneself not to smoke during a particular time of day.
3. *Take fewer puffs.* Although a smoker may not be able to reduce the total number of cigarettes used, puffing less on each one will reduce the exposure to the total dose of tars, gaseous components, and toxic chemicals inhaled. While this procedure might seem expensive in the purchase of more cigarettes, it is cheaper in the long run as expressed in personal health, working ability, and longevity.
4. *Smoke one-third down.* Regardless of the brand smoked, the major amounts of tars and nicotine are found in the last few puffs of a cigarette. Tobacco acts as a filter and screens out a portion of the tars and nicotine as they pass through it. As a consequence, smoke from the first third of a cigarette contains approximately 2 percent of the total tars and nicotine, while the last third yields nearly 50 percent. Do not smoke all the way down on cigarettes. Those extra puffs can be perilous puffs!
5. *Choose a low-tar and low-nicotine cigarette.* By reducing one's exposure to these constituents of cigarette smoke, health risks are likely reduced but not eliminated. No minimum levels of these substances have been determined risk-free or safe. Cigarette manufacturers reveal the tar and nicotine content of their products because of governmental action and increased public interest. Choosing a less harmful cigarette may be as easy as switching to another brand or to another version of the same brand. In every instance, the buyer should beware!

Anything short of quitting completely is only a compromise, however. While most successful quitters stop smoking immediately and permanently, others—particularly heavy, addicted smokers—find participation in a smoking withdrawal program to be helpful.[45] Stop-smoking programs have been particularly effective, especially those conducted by the American Lung Association, the American Cancer Society., the American Heart Association, Seventh Day Adventist Breathe-Free Plan to Stop Smoking, Smoke Stoppers, and Smokers Anonymous. Local smoking control programs are usually listed under "Smokers' Information and Treatment Centers" in the telephone company's directory of agencies. Community hospitals, counseling programs, health agencies, and health promotion centers often sponsor support groups that prove helpful to some smokers.

For many individuals who are not successful in their own attempts to quit smoking via self-help books, videotapes, E-Z Quit simulated cigarettes, quit-smoking computers, and various other techniques, a drug is available without prescription. Known as *Nicorette,* this nicotine chewing gum decreases the smoker's desire for nicotine and relieves withdrawal symptoms. More effective, practical, and safer than injected and capsule or pill forms of nicotine, the chewing gum allows a low level of nicotine to be absorbed through the mouth's lining directly into the bloodstream.

Developed as a temporary aid to smoking cessation, nicotine chewing gum is most effective in the early phase of withdrawal. However, *Nicorette* is no panacea. Studies of the gum's effectiveness have found mixed results.

Successful quitting appears to depend on more than chewing the nicotine gum. The smoker's motivation to quit, presence or absence of contraindications, awareness of and willingness to tolerate possible side effects of the gum, physician support, and participation in a professionally supervised behavior modification program influence the success or failure of this technique.

It appears that group-based behavioral programs that rely on social reinforcement and follow-up support, in combination with nicotine gum, will likely prove the most effective strategy for most smokers. However, drinking coffee and carbonated beverages tends to interfere with the effect of the prescription gum. Those who use *Nicorette* are well-advised not to chew the gum on their coffee breaks or to eat or drink anything during or immediately before *Nicorette* use.[46] *Nicorette* should not be used by children or pregnant women. People with stomach problems, ulcers, angina, or heart disease should talk to their doctors before using this product.

Even newer forms of medical nicotine are also marketed as the nicotine patch and nicotine nasal spray. Similar to *Nicorette* chewing gum, the patch provides a dose of nicotine that can help relieve the body's craving for this addictive substance. Available without a prescription, Nicoderm, Habitrol, and Nicotrol are small, thin, twenty-four-hour patches that go on a person's upper body and deliver a continuous flow of nicotine through the skin. This nicotine patch—a transdermal (across the skin) system—can reduce nicotine withdrawal symptoms that usually develop with quitting smoking. To reduce the risk of heart attack, however, patients are warned not to smoke while wearing the patches. The patch should not be used by pregnant or breast-feeding women. Patients with angina, diabetes mellitus, peptic ulcer, or hypothyroidism, and those who recently have had a stroke or heart attack, should consult with their doctors before using the patch.

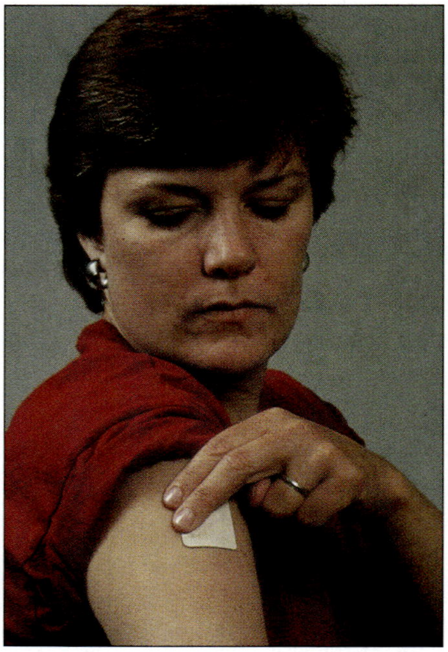

You can be an ex-smoker too, with Nicotine patch, Nicotine gum, or the new, prescribed nasal spray.

© National Cancer Institute

Prescription-only nicotine nasal spray (Nicotrol NS) and the newer Nicotrol nicotine inhaler are available. Like nicotine gum and the patch, the spray and inhaler are promoted as ways to help smokers stop smoking. Nicotine is addictive and it is possible to become dependent on the spray and inhaler, therefore, use of these products is not recommended for more than three months. In 1997, the FDA approved a nicotine-free antismoking pill called Zyban. This prescription antidepressant helps reduce withdrawal symptoms and cravings in smokers who are trying to quit.

Chapter Summary

1. Tobacco, a plant native to America, has become a popular source of mild stimulation. The smoking of tobacco cigarettes is considered the largest single preventable cause of illness and premature death in the United States.
2. Both individuals and the American society are "hooked" on tobacco products. While the federal government supports antismoking programs and research, it also subsidizes tobacco growers.
3. About 30 percent of the adult population smokes. This number represents a declining minority, but there is evidence that adult females are increasing their use of tobacco products as are teenagers.
4. More people are smoking low-tar and low-nicotine cigarettes. However, any such protection from diseases offered by these new tobacco products is negated by compensatory practices—increasing the number of cigarettes smoked, shortening the interval between puffs, increasing the depth of inhalation, and smoking to a shorter butt.
5. Although cigarettes have provided the user with certain personal gratifications, the nonsmoking majority has become assertive in demanding plain, unpolluted air. The nonsmokers' liberation movement and government regulation have resulted in many restrictive practices on smokers' behavior.

6. Smoking is a learned behavior with many psychological rewards, especially for maturing adolescents. Factors in smoking behavior are classified as stimulation, handling/oral gratification, pleasurable relaxation, tension reduction, psychological and physical addiction, and habit.
7. The health consequences of smoking are related to the constituents of tobacco smoke: gases; tar; and nicotine, the physical dependency-producing or addictive component. Additionally, excess mortality and morbidity associated with smoking are dose related; that is, death and disease rates increase with amount smoked, duration of smoking, earlier age of initiation, inhalation of smoke, and higher tar and nicotine content.
8. Passive smoking, the inhalation of environmental tobacco smoke by a nonsmoker, is recognized as having several adverse health effects on the nonsmoking population. Secondhand smoke can cause heart disease, lung cancer, and the increased occurrence of respiratory disability and diseases.
9. Cigarette smoking contributes to coronary heart disease, lung and various other cancers, chronic obstructive lung disease, a variety of chronic and disabling conditions, lower birth weight of infants, increased risk of spontaneous abortion, sudden infant death syndrome, impaired oxygen uptake and exercise tolerance, age-related macular degeneration, premature facial wrinkling, and undesirable drug interactions.
10. Nicotine and carbon monoxide are the culprits in coronary heart disease and other cardiovascular diseases; tobacco tars are responsible for triggering lung cancer (often through genetic mutations) and its precursors of tissue changes: hyperplasia; loss of ciliary function in columnar cells; and carcinoma *in situ*. Chronic obstructive lung disease is a response to inhalation of smoke irritants and is manifest as pulmonary emphysema and chronic bronchitis.
11. Use of chewing tobacco and snuff represents a significant health risk. Smokeless tobacco is not a safe substitute for smoking cigarettes. It can cause cancers of the mouth and throat, gum damage, loss of teeth, and can lead to nicotine addiction and dependence.
12. Smoking of tobacco is often portrayed as a reward versus risk practice. The psychosocial and short-term rewards of smoking are perceived as more important than the long-term risks of diseases and premature death.
13. Although there is no safe, risk-free cigarette and no safe level of smoking, a smoker can reduce the risks associated with tobacco use by inhaling less smoke; smoking fewer cigarettes; taking fewer puffs; smoking only one-third down on each cigarette; and choosing a low-tar, low-nicotine, and low-carbon-monoxide yielding product.
14. The benefits of smoking cessation via the self-initiated "cold-turkey" approach, group-based smoking withdrawal programs, the use of *Nicorette* or the nicotine skin patch, or taking the antismoking pill, *Zyban*, are significant. Quitting smoking reduces the risk of heart disease, lung cancer, and various other cancerous diseases, stroke, chronic obstructive pulmonary (lung) disease, and low-birth-weight babies.

World Wide Web Sites

Action on Smoking and Health

www.ash.org

Agency for Health Care Policy and Research

www.ahcpr.gov

National Center for Tobacco-Free Kids

www.tobaccofreekids.org

Review Questions and Activities

1. Where did smoking of tobacco leaves begin?
2. Why is smoking considered "suicide in slow motion"?
3. What contradictions are apparent in the puzzling phenomenon known as tobacco smoking?
4. Survey your class, friends, and/or neighbors to determine the prevalence of smoking. How do these results compare with national statistics cited in the text?
5. What factors may be responsible for the continuing increase in smoking among young females.
6. Determine if chewing tobacco or "snuff dipping" is popular among your friends and acquaintances. What reasons do they give for such practices?
7. Why is smokeless tobacco not considered a safe substitute for smoking cigarettes?
8. Explain how compensatory smoking can negate the benefits of low-yield cigarettes.
9. What motivational appeals do cigarette advertisers use to promote smoking?
10. What are some of the psychological rewards associated with smoking?
11. What factors likely influence teenagers to begin smoking?
12. Explain the following terms in relation to cigarette smoking: *stimulation, handling/oral gratification, relaxation, tension reduction, craving,* and *habit.*
13. What components of tobacco smoke are thought to be responsible for the major diseases associated with smoking?
14. In what way is *nicotine* responsible for the continuation of smoking?

15. Is tobacco use psychologically or physically dependency producing?
16. Summarize the major research findings linking cigarette smoking and passive smoking with excess mortality and morbidity.
17. In what way is benzo (a) pyrene, one of the chemicals in cigarette tars, related to the development of lung cancer?
18. How is smoking thought to contribute to heart and blood-vessel diseases?
19. What are three smoking-induced cellular changes that are considered as precursors of lung cancer?
20. How does smoking contribute to chronic obstructive lung disease?
21. Contrast pulmonary emphysema with chronic bronchitis.
22. Explain smoking behavior in terms of a rewards versus risks phenomenon.
23. In what ways can a smoker reduce the health risks often linked with tobacco use?
24. What specific resources are available in your community to help smokers quit their use of tobacco products?

References

1. Avram Goldstein, *Addiction: From Biology to Drug Policy* (New York: W. H. Freeman, 1994), 101–17.
2. Antonia C. Novello, preface to *Health Benefits of Smoking Cessation,* a report of the Surgeon General, executive summary, USDHHA Publication No. CDC-90-8416 (Washington, D.C.: GPO, 1990), xi.
3. H. Thomas Milhorn, *Drug and Alcohol Abuse* (New York: Plenum Press, 1994), 293.
4. David Krogh, "Smoking: Why Is It So Hard to Quit?" *Priorities,* (spring 1992): 29–31.
5. American Cancer Society, *Cancer Facts and Figures—1996* (Atlanta: American Cancer Society, 1996), 24–25.
6. "Hooked on Tobacco: The Teen Epidemic," *Consumer Reports.* 60, no. 3 (March 1995): 142–47.
7. Institute for Health Policy, Brandeis University, *Substance Abuse: The Nation's Number One Health Problem* (Princeton, N.J.: Robert Wood Johnson Foundation, 1993), 13.
8. American Cancer Society, *Cancer Facts and Figures—1996,* 25.
9. Barry Stimmel and the editors of Consumer Reports Books, *The Facts about Drug Use: Coping with Drugs and Alcohol in Your Family, at Work, in Your Community* (New York: Haworth Medical Press, 1993), 216–18.
10. Ronald Davis, "The Ledger of Tobacco Control: Is the Cup Half Empty or Half Full?" *Journal of the American Medical Association* 275, no. 16 (24 April 1996): 1281–84.
11. Stanton Glantz, John Slade, and Deborah Barnes, *The Cigarette Papers* (Berkeley, Calif. University of California Press, 1996), 103–05, 436–42.
12. U.S. Department of Health and Human Services, *Preventing Tobacco Use among Young People,* a report of the Surgeon General, executive summary (Atlanta: U.S. Department of Health and Human Services, Public Health Service, Centers for Disease Control and Prevention, Office on Smoking and Health, 1994), 5–6.
13. This section is based on the following Public Health Service (USDHHS) reports of the Surgeon General (all available from the U.S. Government Printing Office): *Smoking and Health; The Health Consequences of Smoking for Women; The Health Consequences of Smoking; The Changing Cigarette; and The Health Consequences of Smoking: Cancer.*
14. Robert Julien, *A Primer of Drug Action,* 7th ed. (New York: W. H. Freeman and Company, 1995), 168–69.
15. Gesina Longenecker, *How Drugs Work* (Emeryville, Calif.: Ziff-Davis Press, 1994), 88–89.
16. Anastasia Toufexis, "How Smokers Get Hooked," *Time* 147, no. 11 (11 March 1996): 60.
17. C. Everett Koop, *The Health Consequences of Smoking: Nicotine Addiction,* a report of the Surgeon General (Washington, D.C.: GPO, 1988), 9.
18. Stanton Glantz and others, "Looking Through a Keyhole at the Tobacco Industry," *Journal of the American Medical Association* 274, no. 3 (19 July 1995): 219–24; John Slade and others, "Nicotine and Addiction: The Brown and Williamson Documents," *Journal of the American Medical Association* 274, no. 3 (19 July 1995): 225–33; Richard Kluger, *Ashes to Ashes* (New York: Alfred A. Knopf, 1996); and Philip Hilts, *Smoke Screen* (Reading, Mass.: Addison-Wesley Publishing Company, Inc., 1996).
19. Margie Patlak, "New Devices Aim at Improving PAP Test Accuracy," *FDA Consumer* 30, no. 8 (October 1996): 9–13; Edward Giovannucci and others, "A Prospective Study of Cigarette Smoking and Risk of Colorectal Adenoma and Colorectal Cancer in U.S. Women," *Journal of the National Cancer Institute* 86, no. 3 (2 February 1994): 192–99; and Edward Giovannucci and others, "A Prospective Study of Cigarette Smoking and Risk of Colorectal Adenoma and Colorectal Cancer in U.S. Men," *Journal of the National Cancer Institute* 86, no. 3 (2 February 1994): 183–91.
20. "The Eighteen-Year Gap," *University of California at Berkeley Wellness Letter* 7, no. 4 (January 1991): 2.
21. Johanna Seddon and others, "A Prospective Study of Cigarette Smoking and Age-Related Macular Degeneration in Women," *Journal of the American Medical Association* 276, no. 14 (9 October 1996): 1141–46; and William Christen and others, "A Prospective Study of Cigarette Smoking and Risk of Age-Related Macular Degeneration in Men," *Journal of the American Medical Association* 276, no. 14 (9 October 1996): 1147–51.
22. Denise Kandel, Ping Wu, and Mark Davies, "Maternal Smoking during Pregnancy and Smoking by Adolescent Daughters," *American Journal of Public Health* 84, no. 9 (September 1994): 1407–13.
23. Joel Coste, Nadine Job-Spira, and Herve Fernandez, "Increased Risk of Ectopic Pregnancy with Maternal Cigarette Smoking," *American Journal of Public Health* 81, no. 2 (February 1991): 199–201.
24. Bengt Haglund and Sven Cnattingius, "Cigarette Smoking As a Risk Factor for Sudden Infant Death Syndrome: A Population-Based Study," *American Journal of Public Health* 80, no. 1 (January 1990): 29–32.
25. Alexander Glassman and others, "Smoking, Smoking Cessation, and Major Depression," *Journal of the American Medical Association* 264, no. 12 (20 September 1990): 1546–49; and Robert Anda and others, "Depression and the Dynamics of Smoking," *Journal of the American Medical Association* 264, no. 12 (26 September 1990): 1541–45.
26. Diane Gold and others, "Effects of Cigarette Smoking on Lung Function in Adolescent Boys and Girls," *New England Journal of Medicine* 335, no. 13 (26 September 1996): 931–37.
27. National Center for Health Statistics, "Relationships between Smoking and Other Unhealthy Habits: United States, 1985," *Advancedata* 154 (27 May 1988): 6.
28. Donald Kadunce and others, "Cigarette Smoking: Risk Factor for Premature Facial Wrinkling," *Annals of Internal Medicine* 114, no. 10 (15 May 1991): 840–44.
29. James Pirkle and others, "Exposure of the U.S. Population to Environmental Tobacco Smoke," *Journal of the American Medical Association* 275, no. 16 (24 April 1996) 1233–40.
30. U.S. Environmental Protection Agency and U.S. Department of Health and Human Services, *Respiratory Health Effects of Passive Smoking: Lung Cancer and Other Disorders,* a report of the EPA, NIH Publication No. 93-3605 (Bethesda, Md.: National Institutes of Health, 1993), 3–17.
31. Dwight Janevich and others, "Lung Cancer and Exposure to Tobacco Smoke in the

Household," *New England Journal of Medicine* 323, no. 10 (6 September 1990): 632–36.

32. Elizabeth Fontham and others, "Environmental Tobacco Smoke and Lung Cancer in Nonsmoking Women," *Journal of the American Medical Association* 271, no. 22 (8 June 1994): 1752–59.
33. Stanton Glantz and William Parmley, "Passive Smoking and Heart Disease," *Journal of the American Medical Association* 273, no. 13 (5 April 1995): 1047–53.
34. Stanton Glantz and William Parmley, "Passive Smoking and Heart Disease: Epidemiology, Physiology, and Biochemistry," *Circulation* 83, no. 1 (January 1991): 1–12 and "Is Secondhand Smoke a Hazard?" *Consumer Reports* 60, no. 1 (January 1995): 27–33.
35. Fernando Martinez, Anne Wright, and Lynn Taussig, "The Effect of Paternal Smoking on the Birthweight of Newborns Whose Mothers Did Not Smoke," *American Journal of Public Health* 84, no. 9 (September 1994): 1489–91.
36. American Heart Association, *Heart and Stroke Facts* (Dallas: American Heart Association, 1995), 19–20.
37. American Cancer Society, *Cancer Facts and Figures—1996,* 10.
38. Mikhail Denissenko and others, "Preferential Formation of Benzo [a] pyrene Adducts at Lung Cancer Mutational Hotspots in P53," *Science* 274, no. 5286 (18 October 1996): 430–32.
39. Unless otherwise indicated, the information in this section is derived from the following sources: Public Health Service, *The Health Consequences of Using Smokeless Tobacco,* a report of the Advisory Committee to the Surgeon General (Washington, D.C.: GPO, 1986); and U.S. Department of Health and Human Services, Public Health Service, *Smokeless Tobacco or Health: An International Perspective.* NIH Publication No. 93-3461 (Bethesda, Md.: National Institutes of Health, 1993).
40. Virginia Ernster and others, "Smokeless Tobacco Use and Health Effects among Baseball Players," *Journal of the American Medical Association* 264, no. 2 (11 July 1990): 218–24.
41. "College Athletes." *Monday Morning Report* 14, no. 23 (25 March 1991): 1.
42. *Smokeless Tobacco.* Datafax Information Series (Tempe, Ariz.: Do It Now, 1990), 2.
43. Antonia C. Novello, preface to *Health Benefits of Smoking Cessation,* v–xii.
44. S. Goya Wannamethee and others, "Smoking Cessation and the Risk of Stroke in Middle-aged Men," *Journal of the American Medical Association* 274, no. 2 (12 July 1995): 155–60.
45. Thomas Glynn. "Methods of Smoking Cessation—Finally, Some Answers," *Journal of the American Medical Association* 263, no. 20 (23–30 May 1990): 2795–96; and Michael Fiore and others, "Methods Used to Quit Smoking in the United States," *Journal of the American Medical Association* 263, no. 20 (23–30 May 1990): 2760–65.
46. Jack Henningfield and others, "Drinking Coffee and Carbonated Beverages Blocks Absorption of Nicotine from Nicotine Polacrilex Gum," *Journal of the American Medical Association,* 264, no. 12 (26 September 1990): 1560–64.

Chapter 9

Cocaine and other "chemical uppers"

KEY TERMS

Amphetamines
Anorectic
Antidepressant
Attention Deficit-Hyperactivity Disorder
Caffeine
Caffeinism
Cocaine
Cocaine Psychosis
Crack Cocaine
"Crashing"
Dextroamphetamine
Ephedrine
"Flash"
Fluoxetine (Prozac)
Formication
Freebasing
"Ice"
Khat
MAO Inhibitors
Mariani's Wine
Methamphetamine
Methcathinone
Narcolepsy
"Rush" Reaction
"Speed"
Speedball
Speed Runs
Toxic Syndrome
Tricyclic Compounds

chapter objectives

After you have studied this chapter, you should be able to do the following:

1. Define the key terms.
2. Describe several general effects of behavioral stimulants, such as cocaine and the amphetamines.
3. Explain why using CNS stimulants frequently becomes a compulsive drug-taking behavior.
4. Discuss the historical influences that have been responsible for cocaine's initial popularity as a recreational drug.
5. Distinguish among the various use patterns of cocaine consumption.
6. Compare the relative hazards involved in snorting, injecting, and freebasing cocaine.
7. Describe the unique features of "crack," including its addictive nature.
8. Explain the attraction and the dangers of combining cocaine with CNS depressants or sedatives.
9. Describe the probable effects of cocaine use in relation to light or moderate use, to use of relatively high doses, and to long-term use.
10. List the similarities and differences between cocaine and the amphetamines in terms of origin, specific effects, duration of effects, reasons for abuse, and frequently associated risks to health.
11. Compare and contrast the effects of "crack" with those of "ice"—the smokable form of methamphetamine.
12. Name three current medical uses of the amphetamines.
13. Describe the general effects and therapeutic uses of MAO inhibitors, tricyclic compounds, and fluoxetine (Prozac).
14. Identify the commonly experienced drug effects of caffeine.
15. Distinguish the condition of caffeinism from the phenomenon of caffeine dependence.
16. Explain how individuals can reduce their intake of caffeine-based beverages and medications containing caffeine.
17. Compare and contrast the origins, motivations for use, and effects of methcathinone and ephedrine.

Introduction

In chapter 8, nicotine—one addictive and toxic stimulant—was described in detail. In this chapter, the focus is on the other "chemical uppers"—cocaine; amphetamines; caffeine; and various plant stimulants, including khat. These psychoactive drugs tend to speed up, excite, and activate various body functions and parts.

The underlying reasons for using "chemical uppers" are complex. On occasion, most people have sought some type of physical or mental "uplifting." To some extent, the reduction of fatigue, the prevention of sleep, and the elevation of mood have been achieved temporarily through the use of drugs called central nervous system (CNS) stimulants.

There are several types of CNS stimulants. In this chapter the major emphasis will be on the so-called behavior stimulants (such as cocaine and the amphetamines) that increase mental and physical activity and elevate mood in healthy individuals. The clinical antidepressants that have no pharmacological effects in healthy people will then be explained, as well as the common stimulant found in coffee, tea, chocolate, and certain medications. The chapter then concludes with a brief overview of various plant stimulants.

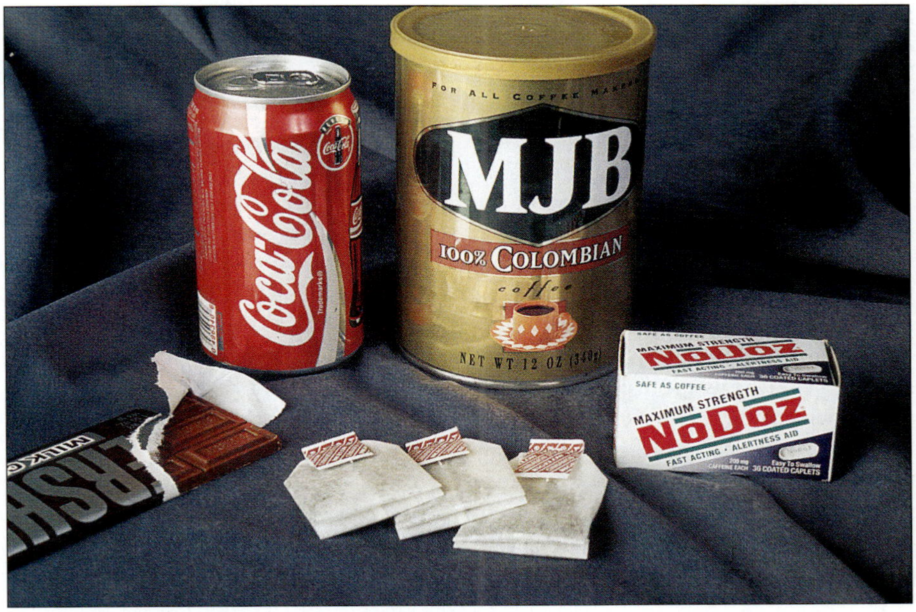

All of these products contain a legal stimulant, caffeine.

© Jonathan Nourok/PhotoEdit

Chemical Uppers

As in other "drug families," psychoactive stimulants share several common features and similarities, discussed in the following sections.[1]

Basic Perspectives

Drugs classified as CNS stimulants increase alertness, physical activity, and excitement by speeding up the body's processes. Often called "uppers" or "ups," these stimulating drugs increase behavioral activity and psychomotor functions.

Unlike the depressant-type drugs, or "downers," all of which cause a general sedation, the stimulants display a diverse pharmacology. For instance, the convulsions produced by strychnine—a CNS stimulant better known as a rat poison ingredient—are different from the euphoria and improved performance induced by an amphetamine, another common stimulant drug.

Of all the abused drugs, cocaine, the amphetamines, and caffeine are among the most powerfully reinforcing. That is, the pleasurable effects experienced from taking these CNS stimulants compel the users to engage in repeated, often compulsive consumption of such substances. As addiction to these drugs occurs—especially cocaine and the amphetamines—the repeated use of these psychoactives will likely continue, despite many harmful and self-destructive consequences.

Among the most widely used stimulants are **caffeine** and nicotine—two substances rarely perceived as drugs until recent times. Caffeine is still considered relatively harmless and millions of children consume large amounts of this drug in cola drinks.[2] In addition, caffeine is the active ingredient in coffee and tea. These beverages are often used as mild "pick-me-up" or wake-me-up" substances. Caffeine is also the active ingredient of nonprescription sleep prevention medications.

Use of either caffeine or nicotine can result in a drug dependency, but neither causes serious psychiatric symptoms nor severe impairment of work or family life—except for the adverse consequences of long-term tobacco use.

Other CNS stimulants are more potent and have an even greater potential for producing a drug dependency. Available by prescription or only for medical research, drugs such as cocaine and amphetamines are controlled medications (Schedule II) under provisions of the Controlled Substances Act. Cocaine and various amphetamines are also available on the illicit street market, especially because their medical uses have been curtailed in the United States.

Common Effects

Use of "chemical uppers," especially stronger stimulants such as cocaine and amphetamines, forces the body to release its natural stimulants—neurotransmitter substances, primarily norepinephrine and dopamine, but also serotonin. Cocaine, amphetamines, caffeine, and certain antidepressants potentiate the actions of norepinephrine.

At low doses, stimulants mimic the actions of these specific neurotransmitters. The results include a behavior-arousal response with increased alertness, a perceived surge of energy, the shifting of blood flow from the skin and internal organs to the muscles, and an increase in levels of oxygen and blood sugar. Such reactions represent an exaggerated mobilization of the normal, human fight-flight-fright response.[3]

Other actions of the stimulants include increased heart rate and blood pressure and energized muscular activity. Overstimulation may surface as irritability, restlessness, and insomnia. When long-term or excessive high-dose use of stimulants depletes the body's natural supply of energy-producing neurotransmitters, various body systems begin to shut down, resulting in physical collapse and mental depression.

Psychological reliance upon the stimulants is common because they tend to make users feel stronger, more decisive, and self-possessed. These stimulants also produce a euphoria along with a decreased perception of fatigue, a decreased need for sleep, and a decreased appetite. (See box 9.1 for a description of the effects of stimulants on driving.) Some nonmedical users also believe stimulants increase the desire for and pleasurable aspects of sexual behavior.

However, while cocaine, amphetamines, and plant stimulants such as methcathinone and ephedrine tend to elevate mood and stimulate the behavior of healthy people, the antidepressants have no significant effect on people without mental or chemical disorders. Reflecting their unusual pharmacological characteristics, the antidepressants produce their desirable effects only in psychologically depressed individuals.

Box 9.1 Cocaine, Amphetamines, Caffeine, and Driving:

Why Take the Risk?

Cocaine, amphetamines, and other stimulants including phenylpropanolamine, ephedrine, and caffeine (found in specific nonprescription medicines) stimulate the central nervous system. Small amounts of these drugs usually make people who are tired feel more alert.

Studies reveal that small doses of amphetamines, given to subjects for a limited time, usually improve performance of several driving skills. However, these subjects tend to overestimate their performance and take more risks. Actual driving records indicate that people who take amphetamines are slightly more accident prone, probably for these reasons.

While heavy amphetamine use and repeated use of other stimulants to combat fatigue will tend to keep drivers awake and active for long stretches of time, these stimulants will also make the drivers edgy, less coordinated, and more likely to be involved in traffic accidents. One accident study found that amphetamine users were four times more likely to be involved in car crashes than nonusers.

Presently, there is only limited information about cocaine's effects on psychomotor driving skills. Research does show that typical so-called social amounts of inhaled cocaine can produce lapses in attention and concentration. Although users often report that cocaine, like other stimulants, increases their concentration and improves performance on a variety of tasks, there is no objective evidence supporting these reports. Moreover, cocaine is a short-acting drug, and within an hour the user feels not only less alert but more anxious, tired, or depressed than before.

Regular users sometimes report feelings of restlessness, irritability, and anxiety, but even low doses may create psychological problems. These adverse effects are minor in comparison with the consequences of combining alcohol with cocaine, a practice known as "speedballing." Used in such a combination, cocaine tends to mask alcohol's effect, so that an individual who feels sober enough and sufficiently alert to drive will become intoxicated as the effects of cocaine wear off.

Although caffeine can help the drowsy driver stay alert, coffee can't make the drunk driver sober. Studies show that ordinary amounts of caffeine do not improve an inebriated person's driving skills.

Driving requires a combination of thought and motor skills, a great deal of common sense, and a concern for the safety of everyone on the road. Safe driving requires an observant eye, a steady hand, and a clear head. By mixing drugs with driving, you are only asking for trouble. Why take the risk?

Source: Modified from the National Institute on Drug Abuse.

Various Use Patterns

These chemical "eye openers" are used in various recreational or nonmedical ways to achieve a feeling of well-being and increased alertness. Until recently, the most common patterns involved periodic oral and nasal use of stimulants, such as swallowing amphetamine capsules and inhaling (snorting) cocaine. Occasionally, these stimulants have been used in combination with depressant drugs, including alcohol, barbiturates or other sleeping pills, tranquilizers, marijuana, and various psychedelics.

When used alone in large doses, stimulants often induce a temporary sense of exhilaration with superabundant energy, increased activity, extended wakefulness, and loss of appetite. At this dosage level, the user may also experience dizziness, tremors, confusion, headaches, flushing or sweating, nausea, chest pain, and the sensation of a racing heart.

With only infrequent use of stimulants, however, the condition of tolerance does not usually develop.

Another major pattern of stimulant use is intravenous injection, usually of a specific amphetamine (methamphetamine, or "speed") or cocaine. Such a use pattern often develops after extended oral use of amphetamine or cocaine inhalation.

After the injection, users typically report an initial **"flash"** or **"rush" reaction.** This "flash" effect is a short, intense, generalized sensation similar to a sudden splash of cold water or a total body orgasm. Almost instantaneously, complete well-being is experienced and feelings of boredom and depression vanish.

Users also perceive a marked enhancement of their physical strength and mental abilities. Sometimes, though, CNS stimulant abusers also experience irritability, anxiety, and apprehension, and some even display hostile, aggressive behavior.

Due to the cumulative effects of these stimulant-type drugs, long-term users sometimes develop a pattern of stimulant use during the day and depressant (alcohol and sleeping pills) use at night. This chemical rotation—"speeding up" followed by "slowing down"—interferes with normal body processes, which can lead to serious illness.

Yet another form of stimulant use was introduced in the late 1970s with the appearance of freebase, a form of cocaine that could be smoked. This first form of smokable cocaine involved a rather dangerous process of converting "street cocaine" to freebase crystals that were then smoked through a water pipe.

Then, in the mid-1980s, a newer form of cocaine, called "crack," emerged. Relatively low in cost and available in ready-to-smoke form without fancy paraphernalia, crack is considered to be the most addictive form of cocaine. Crack is intensified cocaine. Its effects are amplified, sharper, meaner, and uglier than those of plain cocaine. Many experts believe that crack accounted for much of the cocaine-abuse epidemic that began in the United States in 1985 and still continues.

Drug Dependence and Compulsive Behavior

Tolerance to the euphoric and the appetite-suppressant effects of stimulants develops rapidly with intravenous injection. Extremely high dose levels are sometimes accompanied by paranoid feelings. In addition, the user may engage in endless compulsive activities such as grinding the teeth and touching and picking the face and extremities. These peculiar behaviors are often referred to as hypomania or knick-knacking.

There may also be a preoccupation with one's own thoughts; a general suspiciousness; and eventually a **toxic syndrome,** consisting of tremors, agitation, hostility, panic, headache, flushed skin, chest pain, excessive perspiration, vomiting, and abdominal cramps. If there is no medical intervention, high fever, convulsions, and heart and blood-vessel collapse may be followed by death.

A desire to reexperience the "flash" and to avoid the loss of the stimulant's effects and the onset of "withdrawal symptoms" compels some long-term users to engage in **speed runs** or binges. These are several days of nearly continuous stimulant use during which a solution of amphetamine is injected or cocaine is smoked at frequent intervals. Such binging on stimulants is a frequent use pattern. In time, such compulsive use leads to the exhaustion of the user, who is tense and completely disorganized mentally.

When this individual finally stops taking the drug—often to end an unpleasant "speed run"—he or she experiences a disturbing period of depression. This sudden mental "low" is referred to as **crashing.** Such rebound depression is in sharp contrast with the mental "high" induced by the stimulant.

Now the person sleeps for as long as forty-eight hours, then awakens with a huge appetite. However, the individual feels quite lethargic for several days to several weeks. Panic reactions, continued depression, irritability, and assaultive and suicidal behavior are common. These reactions to discontinued amphetamine use are indicative of a withdrawal phenomenon.

In the past, scientists have disagreed about the capability of CNS stimulants to cause a true physical dependence. There is now widespread agreement that cocaine, amphetamines, and caffeine are addictive. Although not all users become dependent, addiction is still considered the most common complaint of the major stimulants.[4] Tolerance occurs and a withdrawal reaction is demonstrated, although the symptoms are not as severe as the physical withdrawal seen in heroin and alcohol dependency.

Compulsive drug-taking is often displayed, though stimulant use tends to be more irregular than the use patterns associated with the opioids, alcohol, and nicotine. Stimulant addicts do not need a daily dose to satisfy a strong physical need.[5] But such stimulant-dependent persons may also have a strong psychological need to continue taking their "chemical uppers." Cocaine and amphetamines are among the most powerful agents of psychic reward and reinforcement that provide the foundation of drug dependency.

Cocaine

The major psychoactive ingredient extracted from the leaves of the coca plant *(Erythroxylon coca),* **cocaine** is the most powerful CNS stimulant of natural origin.[6]

Unique Characteristics

The U.S. Pharmacopeia compound consists of white, odorless crystals or crystalline powder derived from a coca leaf paste. A vegetable alkaloid chemically labeled *benzoylmethylecgonine (methylbenzoylepgonine),* cocaine is better known as "coke," "C," "snow," "blow," "toot," "leaf," "flake," "freeze," "happy dust," "Peruvian lady," and "white girl."

Sold on the street, this drug is a mixture of the pure cocaine substance (cocaine hydrochloride) and various adulterants added to increase the quantity, typically for the seller's profit. Common adulterants include various sugars (lactose, inositol, and mannitol) and local anesthetics such as lidocaine.

The purity of cocaine varies from a low of about 15 percent to a high of nearly 95 percent, depending upon the amount of adulterants in any particular sample. Usually, samples of cocaine powder are about 83 percent pure cocaine or higher today, whereas comparable samples several years ago were only about 27 percent pure cocaine. Smokable crack cocaine now averages from 75 to 90 percent pure, up significantly from only 34 percent purity in the late 1980s.

Since enactment and enforcement of the Harrison Narcotic Act of 1914 and its amendments, cocaine has been classified with the narcotics and subjected to the same controls as opium, morphine, and heroin. In 1922, the coca leaf derivative was defined legally as a narcotic drug, although cocaine is not a narcotic in the pharmacological sense. This narcotic definition still applies, despite cocaine's differing drug effects.

Medical Uses

For hundreds of years, the Inca tribes of South America have chewed coca leaves for mild refreshment and relief from fatigue. During the last quarter of the nineteenth century, cocaine was a recommended therapy for depression and other mental illnesses, digestive disorders, degeneration of tissues, morphine and alcohol addiction, and asthma, and as an aphrodisiac and local anesthetic.

Presently, cocaine has only limited therapeutic uses because of its toxicity and potential for abuse.[7] One clinical application is related to its unique characteristics as a local anesthetic. When applied to the surface of mucous membranes, cocaine produces anesthesia and vasoconstriction (a narrowing effect on blood vessels). This vasoconstriction action reduces bleeding during surgery. As such, cocaine has been a valuable drug to both patient and surgeon when applied to the nose, throat,

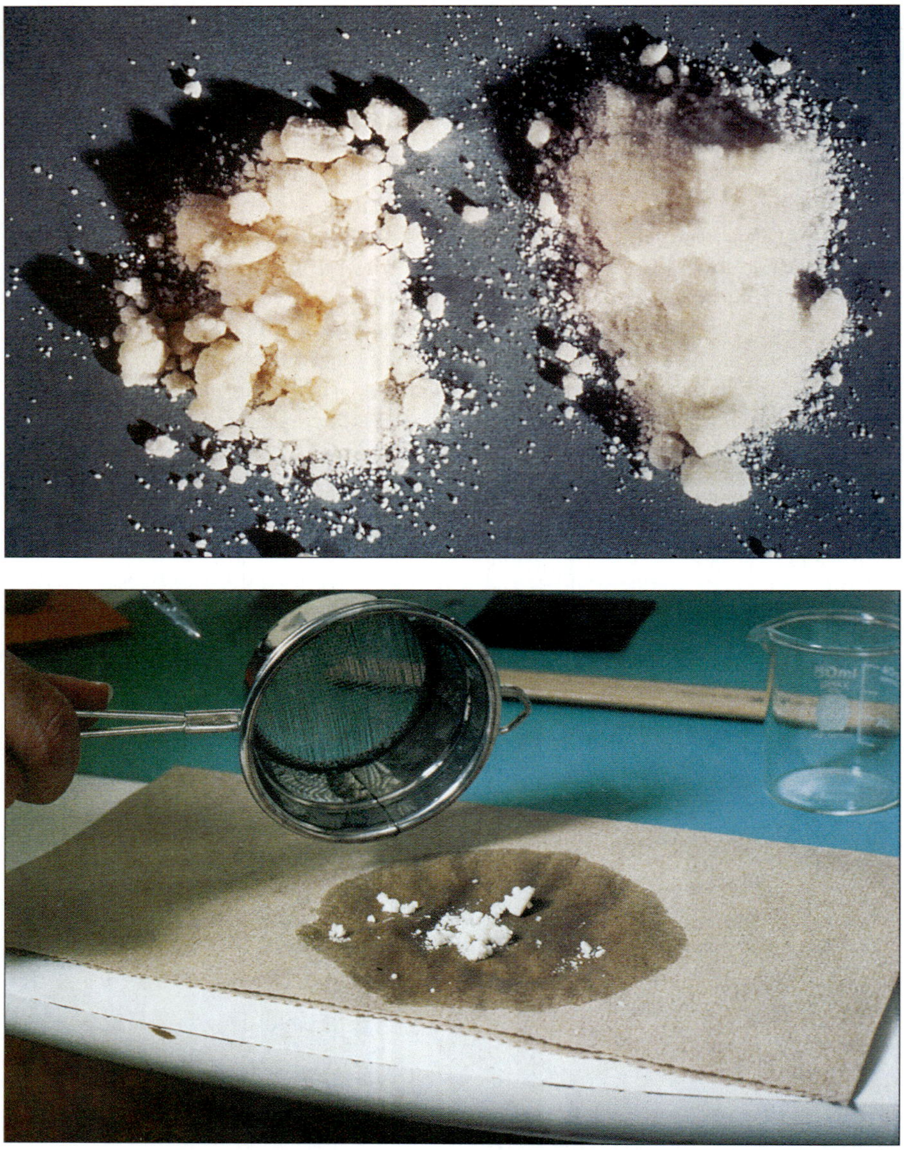

(Top): Pure cocaine, known as cocaine hydrochloride, appears as a white crystalline powder. (Bottom): Crack cocaine, the most addictive form of cocaine, appears as white gravel, slivers of soap, or tiny chunks known as "crack rocks."

Drug Enforcement Agency

larynx, or lower respiratory passages in intranasal surgery.

However, even this use may be accompanied by severe toxicity. At one time, cocaine was used extensively in eye surgery, but even this therapeutic application has become obsolete with the introduction of safer drugs as local anesthetics.

Another therapeutic use, until recently, has been in conjunction with *Brompton's cocktail.* A solution of cocaine, methadone, and alcohol, the special "cocktail" was first used for the relief of pain in terminally ill patients. The legal use of cocaine in Brompton's cocktail increased, especially in England, because of the proliferation of hospice services in which controlling patients' pain without causing stupor or unconsciousness is highly desirable. This liquid analgesic was administered in low doses at regular intervals or upon demand by patients. Thus, the dying were maintained as pain-free as possible, awake, alert, and fully conscious until the final moments of their lives.[8] However, nearly all hospices reformulated their painkillers without cocaine and now rely instead upon a combination of morphine and alcohol, the standard in such caregiving institutions in the United States.

Historical and Legal Aspects

Although the precise origin of chewing coca leaves for euphoric effects has not been determined, many authorities date its widespread practice to the pre-Colombian South American Indians who inhabited the Andes Mountains.[9] Early myths and legends suggest that the coca plant was of divine origin and was frequently associated with sexual behavior.

It is likely that some South American tribes chewed coca leaves as early as A.D. 600 to 800 However, by the thirteenth century a definitive role had been established for the coca plant in the religious and political structures of the early Inca Empire. To guarantee a safe crossing of the Andes Mountains, individuals offered coca leaves to the gods. Later, the Incas employed the leaves in their sacrificial rituals. The cultivation of the coca bush eventually became a state monopoly, and the use of coca leaves evolved as an exclusive privilege of the ruling class.

At the time of the Spanish conquest of the Inca Empire in the sixteenth century, coca leaves were no longer a symbol of political authority or social status. Nevertheless, the Spanish soon realized the profit potential of trading coca leaves with the Incas for their gold and silver. After their conquest, the Incas increased their coca leaf chewing, possibly because of a decline in the food supplies, the institution of formal labor by the Spanish, and the euphoric feeling induced by the drug.

Although the chewing of coca leaves never became popular in either Europe or North America, various drinks made from the coca leaf were introduced into Europe. One of them, **Mariani's wine,** became most successful with endorsements from notable artists and religious leaders. In the United States, John Styth Pemberton introduced a product similar to Angelo Mariani's wine in 1885 and

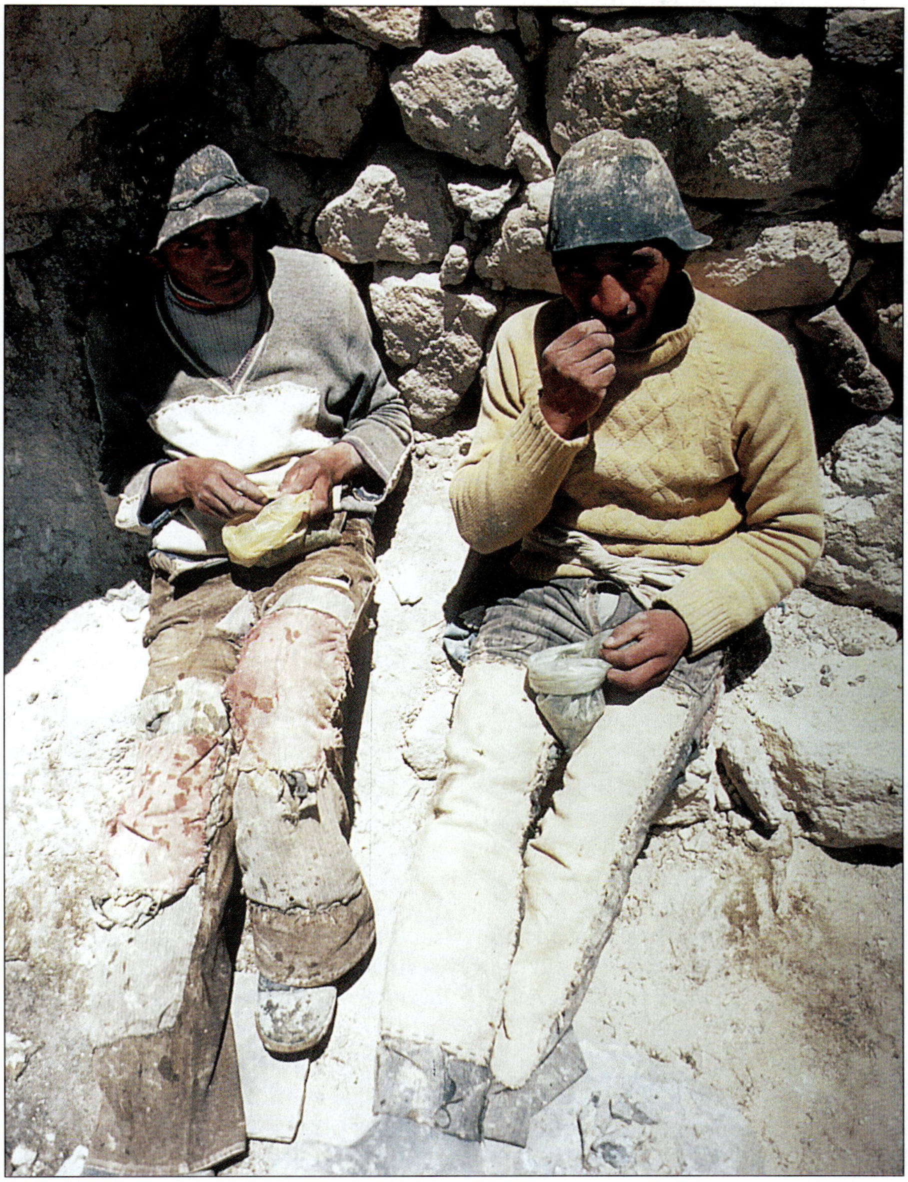

In Bolivia, these miners are chewing coca leaves as a social ritual and for mild stimulation during a workbreak.

© Jeffrey L. Rotman/Peter Arnold, Inc.

promoted the new French Wine Cola as a nerve and tonic stimulant.

The next year, Pemberton concocted another coca product, a syrup that he named Coca-Cola. This new "remarkable therapeutic agent" and "sovereign remedy" contained coca leaf flavoring (cocaine) and caffeine, an extract of the kola nut. Eventually, all references to Coca-Cola's medicinal properties were dropped, and by the time the Pure Food and Drug Law was passed in 1906, Pemberton's successors had removed the cocaine. The reformulated drink was flavored with decocainized coca leaves and caffeine.

It was not until 1844 or later that cocaine was first isolated in pure form from coca leaves. Early investigations by European and American physicians suggested that cocaine had great potential as a therapeutic agent. One of the stimulant's most noted advocates was Dr. Sigmund Freud, who used cocaine presumably to cure his own depression and promoted its use for numerous physical and mental disorders.

Such initial enthusiasm supporting the therapeutic applications of cocaine soon diminished with mounting evidence of its health liabilities. Nevertheless, between 1890 and 1906—the "golden age of patent medicines"—cocaine was a basic ingredient of numerous ointments, powders, lozenges, and wines. These products were advertised as cures for asthma, colds, corns, eczema, neuralgia, opiate and alcohol addiction, and even venereal disease.

By the turn of the century, the federal government and the medical profession became concerned with the widespread misuse and abuse of proprietary medicines. Influenced by horrible tales of cocaine-crazed individuals committing mass rapes and murders, public opinion also turned against cocaine. The national hysteria resulted first in the Pure Food and Drug Law of 1906 (which regulated labeling the patent medicines) and later in the Harrison Narcotic Act of 1914, which ended cocaine's use in patent medicines and established penalties for violations of regulated uses. This loss of respectability, together with the high cost of illegal cocaine, led to reduced cocaine use among Americans.

The reemergence of cocaine as a recreational drug in the mid-1960s began when the federal government initiated a campaign to crack down on the production and use of amphetamine, another CNS stimulant. Physicians were warned about overprescribing stimulant drugs, and the battle against illicit "speed" labs was stepped up. As the supply of one stimulant decreased, the smuggling of illicit cocaine suddenly became profitable.

Portrayed as the "caviar of drugs," in the 1970s, cocaine developed its appeal based on pharmacologic effect and symbolism. Indeed, cocaine became an emblem of wealth and status, and a "black market" for the stimulant evolved rapidly and continues to flourish as a profitable enterprise. But cocaine's initial acceptance was also related to the intense "high" it produces, the false perception that cocaine is not dangerous, and the mistaken belief that the drug is not addictive.

Most of the world's coca leaves come from the mountainous regions of Peru and Bolivia. Coca paste is refined in Colombia, and the final product is then smuggled into the United States, typically by either plane or boat. For several years, the main port of entry was south Florida. Now there are several others, especially on the Mexican border and the islands of the eastern Caribbean, including Puerto Rico.[10]

Although Americans are continuing their romance with cocaine at a somewhat lower level, exposure to the drug's risks still results in more than 140,000 emergency room episodes of cocaine abuse each year. Use of this drug in the United States is declining because of the numerous instances of overdose and the widely publicized deaths of prominent athletes due to cocaine's effects. About 1.5 million Americans currently use cocaine, which is a significant decline from a peak of 5.7 million in 1985.[11]

Patterns of Using Cocaine

Several distinct use patterns have developed among those who consume cocaine. Some of these patterns, such as chewing and snorting, may be considered traditional, whereas the somewhat newer techniques involve injecting and smoking cocaine derivatives. The use patterns described in the following sections reflect the various methods of administering cocaine.

Oral Use

Oral use of cocaine can still be found, especially in Peru, where Andean Indians chew coca leaves as a social ritual and for mild stimulation. Used in this way, cocaine evidently causes no serious health hazards or social problems.

Members of the upper socioeconomic classes in Peru also brew tea made from coca leaves. While not a typical use pattern in the United States, expanded interest in coca leaf chewing among counterculture groups has occurred as part of a trend toward organic or natural drugs.

Snorting

When extracted from other chemicals in the coca leaf, cocaine is isolated as a hydrochloride salt, known as cocaine hydrochloride. This form of cocaine usually appears as a white, crystalline powder. Dissolved in water, the cocaine can be mixed easily with other fluids and sold as "refreshing beverages" or injected directly into the veins.

Nevertheless, the modern epidemic of cocaine use featured neither drinking nor injecting, but a procedure referred to as snorting. Sometimes known as tooting or blowing, snorting involves sniffing cocaine powder directly into the nostrils, where it is absorbed into the bloodstream through the nasal mucosa (lining).

Typically, the user finely chops the "coke" powder with a razor blade on a hard, flat surface and then arranges the powder into thin lines or columns, approximately 3 to 5 centimeters long. The user than inhales intranasally a line of cocaine, often through a rolled dollar bill or a straw or from a "coke spoon." The inhaled cocaine penetrates the mucous membranes of the nasal lining, enters the bloodstream, and is circulated to the brain within 3 to 5 minutes. One line usually provides the user with 20 to 40 minutes of stimulation and mild euphoria.

Absorption through other mucous membranes is an alternative use pattern employed by a minority of cocaine users. Some people rub cocaine on their gums, palates, or the underside of their tongues, or have the powder blown from a straw onto the mucosal surface of the back of the throat.

Another uncommon absorption technique involves the topical application of the powder to the mucosa of the vagina or the male genitalia. Some users report that this prolongs intercourse and intensifies orgasm. However, some males claim that using cocaine by any route of administration causes temporary impotence.

A number of cocaine users "snort" almost on a daily basis but manage to avoid tolerance. They claim they can stop anytime. While the phenomenon of psychological dependence is not fully understood, regular cocaine use often produces the compulsive user, the cocaine addict.

Intravenous Injection

Intravenous injection of a cocaine solution, whether alone or in combination or alternation with another euphoriant, usually induces an intense, initial "rush" or "flash" not often experienced when cocaine is taken orally or snorted. A relatively short-lived experience of pure pleasure, the "rush" lasts about ten minutes. After this phenomenon, described as feeling as if electricity is running through one's brain, the user craves yet another shot before undergoing the unpleasant experience of "crashing."

Some cocaine "injectors," and addicted heroin "injectors," have switched to smoking a cocaine derivative, because of the real danger of contracting AIDS (acquired immunodeficiency syndrome). Injecting cocaine carries additional hazards of other serious infections, formation of blood clots, and possible adverse reactions to impurities in the injected mixture.

Combined Use with Depressants

Combined use of cocaine with certain depressant drugs has become a fairly common practice, especially among long-term compulsive users. Sometimes a mixture of cocaine and heroin—referred to as a **speedball**—is taken. Such combined or even sequential use of cocaine and a depressant smooths out the stimulant's effects, reduces nervousness and excitability, and softens "crashing" after an extended cocaine binge.

Nonetheless, speedballing does increase the risks of drug dependency, toxic overdoses, and financial disaster, as well as deeper involvement with the law. John Belushi, a famous comedian, allegedly died because of speedballing—multiple injections of a cocaine-heroin mixture—which resulted in a sudden buildup in one or both drugs of toxins that proved deadly.

Contrary to widespread belief, CNS stimulants and depressants reduce respiratory activity and produce a temporary lapse of breathing. Furthermore, the combination stimulant-depressant speedball is not an antidote for either drug. Though a small amount of cocaine reduces the depressant effect of heroin, equal amounts of the two drugs potentiate the effects of heroin. When heroin is not available, alcohol or barbiturates are sometimes substituted for the opioid after snorting or intravenous injection of cocaine.

Freebasing

A new cocaine danger called **freebasing** surfaced in the 1970s. Through an elaborate "do-it-yourself" chemical process, cocaine hydrochloride powder is changed into a smokable and more potent substance called "base" or "freebase." The procedure, which is extremely dangerous, involves treating the cocaine powder with a strong alkali and then ether. (See figure 9.1.) Former comedian Richard Pryor apparently was involved in a freebasing accident that set fire to his clothing and left him with third-degree burns on the upper half of his body.

The "freebase" is then smoked in a water pipe or sprinkled on a marijuana or tobacco cigarette. Within a few minutes, the stimulant reaches the brain and produces a sudden and intense high. This euphoria subsides quickly and is often followed by an uncomfortable restlessness, irritability, and depression. To maintain the high and avoid the crash, freebase smokers sometimes continue smoking until they are either exhausted or have run out of cocaine.

During the early 1980s, more cocaine users began freebasing and injecting intravenously. These routes of administration result in quicker and more direct absorption of the drug and, therefore, provide a more immediate and intense euphoria.

At the same time, though, freebasing and intravenous injection increase the possibility of acute toxic reaction—visual disturbances, nervousness, tremors, convulsions, irregular heartbeat, and stoppage of breathing. Increasing prevalence of freebasing also resulted in greater incidence of lung damage, psychosis, chemical poisoning, and explosion-type burns.

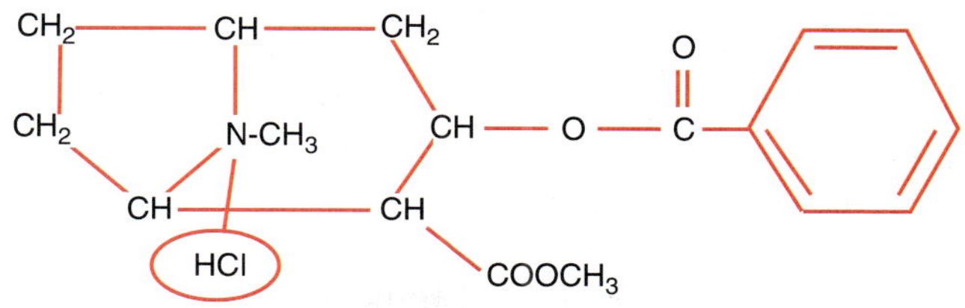

Cocaine hydrochloride

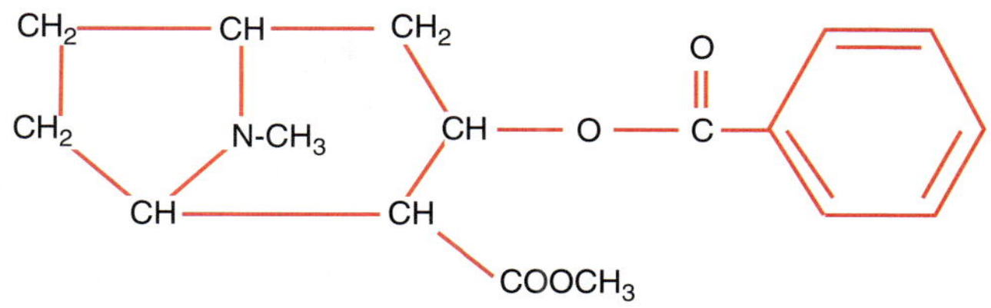

Freebase cocaine – without the HCl or hydrochloride molecule, also known as a "base." Consequently this is cocaine without the "base."

figure 9.1

Comparative molecular structures of cocaine used in snorting and injection with freebase cocaine.

Crack Smoking

In 1985, another form of smokable cocaine emerged and dramatically changed the drug scene in America. **Crack cocaine** is also derived from cocaine hydrochloride. But unlike the dangerous ether procedure used in making freebase, the conversion process for making crack is somewhat safer and uses ammonia or baking soda and water. The name *crack* describes the sounds that occur when this form of processed cocaine is smoked.

Crack resembles hard shavings that are similar to slivers of soap, and it is often sold in small vials, in folding papers, or in heavy tinfoil. Sometimes the crack material is broken into tiny chunks that are sold as "crack rocks." Unlike freebase, which requires the use of elaborate paraphernalia, crack can be smoked either in a pipe or mixed with marijuana. On occasion, crack cocaine also contains a small amount of PCP, a particularly hazardous "dissociative anesthetic" known as "angel dust."

An intensified form of cocaine, crack is considered one of the most addictive substances ever known, more so than heroin, barbiturates, and alcohol. Its vapors are inhaled, therefore crack is quickly absorbed through the lungs into the bloodstream and reaches the brain within a matter of seconds. This action is faster than when cocaine is snorted or injected. Once within the brain, crack produces a short, intense, electrifying feeling of euphoria.

Then, within several minutes of the pleasant high, a smoker usually develops a severe crisis-like "hangover" characterized by a deep depression, extreme sadness, irritability, occasional feelings of paranoia, and an overwhelming craving for more of the drug. However, it is the withdrawal hangover, not the euphoric high, that makes crack so addictive. Smoking crack is the most common form of cocaine use.

Crack users have become innovative in their simultaneous use of smokable rock with other psychoactives. Sometimes crack smokers place rocks of freebase in marijuana to produce "champagne" or "caviar"—crack-laced joints. Frequently, crack users will smoke "geekjoints" or "blunts"—cigarettes or cigars filled with tobacco and crack. Smokable speedballs ("hot rocks") are combinations of crack and "tar" heroin. To concoct "space base," some users mix PCP (phencyclidine) with crack, while others prepare "crack coolers" by adding crack or regular cocaine to wine coolers.

Still another form of smokable cocaine, *basuco,* has surfaced in Miami, Florida, and New York City. Cocaine basuco (or "bazuko") is sometimes called cocaine sulfate, coca paste, or just simply "base." A crude form of cocaine, basuco is highly contaminated with lead and petroleum by-products. The drug is typically mixed with tobacco or marijuana and smoked as a cigarette.

Effects of Cocaine

As with other drugs, the effects of this CNS stimulant are dependent upon the dose, the drug's purity, the user's mindset, the psychosocial setting, and the route of administration. The initial euphoric effects are intense but subside quickly. Users report an increased feeling of self-confidence and supercharged energy. They also experience wakefulness, talkativeness, increased heart rate and blood pressure, dilation of the pupils of the eyes, a rise in body temperature, constriction of blood vessels, and a reduction of appetite. Other responses include a reduction of fatigue (masked by stimulation of the central nervous system), enhanced mental alertness, and increased sociability.

Mechanism of Action

The physical and mental effects of cocaine are produced by increasing levels of specific neurotransmitters. Cocaine potentiates norepinephrine neurotransmitter. Such an action mimics the natural release of adrenaline, a body hormone that is a powerful stimulant of the sympathetic nervous system. This electrochemical chain reaction produces an increased heart rate, blood pressure, and cardiac output, and a general alerting response in the body.

Increased levels of dopamine neurotransmitter in the brain's reward circuit are also caused by cocaine. This change results in the intense pleasure or euphoria often associated with the use of this stimulant and thereby sets the stage for reinforcing drug-taking behavior.

But cocaine also blocks the reuptake and reuse of these same neurotransmitters. Temporarily, the neurotransmitter levels are increased in the synapse and their effects are prolonged. However, this excess of dopamine causes a downsizing of dopamine receptors in a complex process known as "down regulation." Eventually, the result is a bankruptcy of dopamine, when cocaine is no longer taken or when the supply of the drug has been exhausted.

With lower levels of dopamine, the user experiences an emergency craving to replenish these natural brain chemicals. The cocaine abuser mistakenly interprets the cravings as a need for more cocaine. Soon, as in the case of crack cocaine, getting more crack, smoking crack, and experiencing crack become more important than anything else.

Major Influencing Factors

There is considerable evidence that the frequency of using cocaine and the route of administration or use are important factors that influence the effects of cocaine in the human body. For instance, *occasional light use* is associated primarily with pleasurable psychological effects. However, researchers familiar with the cocaine "street scene" have concluded that laboratory experiments and surveys of users often underestimate the number and the severity of the undesirable effects, especially the depression and irritability of crashing, and the overwhelming desire for more of the drug.

Regular users sometimes report feelings of restlessness, irritability, anxiety, and even sleeplessness. In addition, even low doses of cocaine can create various psychological problems and "mood swings," while long-term use can result in hallucinations of touch, sight, taste, or smell. *Prolonged snorting* tends to dry out the mucous membrane linings of the nose until they crack, bleed, and develop ulcer-like sores. *Long-term use* also produces coldlike symptoms, with a runny nose; results in a dull headache; and may erode the cartilage separating the nostrils.

Regardless of the route of administration, prolonged use of cocaine often results in malnutrition because appetite is impaired. In time, chronic abusers often lose weight and develop a variety of vitamin deficiencies. Long-term use also contributes to a variety of sexual problems, including a loss of interest in sexual interaction, erectile difficulties, and greater insensitivity.[12] Moreover, it appears that prolonged use of cocaine is also linked with low sperm count and infertility in males.

Some Undesirable Effects

Among the more alarming effects of prolonged cocaine use are confusion, anxiety, and **cocaine psychosis,** characterized by paranoia and hallucinations of a tactile, visual, olfactory, and auditory nature. This severe psychotic reaction can occur while the user is still taking cocaine.

One hallucination that is particularly frightening is referred to as **formication.** Also known as parasitosis, formication is the false perception that bugs (insects such as ants) or snakes are crawling under one's skin. This feeling may be so intense that some individuals may scratch and pick their skin into open sores and gouge themselves with a knife to cut out the imaginary invaders.[13]

Continued use of cocaine may also make the brain more sensitive to the drug (the so-called *kindling effect*), so that even low doses of cocaine may bring on seizures and eventually sudden death. In this case, no dose can be considered safe.

In addition to the most serious health effects associated with snorting and injecting, freebasing and crack-smoking can also lead to lung damage that is similar to emphysema and interferes with efficiency of lung function and breathing.

Cocaine-Exposed Babies

Sometimes cocaine abuse can have adverse effects on nonusers as well. For instance, if women use cocaine heavily during pregnancy, there is the distinct possibility that their children will be born as "cocaine" or "crack"-exposed babies. The mothers tend to experience higher rates of premature births and miscarriages, while their babies are typically small at birth. In addiction, such prenatally cocaine-exposed infants tend to have a higher than average rate of minor congenital abnormalities. Some may suffer brain damage due to cocaine's constriction of blood vessels that supply fetal oxygen. However, there is no clear evidence of a cocaine-exposed baby syndrome as serious or as common as fetal alcohol syndrome.

Many children of heavy cocaine users suffer from attention deficit disorder (hyperactivity) and experience signs of tension, muscle stiffness, poor reflexes, and delayed motor development. However, most of the symptoms disappear by age three. Though mothers' cocaine use during pregnancy has undesirable influences on their children, in most cases it seems to have caused no serious, lasting brain injury.

Life-Threatening Consequences

Although many physicians have long recognized the deadly potential of using cocaine, until recently the general public has been largely unaware of this drug's lethal characteristics (see fig. 9.2). Contrary to the once-held belief that using cocaine was safe, it should be emphasized that this psychoactive drug is highly dangerous and in pure form can kill in minutes.

With the smoking of freebase and crack, *the first dose of cocaine can cause strokes, heart attacks, and sudden death.* Cocaine can kill through various physiological mechanisms.[14]

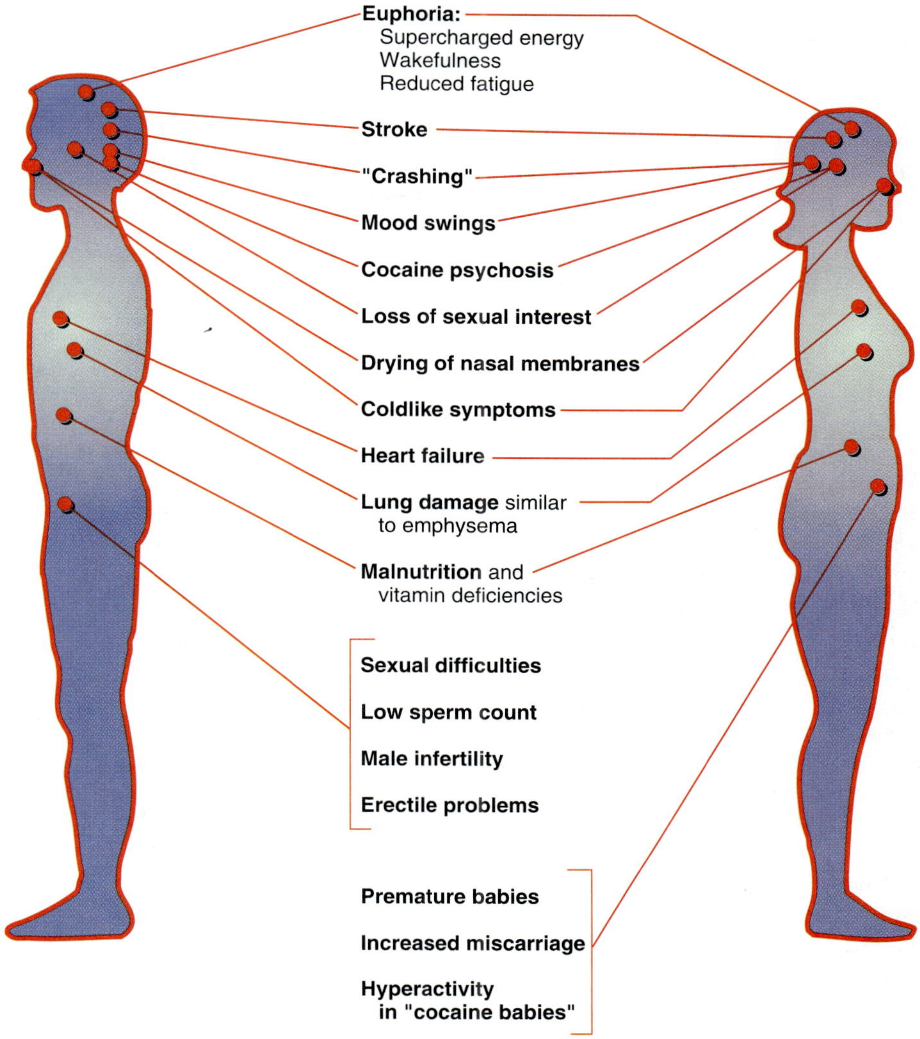

figure 9.2

Effects of cocaine use. Effects depend on dosage, frequency of use, and method of self-administration.

- Regardless of the dosage level, the livers of some users cannot produce an essential enzyme necessary to detoxify cocaine. The continuing presence of unmetabolized cocaine might result in fatal complications, detailed here, that would not otherwise occur in individuals with normal functioning livers.
- Even when cocaine can be detoxified by the liver, death might result from uncontrolled body seizures following use or from paralysis of breathing muscles, due to sudden stimulation of the central nervous system.
- Cocaine can cause such a rapid elevation of blood pressure that a weakened blood vessel in the brain may rupture, resulting in a stroke (cerebrovascular accident) that might kill or paralyze.
- Death through heart failure is related to cocaine's ability to cause damage to the heart muscle by disrupting the blood supply to cardiac muscles, resulting in a myocardial infarction, or heart attack.
- Injected, snorted, and smoked cocaine can cause irregularities in the heartbeat, which can be fatal; heart attacks; and even sudden death from cardiac arrest. There might develop a pattern of abnormally fast contractions of the heart's lower chambers—the ventricles—often in excess of 150 contractions per minute, which can rapidly prove deadly. For more information on cocaine, contact:

Cocaine Anonymous World Services
3740 Overland Ave., Suite H
Los Angeles, CA 90034

Box 9.2 Speed: Yesterday and Today

During the 1960s, a new form of amphetamine abuse developed when massive-dose, intravenous injections of methamphetamine ("meth" or "speed") became popular. The sudden electrifying impact of speed—or "crystal," as it is often called—was usually felt before the needle was removed from the arm of the user.

Even today, those who inject crystal compare the "rush" or "flash" effect with the intense pleasure of physical and psychological exhilaration. In addition to this full-body feeling of well-being, some users also report an awareness of more rapid thinking, an experience of more efficient thought and action, and marked enhancement of sexual performance.

Methamphetamine is manufactured and available as the prescription drug, Desoxyn.[a] However, "street meth" or "street crystal" has emerged in a major way in the United States and Canada. The illegally made drug is produced either in makeshift labs in the United States or smuggled into this country from Mexico. This form of speed is a powder that can be injected, inhaled, or swallowed. Another form of methamphetamine, "crank," sometimes comes packaged in pill form.

Regardless of its nickname or street preparation, methamphetamine is still dangerous and potentially lethal. Continued use places the abuser at risk for the hazards associated with amphetamines. Needle users are especially vulnerable to skin abscesses, hepatitis, tetanus, and even AIDS—common penalties for injecting dirty or shared needles.

When a smokable form of methamphetamine first emerged in Hawaii in the late 1980s and then on the West Coast of the mainland United States, there was great concern that ice would soon become the latest drug menace to sweep across the nation. Highly addictive, "ice" is smoked like crack cocaine and provides a high lasting several hours.

While smokable methamphetamine has spread beyond the West Coast, the anticipated epidemic—the "ice storm"—has not yet materialized nationwide.

The once popular slogan "Speed kills," originally described the death of the personality or spirit of the user who entered a state of limbo, neither physiologically dead nor psychologically alive. But speed can kill physically, because prolonged use can wear out and tear down the human body through vitamin and mineral deficiencies—resulting from poor nutrition—and lowered resistance to disease.[b] Under a general state of stress, the speed freak's body literally begins to burn itself up. Highly energized and denied the benefits of rest, recovery, and even food, the individual undergoes a rapid deterioration of physical and psychological health. Eventually, damage to major organs of the body (lungs, liver, and kidneys) occurs. In this sense, speed can kill!

When controls on the production and distribution of legally produced amphetamines reduced their availability, the speed scene became flooded first by *look-alikes* and then by *act-alikes.* Look-alikes are drugs that are manufactured to look like real amphetamines and mimic their effects. However, the amphetamine look-alike tablets and capsules contain varying amounts of legal nonprescription stimulants, decongestants, and antihistamines, such as caffeine, phenylpropanolamine, and ephedrine. These three legal substances are relatively weak stimulants often found in over-the-counter drugs.

More recently, new single-ingredient drugs called act-alikes have been produced to circumvent state laws that prohibit look-alikes. These act-alikes contain the same ingredients as the look-alikes, but they do not physically resemble any prescription or over-the-counter drugs. Sold on the street as speed and uppers, these drugs are expensive even though they are not as strong as amphetamines. They are typically sold to young people, who are told they are legal, safe, and harmless. This is a major reason why they are abused.

Effects of look-alikes and act-alikes. When taken in large doses, these drugs are similar to amphetamines in their effects, which include anxiety, restlessness, weakness, throbbing headache, difficult breathing, and a rapid heartbeat. Severe high blood pressure can occur and lead to cerebral hemorrhaging (stroke) and death.

Dangers of look-alikes and act-alikes. Look-alikes and act-alikes are not as strong as real amphetamines, therefore they are extremely dangerous for people who, deliberately or accidentally, take the same amount of real amphetamines as act-alikes. For example, people who buy act-alikes on the street might unknowingly buy real amphetamines and take enough to cause an overdose. Also, people who have abused amphetamines might underestimate the potency of the act-alike drugs and take excessive amounts that can result in a toxic reaction.

a. United States Pharmacopeia, *Complete Drug Reference,* 1996 ed. (Yonkers, N.Y.: Consumer Reports Books, 1995), 183.

b. Jim Parker, *Crystal, Crank, and Speedy Stuff* (Tempe, Ariz.: Do It Now, 1994), 4.

Amphetamines

Commonly referred to as "uppers," "pep pills," "bennies," "whites," "dexies," "hearts," **"speed,"** "meth," "crystal," "crank," and "ice," the **amphetamine** drugs are powerful CNS stimulants with cocainelike effects. Unlike naturally occurring cocaine, the amphetamines are synthetic, chemically manufactured substances. But like cocaine, amphetamines also affect those areas of the brain that control blood pressure, heart action, breathing, and metabolic rate, all of which are increased.

When amphetamines are used, appetite is markedly decreased and fatigue is effectively, though artificially, masked. In general, the human senses are hyperalert and the body is in a state of stress. These stimulant drugs enable the users to work harder than necessary and last longer than expected. Unlike those of cocaine, the effects of amphetamines typically last for several hours after taking the drug.

Amphetamine is a collective term for at least four closely related drugs:

1. *Amphetamine* or levoamphetamine (Benzedrine);
2. **Dextroamphetamine** (Dexedrine);

3. **Methamphetamine** (crystal, "meth" or "speed"); and
4. *Dextrometamphetamine* ("ice")

For oral use, these stimulants are manufactured as tablets or capsules that come in various decorator colors and basic white. Powdery or crystalline amphetamine can be snorted or, after being mixed with water, injected intravenously (see box 9.2). A smokable and purified form of crystal methamphetamine—known as **"ice"**—has emerged as the latest variety of amphetamine drugs.

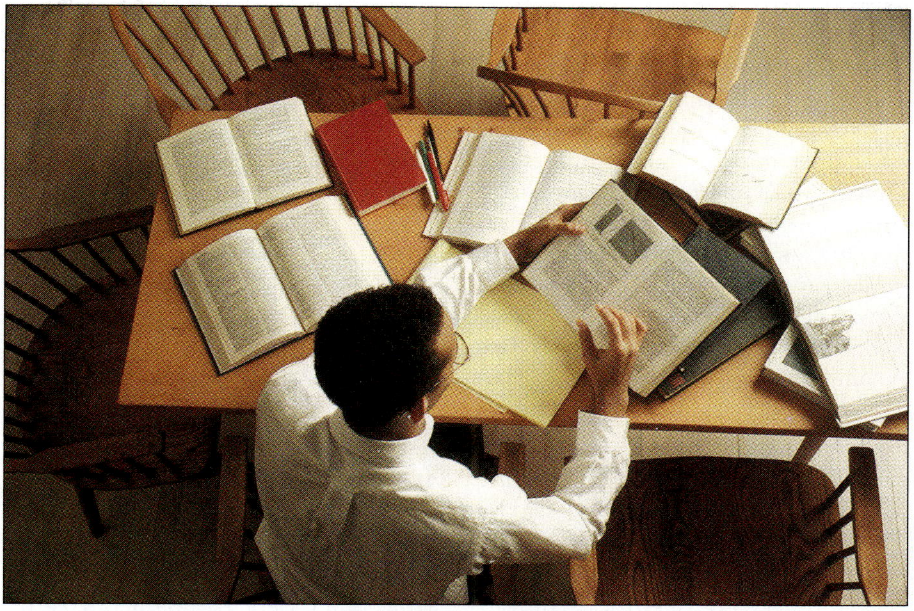

Cramming all night for an exam may be a sufficient, though hardly necessary, reason for using amphetamines.

© Llewellyn/Uniphoto Picture Agency

Effects of Amphetamines

The several amphetamine "chemical cousins" are similar in the effects they induce. In typical therapeutic doses, the amphetamines produce wakefulness and alertness, elevate mood and self-confidence, reduce feelings of fatigue, depress the appetite, enhance concentration powers, induce a mild euphoria, and increase the desire and capacity to work. There is also a noticeable increase in motor and speech activity, respiration, and blood pressure.[15]

Amphetamines tend to be a favorite of those who wish to exert themselves beyond their normal physiological limits. Workers trying to maintain alertness during the night shift, truckers attempting to drive a long distance without stopping for sleep, students cramming all night for an examination, and athletes—including bikers—desiring to enhance their performance often fall into this category of drug abuse. They have discovered that the length of adequate performance is prolonged, while the effects of fatigue are at least partially reversed. (Although the need for sleep can be postponed, it cannot be avoided indefinitely.)

Sporadic or infrequent use rarely leads to major health problems, although an amphetamine injection tends to produce a sudden increase in blood pressure that can cause death from stroke, high fever, or heart failure. In such a case, the entire cardiovascular system (heart and blood vessels) is stressed. Injectors also risk the consequences of using contaminated needles.

Users might also experience dryness of the mouth, sweating, headaches, blurred vision, dizziness, sleeplessness, and anxiety. Higher doses intensify these effects, while long-term heavy use can lead to mood swings, mental confusion, delusions, hallucinations, skin disorders, ulcers, and various diseases that come from vitamin deficiencies. Lack of sleep, weight loss, and depression can also result from persistent use.

When "crystal meth" or "ice" is smoked, users often claim that the drug's euphoric effects are similar to those of cocaine, but without the distortion of mental states. Ice is absorbed through the lungs, so the effects are felt intensely and rapidly—a flash of euphoria followed by an extended period of energized alertness. These effects are identical to those produced by injecting speed, but are delivered without the hazards of using needles.[16] As the high fades, some ice-smokers seek to reexperience the euphoria by increasing their intake. This might involve repeated smoking for days or weeks with only a minimum of food and sleep—not unlike a "run" or binging period of persistent heavy use of speed by meth injectors. In both instances, tolerance tends to build rapidly as huge dosages are consumed.

Whether as extensions of therapeutic action or as a result of overdose, toxic effects can also include involuntary shaking of the body, tenseness, hyperactive reflexes, and assaultiveness. Panic states are common, and suicidal or homicidal tendencies sometimes develop, especially in mentally ill patients. Heavy, frequent doses can even produce brain damage that can result in speech disturbances and difficulty in turning thoughts into words.

Perhaps the most dramatic consequence of amphetamine abuse is the experience of stimulant-induced toxic psychosis. This bizarre phenomenon is characterized by feelings of persecution, delusions, and hallucinations, similar to the cocaine-induced paranoid schizophrenia-like state. During such an episode, the amphetamine abuser is capable of thinking clearly and can recall relevant and extraneous facts. However, such an individual is often preoccupied with *formication*—the perceived sensation of having "crank bugs" crawling under one's skin. Compulsively, the abuser begins picking at his or her skin and, in doing so, creates multiple ulcerations. People sustaining *amphetamine psychosis* frequently exhibit other forms of equally strange and even violent behavior.[17]

Amphetamine Dependence

There is a great similarity in the patterns and symptoms of amphetamine and cocaine dependency. Taking large amounts of amphetamine on a continuing basis typically leads to drug dependence or addiction. Tolerance to the euphoric and appetite-suppressant effects of amphetamines usually develops rapidly after repeated oral, smoked, and injected doses, necessitating increased dosage levels to obtain the desired effects.

When the regular use of amphetamines is stopped suddenly, the individual commonly experiences severe mental depression, fatigue, irritability, long periods of sleep, and extreme hunger. These withdrawal symptoms are considered as evidence of physical dependency by medical authorities. There is no doubt, moreover, that amphetamines are capable of producing a psychological dependence even at low-dose levels.

Amphetamine abusers, though they may stop for a while, usually revert to continued abuse because amphetamine-induced power, self-confidence, and artificial exhilaration are so pleasant, and because of the fear of experiencing the depression and fatigue of "crashing."

Historical and Legal Aspects

Amphetamines were first synthesized in Germany in 1887. However, it was not until 1927 that physicians discovered the drugs' ability to stimulate the central nervous system, alleviate fatigue, and relieve congested nasal passages. Then in 1935 the first clinical use of the stimulant was in the treatment of **narcolepsy,** a condition of uncontrolled sleeping. In 1937, amphetamines were found to have a paradoxical calming effect on children with hyperkinetic disorders (extreme activity and impulsivity).

During World War II, the military services of both the Axis and the Allies used amphetamines to combat soldiers' fatigue, elevate mood, and prolong endurance.[18] In combat situations, amphetamines proved superior to cocaine because they could be taken by mouth rather than by sniffing, and their effect lasted for several hours, not just several minutes.

After World War II, methamphetamine or methedrine was introduced, and nonprescription Dexedrine inhalers for nasal decongestion became almost a fad among the American population. Eventually, the inhalers were removed from the market, but the nonmedical use of amphetamines spread like wildfire.

The modern day "speedball"—an injectable combination of amphetamine and heroin—was originated by military servicemen stationed in the Far East in the early 1950s. (The meaning of the term *speedball* has been expanded to include the combination of any CNS stimulant and depressant.)

For the next twenty years, amphetamines were prescribed widely for the control of depression and as an aid in dieting. They were also used in treating epilepsy, asthma, sedative overdose, and nausea in association with pregnancy.

In 1970, the Controlled Substances Act placed amphetamines under Schedule II and thus restricted severely the manufacture and distribution of these CNS stimulants. Within a short time, legitimate production of these drugs fell by an estimated 80 percent. Many amphetamine tablets and capsules were then diverted from legitimate producers and often manufactured in secret "speed" labs and sold illegally on the street market. Today, illicit amphetamine is more popular than ever, especially on the West Coast and parts of the South and Midwest. The increase in domestic production and distribution of this drug has resulted in greater purity, lower purchasing price, and increased availability. Law enforcement officials call it the "fastest growing drug threat in America."[19]

The stimulant is known as "crystal" and "crank" methamphetamine. When injected, *crystal* (the most powerful of the different forms of speed) produces an intense wave of physical and psychic exhilaration—the "rush" or "flash" reaction. The rush associated with crystal is a potent reinforcer that induces people to continue using the drug, despite serious physical and psychological damage that can result from long-term abuse.

Crank is a common nickname for another form of methamphetamine, usually of the pill variety. However, crank can also refer to pharmaceutical amphetamine and various bootleg amphetamines.

In 1988, another version of speed surfaced in Hawaii as smokable methamphetamine, or "ice." Originally smuggled into the United States from South Korea, Hong Kong, and the Philippines, ice is made cheaply and easily in the same secret labs that produce illegal crystal and crank.

Although ice provides a rapid feeling of intense pleasure that lasts for several hours, in comparison with crack cocaine's fifteen-minute high, this smokable methamphetamine is also responsible for a deep, post-use depression, with symptoms of severe paranoia, hallucinations, and delusions. These unfavorable experiences might prevent the expected epidemic of ice use and contribute to a decline of the drug's initial popularity.

Medical Uses of Amphetamines

The use of prescribed amphetamines for the control of obesity has been one of the more popular applications of these CNS stimulants. In the medical world, amphetamines and amphetamine-like drugs that tend to curb the appetite are referred to as **anorectics.**

In an extensive review of anorectics, the U.S. Food and Drug Administration concluded that patients receiving such drugs will lose more weight than those who are not treated with them. But patients who take these drugs and also diet will lose only a fraction of a pound more each week than those who rely only on dietary restriction. Thus anorectics were found to have only a limited usefulness in treating obesity. Moreover, the rate of weight loss was found to be greater during the early stages of taking diet pills, and combinations of anorectics with barbiturates and tranquilizers were no better than anorectic drugs alone.

While the usefulness of amphetamines in treating obesity was being challenged, it also became apparent that the nonmedical use of prescribed anorectics was skyrocketing. Patients soon discovered the "pep-pill" effect of the amphetamines and increased their use as tolerance and dependence developed. Some people also experienced bizarre and even psychotic behavior as amphetamine anorectics were abused with alarming frequency.

For these reasons, the Food and Drug Administration began urging physicians in the late 1960s to exercise extreme caution in prescribing anorectics, and the FDA was instrumental in decreasing the legitimate production of these stimulants. Obesity contributes significantly to mortality, so the selective and discriminating use of anorectics has been considered as preferable to a ban on such drugs. Nevertheless, many physicians usually reject these medications for treating obesity, because they tend to increase the risk for addiction, sometimes accompanied by paranoid delusions. Concurrently, there was also a noticeable decline in the prescription of amphetamines for improving mood, increasing attention, and overcoming fatigue.

Several other appetite-suppressant drugs have been developed as replacements for the amphetamines. Known collectively as *amphetamine congeners* or *surrogates,* two of these (fenfluramine and phentermine) proved remarkably effective when used as part of a weight-loss program that included a diet-and-exercise regimen and a change in eating habits.[20]

Then, in 1996, the U.S. Food and Drug Administration approved the first new antiobesity drug in more than twenty years. Marketed under the name of Redux, this prescription drug (dexfenfluramine) is a refined version of fenfluramine and works by stimulating the production and release of serotonin neurotransmitter in the brain. Among its various functions, serotonin creates the physical and emotional sensations of having had enough to eat and of being full.[21] However, because of several reports of valvular heart disease in association with the use of these drugs, the manufacturer voluntarily withdrew fenfluramine and dexfenfluramine from the market in September of 1997.[22]

Although somewhat controversial, amphetamines are still medically approved in the United States for treatment of two types of disorders:

1. **Narcolepsy** is a neurological disorder characterized by recurrent episodes or attacks of sleep. These episodes are usually induced by emotional excitement. Large doses of amphetamines prevent such attacks and help patients maintain wakefulness.
2. **Attention deficit-hyperactivity** (hyperkinetic) **disorders** in children are distinguished by extreme hyperactivity or motor restlessness, poor attention span, and impulsive and sometimes disorderly behavior. Dextroamphetamine and another related CNS stimulant, methylphenidate (Ritalin), are effective in managing this disorder.

Aggressive and impulsive behaviors are reduced; the child begins to engage in greater goal-directed behavior and improves attention span. Why these CNS stimulants produce such calming and sedating effects in children is not fully known. Equally mysterious is that amphetamines and methylphenidate do not induce euphoria or overstimulation in hyperkinetic children.

Box 9.3 Antidepressants

Three major types of **antidepressant** drugs—the **MAO inhibitors,** the **tricyclic compounds,** and **fluoxetine (Prozac)**—are used to elevate mood and relieve certain types of mental depression. The CNS stimulating action is related to the drugs' enhancement of various neurotransmitter substances in the brain.

The monoamine oxidase (MAO) inhibitors block a specific brain enzyme that usually breaks down excitatory neurotransmitters, thereby raising norepinephrine levels within the brain. By contrast, tricyclics prevent the reuptake by brain cells of excitatory neurotransmitters and thus prolong their stimulatory effect on the brain.

The antidepressant, Prozac, blocks the reabsorption of serotonin and keeps this excitatory neurotransmitter in circulation where it can continue to stimulate brain cells. Increased levels of serotonin improve mood and ease emotional depression. Despite continuing allegations that Prozac also causes violence and suicide, this medication is one of the top ten prescribed drugs in the United States, surpassing the tricyclics with their unwanted side effects of sleepiness, blurred vision, constipation, dizziness, dry mouth, and weight gain.

MAO inhibitors, including tranylcypromine (Parnate) and phenelzine (Nardil); the tricyclics, such as imipramine (Tofranil) and amitriptyline (Elavil); and fluoxetine (Prozac) are potent drugs and should be used only under close medical supervision.

The precaution about supervised and informed use also applies to the MAO inhibitors. Several years ago, patients who were on prescribed MAO inhibitors for the relief of depression often sustained high-blood-pressure crises that sometimes resulted in death. Research indicated that the afflicted people had a common preference for aged cheese. The MAO inhibitors had reacted with a substance called tyramine, common in aged cheese, and forced the blood pressure to dangerous levels, resulting in severe headaches; brain hemorrhage; and, in extreme cases, death.

To prevent similar medical emergencies, people taking prescribed MAO inhibitors should avoid foods rich in substances that could cause the release of norepinephrine. Such foods include aged and fermented foods, for example: pickled herring, fermented sausages (salami and pepperoni), sharp or aged cheeses, yogurt and sour cream, beef and chicken livers, broad beans (fava beans), canned figs, bananas, avocados, soy sauce, active yeast preparations, beer, Chianti wine, sherry, and other wines in large quantities. Also suspected of reacting adversely with MAO inhibitors are cola beverages, coffee, chocolate, and raisins.

While the MAO inhibitors can be dangerous in combination with certain foods, and while 1 to 4 percent of patients treated with any antidepressant will develop suicidal tendencies after treatment starts, none of these prescribed medicines affects behavior in healthy individuals. These drugs produce their mood-elevating effects only in depressed individuals. Therefore, they have not become abused or controlled drugs, as have other psychoactives.

Caffeine

Usually considered a nondrug because it is taken invisibly into the body under the guise of various beverages, candies, and confections, caffeine is probably the most widely used social drug in the world. A bitter tasting, odorless compound, caffeine is a natural constituent of various plants that are the sources of coffee, tea, kola nut extracts, cocoa, and chocolate. Numerous medications also contain caffeine, including certain over-the-counter analgesics and stimulants.

The most important source of caffeine in the American diet is coffee, an extract from the fruit of the *Coffea arabica* plant and related species. It is estimated that the average American coffee drinker consumes about one thousand cups of coffee each year.

Another popular source of caffeine is the cola-flavored soft drinks people consume so heavily. Children, because of their physical size, are more likely than adults to be affected by caffeine.

Many people consume a surprising and alarming amount of caffeine. Depending upon product, brand, and method of preparation, each cup of coffee has an average caffeine dose of at least 70 milligrams (mg) and as much as 215 mg. Regular cola and pepper drinks range in caffeine content from 40 mg to 54 mg per twelve-ounce serving. Nonprescription alertness tablets contain from 100 mg to 200 mg each, and some analgesics deliver 32 to 65 mg per tablet.

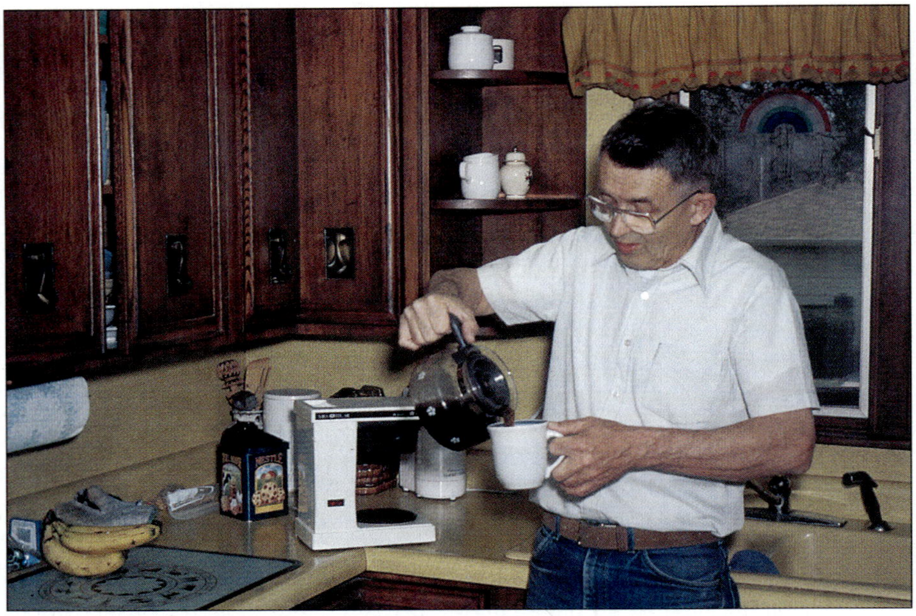

Many people drink coffee to "jump-start" their morning activities and to keep going throughout the day. Caffeine may be one of the most frequently used drugs in the world. No study has related any significant health problems to drinking three cups of coffee or fewer per day.

© James L. Shaffer

Historical Aspects

The precise origin of caffeine use cannot be determined because of the drug's natural occurrence throughout the world. Nevertheless, it is assumed that in one form or another, caffeine has been consumed for thousands of years. It is probable that *coffee* was brought to Europe from Arabia and Turkey; *tea* was introduced into the Western world from China; the *kola nut* was used commonly in West Africa and later became an ingredient in cola drinks; the *cacao tree,* from which chocolate is derived, was found in Mexico and much of Central and South America; the *ilex plant,* source of maté, or Paraguayan tea, is native to Brazil; and *cassina,* the Christmas berry tree, was often used as the source of a caffeine beverage among Indians in colonial America.[23]

Opposition to caffeine beverages began early in history. Coffee was condemned as an intoxicant in certain cultures. Coffee sales were prohibited in Egypt when the beverage was first introduced in the sixteenth century. In Europe, attempts were made to outlaw the drink, while physicians attacked coffee as harmful. Despite these warnings and prohibitions, coffee eventually became an integral part of European and American culture. Today, coffee is a domesticated drug willingly consumed in vast quantities. However, as America becomes more health conscious, more people are drinking decaffeinated coffee. Caffeine in coffee is removed through a process using the chemical methylene chloride. Decaffeinated coffee contains about 4 milligrams of caffeine compared to about 100 milligrams in a cup of brewed coffee. Few people realize that coffee or caffeine is a drug; fewer yet consider caffeine as a potentially dangerous drug. As a poison, it is relatively safe, only because it is used typically in a dilute form.

Effects of Caffeine

Caffeine is a "mild" CNS stimulant whose desirable effects are similar to those of the amphetamines and cocaine. The major pharmacological actions, due to caffeine-induced higher rates of cellular activity and increased synthesis of norepinephrine, are demonstrated primarily in the central nervous system, the kidney, and the cardiovascular system. Depending upon the individual user and the amount taken, effects typically include an immediate increase in body temperature, blood pressure, and body chemistry.

As a stimulant of the CNS, caffeine induces clearer thought, less drowsiness, shortened reaction time, improved intellectual effort, and increased motor activity, respiratory rate, and reflex excitability.

In the cardiovascular system, caffeine increases the rate and force of the heart's contraction, and it produces a general vasodilation of systemic blood vessels, including the coronary arteries, resulting in an increased blood flow. This vasodilation is short-lived and is accompanied by a vasoconstriction (narrowing) of the blood vessels in the brain. Such vasoconstrictive action in the cerebral blood vessels provides some relief from hypertensive and certain types of migraine headaches.

In addition, caffeine speeds up the production of urine, increases the capacity for muscular work, and augments the volume and acidity of gastric secretions (pepsin and acid).

Caffeinism

The popularity of coffee and other products containing caffeine is related to their stimulating actions accompanied by a lessening of drowsiness, a reduction in fatigue, and a more rapid and clearer flow of thought.[24] The amount of such stimulation takes several forms and varies considerably from person to person. Some individuals are able to "sleep like a log" after drinking several cups of coffee, while others may experience a toxic response with a single cup.

Overindulgence in caffeine can lead to a stimulated condition of chronic "caffeine intoxication" or poisoning known as **caffeinism.** Common but often unrecognized, caffeinism is characterized by mood changes, anxiety, disruption of sleep, various bodily complaints, and sometimes the manifestation of other medical and psychological problems. Caffeinism often develops in individuals who consume four or more cups of coffee each day.

Frequent symptoms of this toxic condition include restlessness, nervousness, excitement, insomnia, flushed face, diuresis (increased urine production), gastrointestinal disturbance, muscle twitching, rambling flow of thought and speech, periods of inexhaustibility, excessively rapid heart beat, and psychomotor agitation.[25]

Fatal doses of caffeine are rare but have occurred in adults when doses of the stimulant have exceeded 5 to 10 grams—the equivalent of drinking fifty to a hundred cups of coffee in a brief time!

Caffeine Dependence and Tolerance

The consumption of caffeine in various beverages and products is a culturally reinforced and socially encouraged practice.

The drug's stimulating effects—the sense of well-being, the morning "lift," the alleged increase in efficiency—are the significant reinforcers for continuing use. Assuming that caffeine activates the brain's pleasure centers, it is not surprising that it is so difficult to "kick the caffeine habit."

There is no doubt that caffeine use can lead to psychological dependence, though until recently the existence of pharmacological tolerance has been disputed. Studies indicate that in some people who report trouble staying away from caffeine, a definite chemical syndrome of caffeine dependence can be detected.[26]

Criteria for such a diagnosis include continued use despite knowledge of a persistent physical or psychological problem that is likely caused or made worse by caffeine use, persistent desire or unsuccessful efforts to cut down or control use, a tolerance marked by increasing doses of this drug-beverage, and withdrawal. Common withdrawal symptoms include headache, irritability, lethargy, apathy, difficulty in concentration, decreased work efficiency, nervousness, restlessness, and mild nausea—all usually mild in intensity and tolerable until they subside.

Unfortunately, caffeine withdrawal headaches often lead to unnecessary use of pain relievers, some of which contain caffeine along with an analgesic. The treatment unwittingly contributes to the desire for more caffeine.

Caffeine, Pregnancy, and Birth Defects

Research indicates that heavy coffee use—defined as more than three cups per day—tends to inhibit the process of conception. Such high levels of consumption often delay getting pregnant by at least a year.

Like many other psychoactive substances, caffeine is known to cross the placenta. Caffeine has also been detected in the milk of mothers who breast-feed their infants. Nursing mothers who drink large amounts of coffee on a daily basis report that their babies are often sleepless and irritable. In addition, the CNS stimulant has been proven capable of inducing chromosomal abnormalities in plant and animal cells. Such findings have given rise to concern about caffeine's ability to endanger the human fetus and cause various birth defects.

Scientists investigating women who engaged in heavy caffeine consumption beyond the sixth week of pregnancy found an increased risk for both retarded fetal growth and low birth weight of newborns.[27] This study concluded that women should reduce their caffeine intake to less than 300 mg daily early in pregnancy.

Additional research reveals that caffeine intake before and during pregnancy is also associated with an increased risk of fetal loss (spontaneous abortion or miscarriage).[28] Consequently, most medical authorities advise women to be cautious about using any drug, including caffeine and caffeine beverages, during pregnancy.

Until further studies determine what precise role caffeine plays in causing birth defects and fetal loss, the U.S. Food and Drug Administration believes that pregnant women should also be alert to products other than coffee and tea that have caffeine in them, and avoid them entirely or use them only sparingly under medical supervision.

Caffeine and Diseases

In addition to the possible relationship between caffeine use during pregnancy, and birth defects, some scientists have expressed concern about the effects of the CNS stimulant on the occurrence of specific diseases, particularly cancer and heart disease. However, research indicating that coffee or caffeine has an adverse effect on health status is somewhat controversial and still hotly debated.

Usually, studies indicate that a person who drinks only a few cups each day will probably not develop any serious health risks.[29] No study has related any significant health problem to drinking three cups of coffee or fewer per day.

While it is recognized that coffee can cause irregularities in heartbeat, especially in people with preexisting heart conditions, most studies have failed to demonstrate that small amounts of coffee contribute to heart disease in healthy

table 9.1 Common Sources of Caffeine

Beverages and Foods	Milligrams Caffeine Average	Milligrams Caffeine Range
Coffee (6-oz. cup)		
Brewed, drip method	100	70–215
Brewed, percolator	80	40–170
Instant	70	35–160
Decaffeinated, brewed	4	2–8
Decaffeinated, instant	4	2–8
Tea (5-oz. cup)		
Brewed, major U.S. brands	50	25–110
Brewed, imported brands	60	25–110
Instant	30	25–50
Iced (12-oz. glass)	70	67–76
Cocoa beverage (5-oz. cup)	5	2–25
Chocolate milk beverage (8 oz.)	5	2–7
Milk chocolate (1 oz.)	6	1–15
Dark chocolate, semisweet (1 oz.)	20	5–35
Baker's chocolate (1 oz.)	26	26
Chocolate-flavored syrup (1 oz.)	4	4
Soft Drinks		
Regular		
Cola, pepper		40–54
Decaffeinated cola, pepper		0–0.09
Cherry cola		18–23
Lemon-lime (clear)		0
Orange		0
Other citrus		0–32
Root beer		0
Ginger ale		0
Tonic water		0
Other regular		0–22
Juice added		less than 0.24
Diet drinks		
Diet cola, pepper		0.3
Decaffeinated diet cola, pepper		0–0.1
Diet cherry cola		0–23
Diet lemon-lime		0
Diet root beer		0
Other diets		0–35
Club soda, seltzer, sparkling water		0
Diet juice added		less than 0.24

Selected Medications	Per Tablet or Capsule
Prescription medicines	
Cafergot (migraine headache)	100
Norgesic Forte (muscle relaxant)	60
Norgesic (muscle relaxant)	30
Fiorinal (tension headache)	40
Fioricet (headache pain relief)	40
Darvon compound (pain relief)	32.4
Synalgos-DC (pain relief)	30
Synalgos-DC-A (pain relief)	30
Nonprescription medicines	
Alertness tablets	
NoDoz	100
Vivarin	200
Pain relief	
Anacin, Maximum Strength Anacin	32
Vanquish	33
Excedrin	65
Midol	32.4

Note: The makers of nonprescription appetite suppressants and cold/allergy capsules have removed caffeine from their products.

Source: U.S. Food and Drug Administration.

individuals. It is likely, however, that cigarette smoking and consumption of saturated fats contribute more to the development of cancer and heart disease than does caffeine.

Reducing Caffeine Intake

Persons concerned about caffeine dependence and other potential health hazards can reduce or eliminate this drug from their diets. Here are several suggestions:

1. Before switching from coffee to another beverage, be aware that caffeine is present in many other drinks, including tea, cocoa, and many carbonated soft drinks.
2. While tolerance to caffeine apparently varies from one person to another, remember that the elderly usually have a decreased tolerance to drinks containing caffeine.
3. Aside from the nicotine in tobacco products, caffeine is the major nonprescription stimulant available in the United States. An ingredient in nearly a thousand prescription drugs, caffeine is also added to numerous over-the-counter medicines, including aspirin and other analgesics.
4. Switch your coffee use from beverages prepared by the drip and percolator methods to those that are prepared with instant and freeze-dried products (which contain less caffeine). Some brands of coffee—and tea—are decaffeinated and are 97 percent caffeine-free.
5. The amount of caffeine in "regular" coffee depends on how long the coffee is brewed (the longer it is brewed, the more caffeine) and how finely the beans are ground (the finer the grind, the greater the amount of caffeine). To cut back on caffeine, reduce the number of cups of coffee consumed daily, grind your coffee less finely, and do not brew your coffee for a long period.
6. Switch to soft drinks that are caffeine-free, including most root beers and caffeine-free versions of the popular cola drinks.
7. Become familiar with the caffeine content of various beverages and over-the-counter medicines as listed in table 9.1 Then, restrict yourself to

less than 300 mg of caffeine per day. By limiting your caffeine intake, you can still enjoy that first cup of coffee in the morning.

Methcathinone

One drug of abuse in the United States, **methcathinone** has been gaining in popularity in parts of the Midwest and the Northwest. This homemade drug, known as "cat," is a powerful stimulant that resembles cocaine (in appearance and potency) and amphetamine.

Methcathinone was originally investigated years ago by the drug manufacturing industry for possible use as a diet pill. Methcathinone was dropped as a possible medication because of its destructive side effects—addictiveness, paranoia, and intense anxiety.[30] Chemically, this drug is derived from and similar to cathinone, a natural amphetamine-like substance found in the leaves of the East African **khat** or kat shrub, *Catha edulis*.[31] For many centuries, dried khat leaves have been chewed by native populations in the Middle East, Ethiopia, and Somalia as a stimulant and a social facilitator.[32]

Effects of Methcathinone

Typically snorted like cocaine, cat can also be smoked, liquefied and then injected by needle, or consumed orally in mixture with a beverage. The attraction of this drug is the burst of energy it produces, along with a lasting feeling of extreme well-being or euphoria.[33] Such a high is often described as being greater than the high achieved through cocaine; it is so intense that users must sometimes combine cat with large doses of alcohol or marijuana tolerate the intensity of energized feeling.

According to the Drug Enforcement Administration, some cat users binge on this drug for several days, during which they become engulfed in paranoia (delusions of persecution), experience excruciating nervousness, and suffer hallucinations.[34] Appetite decreases significantly or disappears entirely during such a binge, and this often leads to long-term weight loss. Dehydration can occur, along with severe pounding of the heart, headaches, stomachaches, and even the "shakes." When the binge is over, usually because the supply of methcathinone has been exhausted, a deep depression overwhelms the user, who becomes irritable and argumentative. This crash is often followed by a lengthy period of sleep, which does not always restore a sense of normal well-being.

Manufacture and Control of Cat

One of the more alarming concerns regarding homemade methcathinone is the easy availability and low cost of its chemical ingredients. The key component is ephedrine, a legal, over-the-counter asthma medication. Other easy-to-obtain components include drain cleaner; battery acid; paint thinner; Epsom salts; lye; and muriatic acid, sometimes used by construction workers to scrub dried mortar off the face of bricks. When mixed these ingredients can produce fatally poisonous phosgene gas during the production process in secret backroom or basement labs.

Methcathinone has already been banned by the federal Drug Enforcement Administration and listed as a Schedule I controlled substance; other measures emphasize also limiting the availability of ephedrine.[35] Without ephedrine, there can be no cat. Persons who manufacture methcathinone or help others in doing so may be prosecuted under various federal statutes. Manufacturing or possession with intent to distribute is a violation of the U.S. Code and is punishable by a prison term of up to twenty years and a fine of up to $1 million.

Ephedrine

A natural extract of the *Ephedra sinica* shrub, **ephedrine** is another close relative of the amphetamines. The leaves of the ephedra shrub have been used in stimulant teas and in centuries-old Chinese herbal medicines, such as Ma Huang. It helps to open or dilate bronchial tubes in the human respiratory system, therefore ephedrine was originally used to treat asthma. The FDA has also approved its use as a decongestant. Some studies indicate that ephedrine in combination with caffeine can help overweight people lose unwanted pounds.

However, ephedrine is advertised widely as a "thermogenic aid" that temporarily boosts the human body's metabolic rate.[36] Sold over the counter in health-food stores and at truck stops, ephedrine pills and capsules appear under the names of Diet Max, Diet Pep, Herb Trim, Escalation, and Mega Trim. Ephedrine is also an active ingredient in illicit drugs alleged to be amphetamines.[37]

Ephedrine has been heavily promoted as *Herbal Ecstacy* and lesser known products, such as Cloud 9, Ultimate Xphoria, and Rave Energy. Considered as dietary supplements, and therefore not regulated by the Food and Drug Administration, these ephedrine-based concoctions are often marketed as safe, legal, natural, or organic alternatives to MDMA. Known better by its street name of *Ecstasy*, MDMA is an illegal drug of abuse with characteristics of methamphetamine and the psychedelic mescaline.

Unsupervised use of this central nervous system stimulant as a pep pill or a diet pill has been linked with fatal strokes, because ephedrine increases heart rate and blood pressure and tends to constrict blood vessels. These drug actions create the conditions for a cerebrovascular accident (stroke) and a heart attack. Minor side effects include restlessness and insomnia, while serious adverse consequences include nerve damage, rapid and irregular heartbeats, psychotic episodes, and loss of memory.

Although some states have attempted to restrict ephedrine, the FDA has not yet taken action to control the abuse of this common stimulant. This substance is banned for Olympic competition and international soccer because of its frequent use as an ergogenic aid to enhance athletic ability.

At least four hundred reported adverse reactions involving liver failure, elevated blood pressure, strokes, and heart attacks, plus fifteen deaths, have already been recorded. The addition of caffeine to some of the ephedra-based products further increases the potential for harmful effects.[38] Despite these possible, undesirable side effects, Herbal Ecstacy has become wildly popular at rave concerts. At these social happenings, young people often use this druglike "dietary supplement" for euphoric stimulation, mood elevation, and enhanced sexual sensations without a hangover.

Other Plant Stimulants

Other stimulant drugs occasionally consumed in the United States are derived from numerous plants and have been used for centuries by millions of people either for recreation or medicine or both. Two of these plant derivatives are betel nuts and yohimbe.

Betel nuts are widely used in Asian countries and in the island nations of the Indian and Pacific Oceans. They are typically consumed as betel morsels—nuts from the areca palm tree, gum from the acacia tree, and burnt lime, all wrapped in a betel leaf. This small morsel is placed in the cheek or under the tongue and sucked for two or more hours.

A mild stimulation of the central nervous system is the primary drug effect, although a pleasant feeling and reduction of fatigue are often reported. Some people also chew betel nuts for their alleged aphrodisiac effect. Undesirable consequences of using the morsels include a dark red staining of the teeth, mouth, and gums; a toxic condition in the body; and increased risk of cancer of the mouth and esophagus.[39]

Yohimbe, an extract from the tropical yohimbe tree found in West Africa, is used to brew a mildly stimulating tea often used for its aphrodisiac effect. A preparation of ground yohimbe bark can also be used as snuff for quicker results. A feeling of nausea is often the first effect; this is soon followed by a pleasant, euphoric state not unlike the initial stage of an LSD-induced hallucination.

Penile erection is frequently reported because the drug also affects the user's peripheral blood flow. Both males and females claim enhancement of their sexual experiences. Similar to hallucinogenic drugs, yohimbe is used primarily for its stimulating effect. At present, yohimbe is available in the United States in various natural food and herbal stores.

Chapter Summary

1. CNS stimulants, such as cocaine and the amphetamines, usually increase mental alertness, physical activity, and excitement. They are known as "ups" or "uppers."
2. Cocaine and amphetamines—the more powerful stimulants—produce euphoria; decreased perception of fatigue; decreased need for sleep; a decreased appetite, and make users feel stronger, more decisive, and self-possessed.
3. Dependence on CNS stimulants is based upon the desire to repeatedly experience the intense pleasurable feelings of the "flash" or "rush" following injection, tolerance to the euphoric and appetite-suppressant effects of the drugs, and avoidance of mental depression (crashing) after drug use stops.
4. Cocaine is the most powerful CNS stimulant of natural origin and for years enjoyed an unjustified reputation as a user-friendly drug.
5. Derived from coca plant leaves, cocaine has only limited medical uses.
6. Cocaine is snorted or sniffed, injected intravenously, smoked, freebased, and combined with CNS depressants ("speedballing"). The more serious health risks—toxic syndrome, drug dependency, lung damage, cocaine psychosis, formication, blood clots, infection, and burns—tend to be associated particularly with cocaine injection, freebasing, speedballing, and smoking crack. Crack, an intensified form of cocaine, is considered one of the most addictive of drug substances.
7. Using cocaine can result in death by sudden stimulation of the CNS, interference with normal heartbeat, and changes in heart action and blood pressure that can lead to heart attack and/or stroke.
8. Amphetamines (Benzedrine, Dexedrine, "meth" or "speed," and smokable "ice") are powerful, synthetic CNS stimulants with cocainelike effects. Although some of these stimulants have legitimate medical uses, amphetamines are often abused by those who want to extend themselves beyond their normal physiological limits.
9. Prolonged use of amphetamines sometimes leads to toxic conditions, mental confusion, assaultive behavior, amphetamine psychosis, and formication. Psychological dependence develops at low-dose levels; tolerance to the euphoric and appetite-suppressant effects builds rapidly with repeated oral, injected, and smoked dosages; and serious withdrawal symptoms of mental depression and fatigue are evidence of a physical dependence.
10. Amphetamines are used medically as anorectics and in treating narcolepsy and hyperkinetic disorders.
11. MAO inhibitors, tricyclics, and Prozac are antidepressant medications used to elevate mood and relieve mental depression. They are effective only with depressed people.
12. Caffeine is a widely used CNS stimulant present in coffee, tea, chocolate, and many nonprescribed medications.
13. The stimulating effects of caffeine are often perceived as beneficial, but some people experience unpleasant effects such as a toxic response, caffeinism with overindulgence, and caffeine dependence.
14. Two drugs of abuse that have surfaced in the United States are methcathinone (cat) and ephedrine; both have a stimulant effect.

World Wide Web Sites

Caffeine Archives

www.caffeinearchive.com

Cocaine Anonymous World Services

www.ca.org

Fact Sheet on Amphetamines

www.arf.org/isd/pim/amph.html

Review Questions and Activities

1. What are the general drug actions or effects of the behavioral stimulants?
2. Why does intravenous injection of a CNS stimulant usually involve a greater potential health risk than taking the same drugs by mouth?
3. How does a CNS stimulant "flash" or "rush" differ from a CNS stimulant "crash"?
4. Explain why cocaine has often been perceived as a "safe" drug, despite its considerable potential for threatening health and life.
5. Read Bob Woodward's *Wired: The Short Life and Fast Times of John Belushi* (New York: Simon & Schuster, 1984) and identify several factors you think contributed to Belushi's involvement with and death due to cocaine and other drugs.
6. What is the significance of the 800—COCAINE hotline? Contact local substance-abuse programs or clinics for information on this national service.
7. Explain the meanings of the following terms associated with cocaine use: *snorting, intravenous injection, speedballing, freebasing,* and *crack-smoking.*
8. Why is crack cocaine considered to be such a serious threat to the health of users?
9. Compare cocaine dependence with opioid dependence to reveal similarities and differences.
10. Why do you think people try amphetamines and continue to use these cocaine-like CNS stimulants?
11. How is "ice" similar to and different from "crack"?
12. What are the approved medical uses of amphetamine drugs?
13. Explain why antidepressants are not among the commonly abused drugs.
14. Identify ten common sources of caffeine that might be found in many American households.
15. In what ways does caffeine act as a CNS stimulant in the human body?
16. Survey several coffee drinkers. Determine if any of them have ever experienced caffeinism.
17. Do you think there is such a condition as caffeine dependence? What evidence have you observed or experienced that would support your answer?
18. Under the brand names Zoom and Zing, tablets of guarana powder derived from seeds of a jungle shrub have begun appearing for sale in some health-food stores. What are the drug effects of Zoom and Zing? How are these products advertised?

References

1. Basic descriptions of these stimulants are derived from the Drug Enforcement Administration, U.S. Department of Justice, *Drugs of Abuse* (Washington, D.C.: GPO, 1989), 37, 40.
2. Lester Grinspoon and James Bakalar, *The Harvard Medical School Mental Health Review: Drug Abuse and Addiction* (Boston: Harvard Mental Health Letter, 1993), 15.
3. Robert Julien, *A Primer of Drug Action.* 7th ed. (New York: W. H. Freeman and Company, 1995), 125.
4. Charles O'Brien, "Drug Addiction and Drug Abuse," chap. 24 in *Goodman & Gilman's The Pharmacological Basis of Therapeutics,* 9th ed. (New York: McGraw-Hill Health Professions Division, 1996), 570–71.
5. Grinspoon and Bakalar, *The Harvard School Mental Health Review,* 18.
6. U.S. Department of Justice, Drug Enforcement Administration, *The Cocaine Threat to the United States* (March 1995) 2. (Republished in "Cocaine Facts and Figures," *Drugs & Crime Data* [Office of National Drug Control Policy, Drugs and Crime Clearinghouse, 1996]).
7. William Catterall and Kenneth Mackie, "Local Anesthetics," chap. 15 in *Goodman & Gilman's The Pharmacological Basis of Therapeutics,* 9th ed. (New York: McGraw-Hill Health Professions Division, 1996), 338.
8. Elisabeth Kübler-Ross, *To Live until We Say Goodbye* (Englewood Cliffs, N.J.: Prentice-Hall, 1978), 22–23.
9. Nannette Stone, Marlene Fromme, and Daniel Kagan, *Cocaine: Seduction and Solution* (New York: Clarkson N. Potter, 1984), 6.
10. Cathy Booth, "Caribbean Blizzard," *Time* 147, no. 9 (26 February 1996): 46–48.
11. Substance Abuse and Mental Health Services Administration, *Preliminary Results from the 1997 National Household Survey on Drug Abuse* (Washington, D.C., Department of Health and Human Services and the National Clearinghouse for Alcohol and Drug Information, 1998).
12. Patrick Macdonald and others, "Heavy Cocaine Use and Sexual Behavior," *Journal of Drug Issues* 18, no. 3 (summer 1988): 437–55.
13. Tibor Palfai and Henry Jankiewicz, *Drugs and Human Behavior* (Dubuque, Iowa: Brown & Benchmark, 1991), 305.
14. Harold Doweiko, *Concepts of Chemical Dependency,* 2d ed. (Pacific Grove, Calif.: Brooks/Cole, 1993) 88–89.
15. Brian Hoffman and Robert Lefkowitz, "Catecholamines, Sympathomimetic Drugs, and Adrenergic Receptor Antagonists," chap. 10 in *Goodman & Gilman's The Pharmacological Basis of Therapeutics,* 9th ed. (New York: McGraw-Hill Health Professions Division, 1996), 219.
16. Christina Dye, *Ice: Speed, Smoke and Fire* (Tempe, Ariz.: Do It Now, 1991), 2–3.
17. Bertram Katzung, ed., *Basic and Clinical Pharmacology,* 4th ed. (Norwalk, Conn.: Appleton & Lange, 1989), 387–88.
18. Edward M. Brecher and the editors of Consumer Reports Books, "The Amphetamines," in *Licit and Illicit Drugs* (Mount Vernon, N.Y.: Consumers Union, 1972), 279.
19. Methamphetamine—A Growing Domestic Threat," *Police Chief* 63, no. 3, (, 1996): 24–28.
20. "A New Look at Diet Pills." *University of California Wellness Letter* 9, no. 1 (October 1992): 1.
21. "New Weight-Loss Drug," *FDA Consumer* 30, no. 6 (July–August 1996): 4–5; and Michael Lemonick, "The New Miracle Drug?" *Time* 148, no. 15 (23 September 1996): 61–67.

22. Prescription Medications for the Treatment of Obesity," National Institutes of Health Publication, no. 97-4191, (Washington, D.C., March 16, 1998).
23. Brecher and others, "The Amphetamines," 196.
24. William Serafin, "Drugs Used in the Treatment of Asthma," chap. 28 in *Goodman & Gilman's The Pharmacological Basis of Therapeutics,* 9th ed. (New York: McGraw-Hill, Health Professions Division, 1996), 674.
25. American Psychiatric Association, *Diagnostic and Statistical Manual of Mental Disorders,* 4th ed. (Washington, D.C.: American Psychiatric Association, 1994), 212–13.
26. Eric Strain and others, "Caffeine Dependence Syndrome," *Journal of the American Medical Association* 272, no. 13 (5 October 1994): 1043–48.
27. Laura Fenster and others, "Caffeine Consumption during Pregnancy and Fetal Growth," *American Journal of Public Health* 81, no. 4 (April 1991): 458–61.
28. Claire Infante-Rivard and others, "Fetal Loss Associated with Caffeine Intake before and during Pregnancy," *Journal of the American Medical Association* 270, no. 24 (22–29 December 1993): 2940–43.
29. "Coffee and Health," *Consumer Reports* 59, no. 10 (October 1994): 650–51.
30. "Use of Cat, Potent New Stimulant, Called Epidemic in Michigan," *Substance Abuse Report* 24, no. 23 (1 December 1993): 8.
31. Avram Goldstein, *Addiction: From Biology to Drug Policy* (New York: W. H. Freeman, 1994), 157.
32. Gesina Longenecker, *How Drugs Work: Drug Abuse and the Human Body* (Emeryville, Calif.: Ziff-Davis Press, 1994).
33. Paul Glastris, "The New Drug in Town," *U.S. News and World Report,* (26 April 1993), 20–21.
34. Drug Enforcement Administration, *You Can't Trust Cat* (Washington, D.C.: U.S. Department of Justice, Drug Enforcement Administration, 1993), 2.
35. "New Law Attempts to Stop Spread of Cat," *Prevention Pipeline* 7, no. 2 (March–April 1994): 26.
36. "The Scoop on Ephedrine and Ma Huang," *University of California at Berkeley Wellness Letter* 10, no. 12 (September 1994): 6–7.
37. Julien, *A Primer of Drug Action,* 151
38. Geoffrey Cowley, "Herbal Warning," *Newsweek* CXXVII, no. 19 (6 May 1996): 60–64, 67–68.
39. Darryl Inaba and William Cohen, *Uppers, Downers, All Arounders,* 2d ed. (Ashland, Ore.: CNS Productions, 1993).

Part Four

The Mind-Expanding Euphoriants

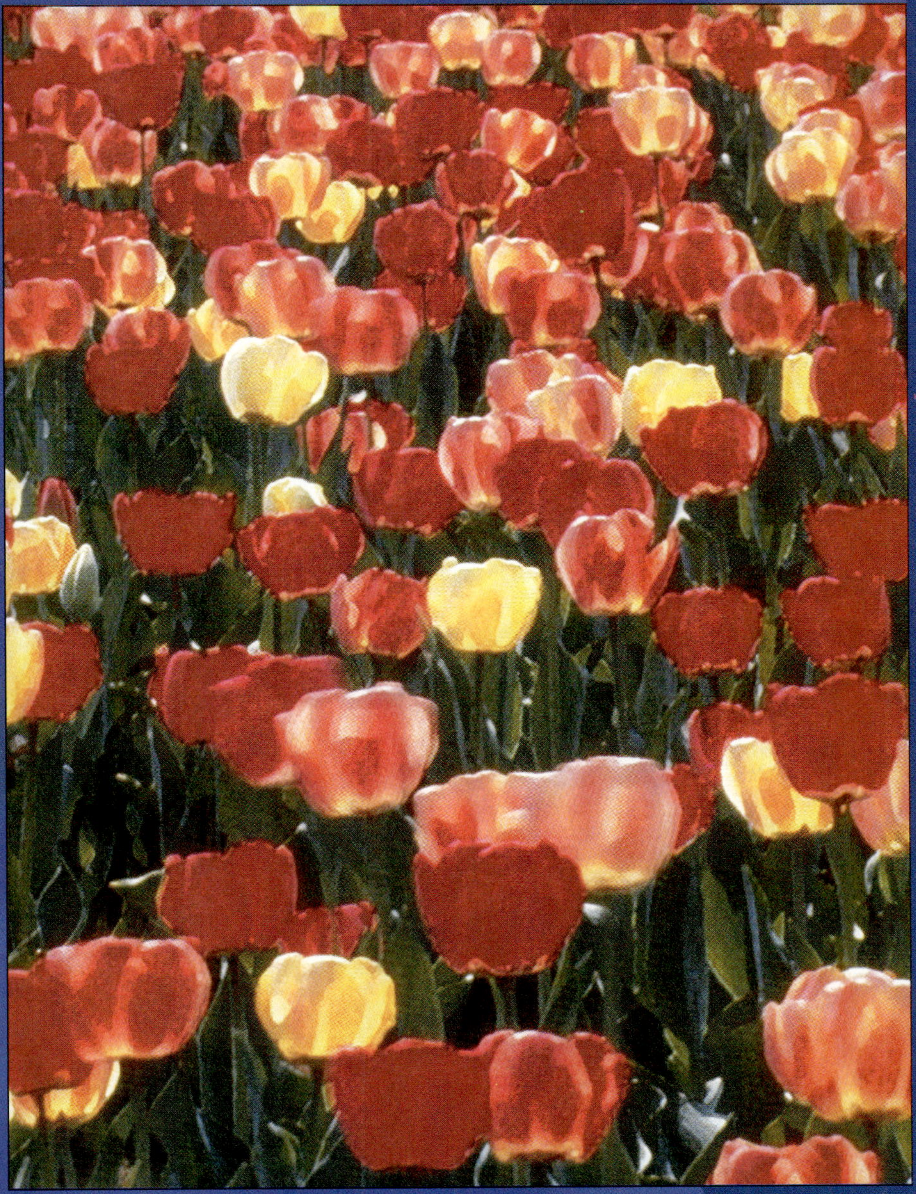

Questions of concern

1. What would likely occur in our society if marijuana were legalized and sold for general consumption at relatively low cost and under strict government controls?
2. Why are the mind-expanding effects of the psychedelics so often feared by nonusers and many potential users?
3. How does the level of social acceptability of psychedelics, particularly LSD and peyote, compare with that of other mind-altering drugs, such as alcohol, tobacco cigarettes, and even marijuana?

Chapter 10

Psychedelics and phencyclidine

KEY TERMS

Aesthetic Experience
Cognitive Experience
Designer Drug
Ecstasy
Hallucination
Hallucinogen
Illusion
Lysergic Acid Diethylamide
Mescaline
Mind Expansion
Peyote
Phencyclidine
Psilocybin
Psychodynamic Experience
Psychotic Experience
Synesthesia
Transcendental (Mystical) Experience
Trip

chapter objectives

After you have studied this chapter, you should be able to do the following:

1. Define the key terms.
2. Describe the major characteristics of the psychedelic state.
3. Distinguish among the following types of psychedelic experiences: psychotic, psychodynamic, cognitive, aesthetic, and transcendental.
4. Differentiate between the terms illusionogenic and hallucinogenic in describing the effects of psychedelics.
5. Identify several commonly experienced, physical side effects of psychedelic drugs.
6. Discuss the historical factors responsible for the beginning of the modern psychedelic era.
7. Explain the basis of the increase in the recreational use of LSD after several years of declining use.
8. Describe several mind-altering effects often experienced on an LSD "trip."
9. Identify three potential hazards associated with using LSD.
10. Compare the psychedelic effects of mescaline and psilocybin with those of LSD.
11. Name and describe the origins and effects of at least four psychedelic substances in addition to LSD, mescaline, and psilocybin.
12. Explain why the designer drug MDMA is often called Ecstasy.
13. Describe the possible range of drug effects associated with use of PCP.
14. Discuss the continuing appeal of phencyclidine despite its notorious reputation as a dissociative anesthetic.
15. Identify two so-called "club drugs" being used primarily for their psychedelic effects.
16. Relate specific health risks with the use of various herbal products.

Introduction

Both an ancient and a contemporary undertaking, the expansion of consciousness continues to be a unique and persistent human endeavor. This search for the "beyond within" has led many to rely upon psychoactive drugs for personal insight and comprehension. Substances most often used for such elusive purposes have come to be identified popularly and legally as hallucinogens—generators of hallucinations.

Distinguished more by their ability to produce states of altered perception and thought than by hallucinations, the various psychedelic drugs—as they will be called in this chapter—include both natural and synthetic compounds. Though not the original psychedelic, LSD will be considered as the prototype and most powerful of these drugs. The abuse of these drugs is the major concern of this chapter.

Another psychoactive drug, phencyclidine (PCP), will also be examined. Distinct from the psychedelics, PCP resembles the mind-expanders and the sedative-hypnotics. Yet PCP is in a class of its own, and it is possibly the most potentially dangerous of the "street" drugs.

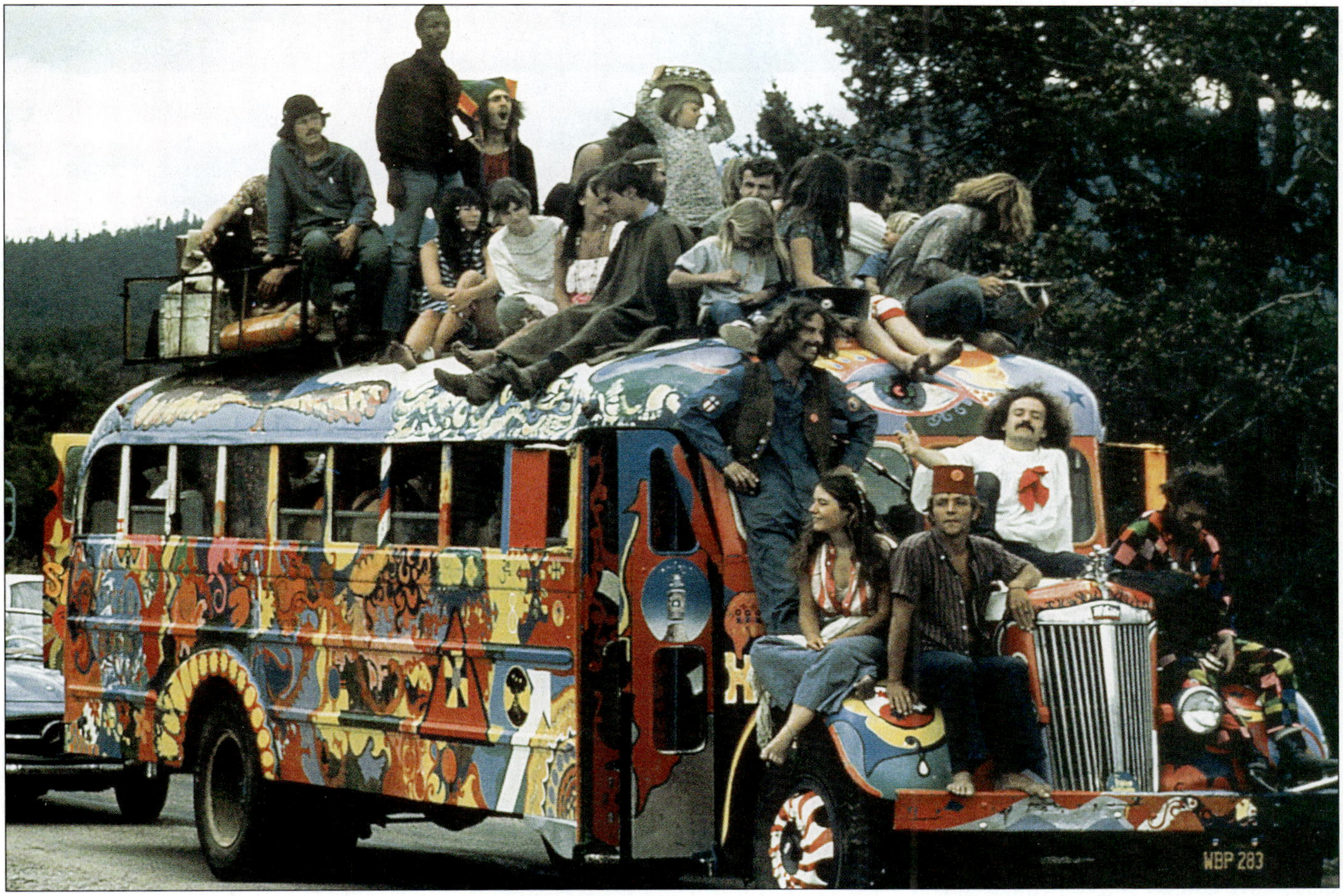

Psychedelic drugs had a significant impact on the counterculture of the 1960s as evidenced in clothing styles, hair lengths, music, language, and use of color. The school bus in the photo could be described as having a psychedelic paint job.

© Lisa Law/The Image Works

The Psychedelic State: Mind Expansion

The major focus of this chapter is the psychedelics, which cause dose-related changes in perception, thinking, emotions, arousal, and self-image.

The terms used to describe the psychedelics include **hallucinogens** (inducers of **hallucinations**), *psychotomimetics* (drugs that mimic psychosis), *psychodysleptics* (substances that are mind-disrupting), and *psycholytics* (dissolvers of the psyche, or mind-looseners).[1]

Drugs such as lysergic acid diethylamide (LSD), mescaline, and psilocybin may function in such bizarre ways. But each of these special labels, based upon a single pharmacological action, refers to only a limited part of the wide range of psychological effects of the drugs.

Major Characteristics

A more inclusive term, *psychedelic* refers to **mind expansion** or *mind manifestation*—the ability of the mind to perceive more than it can tell and to experience more than it can explain. The major characteristics of the psychedelic state are:[2]

- Heightened awareness of sensory input, experienced as a flood of sensation
- Especially vivid but unreal imagery, typical of one's childhood
- An enhanced sense of clarity
- Diminished control over what one experiences
- A persistent feeling that one part of the self is a passive observer—the spectator ego phenomenon—while another part of the self participates and receives unusual sensory experiences
- Replacement of the user's inward-focused attention by the seeming clarity and expansiveness of his or her thinking process, often accompanied by the inability to express or explain these thoughts
- Assignment of profound meaning to the slightest of sensations
- A lessened capacity to distinguish the boundaries of one object from another and of the self from the environment
- The development of a sense of union with humankind or the cosmos

As a group, psychedelics tend to distort the user's perception of objective reality, decrease logical thought, heighten sensation, and change or modify the user's state of consciousness. These drugs invariably bring about a central nervous system excitation that affects the senses—especially time sense—feelings, moods, experience, and mental processes. Stimulation of the sympathetic nervous system (described in chapter 3) also results in increased heart rate and blood pressure, sweating, loss of appetite, and sleeplessness.

In large or toxic doses, psychedelic drugs also produce hallucinations (groundless or mistaken perceptions having no real external cause) and delusions (false beliefs that cannot be corrected by reason), although these are relatively rare. More commonly produced are **illusions** (erroneous perceptions of reality) and "pseudohallucinations" (misperceptions recognized as misperceptions). As a consequence, some people prefer to describe the psychedelics as illusionogenic rather than hallucinogenic.

While mimicking some naturally occurring neurotransmitters of the brain and disrupting others, individual psychedelics have unique, and sometimes subtle, effects that are especially attractive to users. These may include speed of onset, duration of the psychedelic "high," and the particular sense that seems to be altered more than others, whether it is visual or auditory.

Commonly shared properties are also part of the psychedelic allure. One of these is **synesthesia.** In this drug-related effect there is a mingling of the senses, in which one sensation may be translated into another. For example, sounds might be seen, smells might be felt, and colors might be heard.

Box 10.1 Psychedelics, PCP, and Driving *Why Take the Risk?*

LSD, PCP, and other psychedelic or hallucinogenic drugs tend to distort judgment and reality and cause confusion and panic. They can also produce severe mental problems, resulting in strange and violent behavior. Individuals under the influence of these kinds of drugs should not drive.

Psychedelics are particularly hazardous because their effects are unpredictable. In addition, sensations and feelings are likely to change. Users may feel several different emotions at once or swing rapidly from one emotion to another. On occasion, an individual's sense of time and self changes, and the user may experience sensations that seem to "cross over," giving the perception of hearing colors and seeing sounds. These changes can be frightening, and they might cause panic.

PCP use, especially on a regular basis, can affect memory, perception, concentration, and judgment. Signs of paranoia, aggressive behavior, and a general disturbance of the user's thought processes may also appear. These distortions of normal mental functioning disqualify those who use PCP from attempting to drive an automobile.

Driving requires a combination of thought and motor skills, a great deal of common sense, and a concern for the safety of everyone on the road. Safe driving is based on observant eyes, steady hands, and a clear head. By mixing drugs with driving, you are only asking for trouble. Why take the risk?

Source: Modified from the National Institute on Drug Abuse.

Psychological Hazards

Although the changes in perception, mood, and thinking usually are interpreted as euphoric, sometimes undesirable psychological effects occur. Among these are acute anxiety and panic reactions, or *bad trips*—the most frequent adverse effect—characterized by terror, confusion, dissociation, and fear of losing control over oneself.[3] Perception of time and space often become disoriented and users lose a sense of reality, which can be mentally disturbing and physically dangerous. Such reactions last less than twenty-four hours in most instances, but occasionally they persist for days and eventually progress into a chronic, toxic psychosis. In some instances, depersonalization and depression become so severe that suicide is a distinct possibility.

Another psychological hazard is the *flashback reaction.* This response is described as the *hallucinogen persisting perception disorder* or HPPD.[4] Long after psychedelics have been eliminated from the body, one might experience partial recurrences of psychedelic effects, such as the intensification of a perceived color, the apparent motion of a fixed object, or the mistaking of one object for another.

This sometimes alarming situation can be either spontaneous or triggered by physical or psychological stress, by medicines, or by use of marijuana. While the precise cause remains obscure, flashbacks are probably psychological and might involve a "conditioned response" to a previous panic attack.

Psychological effects of the psychedelics, especially LSD, are influenced primarily by the size of the dose taken and by the personality of the user, his or her expectations, previous experience with LSD and other psychedelic drugs, attitudes toward the use of LSD or other illicit drugs, motivations for using the drug, the setting in which the drug is administered, and the persons with whom the user interacts during the LSD experience.[5]

Dosage is a primary concern in relation to the effects of any particular drug. Nearly all LSD comes from illegal domestic laboratories so the quality of the drug will likely vary. Many street samples of LSD contain impurities and adulterants, and thus the amount of the drug per dose is often a surprise and a mystery.

Types of Psychedelic Experiences

Emotional responses to psychedelics can vary from a miserable, hopeless dysphoria (anxiety, restlessness, and depression) to an ecstatic, blissful sensation of well-being and pleasure. This latter response is referred to as euphoria. The expectation of this euphoria, or high, and the likely experience of sensory changes are the most common reasons for taking psychedelic drugs.

The Range of Responses

Researchers have identified at least five major types of potential psychedelic responses, described subjectively by those using mind-expanding drugs. Included are the following types.[6]

> The **psychotic experience** is characterized by intense fear, panic, paranoid suspicion or delusions of grandeur, confusion, impairment of abstract reasoning, remorse, depression, and isolation or bodily discomfort or both. These experiences can be powerful.
>
> The **cognitive experience** is marked by astonishingly lucid thought. Various problems can be seen from a unique perspective in which inner relationships of many levels or dimensions can be viewed simultaneously.
>
> The **aesthetic experience** is defined by a change and intensification of sensory input, including sight, sound, smell, taste, and touch. Fascinating changes in sensations and perceptions can occur, such as synesthesia, apparent lifelike movements in inanimate objects, the appearance of great beauty in ordinary things, an experience of powerful music, and extremely beautiful mental images.
>
> The **psychodynamic experience** occurs when material that was previously unconscious or forgotten emerges in one's consciousness. A release of the tension or conflict from repressed emotions is sometimes reported subjectively as a reliving of incidents from the past or a symbolic portrayal of important struggles between hostile forces in the psyche.

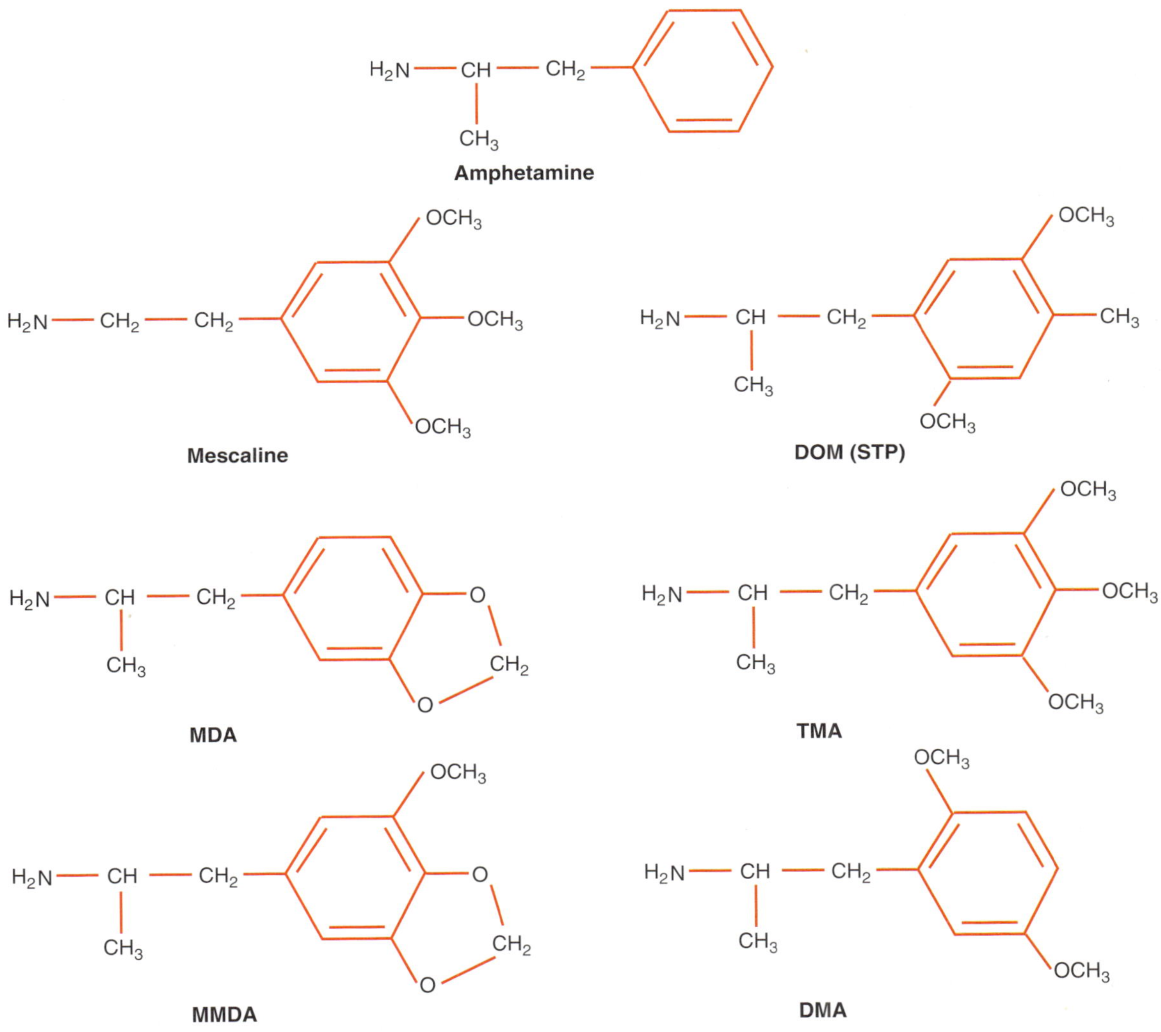

figure 10.1

Structural formulas of amphetamine and six psychedelic drugs. These drugs are related and produce similar effects. The six "catecholamine-like" psychedelics act on norepinephrine and dopamine receptors in the nervous system. There is usually a body-stimulating effect similar to the release of adrenaline. This is followed by the sensory and psychedelic effects related to changes in the amount of serotonin neurotransmitter.

The **transcendental,** or **mystical, experience** is often referred to as the "psychedelic peak" and involves the development of a sense of unity or oneness; transcendence of time and space; deeply felt moods of joy, peace, and love; a sense of awe, reverence, and wonder; meaningfulness of psychological or philosophical insight or both; and the inability to describe the experience of cosmic-type happenings in ordinary words.

A psychedelic experience rarely fits neatly into one category. Aspects of all five are likely to occur in each "trip." Nevertheless, the clear-cut types may be the result of biochemical actions that captivate the mind at any one time.

Pharmacological Effects

If the psychological effects of the psychedelics can be described as exciting, then the physical reactions are somewhat dull by comparison. The pupils of the eyes dilate, body temperature and blood pressure rise, heart rate increases, reflexes are increased above normal, and muscle weakness and tremors sometimes occur. Some "body trips," especially those induced by morning glory seeds and peyote, involve nausea, vomiting, diarrhea, and muscle tension.

Continued, everyday use of the psychedelics leads to tolerance. For instance, after only three or four daily doses, the amount of LSD required to produce desirable psychological effects is increased markedly. However, sensitivity to lower doses returns after a comparable period of abstinence. There is a considerable degree of cross-tolerance among LSD, mescaline, and psilocybin, but none between LSD and such drugs as amphetamines and THC—the active ingredient in marijuana.

When the psychedelic drugs are withdrawn from a person, there is no detectable evidence of physical dependence. Whereas repeated use may result in psychological dependence in some instances, regular, compulsive daily use is somewhat rare. There are several reasons why psychedelic drugs are not used addictively. Psychedelics develop a rapid tolerance so that a user cannot remain high day after day. Also, psychedelic trips are unpredictable, so the user cannot always depend on a pleasurable effect, psychedelic experiences cannot be controlled. Once a user is high, he or she cannot come down until the drug effect wears off. Episodic use of these substances tends to be the pattern of abuse.

Historical Aspects

Many plants containing psychedelic drugs have been known and used for their mind-altering effects since prehistoric times.

Early Use of Mushrooms

It is probable that the mushroom *Amanita muscaria,* neither deadly nor commonly eaten as food, was used medically and recreationally by people in the early Aryan culture of present-day Afghanistan. It is likely that this particular mushroom was the "Soma" described in 3,500-year-old Indian holy books.

Another variety of mushroom containing psilocybin, called "God's Flesh," was employed in the religious rituals of certain Mexican Indians. It is now presumed that the ancient Mayans of Mexico and Guatemala engaged in the worship of these mushrooms as long ago as 1000 B.C.

Religious Use of Peyote

Meanwhile, other tribes of prehistoric Mexican Indians and the Aztecs used the peyote cactus as a religious sacrament. Peyote was still widely used centuries later at the time of the Spanish conquest. Eventually, its use spread northward into America, where several Indian tribes adopted the "peyote cult" with its mystical setting and religious rituals.[7]

An estimated quarter million members of the Native American Church continue to use peyote legally as part of the church's ritual. This church has been exempted from specific provisions of the Controlled Substances Act of 1970. Nevertheless, a 1990 United States Supreme Court ruling declared that there is no constitutional right to take illicit drugs for religious reasons. Individual states are still free, however, to allow religious use of illegal substances, specifically peyote, although more than twenty states forbid any use of peyote.

Sometimes the ancient Aztecs could not obtain or preferred not to use peyote. Then they considered sacred the seeds of the morning glory plant *(Rivea corymbosa),* which contain a relatively mild psychedelic substance chemically similar to LSD. More-modern Europeans employed *Atropa belladonna,* the deadly nightshade plant, as medicine and a poison. Later, the early white settlers in the New World accidentally discovered the psychedelic effects of *Datura stramonium,* the "Jamestown weed," soon shortened to "Jimsonweed" and also known as "loco weed."

Laboratory Synthesis

It is fairly certain, then, that the use of plants with LSD-like effects was prevalent in religious and therapeutic contexts long before Dr. Albert Hofmann and Dr. W. A. Stoll first synthesized lysergic acid diethylamide (LSD) in 1938. It was not until five years later, in 1943, that Dr. Hofmann took his first "acid trip."

Working with the twenty-fifth compound in the lysergic acid series, Dr. Hofmann accidentally ingested a small amount of the untested LSD-25 substance in his Swiss laboratory. He experienced dramatic effects of restlessness, dizziness, and delirium, characterized by excited fantasies and fantastic visions of extraordinary realness, accompanied by an intense kaleidoscopic play of colors.[8] It was this single event that ushered in the modern Psychedelic Era. A few days later, Hofmann took another small dose of LSD and had his assistant record the psychedelic experience. This description was the first account of the effects of LSD.

At first, psychiatrists and scientists felt that the LSD-25 drug would assist the medical community in the study and treatment of mental illness. Some even thought that this strange compound would produce a temporary "model psychosis" that would help science better understand the mechanism of mental disease.

Many experiments were conducted with patients to determine if the psychedelic experience would help them overcome their mental conditions. In conjunction with psychotherapy, closely supervised research with LSD continued into the 1950s. At the same time, the use of this synthetic psychedelic spread from the medical community to the intellectual community, where the mystical potential and possible creative power of LSD were valued.

Nonmedical Use

When the initial reports of LSD's therapeutic value were being questioned, the popularization of the drug was well under way. Students, writers, and philosophers became intrigued with LSD's mind-altering and nonaddicting qualities.

Within a few years, nonmedical use of the drug spread to young people, who were being encouraged to join the "psychedelic revolution" of the 1960s. In some ways, LSD ushered in not only the psychedelic phenomenon but also the whole modern wave of nonmedical drug use. The "psychedelic 1960s" also gave birth to new forms of popular music, art, and fashion styles. Many of these innovations are still with us as "acid rock" music, special light shows at concerts, and brilliant neon or "day-glo" colors used in decorations and clothing.

Among the leaders of this "revolution" and chief advocates of LSD were Professors Timothy Leary and Richard Alpert of Harvard University. Although they made important contributions to "mainstream" psychology, these professors advised young people to "drop out, turn on, and tune in." "Dropping out" was any specific technique by which individuals detached themselves from the routine, convention, ambitions, and the symbolic rewards of society.

Responding to altered states of consciousness produced by psychedelic drugs was the key to "turning on." Aware of one's own internal processes, a person could then "tune in" to a greater and more philosophical concern with beauty, peacefulness, and the fundamental questions of cosmic design.

After Leary and Alpert, joined by their students, began experimenting with LSD and other psychedelics, they were dismissed by the university in 1963. The resulting media coverage, however, served to increase national interest in LSD.

Illegal and Popular

In reaction to the growing use of LSD and its association with the new permissiveness of the "hippie culture," new laws made the recreational use of the powerful psychedelic drug illegal. When new research was also restricted, the only drug company that had been making LSD stopped its production. As a consequence, almost no LSD-related research was conducted for nearly twenty years, and illicit producers—"kitchen chemists"—soon supplied the demand of the street market.

The U.S. Food and Drug Administration has sought ways to allow limited human studies to test LSD and other Schedule 1 psychedelic drugs for their possible medical usefulness.[9] Scientists are investigating LSD as a treatment for addiction to heroin, opium, cocaine, alcohol, and even sedative-hypnotics. Limited research is also being done to examine LSD as an antidote to drug overdoses and as a pain reliever for cancer patients.

Using LSD involves consuming powder pellets called "microdots"; gelatin chips known as "windowpanes"; or the most common method, thin squares of absorbent paper soaked in

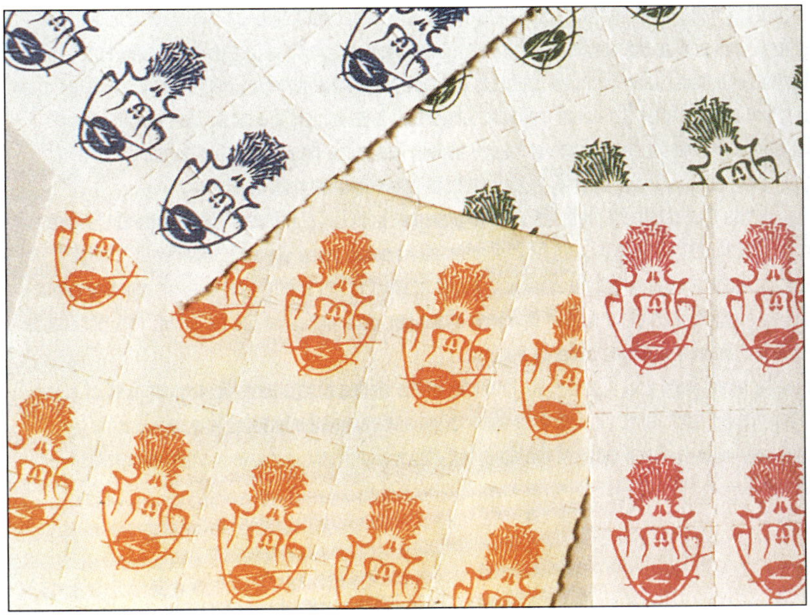

(a)

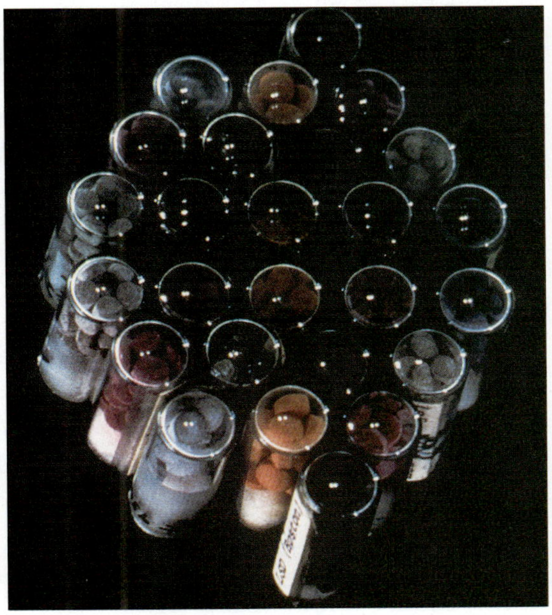

(b)

(a) Today LSD is often eaten in the form of drug-impregnated paper known as "blotter acid." Stamped with distinctive picture designs, blotter acid is printed in books of sheets of 1,000 unit doses. (b) LSD tablets or pellets called microdots were commonly "dropped" during the 1960s.

Drug Enforcement Agency.

liquid LSD—"blotter acid" or "blotter." Supposedly, each square represents one dose. In contrast with bulky carriers (objects and substances containing LSD), such as sugar cubes, animal crackers, gelatin chips, and tiny pellets, "blotter acid" is almost undetectable. Moreover, the potency of today's LSD is not as strong as it was in the "acid" heyday of the early 1970s. LSD tends to produce more-manageable reactions today because of its weaker potency.

LSD's comeback is also related to one of the newest youth fads, "rave parties." These impromptu gatherings consist of young people who meet at designated urban sites, such as abandoned warehouses or vacant racetracks, and party nonstop for several hours or even days. Alcohol is usually banned; the drugs of choice are LSD and another psychedelic, MDMA (Ecstasy), an amphetamine derivative.[10]

There is yet another factor contributing to LSD's resurgence: product packaging. Color-screening and printing on the surfaces of blotter paper, featuring cartoon figures of Mickey Mouse, Snoopy, dragons, stars, and flying saucers, make the "blotter acid" particularly appealing to the younger generation of users—packaging sells.

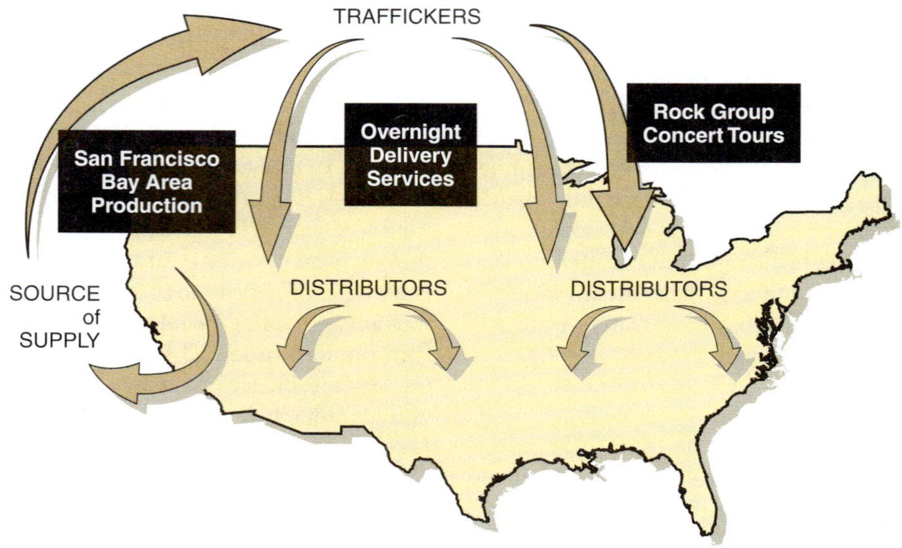

figure 10.2

LSD trafficking from the San Francisco Bay area.

LSD has been and continues to be manufactured in secret laboratories believed to be located in northern California and concentrated in the San Francisco Bay area. At the wholesale production and distribution level, LSD is controlled rather tightly by California-based "syndicates," which have operated with relative impunity for almost twenty years.

Producers of LSD fall into two groups. The first is usually composed of chemists and distributors who work together in close association. This group consists of major manufacturers capable of distributing LSD nationwide. The second type of producer works independently and makes LSD mostly for local consumption.

Lower-level distribution of LSD usually occurs in one of three ways: First, an individual attends a rock concert, meets a source of supply, and exchanges telephone numbers with the source of supply. Second, the individual—deciding to continue to distribute—then calls the source for additional amounts. Typically, the source has either continued on the concert tour or has returned home, which is frequently in northern California. If future communication with the source is difficult, the source provides the telephone number of an associate for future orders. After the initial payment, almost all transactions are made via the public and private mail systems. Payments to a source of supply usually are made through legitimate money wiring services. Third, some dealers travel directly to California to meet their sources of supply.

Reports indicate that shipment methods used to transport both large and small quantities of LSD are often similar, because most of the psychedelic is distributed as small paper squares, often with printed designs, that have been soaked with LSD. The drug-paper product is frequently concealed in greeting cards, cassette tapes, or articles of clothing mailed to a post office box established by the recipient. This post office box usually is listed under a fictitious name or business.

Traditionally, retail-level LSD distribution networks in the United States have been comprised of young adults who have known each other through long association and common interests. This relationship has encouraged not only hand-to-hand sales of the drug, but also a significant increase in mail order sales.

Source: Modified from the U.S. Department of Justice, Drug Enforcement Administration

Lysergic Acid Diethylamide

LSD is derived from the ergot fungus that grows on rye or from lysergic acid amide, as found in morning glory seeds. The name *LSD* is an abbreviation of the German name for **lysergic acid diethylamide.** The best known and probably the most powerful of synthetic psychedelics, LSD has been estimated to be 100 times more potent than psilocybin and 4,000 times more potent than mescaline in producing altered states of consciousness.

LSD doses are measured in extremely small quantities called micrograms, or "mikes" (millionths of a gram) because it is so powerful. Nearly all other drugs are measured in much larger units—milligrams, or thousandths of a gram. The average effective oral dose is about 30 micrograms (mcg); some "street" doses contain as much as 400 micrograms. Currently, the strength of LSD samples from illegal sources ranges from 20 to 80 micrograms LSD per dose.[11]

The amount per dosage unit varies considerably, as does the quality of the psychedelic, due to the illegal sources of the drug; illicit domestic laboratories (see fig. 10.2). Occasionally some samples of LSD are fairly pure, but they may also contain a variety of other psychedelic drugs, strychnine or other toxic stimulants, and even methamphetamine or speed.

The LSD "Trip"

Sold on the street in a variety of forms, LSD is usually taken by mouth. Only rarely is this drug injected. Sometimes LSD is mixed with tobacco and smoked, but the resultant high is typically unsatisfactory.

The mind altering effects brought on by LSD and subjectively interpreted are often referred to as an "acid trip" or simply a **trip.** Although the effects of LSD are unpredictable and vary considerably from one person to another, and from one occasion to the next, several distinct, though somewhat subjective, phases with unique experiences may be anticipated.[12]

In the *first phase,* beginning shortly after taking LSD and lasting up to two hours, the user perceives a release of inner tension. Other characteristics of this phase include laughing or crying, a feeling of intense well-being (euphoria), restlessness, heightened awareness, and enhanced rapport with others.

About thirty to ninety minutes following use of the drug, the *second phase* begins and is usually marked by perceptual distortions, such as visual illusions and hallucinations. One of the more striking and memorable effects is the alteration of visual perception and heightened brightness of colors with halos around objects.[13]

These changes in perception often involve the occurrence of synesthesia—the mingling of senses in which one sensation is translated into another. Common physical effects include dizziness, weakness, drowsiness, nausea, rapid pulse, increased heartbeat and blood pressure, and loss of appetite.

Three to four hours after LSD is taken, the *third phrase* begins. In this part of the trip, the drug user often reports a distorted sense of time—the psychedelic experience seems to move slowly through the past, present, and future, which appear to fuse together. There might also be marked mood swings and a feeling of ego disintegration—that is, a sense of being separate from one's body. LSD users mistakenly believe they possess magical powers of absolute control over their lives. Such false beliefs and loss of contact with reality have resulted in serious injury and even death.

About four hours after initial use, the effects of LSD begin to lessen. "Waves of normalcy" are experienced as the drug taker begins to recover and gradually returns to a nondrugged waking state.

LSD Hazards

A trip that begins in beautiful excitement can suddenly become frightening and take on the characteristics of a "bad trip." Bad trips are the most common adverse effect of LSD and usually take the form of either a sudden, intense panic reaction or one or more psychotic reactions involving serious breaks with reality, persistent hallucinations, and delusions.[14] Sometimes there develops an intense oversuspiciousness leading to the false belief that one is being persecuted or harmed by others.

If a person has suffered from emotional disorders before using LSD, the trip may trigger an emotional breakdown. However, bad trips can occur even among those who have had many earlier good trips.

Bad trips usually end after eight to twelve hours, as the immediate effects of LSD wear off. In most instances, psychiatric help is not needed. The best treatment appears to be protection, companionship, and reassurance throughout the duration of the trip. On occasion, though, physician-prescribed drugs may be required for some LSD users.

Whether LSD or any other psychedelic drug can cause permanent mental illness in otherwise normal, healthy, individuals is an open question. Some heavy users have developed impaired memory and attention span, mental confusion, and difficulty with abstract thinking. Reported periods of emotional imbalance and the experience of dreamlike states while awake may be evidence of structural damage to parts of the brain. But whether these abnormal occurrences are permanent or temporary has not been determined.

While LSD does not appear to cause genetic damage or cancer, street doses of the psychedelic are frequently cut or adulterated with many unidentified drug substances, so that precise effects are uncertain and unpredictable. Consequently, pregnant women should not take this drug. LSD also causes uterine contractions, so this psychedelic poses yet another threat to the pregnancy.

There are other dangers associated with the use of LSD. These can include a terrifying panic, a fear of losing one's mind that might lead to suicide, an unanticipated and terrifying flashback lasting up to ninety minutes, and accidents resulting in injury or death.

Such risks are reduced considerably when LSD is taken in a group situation. A nonuser might volunteer to serve as a guide, assisting those who are having bad trips and preventing users from harming themselves or others (see box 10.2).

The Other Psychedelics

While LSD is the primary example of a psychedelic drug, it is by no means the only one. Over one hundred other substances, both naturally occurring and synthetic, can induce mind-expanding and mind-manifesting effects. Some of these are described in the following sections to highlight the differences and the similarities among these drugs.

Peyote and Mescaline

The peyote cactus, *Lophophora williamsii,* has been used in the religious rituals of Mexican Indians for thousands of years. The ancients were convinced they could communicate directly with their gods without the need for priests because of the visual and kaleidoscopic illusions produced by **peyote.**

Box 10.2 Psychological First-Aid for Psychedelic Panic

Sometimes people who use psychedelic drugs experience a "bad trip" characterized by panic reactions—feelings of terror, confusion, depersonalization, and a fear of losing control over oneself. Rather than medical attention in a hospital emergency room, psychological first aid—"talking down" the person in such a panic situation—is often the best care that a friend can provide. These suggestions are likely to help the person who has sustained such a panic reaction, whether it is drug-related or not, and focus on reassurance, reduction of stimuli, orientation to reality, and use of "alternative-focus" activities.

1. Do no harm to those who are panicked. If you as a "guide" or first-aider become part of the problem by transmitting your fears and apprehension, then you cannot contribute to the solution. Stay calm and smile. Do not yell or shout; do not cry or become hysterical. Do not tell the panicked individual how bad or serious his or her trip has been. In other words, don't make the situation worse!
2. Do not expect immediate or miraculous results. Remember that a bad trip might last several hours. Trippers are often highly suggestible, so you can help by turning a bad trip into a good trip.
3. Reassure individuals that the panic is temporary, that the drug's effects will not persist, and that they will return to normal. The best reassurance is your offer to stay with them as long as you are needed.
4. Help panicked individuals relax. Encourage them to breathe calmly. Tell them to experience the trip as if they were watching a television program or a movie. Advise them to stop fighting the trip.
5. Calm the environment by dimming lights and reducing loud music or other noise. If the environmental setting cannot be altered favorably, then guide the "tripper" to a better one.
6. To orient people to reality, describe familiar objects to them: jewelry, photos, purse or wallet, chair, or toy. Ask them to describe such objects to you. Tell them where they are and, in general terms, what is happening. Remind them that they are not crazy or psychotic, and that their psychic trip is drug-induced. Help them concentrate on controlling breathing and on the rising and falling movements of their stomachs. As their fears tend to subside, tell them about the longer periods of time between waves of fear.
7. When panicked individuals talk about specific problems or concerns, explain that the particular situation has been exaggerated or magnified by a drug, and the problem will appear less threatening after the trip.
8. If you cannot postpone consideration of a problem or divert the tripper's attention to another topic, such as art, music, or sports, then listen patiently in a friendly manner. If the tripper expresses fear or anger, do not be judgmental. Ask the person to explain why she or he is feeling those emotions; then you might provide alternative solutions for the tripper to consider.
9. Direct the tripper's attention to an external focus by suggesting alternative activities, such as taking a shower, going for a walk, eating, listening to music, or watching television.
10. Never give any medication to people experiencing a panic situation, even if you believe a particular drug might cure or reduce a bad trip.
11. If panic, fear, and anxiety do not appear to lessen, or if physical signs or symptoms of distress appear or become worse as time goes on, then take the tripper to a medical facility.

Source: Modified from Jim Parker, *Drug Crisis Response* (Tempe, Ariz.: Do It Now, 1990), 45–46.

The fleshy green cactus tips—the mescal buttons—are dried in preparation for chewing and oral consumption. Rather than endure the bitter taste of the sliced mescal buttons as the Indians of the Native American Church do, some users prefer to smoke the ground-up material. Others brew a peyote tea or swallow capsules containing a powdery form of the cactus buttons. Regardless of the method of administration, peyote tends to cause stomach disorders, nausea, and vomiting. Afterward, psychedelic effects persist for six to ten hours and typically include feelings of weightlessness and depersonalization, perceptual distortions, and synesthesias.

Mescaline is the major psychoactive ingredient of the peyote cactus and is responsible for the mind-manifesting, LSD-like effects of the mescal buttons. In doses of 200 to 500 mg (the equivalent of about twenty mescal buttons), mescaline causes increased heart rate, body temperature, blood pressure, and dilation of the pupils of the eyes, as well as a slowing down of coordination and reflexes, and a diminished ability to concentrate.[15]

The chemical name for mescaline, which can now be synthesized in the laboratory, is *3, 4, 5-trimethoxyphenethylamine.* Available as capsules, tablets, or in liquid form, synthetic mescaline usually produces less intense nausea and vomiting than does peyote, although the psychedelic effects are almost identical to those of LSD. Synthetic mescaline is rarely available on the street, and samples sold as mescaline frequently contain LSD, PCP, or amphetamine.

While mescaline induces altered perceptions, it tends to cause less mental or cognitive disorganization than is caused by LSD. Neither peyote nor its mescaline derivative produces physical dependence.

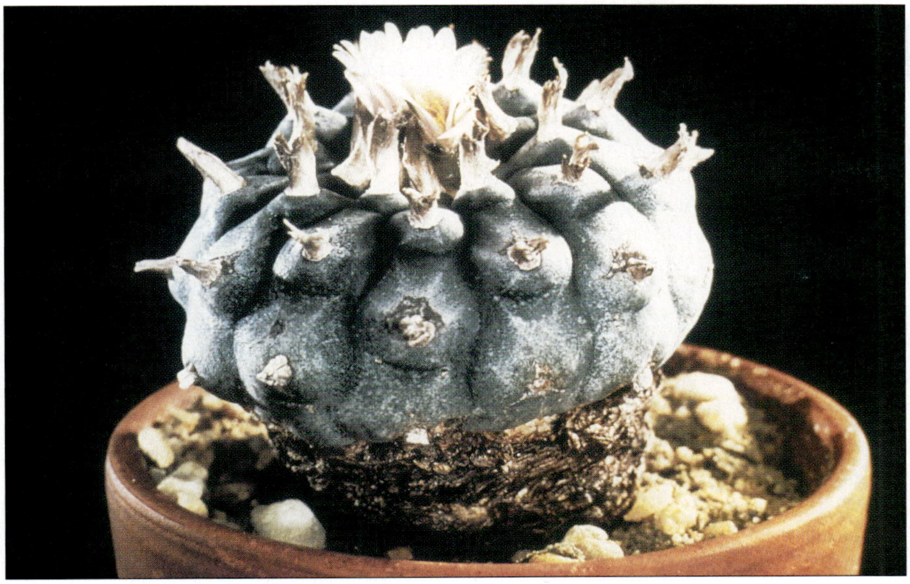

Peyote cacti may be eaten, smoked, or brewed into a tea and produce a psychedelic effect.
Drug Enforcement Agency

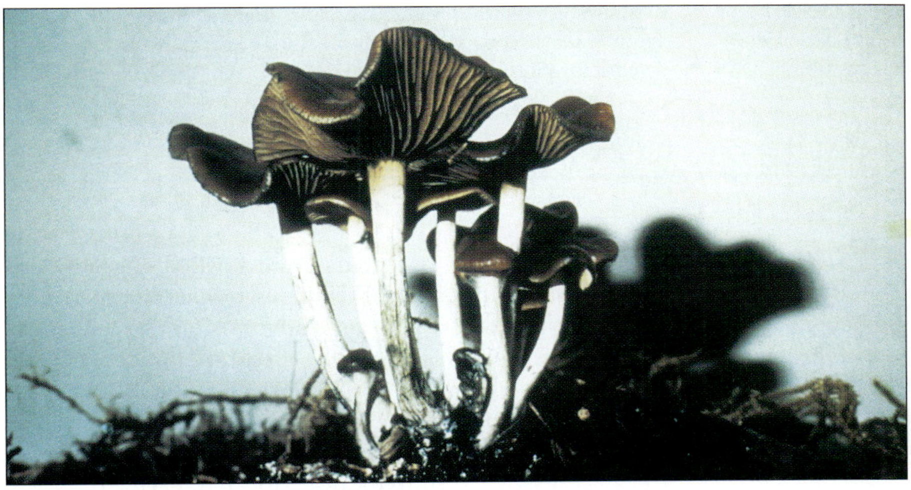

The Psilocybe mushrooms produce effects similar to LSD.
Drug Enforcement Agency

Psychological dependence is rare, but tolerance develops rapidly, often within three days of continual use. Cross-tolerance with LSD and psilocybin exists. Along with LSD and other psychedelics, peyote and mescaline are Schedule I drugs under the provisions of the Controlled Substances Act. However, peyote is legal for members of the Native American Church who use mescal buttons sacramentally in their rituals.

The mescaline derived from mescal buttons is not the source of tequila. A distilled spirit and popular alcoholic beverage, tequila is made from the fermented juice of the cactuslike agave plant, also known as mescal. However, unlike the mescal buttons of the peyote cactus, the mescal-based alcoholic beverage is intoxicating but not specifically psychedelic.

Psilocybin

When Psilocybe mushrooms (*Psilocybe caerulescens, Stropharia cubensis,* and several other members of the *Psilocybe* genus) are eaten, their effects on human perception and cognition are similar to those caused by mescaline and LSD. Before the onset of this drug's unique mental effects—visions perceived with eyes closed and altered states of consciousness—the intake of **psilocybin** may cause nausea, drowsiness, and feelings of numbness.[16]

The psychoactive ingredients of these sacred or "magic" mushrooms are psilocybin and psilocin, both chemically related to LSD. Both of these drugs can be made synthetically in the form of a white crystalline powder, but they may also be contained in mushroom preparations. Much of what is sold on the street, however, consists of LSD and other chemicals. Like mescaline, psilocybin is rarely available on the street, although some users have procured grow-your-own psychedelic mushrooms from special mail-order houses.

For psilocybin to produce psychedelic effects, it must be changed (metabolized) to psilocyn in the body so that it can enter the brain.[17] After 1 to 5 grams of the dried mushrooms are eaten, or a dose of 20 to 60 mg of synthetic psilocybin is taken, effects begin within half an hour and last three to six hours. The duration of the psilocybin trip is considerably shorter than that of an LSD trip. Injection of psilocybin will initiate the trip somewhat earlier.

Usually, the effects are similar to but less intense than those of LSD. Psilocybin has developed a reputation for producing strong visual distortions, and it is believed to produce particularly vivid and colorful illusions. Tolerance to the effects of psilocybin builds rapidly with daily use, although physical dependence does not occur. Though psychological dependence is a possibility, it is thought to be rare.

DMT

A derivative of certain South American shrubs, and a synthetic compound, DMT is a powerful, fast-acting drug that produces psychedelic effects of an extremely short duration. Known chemically as *dimethyltryptamine,* DMT is

Box 10.3 Recreational Use of Herbal Supplements: Buyers Beware!

For many years, a variety of herbs have been used in a recreational way as legal alternatives to illegal psychedelics. For instance, catnip, juniper, and kavakava products have been smoked, and preparations of thorn apple, periwinkle, and mandrake have been brewed as teas for their hallucinogenic effects. These herbal preparations and other so-called "dietary supplements" have never been subject to government regulation, even though they cause druglike effects in the human body.

In 1993, when the U.S. Food and Drug Administration (FDA) proposed to regulate these products, negative congressional reaction was so intense that the Dietary Supplement and Health Education Act of 1994 was passed. This act exempted vitamins, minerals, amino acids, and herbs from regulation by the Food and Drug Administration.

Despite that nearly all of these dietary supplements have drug effects, these products remain largely unregulated and often prove to be harmful, even when directions are followed. While manufacturers are required to inform consumers that the health claims of these products have not been evaluated by the FDA, such claims are typically hidden on the supplement's label.

Three herbal preparations have proved to be especially hazardous. These are:

Ephedra *(Ephedra sinica)*. Often referred to as Ma Huang, ephedra contains ephedrine and pseudoephedrine—stimulants—and is the basic ingredient of Herbal Ecstacy. Marketed as a legal, safe, and natural alternative to MDMA (Ecstasy), Herbal Ecstacy allegedly produces a rapid high and a mild stimulating effect when combined with caffeine. Dangers often associated with the use of ephedra-based products include increased heart rate and blood pressure, seizures, heart attacks, and strokes.[a]

Yohimbe *(Corynanthe yohimbe)*. Obtained from the bark of an African tree, this product is often sold as a male aphrodisiac. However, there is no conclusive proof of its effectiveness. Some people do report that when smoked or used as a tea, yohimbe produces a mild stimulant-hallucinogenic effect. An overdose can result in increased blood pressure, weakness, nervous agitation, paralysis, stomach disorder, seizures of the body, and sometimes death.

Lobelia *(Lobelia inflata)*. This herb is sometimes smoked or brewed as a tea to provide a mild euphoriant effect comparable to marijuana. Known as "Indian tobacco," lobelia acts like nicotine and can produce both a stimulation and depression of the autonomic nervous system. Large quantities cause vomiting, so overdoses are rare. Nevertheless, this herbal supplement can depress breathing, induce coma, and eventually cause death.[b]

[a]Geoffrey Cowley, "Herbal Warning," *Newsweek* CXXVII, no. 19 (6 May 1996): 60–64.

[b]"Herbal Roulette," *Consumer Reports* 60, no. 11 (November 1995): 698–705.

produced in either liquid or powder. Usually DMT is combined with tobacco, parsley, or marijuana and smoked. Sometimes a finely ground powder of DMT is sniffed, eaten, or prepared in a solution for injection, although oral use of this drug does not produce a psychoactive effect.

One of the surprising aspects of DMT is its almost instantaneous impact upon the user. Psychedelic effects often begin and reach their peak of intensity within ten minutes after smoking. The trip lasts only thirty to sixty minutes, and then the visual and time-sense distortions subside rapidly. In essence, a DMT trip is a compact version of an LSD trip, without the side effects of LSD.

As with most other psychedelics, use of DMT soon produces a tolerance, but there is no evidence of physical dependence. Despite its appeal as the "businessperson's trip"—allegedly a DMT trip can be taken during a lunch hour—there is little demand for this drug. Perhaps DMT's action as a MAO inhibitor is its greatest potential hazard. When taken in combination with various foods, liquids, and other drugs, DMT can cause life-threatening changes in blood pressure. (See chapter 9, box 9.4, on antidepressant drugs.)

Morning Glory Seeds

Pulverized seeds of the common morning glory plant (*Ipomoea purpurea* and various species of *Rivea* and *Argyreia*) contain a psychoactive substance, *d*-lysergic acid amide. This psychedelic drug is similar to LSD but is much less potent. A dose of between 200 to 300 seeds will induce LSD-like effects within thirty minutes if taken as a powdery mixture or almost immediately if injected as a liquid preparation. Sometimes the seeds are chewed thoroughly before they are swallowed. The chewing process releases the psychoactive drug for absorption into the bloodstream.

After an initial period of apathy and irritability, the user typically experiences a pleasant state of elation and serenity, similar to the effects of a low dose of LSD. However, "pearly gates" and "heavenly blues," as the seeds are often called, are not ideal psychedelics unless a natural source can be located. Seed producers coat commercially available seeds with a poisonous substance to discourage their use as a recreational drug. Upon ingestion, the toxic substance of the coating induces dizziness, nausea, vomiting, chills, and diarrhea.

Nutmeg

A commercial spice derived from the tropical evergreen *Myristica fragrans*, nutmeg appears as either the whole, dried seed or as a preparation of coarsely ground powder. The seed and the powder can be eaten; the powder is occasionally sniffed. Two to five hours after grated nutmeg is swallowed, a confusional state with mild euphoria and illusions develops. These effects are in response to a chemical identified originally as myristican. However, other psychoactive substances may also be involved. In most instances, nutmeg is used only when more powerful drugs are not available.

Mace, the orange, lacy covering of the nutmeg shell, also contains myristican. Sometimes the ground or whole mace is used as a kitchen spice. When swallowed in quantity, mace induces mild psychedelic effects.

MDA

Nicknamed the "mellow drug of America" and "speed for lovers," MDA has the chemical name *3, 4-methylenedioxyamphetamine.* Derived from various plant oils, including sassafras, MDA can also be synthesized as a white powder. This product can be taken orally (in a capsule), sniffed, or injected as a solution.

Chemically similar to mescaline and the amphetamines, MDA induces an euphoric, peaceful, dreamlike state beginning about an hour after a person takes the drug. The average trip may last nearly eight hours. Though at high doses MDA produces many physical reactions—some requiring emergency medical treatment—the most notable effect seems to be tranquility.

MDMA

Known as **"Ecstay,"** "Adam," "the Big E," and "XTC," MDMA is a chemical cousin of MDA. This psychoactive drug combines some of the hallucinogenic effects of mescaline with the stimulant effects of amphetamines.[18]

Originally synthesized in 1914, MDMA *(methylenedioxyamphetamine)* did not become a significant drug of abuse until the 1970s, when it enjoyed a sudden popularity among American college students. Although taking the drug by mouth is usually preferred, MDMA is inhaled on occasion, but only rarely injected. Derived by chemically engineering MDA, MDMA is considered a "**designer drug**"—an originally legal substance that acts similarly to its illegal cousin (see box 10.4).

Box 10.4 Designer Drugs: Hallucinogens

Illegal drugs are defined in terms of their chemical formulas. To circumvent these legal restrictions, "underground chemists" modify the molecular structure of certain illegal drugs to produce analogues known as "designer drugs." (An analogue is a substance derived from a chemically similar compound.) These chemically engineered analogues can be several hundred times stronger than the drugs they are designed to imitate.

Analogues of amphetamines and methamphetamines cause nausea, blurred vision, chills or sweating, and faintness. Psychological effects include anxiety, depression, and paranoia. As little as one dose can cause brain damage. The analogues of phencyclidine cause illusions, hallucinations, and impaired perception.

Type	What Is It Called?	What Does It Look Like?	How Is It Used?
Analogues of amphetamines and methamphetamines (Hallucinogens)	MDMA (Ecstasy, XTC, Adam, Essence) MDM STP PMA 2, 5-DMA TMA DOM DOB MDEA (Eve) ET (Love Pills, Love Pearls) Nexus	White powder Tablets Capsules	Taken orally Injected Inhaled through nasal passages
Analogues of phencyclidine (PCP) (hallucinogens)	PCPy PCE TCP PHP TPCP	White powder	Taken orally Injected Smoked

Source: Modified from the U.S. Department of Education.

Advocates of MDMA first labeled the drug "the LSD of the 1980s" and then the drug "fashion flash" of the 1990s, because it provides the euphoric rush of cocaine and some of the mind-expanding qualities of psychedelics.[19] As a consequence, MDMA has become a favorite attraction of "rave parties" in the United States (See box 10.5).[20] In more practical terms, perhaps, MDMA is considered the successor to MDA and is often viewed as an aphrodisiac, despite its interference with erection and its inhibition of orgasm in both sexes.

Research indicates that MDMA is somewhat milder and shorter lasting than MDA and exerts amphetamine-like effects on the body (dilated pupils, dry mouth and throat, lower-jaw tension, grinding of the teeth, and overall stimulation). However, many users report a general relaxation effect, decreased use of psychological defense mechanisms, increased empathy for others, promotion of

Box 10.5 Club Drugs: New Psychedelic Highs and Health Risks for the New Century

Each night in various night clubs and raves across the nation, some members of the X-generation are experiencing unusual and often unpredictable effects with so-called "club drugs." These psychedelics promise new versions of expanded self-awareness, but may also deliver some unanticipated side effects and risks to health and life.

Ketamine. Common street names: *Special K* and *Vitamin K.* Identified as a dissociative anesthetic somewhat similar to phencyclidine, this club drug produces fewer unpleasant hallucinations and psychological problems. Still used along with an antianxiety medication to provide satisfactory anesthesia for various purposes, ketamine is especially useful in emergency surgical procedures.[a]

Users undergo major changes in thought and perception and a dissolving of the ego. On occasion, there is a sensation of floating and disconnectedness from the body. Particular hazards of using ketamine include numbness, incoordination, feelings of helplessness, and vomiting when combined with alcohol.

GHB. Common street names: *Liquid X, Easy Lay, GBH,* and *Grievous Bodily Harm.* Promoted as a natural human growth hormone, GHB is an odorless and practically tasteless liquid that can depress the respiratory system, especially when mixed with alcohol. Using this drug or taking it unknowingly often results in unconsciousness and a loss of memory. As such, this club drug masquerades as a dietary supplement and may be replacing Rohypnol as the latest "date-rape drug."[b]

Valued for its psychedelic effects and also used as a sleep aid, GHB can produce headaches, nausea, vomiting, slowed heart beat, amnesia, seizures, and respiratory failure—a stoppage of breathing.

2 C–B. Common street names: *Nexus, Utopia.* Similar to MDMA, this recent arrival on the club-rave scene produces a surge of energy or tremor and visual disturbances and hallucinations, often within one to two hours after use. Those who take this drug report feelings of greater personal insight and heightened emotional awareness and sensitivity. In addition, various sensory effects include a greatly heightened ability to smell, touch, and taste.

To reduce the greatest risk linked with taking this substance, users are cautioned to drink large amounts of water to prevent dehydration.[c]

[a]Bryan Marshall and David Longnecker, "General Anesthetics," chap. 14 in *Goodman & Gilman's The Pharmacological Basis of Therapeutics,* 9th ed. (New York: McGraw-Hill Health Professions Division, 1996), 326–27.

[b]Christine Gorman, "Liquid X," *Time* 148, no. 16 (30 September 1996): 64.

[c]Jim Parker, *Club Drugs* (Tempe, Ariz. D.I.N. Publications, 1996), 4–5.

intimate communications, and enhanced sensual experiences, especially the pleasures of touching.

Some physicians and therapists have found MDMA to be a significant therapeutic aid in dissolving personal anxieties in certain patients.

Although the claimed benefits sound attractive, other investigations have revealed several undesirable effects of MDMA. Recreational users report that over time the desired effects of the drug become weaker, while the negative side effects become more likely.[21] Psychological difficulties reported by users include mental confusion, depression, anxiety, generalized panic, and even paranoia. Common physical problems experienced are increased muscle tension, nausea, blurred vision, rapid eye movements, faintness, and increased heart rate and blood pressure. However, the greatest fears are associated with Ecstasy's potential for acting as a toxic substance within the brain.

There is increasing concern that MDMA causes irreversible brain damage.[22] The production of serotonin neurotransmitter would be adversely affected in that situation. Serotonin is the brain chemical that researchers believe controls mood, appetite, and sexual functioning.

MDMA was temporarily restricted as a Schedule I controlled substance in 1985 and permanently classified in Schedule I in 1988 because of its potential for abuse and its possible neurotoxic effect. Also that year, the Drug Enforcement Administration rejected arguments supporting its treatment value. As an analogue of MDA, MDMA is also illegal as a "designer-recreational" drug.

DOM (STP)

Another synthetic variation of mescaline and amphetamine, DOM *(4-methyl-2, 5-dimethoxyamphetamine)* was first introduced to the drug scene in 1967 as "STP." Named after a motor oil additive—scientifically treated petroleum—the original acronym was soon reinterpreted to "Serenity, Tranquility, Peace."[23]

Usually taken orally, DOM at low doses induces an amphetamine-like euphoria and feelings of enhanced self-awareness. At higher dose levels, LSD-like effects are experienced. Usually less potent than LSD, DOM is not metabolized rapidly, remains in the body much longer than most other psychedelics (from twelve to twenty-four hours), and produces a variety of physical problems, including nausea, sweating, tremors, and convulsions. The length and intensity of the DOM (STP) trip contribute to an unusually high rate of bad trips produced by the drug.

Chemical Variations

An almost endless number of psychedelics have been synthesized by creative "kitchen chemists" for the illegal street market. Some of these, such as DOB *(4-bromo-2, 5-dimethoxyamphetamine)* and MMDA are mescaline-amphetamine variants similar to DOM and MDA, respectively. Other psychedelics with stimulant properties are PMA *(para-methoxyamphetamine)* and TMA *(trimethoxyamphetamine).* DET *(diethyltryptamine)* is similar in chemical structure to DMT.

These drugs differ from one another in terms of speed of onset, duration of action, potency, and capacity to modify mood. They are seldom pure, their capsule dosages are variable, and they are often misrepresented as other psychedelics.

At Issue

Should we legalize all mind-changing drugs?

Point: Why not? We already provide for the legal manufacture, sale, and consumption of alcoholic beverages and tobacco products—sources of our major drug-related health problems in terms of annual numbers of deaths and disease conditions. Continuing the present format of "legal drugs" versus "illegal drugs" seems hypocritical and illogical. Our antidrug policies have resulted in more powerful drugs, increased crime to finance drug abuse, and a literal gold mine for the criminal element of the underworld. Many prominent Americans consider the drug war ineffective, unethical, wasteful, and not capable of being won. Furthermore, experience suggests that marijuana and heroin would be less destructive if they were controlled through legalization or decriminalized.

Counterpoint: Legalization of illegal drugs is an outrageous and intolerable idea that would inevitably encourage more self-destructive drug-taking behavior. Those who support this proposal tend to be irresponsible intellectuals who never have to live or work with drug-dependent individuals, care for crack-addicted babies, or inhabit a neighborhood terrorized by drug gangs and drug-related warfare. History suggests that legalization of drugs speeds up new drug use and spawns an ever-increasing number of long-term drug users who often begin drug use during childhood. Legalization of alcohol and tobacco products did not reduce the many deaths, illnesses, accidents, and crimes associated with these now-legal drug substances. It's about time the American public realizes that the availability and use of mind-changing drugs endanger the capacity to make intelligent decisions and threaten personal health and performance. Moreover, expanded legal drug use is incompatible with normal child development, maturation, and learning. You can't be in favor of more drugs and child health at the same time.

Phencyclidine

Developed in the 1950s as a surgical anesthetic, **phencyclidine,** or PCP, was introduced into medical practice under the trade name Sernyl. In 1965, this drug was taken off the market for human use because it produced unpleasant side effects, including hallucinations, in many patients.

Originally designated a depressant by the federal government, and long considered a psychedelic or hallucinogen by many drug treatment professionals, phencyclidine is a unique drug. It has stimulant, depressant, psychedelic, hallucinogenic, psychotomimetic, analgesic, and anesthetic properties, all of which are dose dependent.

Its precise pharmacological classification has not yet been agreed upon by the scientific community. Perhaps PCP will eventually be considered a "dissociative anesthetic," because during anesthesia this drug appears to make patients insensitive to pain by separating or dissociating their bodily functions from their minds without causing loss of consciousness.[24]

Contrary to popular belief, PCP, known chemically as 1-*(1-phenylcyclohexyl)* piperidine hydrochloride, is not a one-of-a-kind drug. Modifications of the basic PCP manufacturing process have yielded a number of chemically similar compounds referred to as *analogues*. These PCP variants, or analogues, including PCC, PCE, PHP, TCP, and an anesthetic, ketamine, produce similar psychic effects and have already been sold on the illicit street market as PCP.

More commonly, PCP is sold under numerous other names that reflect its bizarre effects, such as "angel dust," "peep," "supergrass," "KJ," "killer weed," "ozone," "embalming fluid," "rocket fuel," "bacon," and "Hog". In the past, PCP was often misrepresented as more attractive drugs, such as THC or other marijuana components, mescaline, LSD, amphetamine, and even cocaine, because of phencyclidine's bad street reputation.

Pure PCP is a white crystalline powder that has bitter taste. It can be mixed with dyes, dissolved in water, and cut with adulterants, and it can contain contaminants resulting from its makeshift manufacture.

Phencyclidine can be inhaled or sniffed, taken by mouth, smoked, and injected intravenously. However, PCP is most commonly smoked on "Sherman" or "More" cigarettes (known as "sherms" and "superkools"), which have thick brown wrappers that absorb liquid PCP and still allow the cigarettes to be smoked. Sometimes PCP powder is placed on parsley or other leaf mixtures and smoked as "angel dust" in cigarettes or joints. Less frequently, liquid PCP is drunk mixed with lemonade or some alcoholic beverage, or injected two to three times a day.

Effects of PCP

The pharmacological actions of PCP depend upon the route of administration and are dose-related.[25] PCP is potent, therefore, the difference between a dose that produces a pleasant loss of sensation (sensory deprivation) and one that results in a bad trip is small. Consequently, the effects of this drug differ widely from one PCP user to the next.

When PCP is eaten, it produces a high lasting five to eight hours; when smoked or snorted, the effects can last three to five hours. Small doses lead first to a mild depression, then to stimulation.

A common initial experience has been described as a drunken state, a floaty euphoria with numbness of the extremities—a result of PCP's anesthetic effect. Users often appear to be "stoned" and display a staggering gait and slurred speech. In addition, the PCP taker experiences a temporary state of depersonalization and detachment from his or her surroundings. Feelings of strength, power, and invulnerability may coexist with this dreamy sense of estrangement.

In moderate doses, analgesia and anesthesia are produced, so that PCP users often do not know when they are being burned, when they have been cut, or when they have strained muscles or broken bones. A confusing psychic state resembling a form of sensory isolation is produced. As a result, the user dissociates, or disconnects from reality, and is no longer aware of what is happening. Changes in body image, disorganized thoughts, drowsiness, and hostile and bizarre behavior also have been recorded.

While heart rate and blood pressure are elevated, the central nervous system undergoes a depression. Increased salivation, sweating, repetitive movements, and muscle rigidity may occur. With increasing dosage, analgesia and anesthesia are more pronounced, and stupor or coma may develop, but the eyes of the PCP taker remain open. In large doses, PCP may produce convulsions.

PCP Overdose

The effects of PCP are often unpredictable because of the level of potency of any given dose. Overdosing is a possibility. The victim of overdose is likely to experience muscular incoordination, oscillating movements of the eyeballs, inability to move from a fixed position, vomiting, skin flushing, noticeable perspiration, generalized anesthesia (loss of sensation), and psychotic episodes.

PCP-induced psychosis may be characterized by hostile and assaultive behavior and body posturing resembling schizophrenia.[26]

The psychotic experience usually progresses through three stages, each lasting about five days.[27] The first stage is often the most severe and is marked by delusions, anorexia (lack of appetite), insomnia, and the possibility that the user will assault others. This is followed by an intermediate, second stage with continued paranoia, restlessness, and intermittent control over one's behavior. In the third stage, the PCP user undergoes a gradual recovery, but social withdrawal and severe depression often persist for months.

PCP can display the harmful properties of a CNS depressant, inducing cardiovascular instability, respiratory depression (stoppage of breathing), seizures, and coma. To prevent death, emergency medical treatment will include life-support measures, isolation of the victim to reduce sensory stimulation, and in some cases where PCP was ingested orally, detoxification by gastric suctioning.

The number of deaths associated with combining PCP with alcohol or with heroin has been higher than expected, reflecting either a users' preference for taking these drugs in combination or some interaction in the effect of the drug combinations. Many of the reported PCP-related deaths, however, were not the result of overdose or drug interaction but rather resulted directly from external events, such as homicides, accidents, suicides, gunshot wounds, strangling, drownings, auto accidents, falls, and cuts.

Historical Aspects

Although the synthesis of PCP was originally described in 1926, it was not until the early 1950s that scientists first studied its potential use as a drug that could produce anesthesia without significant depression of heart and lung function. Clinical use of PCP soon raised serious doubts about its usefulness as an anesthetic, however. Humans sustained numerous postoperative difficulties, ranging from mild to profound disorientation, agitation, manic excitation, delirium, and hallucinations. When subanesthetic doses of PCP were found to induce schizophrenia-like symptoms in normal subjects and to intensify primary symptoms of schizophrenic patients, PCP was restricted to its only legal use at that time, as a veterinary analgesic-anesthetic.

PCP first appeared on the illegal drug scene in 1965, but it did not attract much attention until it emerged as the "PeaCe Pill" during 1967, and as "hog" in New York City's "hippie" community in 1968.

As reports of increased adverse medical and psychiatric effects related to PCP were publicized, and as its recreational use spread throughout the United States, phencyclidine gained notoriety as a major drug menace. In 1977, the National Institute on Drug Abuse started a nationwide campaign to inform both professionals and the public of PCP-abuse hazards. Although today's use of PCP appears to be concentrated predominantly among former users and young adults, some preteens and adolescents are being hospitalized for PCP-related emergencies in some large urban areas.

Legal Prohibition

Responding to the national concern over the abuse of PCP and the severe behavioral toxicity of phencyclidine and its analogues, the federal government temporarily classified PCP as a Schedule II controlled substance. Then, in 1979, PCP was permanently elevated it to Schedule I status.

In 1978, the U.S. Congress enacted the Psychotropic Substance Act. This legislation imposed severe penalties for the manufacture of PCP and its analogues and for possession with intent to distribute them. Legislation was also passed mandating that sales of piperidine (a chemical intermediate in the synthesis of PCP) or its salts and derivatives be reported to the U.S. attorney general and the Drug Enforcement Administration.

Chapter Summary

1. Psychedelics are drug substances that change thinking and perception. Such mind expansion is characterized by heightened awareness of sensory input and sense of clarity, unusual sensory experiences and perceptions of the environment, assignment of profound meaning to the slightest sensation, lessened capacity to distinguish self from the environment, and a sense of cosmic union.

2. Synesthesia is a psychedelic drug-related effect in which there is a mingling of the senses. For example, sounds might be seen, smells might be felt, and colors might be heard.

3. Particular hazards of psychedelics are a "bad trip" (panic reaction) and a "flashback" (repetition of

the drug's effects without using the drug again).

4. The types of psychedelic experiences are distinguished as psychotic, psychodynamic (surfacing of subconscious ideas), cognitive (clearness of thought), aesthetic (fascinating perceptions and sensations), and transcendental.

5. Physical side effects are dull compared to the psychological effects. They involve changes in temperature, blood pressure, heart rate, and reflexes; and include nausea, vomiting, and diarrhea. Repeated use often leads to tolerance and, in some instances, psychological dependence. Physical dependence has not been demonstrated.

6. Though plants with psychedelic effects had been used for many centuries, the synthesis and personal use of LSD by Albert Hofmann in 1943 ushered in the Psychedelic Era.

7. Initially used in the treatment of mental conditions, LSD was soon adopted by students, writers, and philosophers because of the drug's mind-expanding qualities. Eventually, LSD became associated with the "hippie culture," dropping out of conventional society, and antiestablishment social movements. Legal production of LSD was stopped in the mid-1960s.

8. Derived from ergot fungus or from lysergic acid amide, LSD is the most powerful synthetic psychedelic. It is 100 times more potent than psilocybin (derived from sacred mushrooms or synthesized) and 4,000 times more powerful than mescaline (derived from peyote cactus or synthesized).

9. Other psychedelics are DMT, morning glory seeds, and nutmeg (all naturally occurring), and MDA, MMDA, DOM, DOB, and DET (all synthesized).

10. MDMA, a designer drug derived chemically from MDA and often called Ecstasy, has become a popular recreational drug because it tends to combine the rush of cocaine with some of the mind-expanding qualities of psychedelics. MDMA's potential therapeutic value has been rejected by the Drug Enforcement Administration.

11. In a drug class of its own, phencyclidine (PCP) has psychedelic, stimulant, depressant, hallucinogenic, psychotomimetic, analgesic, and anesthetic properties.

12. Introduced as a surgical anesthetic for humans, and then for use in veterinary medical practice, PCP was eventually classified as a Schedule I controlled substance due to its frightening and often violent side effects.

13. Though some users claim to maximize desired psychoactive effects of PCP by means of dose control, the drug's effects are unpredictable and subjectively experienced. A floaty euphoria, anesthesia, sensory deprivation, delusions, hallucinations, violent and assaultive behavior, paranoia, and a severe form of psychosis are possible elements of a PCP trip.

World Wide Web Sites

Toronto Addiction Research Foundation

www.arf.org

Web of Addictions Fact Sheet

www.well.com/user/woa/facts.htm

Review Questions and Activities

1. In what specific ways do psychedelic drugs expand one's mind?
2. Some psychedelics produce psychotic experiences. What types of mind-expanding experiences might be interpreted as more desirable psychedelic effects?
3. How does the phenomenon of synesthesia differ from a flashback reaction?
4. Explain how people achieved psychedelic effects before the synthesis of LSD.
5. What roles did the following individuals play in the modern Psychedelic Era: Albert Hofmann, Timothy Leary, and Richard Alpert?
6. Describe the probable though variable experiences of an LSD "trip" in relation to dosage level, user characteristics, drug-taking environment, and anticipated phases of effects.
7. Compare the following drugs in terms of their origin, their probable psychedelic effects, and their differences in use patterns and duration of action: peyote, psilocybin, DMT, and DOM.
8. What effects of MDMA make this drug, known as Ecstasy, so popular and yet so controversial?
9. Which classification of psychoactive drugs seems most appropriate and most accurate for phencyclidine?
10. Why is PCP often described as a drug menace?
11. Consult a reference text on herbs and herbal preparations and investigate the possible pharmacological effects of broom or Scotch broom, hops, maté, passion flower, prickly poppy, snakeroot, and wild lettuce.

References

1. Lester Grinspoon and James Bakalar, *The Harvard Medical School Mental Health Review: Drug Abuse and Addiction* (Boston: Harvard Mental Health Letter, 1993), 33.
2. Jerome Jaffe, "Drug Addiction and Drug Abuse," chap. 22 in *Goodman and Gilman's The Pharmacological Basis of Therapeutics,* 8th ed., eds. A. G. Gilman and others (New York: McGraw-Hill, 1990), 553.
3. Barry Stimmel and the editors of Consumer Reports Books, *The Facts about Drug Use: Coping with Drugs and Alcohol in Your Family, at Work, in Your Community* (New York: Haworth Medical Press, 1993), 115.

4. Charles O'Brien, "Drug Addiction and Drug Abuse," chap. 24 in *Goodman & Gilman's The Pharmacological Basis of Therapeutics,* 9th ed. (New York: McGraw-Hill Health Professions Division, 1996), 574.
5. Robert Julien, *A Primer of Drug Action,* 7th ed. (New York: W. H. Freeman and Company, 1995), 315.
6. Kenneth Blum, *Handbook of Abusable Drugs* (New York: Gardner Press, 1984), 558.
7. Edward M. Brecher and the editors of Consumer Reports Books, *Licit and Illicit Drugs* (Mount Vernon, N.Y.: Consumers Union, 1972), 338.
8. Avram Goldstein, *Addiction: From Biology to Drug Policy* (New York: W. H. Freeman, 1994), 193.
9. Paula Kurtzweil, "Medical Possibilities for Psychedelic Drugs," *FDA Consumer* 29, no. 7 (September 1995): 25–26.
10. H. Thomas Milhorn, *Drug and Alcohol Abuse* (New York: Plenum Press, 1994), 333.
11. National Institute on Drug Abuse, "LSD (Lysergic Acid Diethylamide)," *NIDA Capsules,* (June 1992), 1.
12. Harold Doweiko, *Concepts of Chemical Dependency,* 2d ed. (Pacific Grove, Calif.: Brooks/Cole, 1993), 144.
13. "Today's Youth In For Bad Trips and Flashbacks: LSD Revisited," *Substance Abuse Report* XXVI, no. 10 (15 May 1995): 8.
14. Christina Dye, *Acid: LSD Today* (Tempe, Ariz.: Do It Now, 1992), 5–6.
15. Jennifer James, *Peyote and Mescaline: History and Use of the Sacred Cactus* (Tempe, Ariz.: Do It Now, 1990), 4.
16. Christina Dye, *Psilocybin: Demystifying the Magic Mushroom* (Tempe, Ariz.: Do It Now, 1991), 4.
17. Gesina Longenecker, *How Drugs Work: Drug Abuse and the Human Body* (Emeryville, Calif.: Ziff-Davis Press, 1994), 104.
18. Harvey Milkman and Stanley Sunderwirth, *Craving for Ecstasy: The Consciousness and Chemistry of Escape* (Lexington, Mass.: D.C. Heath, 1987), 53.
19. Christina Dye, *XTC: MDMA and the Chemical Pursuit of Ecstasy* (Tempe, Ariz.: Do It Now, 1991), 2.
20. Teri Randall, "Medical News and Perspectives: 'Rave' Scene, Ecstasy Use, Leap Atlantic," *Journal of the American Medical Association* 268, no. 12 (22–30 September 1992): 1506.
21. Doweiko, *Concepts of Chemical Dependency,* 150.
22. Robert Mathias, "Like Methamphetamine, ecstacy' may cause long-term brain damage," *Nida Notes,* (November, December, 1996).
23. Tibor Palfai and Henry Jankeiwicz, *Drugs and Human Behavior* (Dubuque, Iowa: Brown & Benchmark, 1991), 315.
24. Leo Hollister, "Drugs of Abuse," in *Basic and Clinical Pharmacology,* ed. Bertram Katzung, 4th ed. (Norwalk, Conn.: Appleton & Lange, 1989), 389.
25. Robert C. Petersen and Richard C. Stillman, "Phencyclidine: An Overview," in *Phencyclidine (PCP) Abuse: An Appraisal* ed. R. C. Petersen and R. C. Stillman (Washington, D.C.: GPO, 1978), 3; Jaffe, "Drug Addiction and Drug Abuse," 557–58; and Grinspoon and Bakalar, *The Harvard Medical School Mental Health Review,* 36.
26. O'Brien, "Drug Addiction and Drug Abuse," 574.
27. Doweiko, *Concepts of Chemical Dependency,* 148.

Chapter 11

Marijuana

Unique and controversial

KEY TERMS

Amotivational Syndrome
Antiparaphernalia Law
Anxiety/Panic Reaction
Cannabinoid
Cannabis
Cannabis sativa
Decriminalization
Glaucoma
Hashish
Hashish Oil
Hemp Plant
Immunosuppressive Effect
Legalization
Marijuana High
Paraquat
Sinsemilla
Teratogen
THC

chapter objectives

After you have studied this chapter, you should be able to do the following:

1. Define the key terms.
2. Identify the natural source of marijuana and name its principal psychoactive ingredient.
3. Name several different uses of cannabis products, other than as a recreational drug, in ancient and modern times.
4. Explain the impact each of the following laws had on marijuana use, misuse, or abuse: Harrison Narcotics Act, Eighteenth Amendment to the U.S. Constitution, Marijuana Tax Act, and the Controlled Substances Act.
5. Distinguish between the concepts of decriminalization and legalization as they pertain to the possession of small amounts of marijuana for personal use.
6. Compare and contrast the major arguments offered for and against the legalization of marijuana.
7. Describe the probable psychological, emotional, and physiological aspects of the marijuana "high."
8. Identify the probable effects of marijuana on motor coordination, reaction time, tracking, cue detection, short-term memory, time sense, and oral communication.
9. Explain the probable effect of social levels of marijuana on driving ability.
10. Describe the conditions of tolerance and dependence as seen in marijuana use.
11. Discuss the amotivational syndrome and its controversial association with marijuana use.
12. Identify the major chronic effects of marijuana use on the respiratory, cardiovascular, and immune systems.
13. List some possible effects of marijuana on male reproduction and sexual function.
14. List some possible effects of marijuana on female reproduction and sexual function.
15. Discuss the therapeutic potential of marijuana in relation to specific diseases or abnormal conditions in humans.
16. Identify developments in the movement to legalize medical marijuana.

Introduction

Marijuana has become a popular psychoactive drug—the most widely used illegal substance in the nation. It has frequently been described as relatively safe despite its illegal status, but it is known to have significant health-threatening effects on users. This chapter examines the history of marijuana and the legal aspects of using it, along with the drug's pharmacology and potential health risks, thereby clarifying some of the uncertainties and myths surrounding this unique substance.

Of all the so-called recreational drugs, pot or grass—as marijuana is commonly called—is the most controversial. Its use has become so widespread in the United States, so those who favor marijuana and its legalization argue that its

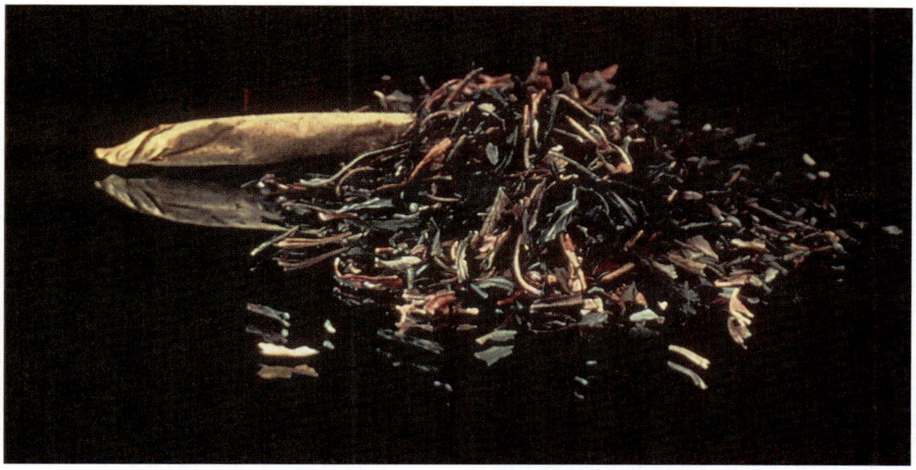

Shown in this photo is a marijuana plant, *Cannabis sativa,* which is cultivated as well as grown wild throughout the world in temperate and tropical areas.

Drug Enforcement Agency

potential risks to health are no greater than those of alcohol or tobacco. Opponents of marijuana insist that its proven and suspected hazards to personal and social health are so potentially harmful that any further legal approval would be unwise and undesirable.

Marijuana: A Brief Description

Marijuana is a prepared mixture of the dried, flowering tops, leaves, and stems of the **hemp plant, *Cannabis sativa.*** (There are two other types of marijuana plants, *Cannabis indica* and *Cannabis ruderalis,* but neither are as common nor psychoactive as *Cannabis sativa.*)[1] Cultivated and grown wild throughout the world in temperate and tropical areas, the leafy cannabis plant grows for one season, dies, and then reproduces through its seed.

Often incorrectly considered a narcotic, marijuana in low to moderate doses typically causes a sedative, dreamlike effect in the user, observed as relaxed, drowsy, and less socially interactive. However, at higher dose levels, marijuana produces effects similar to the mind-expanding psychedelics. As such, marijuana or cannabis shares the characteristics of two major drug classifications.

But unlike the sedatives, marijuana's active ingredient does not produce anesthesia or death. Unlike the powerful psychedelics, there is little cross-tolerance between marijuana and, for example, LSD. So marijuana is a unique psychoactive drug, best described in a class of its own.

Historical and Legal Aspects of Marijuana

Presumably first used by the Chinese as early as 2700 B.C., the hemp plant's fibers were valued highly and used in the manufacture of rope, cloth, and paper.[2] Before any intoxicating or drug effects were associated with the nonfood plant, a commercial application of cannabis was established. Since then, marijuana* seeds have been sterilized and processed for use in animal feed mixtures (the sterilization renders the seeds nonpsychoactive); cannabis fibers have been employed as raw materials in the production of canvas; oil extracts of the hemp plant have been combined with paint pigments.

The ancient Chinese soon discovered the usefulness of cannabis in the medical treatment of a wide variety of ailments.[3] However, the Chinese eventually banned its use because of the plant's unpredictable intoxicating effects.

Upon the introduction of cannabis into ancient India, its mind-altering effects were more generally appreciated. The cultivation of the hemp plant became an agricultural science, and its use eventually became widespread. The early Indian culture accepted the euphoria-producing ability of cannabis as appropriate and as a blessing from the Almighty. In due time, the use of the hemp plant as an intoxicant and as a source of rope and cloth spread throughout Asia, Africa, Europe, and the Americas.

By the time Europeans began exploring the New World, the cannabis plant was a commercial success. During the early seventeenth century, English settlers brought the plant to their colonies in America, where it was the first crop to be introduced in the Massachusetts Bay Colony.[4] Before long, hemp plants were abundant and the hemp fiber industry thrived.

Although the psychoactive properties of the cannabis plant were recognized, the general American public showed relatively little interest in marijuana as a nonmedical, recreational drug. In contrast, the medical uses of marijuana were expanded, and cannabis preparations were prescribed legally for numerous physical and mental ailments until 1940.

When the Harrison Narcotics Act was passed by the U.S. Congress in 1914 in an attempt to control the distribution and use of medical narcotic drugs, cannabis products, including marijuana and hashish, were excluded from the provisions of the act.

In the view of the National Commission on Marihuana and Drug Abuse:

> Marihuana smoking first became prominent on the American scene in the decade following the Harrison Act. Mexican immigrants and West Indian sailors introduced the practice in the border and Gulf states. As the Mexicans spread throughout the West and immigrated to the major cities, some of

* The preferred spelling of this word, *marijuana,* the Spanish variation, will be used throughout the chapter, except in direct quotations or publications containing the English variation, *marihuana.*

Box 11.1 Glossary of Terms for Marijuana-Related Products

1. *Bhang*—the dried leaves and flowering shoots of the cannabis plant, containing smaller amounts of THC; common name for a weak preparation of marijuana used in India and Jamaica.
2. **Cannabis**—a general term for any of the various preparations of the hemp plant, *Cannabis sativa,* and used interchangeably with the term *marijuana.*
3. *Ganja*—the resinous mass derived from the small leaves and brackets of the cannabis plant; common name for a slightly more potent form of marijuana used in India.
4. **Hashish**—the resinous secretions of the cannabis plant collected from the flowering tops, dried, and then compressed into various forms, such as balls, cakes, and cookie-like sheets. This form of cannabis is usually more potent than marijuana, having a THC content ranging from trace amounts up to 20 percent, but averaging between 3 percent and 7 percent. Hashish is the major form of cannabis used in the Middle East and in North Africa. In the Far East, the dried resinous exudate is called *charas.*
5. **Hashish oil**—a dark viscous liquid produced by a process of repeated extraction of cannabis plant materials. A solvent, such as ether or chloroform, percolates through the marijuana mixture, thereby removing more of the existing THC. This extract contains a greater concentration of THC than does hashish, with some samples having a THC content of nearly 60 percent, but averaging about 20 percent.
6. *Marijuana*—a general term descriptive of any part of the cannabis plant, *Cannabis sativa,* or its extract that produces physical or psychic changes in the human. Marijuana is a tobacco-like substance produced by drying the leaves and flowering tops of the hemp plant.
7. **Sinsemilla**—a seedless variety of high-potency marijuana, originally grown in California and prepared from the unpollenated female cannabis plant.
8. *Thai sticks*—a cannabis preparation common in Southeast Asia, consisting of marijuana buds bound onto short sections of bamboo.

Source: Based on definitions and descriptions provided by the Drug Enforcement Administration and the Bureau of Justice Statistics, U.S. Department of Justice.

them carried the marihuana habit with them. The practice also became common among the same urban populations with whom opiate use was identified.[5]

It is also likely that marijuana use increased in popularity as a recreational intoxicant with the enactment of the Eighteenth Amendment to the U.S. Constitution. This prohibition amendment forbade the manufacture, distribution, and sale of alcoholic beverages. Inexpensive and easily available, marijuana was often used as a substitute for ethyl alcohol. During the 1920s, marijuana "tea pads"—late-night smokeries similar to bars—operated in many large cities, including New York.

Allegations of abuse and an association with violence and crime came with the increased use of marijuana. Exaggerated tales of the drug's bizarre effects, especially that it caused murder, rape, sexual excesses, and amnesia, were publicized widely. Marijuana horror stories were portrayed in the Hollywood film *Reefer Madness,* still shown occasionally on college campuses.

By 1935, in reaction to the growing "epidemic" of marijuana smoking most state governments enacted laws against the nonmedical use of cannabis. During this antimarijuana crusade, cannabis and its extracts were inaccurately classified as narcotics in scientific literature and in legal declarations.

The Marijuana Tax Act

In 1937, the U.S. Congress adopted the Marijuana Tax Act, which superimposed a federal prohibitory scheme on each of the state laws banning nonmedical use of marijuana. This federal statute mandated the registration and taxation of both buyers and sellers of marijuana and imposed criminal penalties for violations.

Subsequent federal and state legislation prescribed even harsher penalties, including, in some states, life imprisonment for illegal possession.

Until the early 1960s, the recreational use of marijuana was confined largely to underprivileged socioeconomic groups and certain insulated social groups, including jazz musicians and artists. Such use had little impact on the dominant social order. Nothing changed on the legal scene until millions of middle- and upper-class college youth—and their noncollege counterparts—adopted marijuana smoking as a common form of recreation.

Marijuana became part of the youth and values revolution of the 1960s. Then, under the provisions of the Controlled Substances Act of 1970 (officially known as the Comprehensive Drug Abuse Prevention and Control Act), the U.S. Congress downgraded possession and use of marijuana from a felony to a misdemeanor. Eventually, all fifty states relaxed their severe penalties for simple possession.

Decriminalization and Legalization of Marijuana

In 1973, Oregon became the first state to decriminalize marijuana; that is, the penalties for possession and use of this drug were reduced in severity. By 1980, another ten states had decriminalized the possession of this drug. However, antimarijuana initiatives—including the spraying of paraquat on marijuana crops and the adoption of zero-tolerance standards—were then undertaken by the federal government and the national mood of tolerance toward marijuana began to shift. In 1990, Alaska became the first state to recriminalize

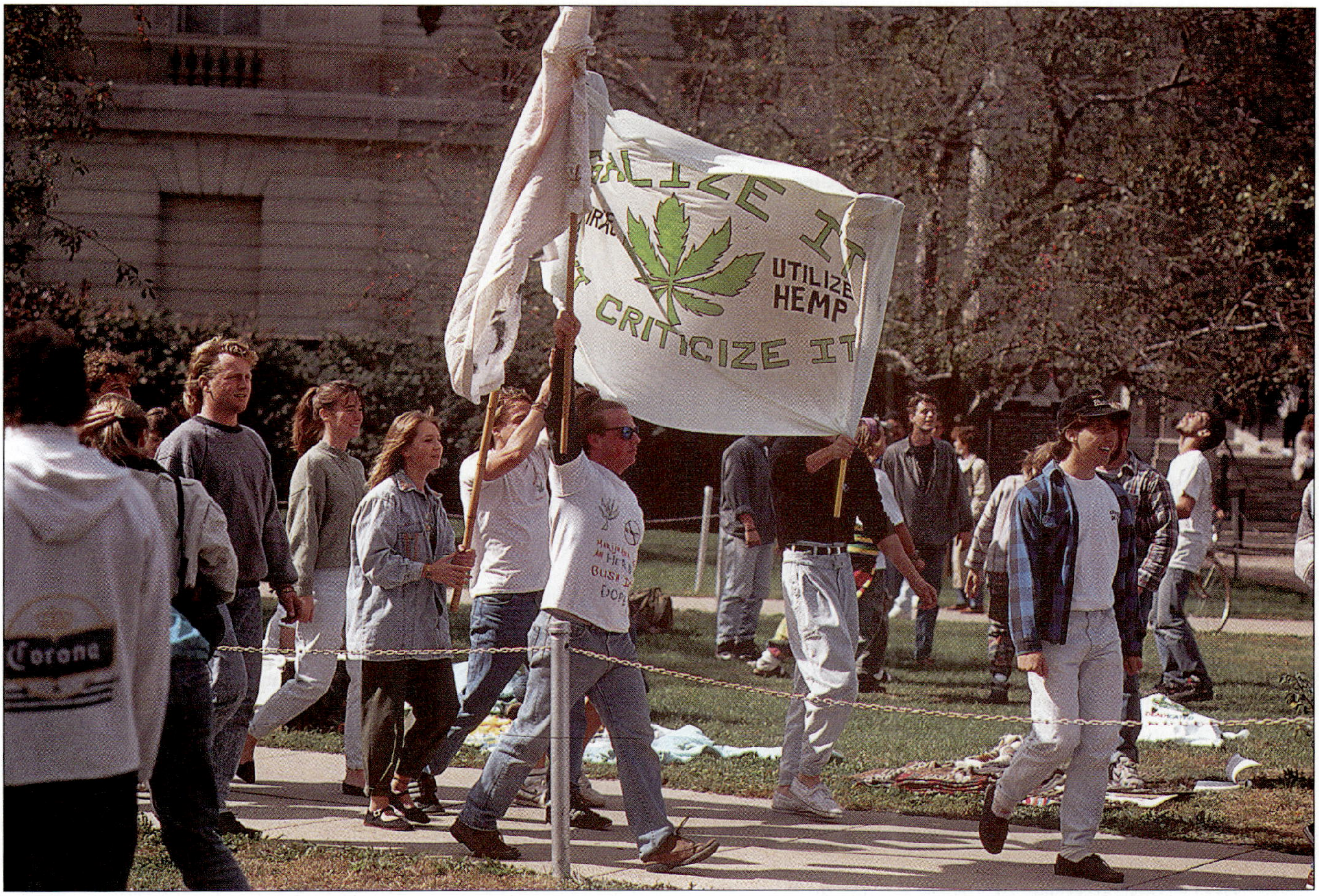

Efforts to legalize marijuana often take the form of peaceful demonstrations both on and off college campuses. Do you think marijuana will be decriminalized or legalized in the near future?
© James L. Shaffer

marijuana possession in a statewide referendum.

Decriminalization

Decriminalization is the legal process of reducing the penalty for a particular behavior still restricted by law. In this instance, the behavior is the possession and use of small amounts of cannabis preparations. The former misdemeanor offense has been downgraded either to a minor misdemeanor—with no permanent criminal record—or to a mere civil offense requiring a civil fine and sometimes also mandating enrollment in a drug education program or involvement in public service instead of a prison sentence.

However, laws forbidding the sale of marijuana remain harsh. In many states, punishment for trafficking in marijuana has increased, while penalties for personal possession have decreased.

The decriminalization procedure is based on the philosophy that harsh criminal penalties are unjustified. Long prison terms and huge fines seem unreasonable and ineffective for punishing marijuana users. Moreover, noncriminal penalties appear to be more appropriate for such drug use that does not usually affect other people or society in general.

By contrast, when criminal penalties are applied, they have often resulted in otherwise law-abiding young people spending time in prison and incurring irreversible damage to their careers and professional advancement. Such consequences apparently cause greater harm to human lives than any effects the drug would have had. As such, criminal penalties appear to be not only harsh and unjust, but counterproductive.

Legalization

Legalization is a legislative declaration approving or authorizing a particular action. In the legalization of marijuana, the state or federal government would not attempt to prohibit or penalize the use of marijuana. However, as in the legalization of alcohol after the period of national prohibition, laws could still regulate the place of use, minimum age of users, time of purchase, production, taxation, and consequences of combining drug use with driving or other public behaviors.

Despite some interest in reform, the federal government has not moved toward legalizing marijuana or any other

At Issue

Shouldn't marijuana be legalized because it is safer than alcohol?

Point: Yes, indeed. Marijuana is relatively safer than alcohol in terms of its drug effects on the human individual and society. Marijuana is a "tamed" drug, and does not cause a hundred thousand deaths each year—as does alcohol—and does not result in cirrhosis of the liver, "marijuanaism," or numerous other health problems related to alcohol abuse. In addition, marijuana is not a contributing factor to half of all highway traffic deaths each year. Nor does pot contribute in any significant way to rape, spouse abuse, absenteeism, or any of the other social problems associated with alcohol abuse in the United States. It is really strange that although marijuana is so much safer than alcohol, the former is illegal, while the latter is still legal.

Counterpoint: Wait just a minute! Such a description of marijuana sounds as if this mind-changing drug is practically harmless. Admittedly, alcohol is the "hardest" drug in terms of its total impact on individuals and society in America. But marijuana is not without serious adverse consequences. And just because alcohol is legal does not mean that society needs or is ready for another legal psychoactive drug. Many people drink alcohol without getting "high," but getting "high" is usually the main purpose of smoking pot! Smoking marijuana presents a clear danger, especially because the potency of the THC content in the 1990s is several times greater than the THC content of samples available in the 1960s and 1970s. Some chronic marijuana users have developed serious lung disease because there are more cancer-causing agents in marijuana smoke than in tobacco cigarette smoke. We know that marijuana can interfere with the body's immune response to various infections and diseases. Even small doses of pot can impair short-term memory function, distort perception, interfere with concentration, and degrade motor skills. Furthermore, long-term marijuana likely causes brain damage and changes in the brain similar to those that occur in aging. Such evidence of harmful consequences of use hardly justifies giving marijuana legal status. It may prove to be more dangerous in the years ahead.

illegal drug of abuse. However, at least twenty-six states have enacted laws or had voter-approved propositions allowing physician-prescribed or recommended use of marijuana in the treatment of serious diseases.

One vocal critic of the federal government's antidrug campaign is the National Organization for the Reform of Marijuana Laws (NORML), based in the nation's capital. NORML has been advocating decriminalization and legalization of marijuana for more than twenty years, but it supports continued prohibition of cocaine. According to NORML, marijuana is a "softer" drug, with lower toxicity potential, than alcohol, cocaine, or heroin. So far, no one has died as a result of a marijuana overdose, and many fewer marijuana-related deaths occur each year in comparison with the huge toll of tobacco-related mortality. In addition, NORML has also spearheaded the challenge to the federal government's ban against the medical use of natural marijuana.

There are many valid counterarguments to the proposal for legalizing marijuana. See the "At Issue" box for a summary of both sides of this argument.

Antiparaphernalia Laws

Reaction to widespread marijuana use by young people has taken the form of **antiparaphernalia laws.** The term paraphernalia refers to items related to the use of illegal recreational drugs, such as pipes, bongs, roach clips, spoons, and roll-your-own cigarette papers. In many communities, local ordinances have been passed controlling or banning paraphernalia sales and the advertising of such accessories, usually sold at specialty shops ("head" shops) and some record stores.

Several states have also passed such antiparaphernalia laws. However, these statutes, along with local ordinances and proposed federal legislation against drug accessories, have been challenged as unjust or ineffective. Critics of such measures argue that these laws are akin to outlawing bottles and glasses to combat alcoholism.

The Current Scene

Marijuana and its use in the United States have undergone some major changes since this drug became popular during the 1960s and 1970s. Five of these changes are described in this section: potency, understanding of effects, age of first use, quantity of use, and amount of domestic production.[6]

Potency Is Up

Although pot smoking is still widespread, the marijuana of today is different from the cannabis available only a few years ago. Improved breeding techniques have resulted in American-grown marijuana many times stronger than the commonly used variety in the 1960s and 1970s. Average potency has increased from 1 or 2 percent nearly twenty years ago to an average THC (tetrahydrocannabinol) concentration of 3 to 8 percent or even 10 percent. (THC is the main psychoactive ingredient in marijuana.) Marijuana cigarettes or "joints" that formerly contained 20 mg of THC now routinely contain 40 mg or more. Hashish samples typically are 100 times more potent than their earlier counterparts.

Effects More Clearly Understood

Much of the early research on the effects of marijuana had been based on users smoking less-powerful varieties of marijuana, therefore many findings and con-

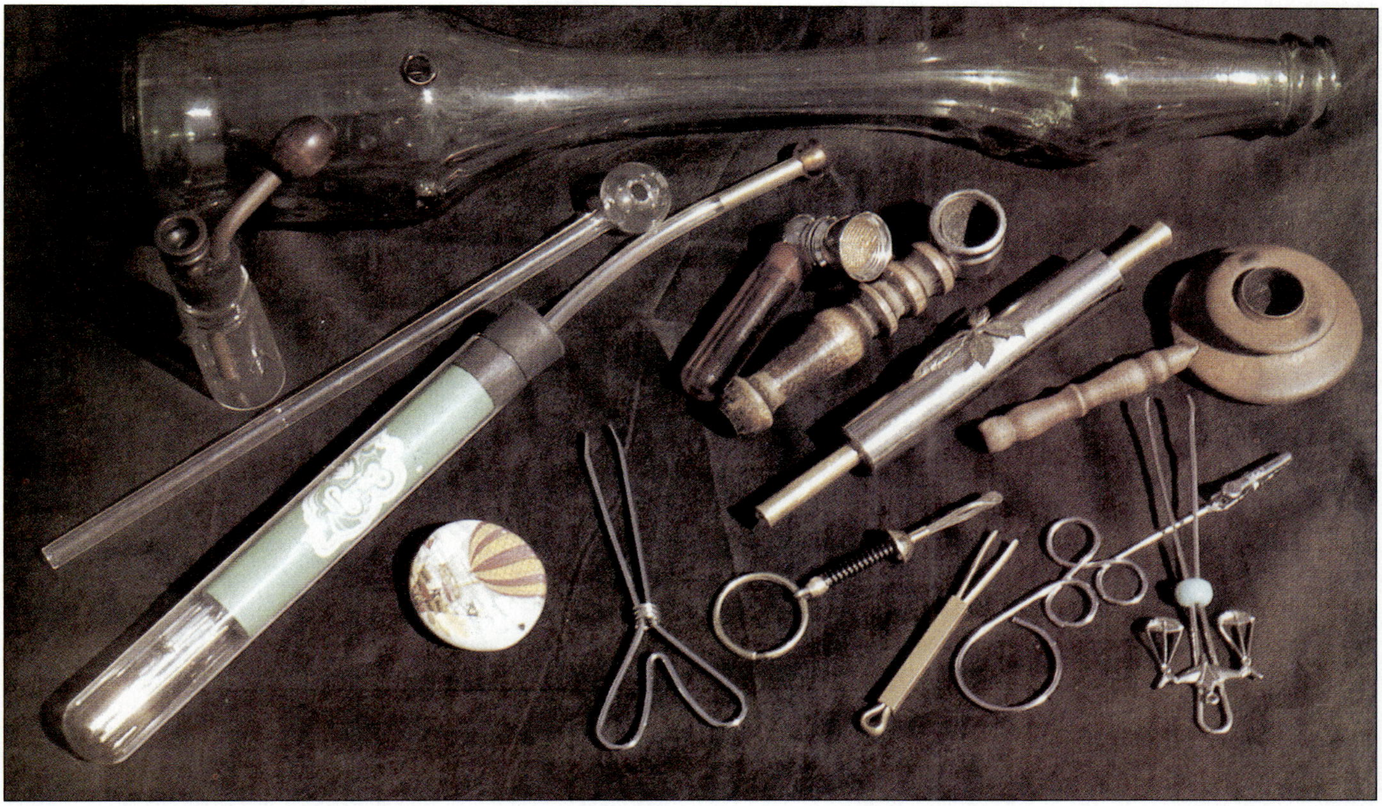

Cannabis paraphernalia, drug equipment or gadgets, sold for use in smoking marijuana.
Drug Enforcement Agency

clusions had little relevance to the use of stronger cannabis now prevalent in the domestic market. Even the hazards of use have been somewhat controversial and ambiguous, because many of the early adverse reactions were studied using an animal model, rather than a human one.

But now, the effects of marijuana on humans are more clearly known, due to extensive research. The scientific community is certain that marijuana reduces coordination; slows reflexes; interferes with the ability to measure distance, speed, and time; and tends to disrupt concentration and short-term memory. In addition, the cancer risks associated with smoking marijuana are recognized as being as great as those related to tobacco smoking. These acknowledged effects will be examined later in this chapter.

Once consider a relatively mild and harmless euphoriant, marijuana is recognized as having a serious potential impact on social functioning and especially on physical health. Moreover, long-term heavy use has often been related to the subsequent abuse of other illegal drugs. Consequently, marijuana is often called a "gateway" drug because its frequent use has been the single best predictor of eventual cocaine use during adolescence.

However, according to prominent drug-abuse experts, there is no convincing evidence for or against this "stepping-stone hypothesis"—that marijuana smoking leads to the use of other illicit psychoactive drugs.[7] Though almost everyone who uses any other illegal drug has smoked marijuana first, most marijuana smokers do not use cocaine or heroin, just as most alcohol drinkers do not use marijuana.

Age of First Use

Marijuana is the number one illegal drug used in America.[8] This psychoactive substance has become a common part of the nation's social scene and is often promoted by music, videos, and clothing that suggest using pot is cool. Millions use marijuana on a monthly basis, and nearly 70 million people have used either marijuana or hashish at least once in their lifetimes.

Young people are increasing their use of marijuana after nearly a decade of declining use rates. The average age of first use is between 16 and 17 years, but drug treatment centers are seeing clients as young as 12- and 13-years-old. Recreational use begins as early as elementary school. (see fig. 11.1)

Quantity of Use

Marijuana use is rising among youth. This is due largely to the many innovative forms of marijuana use that have appeared—combinations of pot and alcohol, and concoctions of marijuana with other illicit drugs, including PCP, cocaine, and opium.

In some communities, marijuana has also been laced with various insecticides and sold on the street as "Wac"—a preparation linked with psychiatric symptoms.

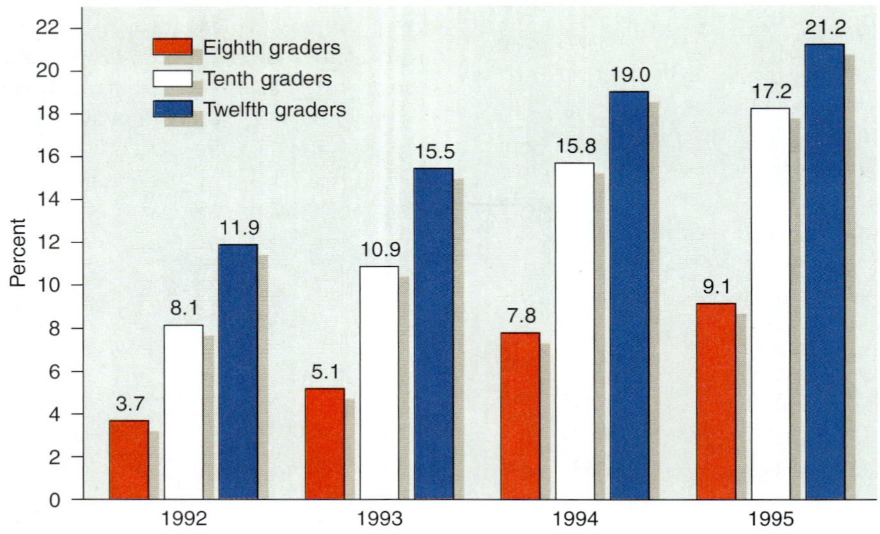

figure 11.1

Past month use of marijuana by eighth, tenth, and twelfth graders, 1992–1995.

After a decade of declining use during the 1980s, marijuana consumption by American youth aged twelve to seventeen years almost doubled between 1992 and 1994. Reports indicate that the rate of marijuana use among youth has continued to climb.

Source: Data from "The Monitoring the Future" study, Institute for Social Research, University of Michigan, and the National Institute on Drug Abuse, as reprinted in The National Drug Control Strategy: 1996.

Marijuana soaked in formaldehyde and allowed to dry—a combination known as AMP—has effects common to both marijuana and PCP or phencyclidine intoxication.

This toxic mixture has produced some serious mental disturbances in users. Marijuana is also laced with cocaine in a unique combination known as "primos."

One alarming result of this increased use and combination use is the 50 percent increase in 12- to 17-year-olds who ended up in hospital emergency rooms in 1994 for smoking pot as in 1993.

Domestic Production

Over the past several years, large-scale production of marijuana in the United States has quadrupled the domestic pot crop. American-grown marijuana accounts for at least 25 percent of marijuana used in this country.[9] However, the bulk of marijuana used still comes from Mexico; Latin America; and countries in Southeast Asia, such as Thailand.

Domestically, marijuana is grown in small plots and frequently in greenhouses by individual growers or in large urban warehouses where plants are cultivated hydroponically (without soil). Outdoor plots are usually located in remote areas and have been found in some of our national parks and forests.[10] Marijuana is one of this country's largest cash crops and enriches the economies of several states.

Marijuana and THC

Typically, cannabis products are smoked in pipes or in loosely rolled homemade cigarettes called "joints." Marijuana and its extracts might be used alone or in combination with other drugs. They might also be taken orally—eaten alone or as an ingredient in food preparations.

Cannabinoids

The several plant parts of cannabis that make up the marijuana mixture are chemically complex.[11] At least 426 individual compounds have been identified, more than 60 of which are specific to cannabis.

Chemical compounds found only in cannabis are referred to as **cannabinoids.** Several of these are routinely measured in identifying cannabis samples.

When marijuana is smoked, some of the chemicals contained in the mixture of dried plant particles are further changed into many other compounds in the process of burning. One of these "new" chemicals, benzopyrene, is known to be cancer-causing and is 70 percent more abundant in marijuana smoke than in tobacco smoke.

Tetrahydrocannabinol

The most active and principal mind-altering ingredient of marijuana is identified as delta-9-tetrahydrocannabinol, or **THC** for short. The amount of this specific cannabinoid is an indicator of the psychoactivity of a drug sample, though other chemicals may eventually prove to be important for their drug effects upon the human body or their interaction with THC.

Though the THC content determines the potency of marijuana, THC occurs in various concentrations in different parts of the plant. Thus the amount of THC in marijuana sold on the street is influenced by the source and selectivity of plant materials, and also by the plant strain, climate, soil conditions, harvesting process, and any added ingredients to the mixture.

THC Content

In the United States, the THC content of marijuana varies from 2 percent to 8 percent, with a high of 15 percent in some strains of sinsemilla—a seedless variety of marijuana with increased resin content rich in psychoactive cannabinoids.

Preparations of such marijuana, with relatively higher levels of THC, contribute to higher levels of intoxication and potentially to more severe and adverse consequences. Therefore marijuana can no longer be viewed as an innocuous drug, the "harmless little giggle" John Lennon referred to during the 1960s.

Paraquat

Some cannabis preparations may have been sprayed with **paraquat.**

Used throughout the world as a powerful herbicide or weed killer, paraquat causes temporary damage to the heart, kidneys, central nervous system, liver, skeletal muscles, and spleen. However, lung damage, caused by continuous smoking of large quantities of paraquat-contaminated marijuana, has proved clinically to be permanent and in some cases severely injurious. The changes in lung tissue after smoking appear to be dose related.

Paraquat has been banned on public land since 1983 because of environmental concerns, but it is still sprayed on private lands by the federal government, and is used in some foreign nations.

Metabolism of THC

When smoked, the THC is rapidly absorbed by the blood in the lungs and transported to the brain in less than thirty seconds. Effects of cannabis also appear quickly, psychologically and physically, and reach their peak about the time smoking is completed.

By contrast, if the same amount of THC were eaten, absorption would take much longer, and effects would develop more slowly (over 2 to 3 hours), would last longer, but could not be controlled after the marijuana had been swallowed.

In a short time, the liver begins to change THC to many chemical byproducts, known as metabolites. However, approximately 25 to 30 percent of the original THC compound, with various cannabinoid metabolites, remain in the human body one week after the initial dose is taken.

Research further reveals that, in a frequent user, complete elimination of a single dose may require at least one month after the last use, during which time marijuana residuals can be detected in urine.[12] THC and other cannabinoids because of their fat solubility accumulate in the fatty tissues and are eliminated slowly from the human body.

Urine Testing for THC

Laboratory tests of urine and other body fluids have been used increasingly by business and industry, drug treatment programs, the military services, and parole and probation officials to determine if individuals have been using marijuana. State-of-the-art marijuana detection procedures reveal the following:[13]

1. Urine screening and confirmatory testing can detect THC metabolites with a fair degree of accuracy and reliability.
2. After smoking a single marijuana cigarette, a positive test can be expected in about 2 to 3 hours, with the highest urinary concentration at 5 to 6 hours.
3. Depending on which concentration of the drug in urine is considered as positive or negative, the detection period for a positive urine test ranges from 1 to 2 days for a "low -dose" marijuana cigarette; from 5 to 7 days for casual use of up to four joints per week; 10 to 15 days for daily use; and 1 to 2 months for chronic heavy use.
4. A positive test has no relationship to marijuana intoxication (because THC metabolites do not usually appear in the urine until nearly two hours after smoking) and cannot distinguish between one time or regular use.
5. Urine tests cannot provide totally accurate results without confirmation.
6. An FDA-approved saliva test and a breath test can detect THC in persons for as long as 3 to 5 hours after they have smoked marijuana. Increasing use of hair analysis will reveal a six-month history of drug use, including marijuana.

Although many problems have arisen with urine testing for marijuana—numerous false-positive test results and drug users who avoid detection by switching temporarily from pot to alcohol or cocaine—the effectiveness of preemployment drug screening for marijuana in predicting employment outcome has been established.[14]

Considerably less than previously estimated, those with marijuana-positive urine samples experienced 55 percent more accidents on the job, 85 percent more injuries, and a 78 percent increase in absenteeism. Moreover, for identified marijuana users, the relative risk for employment turnover was 56 percent. These rates are much less than earlier estimates, but it is evident that preemployment drug screening that is positive for marijuana is associated with unfavorable employment outcome.

The Marijuana High

There is no doubt that the mind-altering effects of marijuana are the bases for its widespread popularity. Low to moderate doses tend to induce a sense of well-being and euphoria and produce a feeling of relaxation, a dreamy state of sleepiness. This individually perceived, favorable response to marijuana intoxication is referred to as the **marijuana high**—peaking about thirty minutes after use and then disappearing in 2 to 4 hours.

Numerous behavioral and psychological effects have been reported, but they are often subjectively interpreted and influenced by several variables: (1) the *drug*—dose, type of preparation, route of administration, and grade or amount of THC present in any given dose; (2) the *marijuana user*—personality, psychological state, motivation, level of expectation or mind-set, and prior experience with the drug; and (3) the physical and psychosocial *setting* in which the use of the drug occurs.

Nevertheless, when low social doses (one or two joints) are used, the effects of the high may go undetected by others, especially unknowing observers. As the THC concentration in marijuana increases, however, a low social dose may have some observable effects.

Common reactions of the "high" focus on changes in sensory perception, including sight, smell, taste, and hearing. The senses seem to become more vivid. These experiences may be accompanied by alterations in thought formation and expression.

Sometimes there may be shifting sensory imagery, rapid fluctuations of emotions, fragmentary thoughts with disturbed associations, and an altered sense of personal identity.[15] For some marijuana users, the body calms down to a quiet period of pleasurable introspection, while others develop a giddiness and gregarious mood and engage in ridiculous conversation and laughter.

During the period of this "high," there is a reduction of mental function, perception, reaction time, learning, and memory. Coordination and the ability to track the movement of an object from one place to another are impaired. Such adverse effects last for several hours beyond the "high."[16]

Cannabis also tends to focus and intensify a person's concentration on the here and now. Additionally, under the influence of marijuana, certain compulsions arise. Frequently reported are obsessive desires for food, especially sweets, and music—the louder and more rhythmic, the better.

While marijuana has not been clinically proven to be an aphrodisiac, there is a widely held belief that marijuana smoking enhances social effectiveness and heightens sexual pleasure. Marijuana use probably can reduce sexual inhibitions and enhance hearing, vision, and skin sensitivity—all of which are conducive to sexual enjoyment. Like ethyl alcohol, too much marijuana can interfere with sexual performance and response, and might result in a loss of interest in sex.

Physical aspects of the high often include a temporary increase in heart and pulse rates, an increase in systolic blood pressure, and a marked reddening of the eyes.[17] Additional effects are a slight drop in body temperature, a decrease in intraocular pressure of the eye, and an increase in blood-plasma volume and in appetite.

Behavioral and Psychosocial Effects

In terms of immediate threat to one's life, marijuana is a relatively "safe" drug. There has never been a documented case of a lethal overdose due solely to marijuana. However, in some situations the pleasant effects of marijuana intoxication can be considered adverse and dangerous. This is true for the distorted perceptions that pose definite risks for driving motor vehicles or operating machinery. But there are other behavioral and psychological effects of using marijuana that pose additional risks for users.

Significantly more youth use alcohol than use marijuana. But unlike current drinkers, many more marijuana users report having bought and smoked this drug at or near school. This situation has raised a major, continuing concern about marijuana's effect on the learning process.

The Role of Neurotransmitters

The mechanism of THC's action is not entirely understood. It is recognized, however, that THC receptors in the central nervous system are numerous, especially in the cerebrum and cerebellum. A compound named anandamide has also been identified as reacting with these THC receptors. It is likely other substances, including neurotransmitters, will eventually be discovered as interacting with the same receptors.

THC's production of euphoria is related to a morphinelike substance, opiopeptin.[18] When THC acts on opiopeptin receptors, an opiopeptin substance is released. This brain chemical acts on dopamine receptors in the brain's reward or pleasure circuit. While dopamine uptake is inhibited, the dopamine neurotransmitter effect in the synapse is enhanced.

In many ways, chocolate and marijuana share a similar brain chemistry. Basic chemicals in chocolate apparently target the same receptors with which THC interacts in the brain.

Acute Effects

Changes in perceptual and psychomotor functions that can be seen after a single dose of marijuana are known as "acute effects." In general, these changes are related to THC's impact on the information-processing center of the brain, the limbic system, and the temporary disruption of the brain's neurotransmitters. Moreover, these effects are dose related; for example, low doses have small effects, whereas higher doses tend to have greater effects. Research has revealed numerous acute effects:[19]

1. *Motor coordination* is impaired; specifically, the drug affects hand steadiness, body sway, accuracy of carrying out body movements, and the ability to maintain postural stability. Although an individual under the influence of marijuana may feel graceful, he or she may become somewhat clumsy.
2. *Reaction time,* the time lag between a signal and a person's response to that signal, may be increased in some individuals, but not all. When intoxicated with marijuana, an individual is often less likely to pay attention to the reaction-time task of the moment.
3. *Tracking,* following a moving stimulus, is significantly and consistently diminished. Tracking impairment often lasts for 4 to 8 hours beyond the feeling of intoxication. Such a disability would interfere seriously with driving and flying skills.
4. *Signal or cue detection,* such as the ability to perceive a brief flash of light, is significantly impaired by low to moderate doses of smoked marijuana. This impairment of visual perception constitutes a major risk for users who operate machinery.
5. *Short-term memory* is slightly diminished by a single moderate dose of marijuana. Remembering a sequence of numbers or memorizing and following a series of directions become more difficult to accomplish. The memory deficit is particularly evident in acquiring and storing information, tasks dependent on attention.
6. *Learning ability and paying attention* are impaired in heavy marijuana users, even after a day of supervised abstinence from the psychoactive drug. These lingering results—the "carryover effect" of using marijuana—persist after the drug is metabolized and no longer affecting the human body. This particular

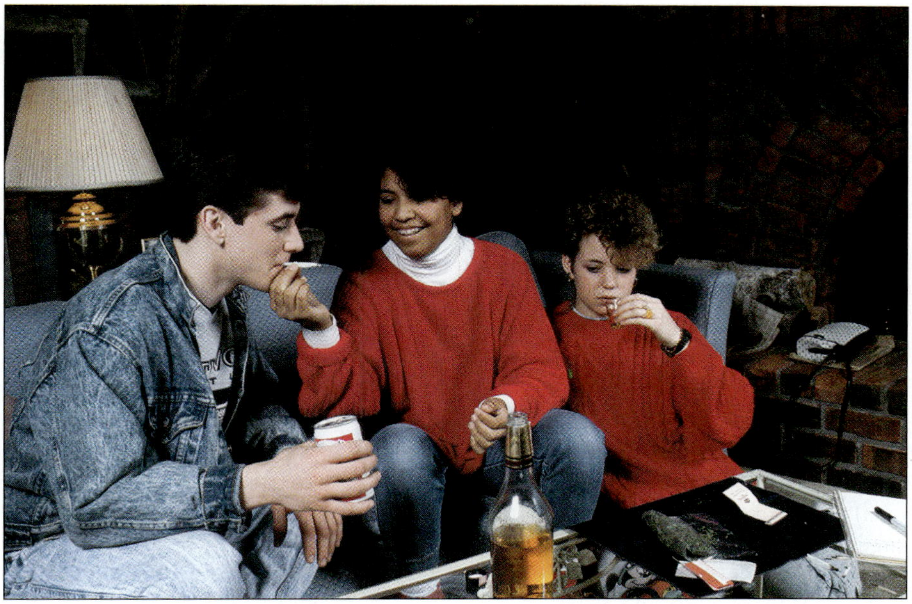

A particularly dangerous recreational activity—the use of marijuana in combination with alcohol—especially if such use occurs prior to driving.

© Mark M. Walker/The Picture Cube

finding disproves the common belief that once the period of marijuana intoxication wears off, mental functions are restored to their normal, predrugged condition.

7. *State-dependent learning* occurs with marijuana. That is, material learned while under the influence of the drug is remembered best in the state of drug intoxication in which it was originally learned. The quality of learning and recall are almost always impaired because the user's ability to acquire the information or skill will be impaired while the user is intoxicated.
8. *Time sense,* the ability to perceive accurately the passage of time, is adversely affected by moderate doses of marijuana. Users consistently overestimate the amount of time that has elapsed.
9. *Oral communication,* even in low to moderate doses, is impaired. Users' ability to conduct a sequential dialogue with others is adversely affected. By impairing short-term memory, marijuana disrupts the continuity of speech. The introduction of irrelevant words and ideas into conversation further interferes with communication skills of speaking.

Automobile Accidents

Teenagers who are inexperienced drivers and who smoke marijuana as often as six times a month are more than twice as likely to be involved in traffic accidents.[20] In a study of accident victims admitted to a shock trauma unit in Baltimore, Maryland, one-third of admitted patients had detectable levels of marijuana in their blood, indicating use of the drug within 2 to 4 hours prior to admission. Reported by the National Institute on Drug Abuse, this study also found that four of every ten persons thirty years of age or younger were under the influence of marijuana at the time of the accident.

Despite the many variables associated with the impact of marijuana on human behavior, there is good evidence that the use of marijuana even at typical social levels definitely impairs driving ability and related skills.

The marijuana user displays the common signs of "marijuana intoxication," a condition of euphoria accompanied by impaired motor coordination, anxiety, sensation of slowed time, impaired judgment, social withdrawal, memory and concentration impairment, psychological confusion, and feelings of fuzziness and dizziness.[21]

Studies of adversely affected driving skills were conducted with laboratory-based driving simulators, on "closed test" driving courses, in surveys of accidents, and in questioning marijuana users. In relation to operating a motor vehicle, the use of social levels of marijuana consistently

> impaired motor coordination, in other words, specific car-handling skills of braking, steering, and tracking;
>
> decreased consciousness of external stimuli, particularly flashing lights and other cues;
>
> impaired judgment and concentration ability;
>
> resulted in marijuana users' receiving higher-than-average numbers of tickets for driving violations and being involved in a higher-than-average number of auto accidents; and caused the user to overestimate amounts of time that had elapsed.

The combination of these effects adds up to a severe reduction in driving abilities. Overconcentration and a shortened memory span will prevent detection of warning signals, and the adverse effects on time sense, and possibly depth perception and reaction time, can create confusion about traffic movement and appropriate drivers' responses.

Just as alarming is the likelihood that the detrimental effects on driving skills may last several hours beyond the time when users experience either euphoria or sleepiness.

Another dangerous practice is the use of marijuana in combination with alcohol prior to or while driving. Such a combination will likely result in greater risks of accident than those posed by either substance alone.

Anxiety/Panic Reaction

Although the mind-altering effects of marijuana make its use attractive, some users report experiencing bad trips—**anxiety/panic reactions** perceived as unpleasant or undesirable. About one-third of regular users have reported that, while intoxicated, they experienced the most common disturbing reaction to marijuana—sudden panic, fears of dying or going insane, and paranoid thoughts (feelings of being ridiculed or persecuted). Hallucinations do not typically develop. While first-time users are more likely to have these adverse reactions, regular users also report that anxiety, fear of losing control, confusion, dependency feelings, and aggressive urges are common occurrences.

Medical treatment is not usually needed, although thousands of people on marijuana seek assistance in hospital emergency rooms each year. People experiencing anxiety/panic reactions need reassurance and calming support from friends or caregivers while waiting out this frightening period. The duration of these incidents ranges from only a few minutes to a few hours. Such undesirable reactions—milder versions of an LSD bad trip—usually decline after use of the drug is stopped.

While truly nightmarish experiences are rare, more-concentrated forms of marijuana have produced occasional psychedelic effects and even prolonged episodes that some describe as a "cannabis psychosis" with hallucinations, delusions, and acute schizophrenia in which thoughts and feelings do not relate to each other logically. More serious reactions have also been observed: (1) dysphoric reaction—severe anxiety, restlessness, and agitation—among the elderly on therapeutic doses of THC; and (2) acute brain syndrome—impaired attention span, memory, perception, and sleep pattern—in people who use cannabis products with extremely high levels of THC.

Tolerance and Dependence

Frequent, continuous use of most psychoactive drugs leads to the condition of *tolerance,* a diminished response to a repeated dose. A state of increased resistance to the drug's effects, tolerance is related to (1) reduced sensitivity of target nerve cells to the drug's effects; and (2) probable increased rate of drug metabolism or elimination, which lowers drug concentrations at sites of action.

Tolerance to marijuana can occur and likely results from an adaptation of neurons to the continuous presence of the drug.[22] Although tolerance appears to develop rapidly, it also disappears rapidly. Moreover, this condition does not seem to be a serious problem with most marijuana users, who appear to endure higher levels of marijuana without experiencing the severe mental and emotional effects often reported by first-time users.

Physical dependence, also the likely result of temporary and compensatory changes in the nervous system, is evident in withdrawal signs and symptoms. The combination of these observable signs and individual complaints is known as the *withdrawal* or *abstinence syndrome* and appears following discontinuation of regular marijuana use.

The withdrawal syndrome is rather mild because marijuana lingers so long in the human body before complete metabolism and elimination.[23] Commonly reported symptoms include restlessness, irritability, mild agitation, decreased appetite, sweating, insomnia, sleep disturbances, nausea, and occasional vomiting and diarrhea. Fortunately, most of these signs and symptoms disappear within two days, and the syndrome is not considered life threatening.

Although physical dependence can develop rapidly, the condition is usually associated with situations in which marijuana or THC doses were maintained at constant levels not typically seen in occasional social use. Cannabis dependence does *not* necessarily equate with compulsive behavior to use more marijuana.

Nevertheless, there is clinical evidence of a condition referred to as "primary marijuana addiction."[24] This disorder is occurring among people who are starting to use marijuana in a chronic, compulsive way, despite negative consequences. But unlike other drug addictions, marijuana does not produce sudden and dramatic personality shifts, and withdrawal rarely requires hospitalization.

Passive Marijuana Smoking

Passive or involuntary smoking—inhaling secondhand, sidestream smoke from the burning tobacco products of others—is associated with increased health risks, including lung cancer, and with indoor air pollution. Research is being undertaken to learn if passive marijuana smoking also contributes to undesirable health and behavioral effects among nonusers of cannabis.

Much of marijuana smoking occurs in closed and poorly ventilated environments, therefore nonsmokers who are present sometimes experience mild forms of involuntary intoxication and discomfort in breathing.

Some nonsmokers who associate with marijuana users might develop a sensitivity to secondhand marijuana smoke, experience a "contact high," and then become nauseated. It is likely that passive marijuana smoking is a potential threat to the safety and well-being of nonsmokers, as it is to pot smokers.

For more information on marijuana, contact:

Potsmokers Anonymous
208 W. 23rd. St., Apt. 1414
New York, NY 10011

American Council for Drug Education
c/o Phoenix House
164 W. 74th. St.
New York, NY 10023

National Organization for the Reform of Marijuana Laws
1001 Connecticut Ave., N.W., Suite 1010
Washington, D.C. 20036

Chronic Effects: Areas of Concern

Described in this section are various changes that can develop after prolonged marijuana use, and those that might continue after use of cannabis preparations has stopped. Such persistent, lasting changes are termed "chronic," which means that they tend to be long-term in their duration.[25]

Amotivational Syndrome

There are few issues related to marijuana use more controversial than the so-called **amotivational syndrome.** Never considered as a specific medical diagnosis or disorder, the syndrome describes a pattern of personality changes observed in some frequent users of marijuana.

Usually characterized by apathy, lack of concern for the future, and loss of motivation, the amotivational syndrome tends to persist well beyond the period of marijuana intoxication. Other aspects of the personality pattern include loss of ambition, loss of effectiveness, dullness, diminished ability to carry out long-term planning, difficulty in concentration, intermittent confusion, impaired memory, and a decline in work or school performance. When regular use stops, the syndrome usually disappears over several weeks.

Clinical observations and self-reports by marijuana users support the common occurrence of this condition. However, interpretation of the evidence linking marijuana to amotivational syndrome is difficult.

This group of symptoms is also observed in nonmarijuana users, and daily use of marijuana is not always associated with loss of motivation. Even if there is an association between the syndrome and use of marijuana, such a relationship does not prove that the drug causes the syndrome.[26]

Persistent concern about amotivation remains something of a chicken-or-egg question.

It has not been definitely shown whether marijuana causes lack of motivation through its drug effects or whether unmotivated people use pot as a symptom of alienation.[27]

Marijuana: Threat to Maturation

Though it is likely that personal qualities and certain drug effects contribute to motivational problems among some frequent marijuana users, the repeated use of any sedating drug, such as marijuana, alcohol, or barbiturates, can be hazardous to adolescents and to adults.

Adolescents are undergoing a period of rapid physical, mental, and emotional change. Their views of themselves and the world are also changing radically. Adolescents are engaged in processes of questioning, searching, and testing that eventually will determine their career and lifestyle choices. They are learning many cognitive, psychological, and social skills. Failure to acquire these skills can impair their maturation.

For the reasons previously cited, and in light of the increasing daily use of marijuana by younger and younger adolescents and preadolescents, hundreds of parents' groups have banded together to form the National Federation of Parents for Drug-Free Youth. Organized and highly vocal, this group has been increasingly influential in the field of drug-abuse treatment and prevention. The major concerns of this group have been to prevent marijuana use among young people and to enact antiparaphernalia laws on the local level. Many parents view marijuana use as psychological escapism that interferes with growing up and becoming mature and responsible individuals (see box 11.2).

Box 11.2 Developmental and Psychosocial Concerns Associated with Using Marijuana

1. Use of marijuana may impair or reduce:
   - short-term memory,
   - comprehension,
   - concentration, and
   - attention span, with adverse effects on learning ability in both young people and adults.
2. While marijuana-intoxicated, users may display indicators of impaired psychological functioning, including:
   - disjointed thinking and fragmented speaking,
   - reduced problem-solving ability, and
   - difficulty with concept formation.

   Most of these effects seem to share in common an impairment of short-term memory, which in turn can lead to a loss in one's train of thought.
3. Marijuana use can contribute to:
   - social withdrawal and
   - general lack of motivation, therefore preteens and adolescents are disabled in forming their personal identities as they disengage from childhood attachments and parental controls to form new relationships and values.
4. As teenagers and young adults begin to experience heightened sexual awareness and develop their gender identities, use of marijuana can disrupt this important developmental process and cause severe sexual anxiety.
5. Many health care providers and medical organizations, including the American Academy of Pediatrics, believe that marijuana, by providing a convenient chemical escape from normal "growing pains," can prevent young people from learning to become mature, independent, and responsible adults.

Source: Derived from the National Institute on Drug Abuse, and *Marijuana: Your Child and Drugs,* 2, American Academy of Pediatrics, 1986.

Flashback

Self-reports indicate that some marijuana users experience an undesirable recurrence of the drug's intoxicating effects with no recent drug intake to explain the altered perceptions and disturbing emotions. This brief, spontaneous phenomenon is called a *flashback,* and it may range from mild puzzlement to full-blown panic. In some instances, marijuana reportedly has triggered LSD-type flashbacks in people with prior LSD experience. Although there is no pharmacological explanation of the flashbacks, reports of these somewhat frightening conditions tend to be consistent. It is probable that these bizarre effects have a psychological origin. Such occurrences might be post-traumatic reactions when the drug user is fatigued or emotionally stressed.

Mental Illness

Available data indicate that marijuana use neither causes nor worsens mental illness. As with several other drugs, though, clinical reports show a temporary association between cannabis products and the return of mental symptoms. Marijuana appears to enhance the resurfacing of *preexisting* mental disorders. Patients with a history of schizophrenia, mood disorders, and depression may be especially sensitive to marijuana's effects. Sometimes the "renewed" emotional disturbances are severe.

The Respiratory System

A major concern about marijuana smoking is its potential for harming the structure and function of the lungs. The unfiltered marijuana smoke is drawn into the lungs by way of the trachea, nasopharynx, bronchi, and alveoli—the "respiratory tree" of airway passages. Within the body, marijuana might be capable of assaulting not only the tissues of the lungs, but also specific self-cleansing and self-protective mechanisms that function in the lungs.

Unlike the tobacco cigarette, the marijuana cigarette often contains contaminants of unknown origin. Almost the entire marijuana cigarette is smoked, and the smoke is held in the lungs for a much longer time than cigarette smoke is. Moreover, the marijuana smoke contains several chemicals similar to tobacco "tars" that contribute to lung cancer. Cigarette for cigarette, a marijuana "joint" contains about 50 percent more cancer-causing hydrocarbons than a tobacco cigarette.

Other than initial coughing, the short-term response to inhaled marijuana is *bronchodilation,* the opening of various airway passages of the lungs. With heavy, daily use of cannabis products, particularly hashish, long-term extensive inflammatory changes can be seen in lung tissue lining, and measurable airway obstruction occurs. Thus chronic exposure to marijuana smoke eventually leads to *bronchoconstriction,* the narrowing of the air passages. Such a condition impairs the lungs' ability to exhale air.

Scientists at the University of California, Los Angeles, have found that the daily use of 1 to 3 marijuana cigarettes appears to produce approximately the same lung damage and potential cancer risk as smoking five times as many tobacco cigarettes. Biopsies of human lung tissues chronically exposed to marijuana smoke revealed abnormal cellular changes suggestive of precancerous and cancerous conditions. Results of this study also suggest that the way smokers inhale marijuana—more deeply, and holding it longer, than tobacco smoke—in addition to its chemical composition, increases the adverse physical effects. Experimental studies also indicate that the combination of tobacco and marijuana smoke is likely to have a greater cancer-causing potential than either substance used alone.

The Cardiovascular System

The term *cardiovascular* refers to the heart and blood vessels. Research indicates that during the marijuana high there are changes in the heart and circulation of the blood that are typical of stress. Marijuana increases the work of the human heart by increasing heart rate as much as 50 percent and by moderately increasing blood pressure in some people. However, research suggests that these changes are without permanently harmful effects on normal hearts and blood vessels. Marijuana's effects on the cardiovascular system are insignificant among healthy people, and even seem to become less severe following long-term exposure. Smoking marijuana while "shooting up" cocaine, however, has the potential to cause severe and rapid increases in heart rate and blood pressure that could overload the cardiovascular system.

Any temporary increase in the workload of the heart poses a definite threat to patients with hypertension, cerebrovascular disease, and coronary atherosclerosis—serious disorders of the cardiovascular system. In individuals with heart disease, the use of marijuana may trigger chest pain (angina pectoris) more rapidly and following less effort than smoking tobacco does.

Reproduction and Sexual Function

The alleged effects of marijuana on human sexual function and reproduction have been widely reported in the media. Some of the research in these areas involved humans, but much of the scientific investigation has been conducted on animals. Thus the application of research findings to human physiology is somewhat uncertain and unclear.

Various studies indicate that marijuana has a suppressive action upon the function of the testes in animals and men. A reduction in the weights of the prostate gland, seminal vesicle, and testis; reduced sperm production; and lowered levels of testosterone (the principal male sex hormone) have been recorded following chronic use of cannabis or THC. Such effects are thought to be temporary and completely reversed one month after use of the drug is discontinued, because long-term reductions in male fertility and sexual performance have not been reported.

Additional research has not confirmed initial findings regarding lowered testosterone levels associated with marijuana use. In some experiments no change in blood levels of testosterone was recorded, whereas other research revealed an increase in hormone levels. Such conflicting and incomplete evidence prevents a definite statement on marijuana's effect upon testosterone. Still other studies have indicated that the sperm of chronic marijuana users are defective and nonfunctional. Decreased male fertility may be more closely related to abnormal sperm structure and impaired sperm movement than to reduced sperm count.

Few studies have been undertaken to determine the hormone profiles and menstrual patterns of women who use marijuana on a long-term and frequent basis. This situation is based on the several ethical issues surrounding research involving females of childbearing age. As a consequence, information on female reproductive and sexual functioning is scarce.

The first controlled study in women on the acute effects of marijuana, reported by the National Institute on Drug Abuse, has shown that smoking marijuana after ovulation decreases the blood plasma level of luteinizing hormone (LH), essential for implantation of the fertilized egg in the uterus. A single dose of marijuana during the luteal phase of the menstrual cycle suppressed the level of luteinizing hormone and suggests the possibility that long-term use of marijuana may adversely affect reproductive functioning in women.

THC is considered a potential **teratogen** (an agent that causes defects in a developing embryo) because it can cross the placenta of a pregnant female. Reports indicate that low birth weight, prematurity, and a specific condition resembling fetal alcohol syndrome—the "fetal substance syndrome"—occur in some children of women who smoke marijuana heavily during pregnancy.

Total abstention from marijuana seems most advisable for women during pregnancy because of the many unproven variables and the potential for harm. Smoking only one joint results in high-risk, prolonged fetal exposure to marijuana.

The Immune System

Various structural, cellular, and chemical defense mechanisms help protect the human body against assault. The mechanism that specifically protects an individual from disease-causing bacteria, viruses, molds, and toxins is the immune system. Animal studies indicate that THC has a mild, adverse, suppressant effect on the immune system, which would reduce the germ-fighting ability of the body. Human studies have produced contradictory results: Some marijuana users demonstrated a mild **immunosuppressive effect,** while other chronic marijuana smokers developed no significant differences in their immune systems in comparison with nonsmoking subjects.

In Conclusion

There is sufficient evidence that marijuana has a broad range of physical, psychological, and behavioral effects, some of which can be harmful to human health. Available information does not indicate how serious the risk may be. Of growing concern is the realization that marijuana, its THC metabolites, and other cannabinoids remain in the human body up to thirty days or longer after smoking. How disruptive and health threatening these residual chemical compounds might be is speculative.

According to the prestigious Institute of Medicine, what little is known for certain about the effects of marijuana on human health—and all that researchers have reason to suspect—justifies serious national concern. Although it does not appear to be as poisonous or lethal as ethyl alcohol, marijuana might eventually prove to be as life threatening as tobacco cigarettes.

Medical Uses of Marijuana

For thousands of years, people have used marijuana for numerous medical purposes. It is probable that the ancient Chinese first employed the cannabis plant as a therapy; other cultures throughout history have followed.

In the United States, until the Marijuana Tax Act of 1937 classified marijuana as an illegal narcotic and made the prescription of cannabis products difficult, marijuana was contained in nearly thirty medical products. As a pharmaceutical product, marijuana also fell into disfavor with the introduction of new, faster-acting, and dose-controlled synthetic drugs.

Modern scientific study of cannabis as a healing agent did not begin until the nineteenth century, but continued despite controversy until the early 1900s, when serious investigation of marijuana's therapeutic value was abandoned. Research was not resumed until cannabis and its derivatives emerged in the 1960s as popular, though illegal, "recreational" drugs.

Synthetic THC

In 1965, THC was synthesized and later proven to be the major psychoactive ingredient of marijuana. Then in 1985 the United States Food and Drug Administration (FDA) approved a version of this synthetic THC, called dronabinol. Marketed under the trade name Marinol, this synthetic THC was approved as a Schedule II controlled substance and prescription drug for relieving nausea accompanying cancer chemotherapy.[28]

More recently, Marinol has also been designated an "orphan drug" by the FDA for use as a medication to stimulate appetite in AIDS patients, who often experience a severe loss of weight. (Orphan drug status is conferred on certain medicines to encourage pharmaceutical companies to develop drug treatments for rare diseases.)[29]

In reaction to both public and political pressure during the 1970s, the FDA and the Drug Enforcement Administration established a tightly controlled, experimental program to make not only THC capsules but also natural, cultivated marijuana cigarettes available to physicians who wanted to use marijuana as an *antiemetic,* a drug that prevents nausea and vomiting.

Though still classified as a Schedule I controlled substance, and therefore still illegal, marijuana is approved for medical use in thirty-six states. However, federal laws have made it difficult for states to implement their own legislation.

Legalization of Medical Marijuana

Legal efforts to give natural pot a legal status continue because the experimental federal program provided free cultivated marijuana to the seriously ill. In 1991, however, the U.S. Department of Health and Human Services began phasing out this approved medical use, because it undercut official administration policy against the use of illegal drugs. Though a small number of patients already receiving marijuana will continue to do so, new applicants have been encouraged to try synthetic THC instead.

Box 11.3 States Take First Step to Legalize Marijuana as Medicine

In 1996, *California* voters approved *Proposition 215*, summarized here, to:

1. Ensure that seriously ill citizens have the right to obtain and use marijuana for medical purposes where that medical use is deemed appropriate and has been recommended by a physician who has determined that the person's health would benefit from the use of marijuana in the treatment of cancer, anorexia, AIDS, chronic pain, spasticity, glaucoma, arthritis, migraine, or any other illness for which marijuana provides relief.
2. Ensure that patients and their primary caregivers who obtain and use marijuana for medical purposes upon the recommendation of a physician are not subject to criminal prosecution or sanction.

In 1996, *Arizona* voters also approved a similar measure, *Proposition 200,* summarized here, to:

Permit doctors to prescribe Schedule I controlled substances such as marijuana to treat disease or to relieve pain and suffering of seriously and terminally ill patients.

Nevertheless, in 1996, voters in California and Arizona approved the legalization of marijuana as medicine (see box 11.3). Apparently, mercy for sick and terminally ill patients outweighed fears over drug abuse.

Federal law still bans the possession, cultivation, marketing, and prescription of marijuana for any purpose, therefore the impact of these new state laws is uncertain. Regardless of state law, those experimenting with marijuana are subject to federal arrest. Physicians prescribing or advising patients to use marijuana risk losing their licenses to use other federally controlled drugs in their medical practice. There will likely be many court challenges to these state laws, because they do not supersede federal law.

Critics of these medical marijuana laws fear that legalization will result in greater cultivation and availability of the drug, easy diversion of the drug for recreational use, more use and abuse of pot, and an increasing threat to public safety.

Therapeutic Value

When smoked, given intravenously, or taken orally, cannabis, THC, and other cannabinoid derivatives appear to have definite therapeutic effects for a number of disorders, including glaucoma, nausea and vomiting, asthma, epilepsy, muscle spasticity, anxiety, depression, pain, reduced appetite, and withdrawal from alcohol and narcotics. While marijuana's potential as a medical drug has been demonstrated in some of these areas, the dose needed to produce the desired therapeutic effect is often close to the amount that produces unacceptable and undesirable side effects.

Many in the medical profession oppose the use of marijuana as medicine, because the drug affects so many organ systems of the human body. As a consequence, marijuana is not an ideal medical treatment. Moreover, in each instance of proposed therapy, other drugs are more consistently effective and have fewer side effects than marijuana

Yet, one of marijuana's greatest therapeutic advantages is its safety factor. There is no known case of lethal overdose. Marijuana is also less addictive than many drugs used as muscle relaxants, hypnotics, and analgesics.[30] Moreover cannabis has been found to exert its beneficial effects through mechanisms differing from those of other drugs. As a consequence, it is possible that some patients not helped by conventional therapies could be treated successfully with marijuana.

Additionally, cannabis might be combined effectively and safely with other drugs to produce a treatment goal, but with each drug used at a much lower dose than would be required if either were used alone.

Glaucoma

The leading cause of blindness in the United States is **glaucoma,** a disease characterized by increased pressure within the eye. This pressure damages the optic nerve and leads eventually to loss of vision. Cannabis, THC, and other cannabinoid derivatives have been found to reduce the vision-threatening intraocular pressure of glaucoma. However, undesirable physical and psychological side effects have been demonstrated, especially among older patients. Synthetic-THC eye drops have undergone testing with the hope that they can reduce unwanted side effects. Despite its beneficial effects for some patients, marijuana neither prevents glaucoma nor improves vision.

Chemotherapy-Caused Nausea and Vomiting

One of the more promising clinical uses of marijuana has been in the treatment of extreme nausea for patients undergoing cancer chemotherapy—the use of drugs to kill cancer cells. Cancer chemotherapy can produce increased survival in patients with certain cancers, so the nausea and vomiting that interfere with a person's willingness to continue therapy, in effect, become life-threatening side effects. THC and other cannabis derivatives have been proven effective in controlling these undesirable symptoms and are considered to be antiemetics—substances that tend to prevent nausea and vomiting. Some patients (especially older cancer patients), though, report having adverse anxiety/panic reactions, while others show little or no favorable antiemetic response.

However, marijuana may be losing ground as an antiemetic with the approval of a new, powerful, and effective antiemetic drug, odansetron, marketed as Zofran.[31] Odansetron produces no adverse side effects on functioning, no impairment of short-term memory, and no impairment of normal operation of a motor vehicle, as are sometimes experienced with medical marijuana.

Additional Medical Uses

Several actions of marijuana and its derivatives are presently being investigated for possible therapeutic applications. These are:

Appetite stimulant—Social users often report that smoking marijuana increases the appetite. Research suggests that there may well be a stimulating influence on food intake in advanced cancer patients who use marijuana as an antiemetic in conjunction with chemotherapy. Such an effect tends to overcome or reduce the severity of debilitating weight loss in such patients and in those with AIDS-related weight loss.

Anticonvulsant action—Limited human studies confirm results of animal research suggesting that specific components of marijuana—cannabinol and cannabidiol—protect against minimal and maximal seizures characteristic of epilepsy.

Antiasthmatic effect—As indicated earlier in this chapter, the long-term smoking of concentrated marijuana produces a constriction or obstruction of the airways. However, oral intake of THC has actually produced a bronchodilation effect in healthy individuals and in patients with bronchial asthma. Cannabinoid compounds, such as cannabinol and cannabidiol, do not produce psychological effects or alterations in heart function commonly seen with marijuana. Therefore, these two compounds are potentially useful for their airway-expanding effect in the treatment of asthma.

Muscle-relaxant action—Limited studies suggest that THC is effective in relieving the muscle spasms or spasticity common in patients with multiple sclerosis.

Antianxiety effect—Although marijuana use often reduces anxiety, it sometimes produces undesirable psychological effects, including panic and anxiety. In addition, there is no indication that marijuana is any more effective or reliable than currently available antianxiety medicine.

Antidepressant effect—There is no controlled research indicating that marijuana reduces depression with any degree of consistency. Widespread use of marijuana for this reason would appear to be inappropriate.

Analgesic action—Test subjects demonstrating marijuana's analgesic (pain-relieving) effects also tended to experience "mental clouding" and other undesirable pharmacological effects. It is not likely that marijuana will be any more effective than currently available noncannabis analgesics.

Treatment for drug abuse—Research has failed to find marijuana useful in treating alcoholism. Moreover, there is no evidence that cannabis is likely to be more effective than currently available treatments for opiate withdrawal.

While marijuana has not been determined to be superior to any existing treatment for any of the conditions identified, the therapeutic potential of cannabis and its derivatives merits continued research.

Chapter Summary

1. Marijuana is a derivative of the hemp plant, *Cannabis sativa*. Marijuana is a unique psychoactive drug because at different dose levels it produces sedative, then psychedelic, effects.
2. Throughout history, the cannabis plant has had a variety of commercial and medical uses, in addition to its status as a recreational intoxicant.
3. The Marijuana Tax Act of 1937 effectively banned the nonmedical possession and use of cannabis preparations in America. Eventually, simple possession was reduced from a felony to a misdemeanor.
4. Several states decriminalized simple possession of small amounts of marijuana, thereby reducing the penalty to a minor misdemeanor or civil offense. However, the penalties for trafficking remain harsh, and one state has already recriminalized possession.
5. Antiparaphernalia laws control or prohibit the sale and/or advertising of marijuana-related items, such as pipes, bongs, roach clips, spoons, and roll-your-own cigarette papers.
6. Hundreds of chemicals have been identified in marijuana, but the principal psychoactive cannabinoid is THC. When marijuana is smoked, THC is readily absorbed by the blood in the lungs and transported rapidly to the brain. The THC content of today's marijuana is many times higher and more potent than that in marijuana samples during the 1960s and 1970s.
7. The marijuana "high" from low to moderate doses is a sense of well-being, euphoria, relaxation, and a dreamlike state. Common reactions include changes in sensory perception; alterations in thought formation, emotions, and personal identity; and pleasurable introspection or gregariousness.
8. Adverse "acute effects" relate to motor coordination, reaction time, tracking ability, cue detection, short-term memory, time sense, and oral communication.
9. The use of marijuana at typical social levels definitely impairs driving ability and related skills.
10. Some users report having bad trips, whereas frequent continuous use develops tolerance and nonlife-threatening withdrawal, sometimes involving compulsive drug-seeking behavior.
11. Areas of concern related to long-term effects of using marijuana include the amotivational syndrome; flashback;

resurfacing of preexisting mental disorders; potential for harming lung structure and function; temporary increase in workload of the heart; and the possible suppressant effect on testes, the male sex hormone, female reproductive function, and the human immune system.

12. Pregnant women are advised to abstain completely from marijuana because THC is also a potential teratogen (an agent that causes defects in embryonic life).

13. Possible medical uses of marijuana include treating glaucoma, chemotherapy-caused nausea and vomiting, and AIDS-related weight loss.

14. The movement to legalize medical marijuana places state laws in conflict with federal law that prohibits the possession, cultivation, marketing, and prescription of this psychoactive drug. Federal law supersedes state law, so there will likely be many court challenges to the legalization of marijuana for medical purposes.

World Wide Web Sites

Marijuana Anonymous World Services

www.marijuana-anonymous.org

National Organization for the Reform of Marijuana Laws (NORML)

www.natlnorml.org

Review Questions and Activities

1. What is marijuana, and how does it differ from cannabis, hashish, and sinsemilla?
2. In what ways was marijuana used among the ancient Chinese, ancient Indians, Americans up to 1940, and Americans after 1965?
3. Do you believe the Marijuana Tax Act of 1937 has been effective in restricting the nonmedical possession and use of cannabis preparations? Support your response.
4. If you could vote to prohibit, decriminalize, or legalize the possession of small amounts of marijuana for personal use, how would you vote? What factors might influence your vote?
5. What are the penalties in your state for possessing small amounts of marijuana for personal use?
6. Define the nature and purpose of antiparaphernalia laws. Are there any such laws in your community or state?
7. Why is the nonmedical use of marijuana so often regarded as a major drug problem and a threat to American society?
8. What is THC and what effect does it have on the marijuana user?
9. What factors influence the nature and intensity of the marijuana high?
10. Do you believe that using marijuana could have an adverse effect upon driving an automobile? Be specific in your response.
11. Explain what is meant by "state-dependent learning." Relate this phenomenon to using marijuana.
12. What evidence exists in support of the amotivational syndrome resulting from use of marijuana?
13. Compare the effects of smoking marijuana on the human respiratory system with the effects of smoking tobacco on the same body system.
14. Discuss the possible adverse effects that use of marijuana might have on human reproduction and sexual function.
15. What specific properties of marijuana make it useful as a therapeutic drug?
16. Based upon your knowledge of your community or school/college, do you believe that the use of marijuana constitutes a major drug problem? What evidence might be offered in support of your response?
17. Can you identify any popular entertainment figures who promote or encourage the use of marijuana or other drugs? Do you think they are successful? What might their motives be?
18. Explain why so many people use marijuana despite its illegal status and controversial reputation.

References

1. H. Thomas Milhorn, *Drug and Alcohol Abuse* (New York: Plenum Press, 1994), 301.
2. Ernest L. Abel, *Marihuana: The First Twelve Thousand Years* (New York: Plenum Press, 1980).
3. Edward R. Bloomquist, *Marijuana: The Second Trip*, rev. ed. (Beverly Hills, Calif.: Glencoe Press, 1971), 14–15.
4. J. Terry Parker, ". . . And the Grass Keeps Growing: A Brief History of Marijuana Use through the 1600s," *Eta Sigma Gamman* 20, no. 2 (spring 1989): 17–19.
5. National Commission on Marihuana and Drug Abuse, *Marihuana: A Signal of Misunderstanding* (Washington, D.C.: GPO, 1972), 29.
6. "Marijuana: Examining the New Pot Culture," *The Bottom Line on Alcohol in Society* 17, no. 1 (spring 1996): 75–78.
7. Lester Grinspoon and James Bakalar, *The Harvard Medical School Mental Health Review: Drug Abuse and Addiction* (Boston: Harvard Mental Health Letter, 1993), 32.
8. "Marijuana: A Recurring Problem," *Prevention Pipeline* 8, no. 5 (September/October 1995): 1–2.
9. Office of National Drug Control Policy, *The National Drug Control Strategy: 1996* (Washington, D.C.: Executive Office of the President, 1996), 35.
10. Office of Justice Programs, Bureau of Justice Statistics, U.S. Department of Justice, *Drugs, Crime, and the Justice System* (Washington, D.C.: GPO, 1992), 50.
11. Tibor Palfai and Henry Jankiewicz, *Drugs and Human Behavior* (Dubuque, Iowa: Brown & Benchmark, 1991), 452.
12. Barry Stimmel and the editors of Consumer Reports Books, *The Facts about Drug Use: Coping with Drugs and Alcohol in your Family, at Work, in Your Community* (New York: Hawarth Medical Press, 1993), 126.
13. Danielle Hain, *Datafax Information Series: Drug Testing* (Tempe, Ariz.: Do It Now Foundation, 1996), 3; Office of Justice Programs, Bureau of Justice Statistics, U.S.

Department of Justice, *Drugs, Crime, and the Justice System* (Washington, D.C.: GPO, 1992), 115–19; and "Window for Marijuana Detection Called Shorter Than Assumed," *Drug Detection Report* 5, no. 14 (20 October 1995): 1–3.

14. Craig Zwerling, James Ryan, and Endel Orav, "The Efficacy of Preemployment Drug Screening for Marijuana and Cocaine in Predicting Employment Outcome," *Journal of the American Medical Association* 264, no. 20 (28 November 1990): 2639–43.
15. Drug Enforcement Administration, U.S. Department of Justice, *Drugs of Abuse* (Washington, D.C.: GPO, 1989), 45.
16. Charles O'Brien, "Drug Addiction and Drug Abuse," chap. 24 in *Goodman & Gilman's The Pharmacological Basis of Therapeutics,* 9th ed. (New York: McGraw-Hill Health Professions Division, 1996), 572.
17. Jerome Jaffe, "Drug Addiction and Drug Abuse," chap. 22 in *Goodman and Gilman's The Pharmacological Basis of Therapeutics,* 8th ed., ed. A. G. Gilman and others (New York: McGraw-Hill, 1990), 550.
18. Gesina Longenecker, *How Drugs Work* (Emeryville, Calif.: Ziff-Davis Press, 1994), 100–101.
19. Council on Scientific Affairs, American Medical Association, "Marijuana: Its Health Hazards and Therapeutic Potentials," *Journal of the American Medical Association* 246, no. 16 (16 October 1981): 1823–27; Committee to Study the Health-Related Effects of Cannabis and Its Derivatives, Institute of Medicine, *Marijuana and Health* (Washington, D.C.: National Academy Press, 1982), 26–27, 112–28; National Institute on Drug Abuse, "Marijuana Update," *NIDA Capsules,* May 1989, 1–3; and Harrison Pope and Deborah Yurgelun-Todd, "The Residual Cognitive Effects of Heavy Marijuana Use in College Students," *Journal of the American Medical Association* 275, no. 7 (21 February 1996): 521–27.
20. Harold Doweiko, *Concepts of Chemical Dependency,* 2d ed. (Pacific Grove, Calif.: Brooks/Cole, 1993), 101.
21. American Psychiatric Association, *Diagnostic and Statistical Manual of Mental Disorders,* 4th ed. (Washington, D.C.: American Psychiatric Association, 1994), 218; and Norman Miller, *The Pharmacology of Alcohol and Drugs of Abuse and Addiction* (New York: Springer-Verlag, 1991), 200.
22. Robert Julien, *A Primer of Drug Action,* 7th ed. (New York: W. H. Freeman and Company, 1995), 349.
23. "Marijuana: Its Uses and Effects," *Prevention Pipeline* 8, no. 5 (September/October 1995): 3–5.
24. "Marijuana Addiction: The Legacy of the '60s?" *Substance Abuse Report* 22, no. 5 (1 March 1989): 1–2.
25. Committee to Study the Health-Related Effects of Cannabis and Its Derivatives, *Marijuana and Health,* 57–106, 124–26.
26. O'Brien, "Drug Addiction and Drug Abuse," 572.
27. Grinspoon and Bakalar, *The Harvard Medical School Mental Health Review,* 31–32; and Christina Dye, *Marijuana: Personality and Behavior* (Tempe, Ariz.: Do It Now, 1994), 3.
28. Jim Parker, *Marijuana: Medical Uses* (Tempe, Ariz.: Do It Now, 1994), 3–4.
29. "Synthetic THC Approved for Treatment of AIDS-Related Weight Loss, *Substance Abuse Report* 22, no. 6 (15 March 1991): 5.
30. Lester Grinspoon and James Bakalar, "Marihuana as Medicine," *Journal of the American Medical Association* 273, no. 23 (21 June 1995): 1875–76.
31. "Survey: Other Drugs Better Than Marijuana and Marinol for Nausea," *Substance Abuse Report* 25, no. 11 (1 June 1994): 7.

Part Five

Medicines

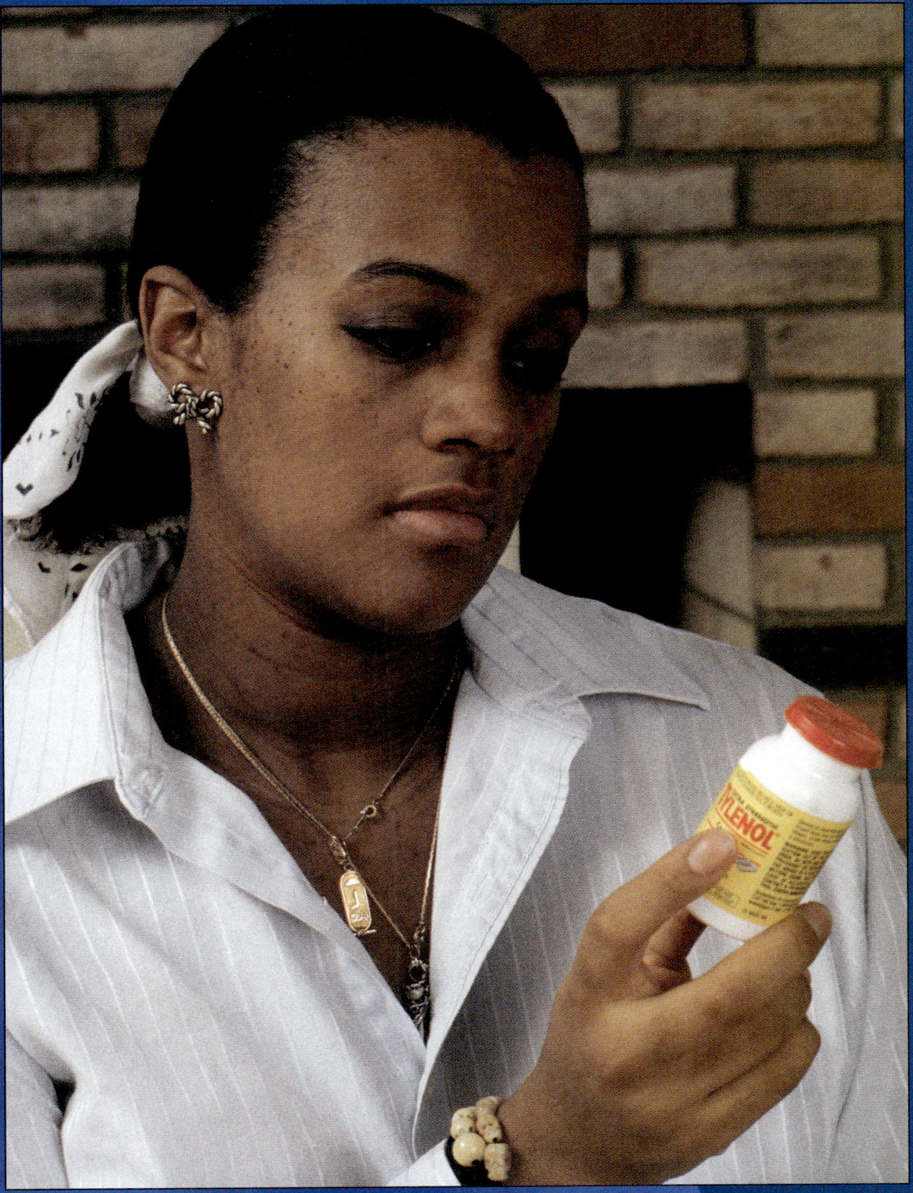

Questions of concern

1. Why do so many people believe so firmly in the concept of fail-safe medication?
2. What factors influence the selection and purchase of specific over-the-counter drugs?
3. How much government control is needed to assure drug-consuming patients that medicines are safe and effective?
4. Why do drug companies set aside a large amount of drug profits for legal costs?

Chapter 12

Over-the-counter drugs

KEY TERMS

Acetaminophen
Adverse Drug Reaction
Analgesic
Antihistamine
Appetite Suppressant
Aspirin
Brand-Name Drug
Fixed-Ratio Combination Product
Food and Drug Administration (FDA)
Generic Drug
Ibuprofen
Ketoprofen
Naproxen Sodium
Nonsalicylates
NSAID
Reye's Syndrome
Salicylates
Salicylism
Self-Limiting Condition
Self-Medication
Side Effect
Sleep Aid

chapter objectives

After you have studied this chapter, you should be able to do the following:

1. Define the key terms.
2. Explain how the use of OTC medications can become a potential hazard to a drug taker's health.
3. List several examples of drug misuse.
4. Distinguish between over-the-counter and prescription drugs in terms of their procurement, conditions of use, powerfulness, and potential for meeting individual needs of patients.
5. Compare and contrast the general drug actions or uses of the following drug classes: anorectal products, antibacterials, dermatologicals, diarrhea preparations, emetics, and nausea medications.
6. List the major anticipated effects of the following types of OTC drugs: analgesics, antipyretics, sleeping aids, stimulants, decongestants, and antihistamines.
7. Describe the similarities and differences between salicylate and nonsalicylate analgesics.
8. List at least eight guidelines for wise and relatively safe use of OTC drugs in the process of self-medication.
9. Distinguish between a drug "side effect" and an "adverse reaction" to a drug.
10. Identify at least eight items of information that must be listed on the labels of OTC medications.
11. Explain why some drugs might remain on the market despite the conclusion of the FDA OTC drug-review process that their effectiveness is doubtful.

Introduction

This chapter provides a consumer's guide to the use of over-the-counter (OTC) drugs in America. In our country the practice of self-medication is common and often beneficial, but because OTC drugs are used so widely, there is also considerable drug misuse in the general population.

Early in the chapter a distinction is made between over-the-counter drugs and those prescribed by a physician. Then a classification of OTC drugs is presented with a description of various drug classes or types, based upon the primary function of drug products in relieving minor symptoms of illness.

Several major OTC drug classes frequently used by adults are examined in detail: analgesics, appetite suppressants, cold preparations, sleep aids, and stimulants. To promote the safe and beneficial use of OTC drugs, several guidelines for sensible use are also provided.

A final section on the safety and effectiveness of nonprescribed drug products offers a special message to people who engage in self-medication and are concerned about their health.

Our Fascination with Drugs

Influenced by advertising on television and radio and in the print media, many individuals firmly believe that some miracle drug is available for almost every human ailment. Many also feel that if a physician's treatment is to be effective, the therapy must include the use of

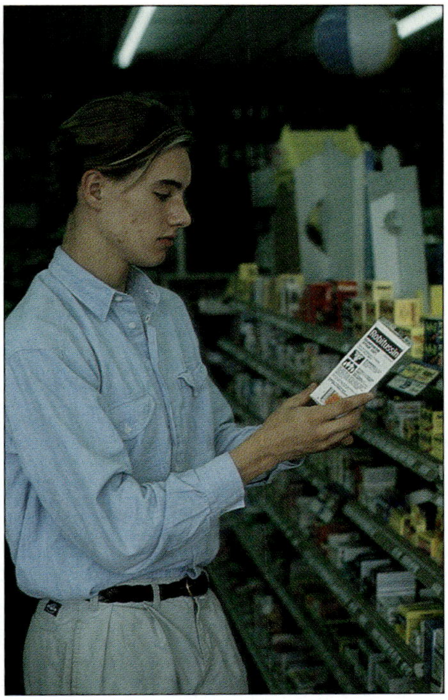

The thousands of over-the-counter medicines present the purchaser with numerous consumer choices in selecting nonprescribed drugs. What factors influence your purchase of OTC medicines?

© Dion Ogust/The Image Works

some drug. These beliefs have achieved the status of national expectations and are reflected in the continuing demand for medicines. Legitimate, reputable drug manufacturers have responded in kind to this persistent demand with hundreds of thousands of drug products designed to treat symptoms, cure, or prevent illness.

In addition to the large quantities of illegally produced and marketed drugs, billions of doses of physician-prescribed medicines and those purchased for self-treatment are used each year. By the mid-1990s, Americans were spending an estimated $50 billion each year on prescription and nonprescription medicines.[1] The price tag for our national "pill-popping" is considerable, and it is even higher when we take into account the human cost of the millions of drug-induced adverse reactions that occur each year in the United States.

Benefits and Risks

Drugs, nevertheless, remain popular because they can have wonderful effects upon the human body and mind. The drugs in medicines can aid in the diagnosis of illness; they can also be used to relieve symptoms of disease, including pain and fever. Some drugs are used to kill or inactivate disease-causing microorganisms; others—vaccines and toxoids—are employed to prevent disease.

Drugs in some medications can slow down or speed-up body functions, and suppress them entirely, as seen in the effect of oral contraceptives on the process of ovulation. While some diseases can be cured by drugs, others, including epilepsy and diabetes, can only be controlled.

However, healing and disease-preventing drugs, especially those taken by mouth, also involve potential risks. Sometimes drugs taken with the intention of restoring or improving health can harm the body and endanger life, as described in earlier chapters. Depending upon their use, certain drugs can act as poisons and intoxicants, alter the effects of other medications, and cause some undesirable and unanticipated side effects, including adverse drug reactions and drug dependencies.

People have continued to spend billions of dollars for nonprescription drugs despite that the U.S. Food and Drug Administration identified—and then banned—over two hundred ingredients as ineffective.[2] In addition, evidence of improper labeling, listing of ineffective drugs as active ingredients, and inadequate warnings about proper use and possible adverse reactions all suggest that safety and effectiveness are not guaranteed absolutely.[3]

Though a drug may be "generally recognized as safe" (GRAS), it isn't necessarily safe for everyone. A drug "generally recognized as effective" (GRAE) is not guaranteed to be completely effective for everyone. Those most at risk are the young, the elderly, pregnant women, and patients being treated for long-term diseases.

Drug Misuse

Equally alarming and life-threatening is the occurrence of *drug misuse,* the widespread inappropriate use of medicines resulting in impaired physical, mental, emotional, or social well-being. Drug misuse involves taking medications in excess of recommended doses, not following directions regarding time intervals between doses or other conditions of use specified on the drug label, and providing personally prescribed medicines to other individuals. (Other examples of drug misuse have been identified in chapter 1.) Sometimes the drug misuser is lucky and no adverse reactions occur. On occasion, though, such drug-misuse practices can have tragic consequences.

Over-the-Counter Versus Prescribed Drugs

As determined by the federal **Food and Drug Administration (FDA),** drugs are classified into two groups: (1) *over-the-counter medicines,* and (2) *prescription medicines.*

Over-the-counter, or *OTC, drugs* include that vast assortment of medications that can be purchased without a physician's prescription. Sometimes these drugs are also known as patent medicines. Nonprescription medicines are regarded as safe if consumers follow the directions and heed the required warnings on the label. In general, OTC drugs have a relatively low risk of causing toxicity (a poisonous condition) and a high margin of safety.

More than 300,000 OTC drugs are on the market, and almost everybody has used them. Typically these drugs are taken or applied on a temporary basis for conditions that do not warrant a visit to a physician.

OTC drugs are sold widely at pharmacies, supermarkets, and department stores. Such drugs include everything from a bar of antibacterial soap to a nighttime sleep aid, headache remedy, or antacid preparation. When directions and warnings on OTC drug labels are followed, most people can use the medicines with relative safety and with beneficial results.

However, OTC drugs rarely, if ever, cure any illness or disease. The major effect of these nonprescription drugs is to relieve minor symptoms of illness, such as headache or menstrual cramping. For example, a cold remedy might make a person feel more comfortable by reducing sniffles and sneezes, but the cold will last as long as it would with no medicine.

In effect, many OTC medicines cover up the signals from the body—the symptoms that usually alert people to take some corrective action. Therefore, OTC drugs should never be used on a regular basis over an extended period. If symptoms persist, an appointment should be made with one's family physician, who can identify and treat the basic problem underlying the symptoms.

Prescription drugs can be obtained only by the direction of a physician. Bearing the *Rx* symbol on their labels, these prescribed drugs can be sold only by a registered pharmacist. Defined primarily as unsafe for use except under professional medical supervision, prescription drugs include certain habit-forming substances and any other drug that is unsafe due to its toxicity or potential for causing a harmful effect, its method of use, or related measures necessary to its proper use.[4]

Classification of OTC Drugs

The following classification of OTC drugs has been established by the OTC drug review process of the FDA. Unless otherwise indicated, examples of specific drug classes were derived from the *Physicians' Desk Reference for Nonprescription Drugs.* Brand names of drugs appear within parentheses, as capitalized, or are referred to specifically as OTC drug preparations.

Allergy relief products—These relieve symptoms of sneezing; watery nose and eyes; itching of the nose, mouth, and throat; headache; irritability; insomnia; and lack of appetite associated with an allergy (a special sensitivity to some ordinary, harmless substance).

Symptoms of allergies are often treated by OTC antihistamines (drugs that block histamine secretion responsible for excess mucus production, tissue swelling, sneezing, and itchy nose and throat), and decongestants (drugs that open stuffed noses). These are among the same drug preparations used in relieving symptoms of the common cold (Actifed, Allerest, Benadryl, Chlor-Trimeton, Contac, Coricidin, Dimetapp, Dristan, Drixoral, Sudafed, Teldrin).

Analgesics—These provide relief of minor aches and pain, and tend to bring down a fever. The most popular of these nonprescription pain relievers are aspirin, acetaminophen, ibuprofen, and naproxen sodium. (This drug class will be examined more fully later in this chapter.)

Anorectal products—These are OTC ointments, creams, foams, and suppositories that provide temporary relief of symptoms associated with hemorrhoids (enlarged, swollen, knotted veins of the lower portion of the rectum and the tissues about the anus) and other anorectal disorders.

Drugs containing a local anesthetic, benzocaine, may relieve pain, irritation, itching, or burning; protectant drugs (calamine and mineral oil) provide a coating over inflamed tissues and relieve itching; counterirritants (menthol in aqueous solution) detract from the sensation of pain; astringent drugs, zinc oxide and witch hazel lotion, relieve irritation and burning; and keratolytics, such as alcloxa, tend to relieve itching. These OTC products are primarily for the relief of symptoms and not the treatment of disease (Anusol, Medicone, Nupercainal ointment, and Preparation H suppositories).

Antacids—These relieve symptoms of heartburn, sour stomach, and/or acid indigestion by neutralizing stomach acid or stopping the production of irritating digestive chemical enzymes. These products are available in tablets, liquids, powders, and capsules and in combinations with pain relievers and antiflatulents (drugs that relieve or prevent the formation of gas or flatulence in the stomach or intestine).

Most of the OTC antacids contain one or more of the following active ingredients: sodium bicarbonate, calcium carbonate, aluminum hydroxide, and magnesium hydroxide. The newer and heavily advertised H_2 antagonistic drugs, such as, Axid, Pepcid AC, Tagamet HB, and Zantac 75, work by suppressing the secretion of stomach acid in the digestive tract.

Antibacterials and antiseptics—These are usually used to treat infections caused by bacteria and include antimicrobial skin cleansers, topical antiseptics applied to the skin to destroy bacteria (Campho-Phenique, Bactine), and topical antibiotics, also applied to the skin as first aid to help prevent bacterial infection in minor cuts, scrapes, and burns (Mycitracin, Neosporin, Polysporin).

Appetite suppressants—These are weight-control preparations, such as diet pills, that reduce an individual's desire to eat food (see pages 262-263).

Arthritis medications—These are used in the treatment of arthritic conditions to reduce the pain and inflammation associated with these illnesses. Many physicians still consider OTC aspirin (acetylsalicylic acid) the drug of first choice for arthritic diseases. Aspirin not only reduces arthritic pain but also reduces inflammation in joint tissues and surrounding structures. The anti-inflammatory action counteracts the cause of pain. In addition to plain aspirin, acetylsalicylic acid also comes in buffered formulas to reduce gastritis (Ascriptin, Arthritis Pain Formula, Bufferin).

By contrast, acetaminophen products relieve pain and reduce fever, but they do not produce the anti-inflammatory effects sought in antirheumatic medications. The anti-inflammatory effects of OTC ibuprofen and naproxen sodium drugs are usually equivalent to those of aspirin.

Asthma preparations—These are drugs that increase or widen the caliber (diameter) of the air passages within the lungs. OTC medications containing bronchodilators, such as epinephrine, epinephrine bitartrate, and racepinephrine hydrochloride, cause tightened air passageways in the lungs to expand, thus relieving shortness of breath and an acute sense of suffocation symptomatic of asthma (Bronkaid Mist, Primatene Mist).

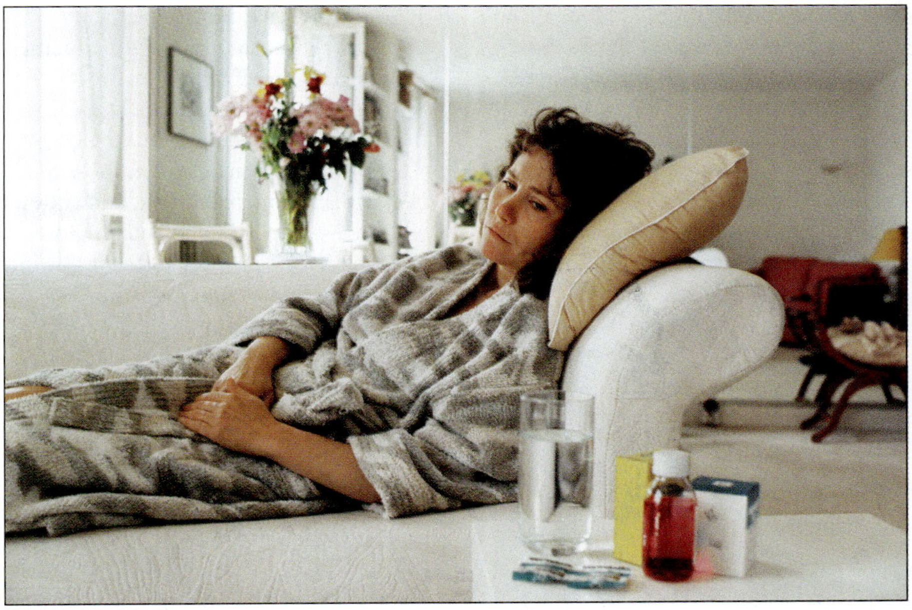

Over-the-counter cold relief medications do not cure the common cold; they merely suppress some of the symptoms.

© Didier Ermakoff/The Image Works

Cold preparations—These provide relief for symptoms of the common cold. Typical OTC remedies include antihistamines; decongestants; and combinations of these medications with analgesics, cough suppressants, and expectorants. However, none of these drugs or combinations can cure a cold. (This drug classification will be examined more fully later in this chapter.)

Contraceptives—These include OTC gels, foams, suppositories, jellies, and vaginal inserts. A related product category includes OTC pregnancy tests (Advance, Clearblue Easy, Daisy 2, e.p.t. Stick Test, First Response).

Cough preparations—These are drugs that suppress coughing; they are referred to as antitussives (Benylin cough syrup, Halls Mentho-Lyptus cough tablets, Robitussin, Sudafed cough syrup, TheraFlu, Vicks Formula 44M multisymptom cough medicine). Some of these remedies for coughing also contain an expectorant that tends to loosen and liquefy mucus in the bronchial airways and thus makes the phlegm easier to cough up (Benylin expectorant, Fedahist, Naldecon, Novahistine, Triaminic expectorant). Some OTC cough preparations are combinations of antitussives, expectorants, antihistamines, and decongestants.

Dental preparations—These include anticavity and antitartar agents, such as toothpastes, gels, fluoride rinses, antiseptic and anesthetic gels, and denture preparations.

Dermatologicals—These are products applied to the skin for relief of various skin disorders, and include facial scrubs, acne preparations (Acnomel,Clearasil), topical analgesics (Americaine, Aspercreme, Icy Hot Cream, Therapeutic Mineral Ice), topical anesthetics (Bactine, Dermoplast, Solarcaine), antiperspirants, bath oils, burn relief medications (A & D Ointment, Nupercainal Pain Relief, Polysporin Spray), dandruff medications and shampoos, dermatitis relief drugs (Aqua Care lotion, Aveeno lotion, CaldeCORT cream, Cortaid lotion, Desitin ointment), fungicides (Cruex, Desenex, Micatin, Tinactin), sunburn preparations, sunscreens, and wound cleansers.

Diarrhea medications—These control or relieve the abnormally frequent passage of watery stools (feces). Diarrhea is usually a self-limiting condition, often without an identifiable cause. Commonly used OTC preparations, such as kaolin and pectin mixtures, are usually less effective than prescribed opioids.[5] These prescription drugs are narcotics or closely related synthetic derivatives.

However, liquid and tablet forms of loperamide (Imodium), an opioid, are available OTC. Although the FDA has not favored the use of bismuth subsalicylate as an antidiarrheal drug, it has been proven somewhat effective in conferring a degree of protection from "traveler's diarrhea"—diarrhea that often occurs when people travel in other countries.[6] Bismuth subsalicylate is the major active ingredient in Pepto-Bismol, an OTC preparation.

Laxatives—These promote or induce defecation or bowel movements, and are usually used to relieve constipation. Most medical authorities, however, recommend nondrug remedies or preventives, including the addition of fiber or roughage to one's diet, increasing liquid consumption, and getting more physical exercise.

Laxatives are usually classified according to their method of action in causing stool evacuation and are marketed as bulkformers, stimulants, salts, hyperosmotics (water attracters), lubricants, stool softeners, and carbon-dioxide-releasing agents.

Mouthwashes—These are oral hygiene aids consisting of antimicrobial or antiseptic mouthwashes or anesthetic sprays, drops, or lozenges that may temporarily reduce bacteria in the mouth, freshen the breath, or relieve mouth and gum discomfort or pain associated with minor sore throat (Chloraseptic Spray, Listerine Antiseptic, Listermint Mouthwash).

Nausea medications—Known as antiemetics, these tend to prevent unpleasant gastric sensations resulting in vomiting, and reduce motion sickness (Dramamine, Emetrol, Pepto-Bismol).

Sleep aids—Originally these were promoted as drugs that would reduce nervousness during daytime and relieve sleeplessness. Presently, these nonprescription medications are used only to help people fall asleep, and they contain antihistamine ingredients that cause drowsiness. (This drug class will be examined more fully later in this chapter.)

Stimulants—These tend to increase physical activity (motor performance) and mental alertness. Most OTC stimulant drugs are composed primarily of caffeine. (This drug class will be examined more fully later in this chapter.)

Vitamins and minerals—These are substances that regulate various normal biochemical reactions within the body. Vitamin supplements (organic substances) might contain one or more of the following nutrients: vitamins A, C, D, E, K, B_1 B_2, B_6, B_{12}, niacin, pantothenic acid, biotin, folic acid, choline, inositol, para-aminobenzoic acid, and rutin.

Mineral supplements might contain one or more of the following inorganic substances: calcium, phosphate, magnesium, iron, zinc, copper, iodine, manganese, molybdenum, chromium, selenium, and cobalt. Also included are various dietary supplements (brewer's yeast, tonics, and liquid diet preparations).

Analgesics

Drugs taken internally to relieve pain without the loss of consciousness are referred to as **analgesics** or *painkillers.* Some OTC analgesics also act as *antipyretics* (agents that reduce fever), and as *anti-inflammatory drugs,* useful in relieving symptoms associated with arthritic diseases—pains, aches, and swelling of joints.

There are two ways of classifying OTC internal analgesics. The first is based on ingredients (the presence or absence of salicylic acid), while the second is determined by a major effect of the drugs (relief or nonrelief of inflammation). In the first classification, OTC pain relievers are identified as either **salicylate** painkillers (such as Bayer Aspirin, St. Joseph Aspirin, and generic aspirin) or **nonsalicylates,** including acetaminophen (marketed as Tylenol, Excedrin, and other brand-name products), ibuprofen (sold OTC as Advil, Motrin IB, and Nuprin), naproxen sodium (available OTC as Aleve), and ketoprofen (marketed OTC as Actron and Orudis KT).

The salicylates and nonsalicylates have been combined with other ingredients, resulting in a variety of cold remedies, antacids, decongestants, antihistamines, buffered analgesics, and medicated gums—all containing a painkiller.

The other major classification distinguishes among the several analgesics according to whether they reduce inflammation—the localized heat, redness, swelling, and pain in a body part that occurs usually in response to some injury or illness. Some of these internal analgesics also act as anti-inflammatory drugs, but not as cortisone-like medications, therefore they are referred to as nonsteroidal anti-inflammatory drugs, or **NSAIDs.**

Aspirin, ibuprofen, naproxen sodium, and ketoprofen are NSAIDs that produce their desirable effects by suppressing or blocking the action of specific prostaglandin chemicals. Such chemicals, produced naturally by the human body, contribute to the perception of pain.

Blocking the action of prostaglandins may prevent inflammation and pain. But prostaglandins also serve a protective role in the stomach. When their formation is blocked, the stomach becomes more vulnerable to irritation and ulceration.[7]

Acetaminophen, in contrast, is not a nonsteroidal anti-inflammatory drug and likely relieves pain by acting on particular nerve endings or pain centers in the brain. While acetaminophen-based analgesics are as effective as aspirin in relieving mild to moderate pain and fever, they do not reduce inflammation.

Salicylates

Until recently, **aspirin** had been the most widely known and used OTC painkiller. Belonging to a family of drugs containing *salicylic acid,* aspirin is so easily available that many people hardly consider it a drug. Others have no idea that aspirin (acetylsalicylic acid) is an active ingredient in such products as Anacin, Bufferin, Alka-Seltzer, Empirin, Ecotrin, and Vanquish. Despite the increasing use of nonsalicylate analgesics, Americans consume nearly 80 billion aspirin-containing tablets each year.

Another salicylate, magnesium salicylate, is the active ingredient in Doan's Caplets and Mobigesic Tablets, also marketed as analgesics. Both salicylates are relatively safe and effective as painkillers, fever reducers, and anti-inflammatory drugs.

However, the FDA has expressed concern about the prolonged use of these OTC drugs for treating symptoms of arthritic diseases without medical supervision. The recommended dosage of these analgesics may relieve the pain and swelling of arthritic conditions but may be insufficient to treat the disease that causes the inflammation. Improperly diagnosed and treated arthritis can lead to crippling and permanent disability.

Versatility of Aspirin

A remarkably useful drug, aspirin is valuable in the treatment of many conditions. As a painkiller, fever reducer, and anti-inflammatory drug, aspirin is present in hundreds of different OTC products on the market. When taken properly, aspirin works best on pain of mild to moderate severity, such as muscular aches, backaches, toothaches, and headaches. Using aspirin as an analgesic does not lead to physical dependency, and it is less toxic than more-powerful analgesics, and much less expensive, too. Aspirin works well for arthritis pain because it reduces swelling in joint tissues and surrounding structures. This salicylate is also helpful in treating rheumatic fever.

Although the precise mechanisms by which aspirin achieves its wide range of effects is not completely known, newly discovered benefits of this analgesic extend far beyond reducing pain, fever, and inflammation. Aspirin is sometimes used in the prevention of heart attacks (see box 12.1).

As popular and versatile as aspirin is, it does have its limitations. Aspirin may no longer be used in topical analgesics applied to the skin. Gargles containing aspirin have no therapeutic effect on a sore throat. Aspirin also has no effect on bacteria or viruses, so it will not cure a cold or the flu, or shorten the duration of either condition. By reducing fever and relieving the pain of headache and muscle aches, aspirin might allow the cold sufferer to become more active prematurely, before the self-limiting disease has run its course in a body that is resting. In this respect, aspirin can do more harm than good.

Box 12.1 New Perspectives About Aspirin and the Prevention of Heart Attack

1. Aspirin appears to prevent heart attacks by interfering with the clotting mechanism in which blood platelets clump together to form clots. Consequently, aspirin inhibits the formation of blood clots in the arteries. However, aspirin does not reverse atherosclerosis in the coronary arteries.
2. Nonaspirin analgesics, such as acetaminophen and ibuprofen, do not share aspirin's clot-preventing action.
3. Some people should not take aspirin under any circumstances, especially those who have an aspirin allergy; hypertension; asthma; or problems with wound healing, including bleeding ulcers.
4. The recommended dose for heart attack prevention might prove to be much less than one regular-strength aspirin every other day. Some researchers believe that the "ideal" daily dose may be as little as one-eighth of an aspirin. Doses larger than recommended may have the opposite effect—the formation of blood clots.
5. After considering age, gender, and other heart attack risks, the prime candidates for using aspirin as a preventive measure appear to be the following:
    a. Any male or female with a family history of heart attack and high cholesterol levels, inactive lifestyle, diabetes, and smoking cigarettes.
    b. Postmenopausal women with one or more risk factors for heart disease.
    c. Males over thirty-five with one or more risk factors besides gender, and those over forty-five with no risk factors except for gender.

Side Effects of Aspirin

Despite their history of therapeutic usefulness, aspirin and the other salicylates are not harmless. These analgesics can produce a variety of undesirable side effects, often affecting the gastrointestinal tract. Commonly reported problems include heartburn, stomach discomfort, nausea, and vomiting. In addition, aspirin may injure the stomach by causing an erosion of and bleeding from the stomach's lining.

Such a condition is evidence of a stomach ulcer, which often occurs in those who repeatedly take high doses of aspirin. To lessen the chances of such side effects, individuals are often urged to take aspirin shortly after meals.

Buffered aspirin, or aspirin coated with or combined with an antacid, may prevent some of the common side effects. The chemical "buffer" makes aspirin dissolve more quickly, thus speeding its absorption into the bloodstream. This buffering effect reduces but does not eliminate the irritating effects of aspirin on the stomach. One form of aspirin has a microfilm coating that protects the tablets from dissolving in the stomach and is less likely to cause stomach irritation. While this "enteric-coated" aspirin is dissolved in the small intestine, pain relief is somewhat delayed. However, less stomach irritation associated with taking enteric-coated aspirin is a special benefit to those on high daily doses.

Pregnant women are cautioned about taking aspirin, especially during the last three months of pregnancy. Aspirin interferes with blood clotting, so it can prolong pregnancy and labor, and cause bleeding before and after delivery. Excessive bleeding tendencies also occur in babies whose mothers use aspirin during their pregnancies.

Reye's Syndrome

Unfortunately, the unsupervised taking of aspirin continues to be a major cause of childhood poisoning, though it is no longer the leading cause of accidental poisoning and poisoning deaths in children since "childproof" containers were introduced.

However, another life-threatening aspect of aspirin use among children and teenagers has been identified. The use of salicylates (aspirin) by young people who have influenza and chicken pox has been associated with **Reye's syndrome** therefore the surgeon general has advised against the use of salicylate preparations for children and teenagers with these diseases.[8]

Reye's syndrome is a rare, acute, brain-damaging, and sometimes fatal condition. It is characterized by vomiting and lethargy that may progress to delirium and coma. The syndrome occurs commonly in young children and teenagers recovering from viral infections.

Salicylism

Salicylism, another undesirable side effect of using aspirin, is poisoning due to acetylsalicylic acid taken in excess. Overdosing with aspirin can result in a condition with symptoms such as nausea, vomiting, ringing in the ear (tinnitus), deafness, or even severe headaches.

These are warning signals that a person has taken too much aspirin. Sometimes hyperventilation, difficulty in hearing, and diarrhea may occur. Such symptoms should be sufficient reminders to stop taking the painkiller or to reduce the dosage.

Even small doses may be too much for the significant number of individuals who are aspirin-sensitive or allergic to aspirin. These people cannot tolerate aspirin; if they ingest it, they may develop minor skin itching, abdominal pain, facial swelling, swelling of the larynx or voice box, and falling blood pressure. Some may develop physiological shock and eventually die.

Nonsalicylates

Drugs that do not contain salicylic acid are known as nonsalicylates. Four common OTC analgesics are so classified and are described in this section.

Acetaminophen

At present, **acetaminophen** is the most popular nonsalicylate drug determined to be safe and effective for the relief of minor pain and as a fever reducer. However, acetaminophen does not reduce inflammation and should not be used in the treatment of arthritic symptoms except under the supervision of a physician. Consequently, its status as the top-selling ingredient of OTC painkillers is being challenged by Advil®, Motrin IB®, and other ibuprofen-based analgesics.

Derived from coal tar, acetaminophen was developed in 1893 but was not promoted widely as an aspirin substitute until the 1970s. Since then, acetaminophen sales have soared under the brand names Tylenol, Datril, Anacin-3, and Paradol. Some analgesics, such as Vanquish caplets, contain combinations of acetaminophen and aspirin.

Until the 1982 poisoning epidemic involving cyanide-laced Tylenol, this medication was the leading brand of nonprescribed analgesic, accounting for one-third of OTC analgesic sales.

Although its capsule form was recalled, Tylenol was not reformulated or renamed. It was reintroduced to the market in triple-sealed, tamper-resistant packages, and it is once again the leading nonprescription pain-killer in terms of market share. In response to the Tylenol tampering, the FDA required nonprescription drug manufacturers to package their products in sealed, tamper-resistant containers to protect consumers from contaminated medicines.

Milligram for milligram, acetaminophen has no advantage over aspirin either as a painkiller or as an antipyretic. The standard tablet for each has 325 milligrams of medication.

However, acetaminophen is less irritating to the stomach than aspirin. The aspirin substitute can be used safely by those allergic to aspirin. Moreover, acetaminophen does not cause stomach bleeding or affect blood clotting and is stable in liquid preparations.

Although acetaminophen is free of most of the side effects of the salicylates, an overdose can result in permanent liver damage. This is especially true in people who combine acetaminophen with alcohol use. Severe and possibly fatal liver disease may occur within two to four days of an acetaminophen overdose, without any warning symptoms of toxicity. Unfortunately, an overdose of this aspirin substitute does not cause a ringing in the ears or any other abnormal condition or easily recognized symptom as experienced in salicylism.

Ibuprofen

A prescription-only pain killer until 1984, **ibuprofen** is now a widely available and effective OTC analgesic. Its popularity is linked to its convenience, because only one or two OTC ibuprofen tablets can reduce inflammation as well as a dozen aspirin tablets. Ibuprofen is designated as a nonsteroidal anti-inflammatory drug (NSAID) because of this particular effect. As a prescribed drug, ibuprofen has been one of the best-selling medications in America.

Consisting of 2-(*p*-isobutylphenyl) propionic acid, ibuprofen has been used extensively in the treatment of rheumatoid arthritis and osteoarthritis and for the relief of mild to moderate pain and for treatment of painful menstruation.

Since the FDA approved lower-dose ibuprofen for nonprescription sale, it has been available under the brand names of Advil, Nuprin, Ibuprin, Motrin IB, and Medipren. These OTC analgesics are promoted as pain relievers and fever reducers.

In addition, these new, nonacetaminophen nonsalicylates have anti-inflammatory effects and are useful in relieving muscular aches, menstrual cramps, backaches, and the minor pain of arthritis. Ibuprofen has become a major competitor to aspirin and acetaminophen.

Compared to aspirin, ibuprofen usually causes fewer side effects and tends to be more gentle to the stomach, though daily use can result in heartburn, indigestion, and gastrointestinal bleeding, even peptic ulcers and perforated ulcers. Consequently, doctors often advise individuals aged sixty and older not to use ibuprofen, because of their increased risk of sustaining such serious and sometimes life-threatening events.[9]

Other adverse reactions may include skin rashes, digestive upsets, or dizziness. People with gout, ulcers, or aspirin allergies should not take ibuprofen products without first consulting a physician. The warning to aspirin-sensitive people applies even though ibuprofen drugs contain no aspirin or salicylates. Cross-reactions may occur in those individuals allergic to aspirin (see box 12.2).

Box 12.2 OTC Analgesics Primer *Aspirin, Acetaminophen, Ibuprofen, Naproxen Sodium, and Ketoprofen*

	Aspirin Products	Acetaminophen Products	Ibuprofen Products	Naproxen Sodium Products	Ketoprofen Products
Analgesic effect	Reduces pain.	Reduces pain.	Reduces pain.	Reduces pain.	Reduces pain.
Antipyretic effect	Reduces fever.	Reduces fever.	Reduces fever.	Reduces fever.	Reduces fever.
Anti-inflammatory effect	Reduces inflammation.	None.	Reduces inflammation.	Reduces inflammation.	Reduces inflammation.
Dosage	325 mg.	325 mg.	200 mg.	200 mg.	12.5 or 25 mg.
Common brands	Anacin, Ascriptin, Bayer, Bayer Plus, Bufferin, Ecotrin.	Anacin-3, Excedrin, Pamprin, Midol, Tylenol.	Advil, Motrin-IB, Nuprin, Pamprin-IB.	Aleve.	Actron, Orudis KT.
Special uses	Often used in treating arthritis and preventing heart attacks, strokes, and cataracts.	Fewer side effects than aspirin; used by those with ulcers or aspirin allergies. Gentler on the stomach than aspirin; reduces fever without risk of Reye's syndrome.	Fewer side effects than aspirin; effective in relief of menstrual cramps. Less toxic in large doses than other pain relievers. May be better for fever and muscle aches associated with a cold.	Often proves effective when other OTC analgesics have not helped. Provides longer-lasting relief.	May prove effective when other OTC analgesics have not helped.
Possible side effects	Nausea, vomiting, stomach irritation, dizziness, diarrhea. Accidental overdose, allergic reactions, salicylism, Reye's syndrome. Prolonged use may cause gastrointestinal bleeding, especially in heavy drinkers; may increase risk of maternal and fetal bleeding and cause complications during delivery if taken in the last trimester.	Upset stomach, nausea, and vomiting. Accidental overdose or long-term use may cause liver damage, hepatitis, reduced white blood cell and platelet count. May cause liver damage in drinkers and those taking excessive amounts (more than 4,000 mg daily) for several weeks.	Similar to those of aspirin; skin rash, sensitivity to sunlight. Accidental overdose, allergic reactions, including anaphylaxis, gastrointestinal bleeding, kidney damage. Gastrointestinal bleeding, especially in heavy drinkers; stomach ulcers; kidney damage in the elderly, people who have cirrhosis of the liver, and those taking diuretics.	Accidental overdose may cause stomach upset and stomach bleeding in some people; not recommended for pregnant women or those with ulcers, asthma, or kidney disease, or for heavy users of alcohol. Gastrointestinal bleeding; stomach ulcers; kidney damage in the elderly, in people who have cirrhosis of the liver, and in those taking diuretics.	May cause or worsen stomach pain and intestinal problems. Should be avoided by children under 16 and by people with high blood pressure, blood clotting problems, and kidney disease. Those consuming 3 or more alcoholic drinks per day or having liver disease should consult their physician about using ketoprofen drugs.
Best for*	Minor, occasional headaches and pain.	Fever reduction, children's pain relief, adults with stomach and intestinal problems.	Reducing inflammation and menstrual cramps.		

Sources: Modified from the U.S. Food and Drug Administration
**Consumer Report on Health.*

Perhaps the most frightening adverse reaction to the use of ibuprofen, including OTC preparations, is the drug's potential for causing damage to the kidney.[10] Even a brief course of ibuprofen may result in acute renal or kidney failure in those individuals who already have mild, asymptomatic (without symptoms) chronic renal failure. Such a serious condition could result in about 1 percent of the people who use ibuprofen, because early kidney failure does not often produce noticeable symptoms.

Naproxen Sodium

Another recently approved OTC analgesic, **naproxen sodium** is marketed under the brand name, Aleve. Like aspirin and ibuprofen, naproxen sodium is an NSAID. It is only the second prescription analgesic (after ibuprofen) to ever be approved for sale over-the-counter.[11]

For many years, naproxen (Naprosyn) and naproxen sodium (Anaprox) have been sold exclusively by prescription as arthritis medications. However, in 1994, because of naproxen's established record as a relatively safe and effective analgesic, the FDA approved naproxen sodium—which works more rapidly than plain naproxen—as a nonprescription pain reliever.[12] In its approval process, the FDA required the drug's manufacturer to change dosage instructions to reflect its new OTC status.

Nonprescription naproxen sodium is sold in tablets containing 200 milligrams of naproxen and 20 milligrams of sodium. It is used for the temporary relief of minor aches and pain associated with the common cold, headache, toothache, muscular aches, backaches, arthritis, or menstrual cramps, and for the relief of fever.

Naproxen sodium provides longer-lasting relief in comparison with other OTC analgesics. Consequently, this analgesic is ideal for use at bedtime. It is also especially effective for menstrual cramps and pain occurring in females after childbirth. However, children under the age of two ought not take naproxen sodium, and those under twelve years old, and pregnant or breastfeeding women, should use this medication only on medical advice.

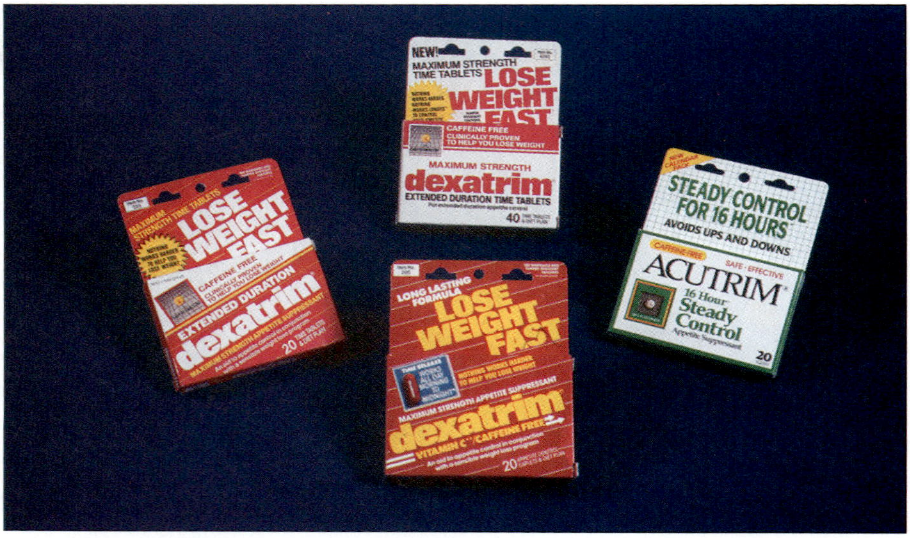

Of limited value in controlling weight, many over-the-counter diet pills contain the same active ingredient. These products feature their caffeine-free content, because caffeine was banned from weight-control products by the U.S. Food and Drug Administration.

© James L. Shaffer

Ketoprofen

Ketoprofen has been available in prescription-only formulations for more than twenty years and is the most recent prescribed analgesic to become available as an OTC drug. It was approved by the FDA in 1995 for nonprescription sale. OTC ketoprofen is distributed as Actron and Orudis KT.

Similar to other analgesics already on the market, ketoprofen products are effective for relief of headaches, body aches, and arthritis. This new OTC drug has been developed for those who fail to get adequate relief from comparable medications already available.

Ketoprofen is another nonsteroidal anti-inflammatory drug like aspirin, ibuprofen, and naproxen sodium. Used for relief of minor aches, pain, and menstrual cramps, this OTC medication also reduces fever, inflammation, swelling, stiffness, and joint pain.

These new OTC analgesics contain either 12.5 milligram or 25 milligram of ketoprofen and are advertised as somewhat more powerful or potent than other pain relievers. Milligram-for-milligram, ketoprofen products are more powerful than other OTC analgesics. Nevertheless, dose-per-dose there isn't much difference in drug effect, because the tablets or caplets are considerably smaller than nonketoprofen OTC pain relievers.

Ketoprofen products are not recommended for children under the age of sixteen, unless taken under the supervision of a physician. In addition, these particular pain killers should be avoided by adults with stomach or intestinal problems, high blood pressure, blood clotting problems, and kidney disease.

Weight-Control Products

The OTC products that help individuals curb their appetites are known variously as *diet aids,* **appetite suppressants,** and *anorectics* or *anorexics.* Though many drugs have been included in diet aids in the past, the U.S. Food and Drug Administration has limited the active ingredients in these products to phenylpropanolamine hydrochloride and benzocaine.[13] Other nonprescription products used in the control of weight, and the regular appetite suppressants, are available in a variety of preparations.

Phenylpropanolamine (PPA) is a mild stimulant and a decongestant often used in shrinking swollen nasal passages. Related to amphetamine, PPA has been

Box 12.3 Eating Disorders and Weight-Control Products

Anorexia nervosa and *bulimia* are two serious eating disorders about which dieters and users of OTC weight-control products should be concerned. Both are food obsessions in which the core symptom is the unending pursuit of thinness.

The anorexic individual finds food to be repulsive and strives to avoid it; the bulimic, by contrast, craves food and indulges in periodic episodes of binge eating that are followed by self-purging. Use of certain weight-control products and diet plans can contribute to both disorders, which often begin in adolescence or young adulthood and mostly affect females.

The person suffering from *anorexia nervosa* has a distorted view of personal body image and body weight. The anorexic rejects food, engaging in a persistent self-starvation process to achieve a desired thinness. After being detected and forced to eat, the anorexic will often induce vomiting in secret and redouble efforts to lose more weight. Frequently, the person becomes so emaciated that hospitalization is necessary.

Bulimia is characterized by a fear of fatness and by "bingepurge" behavior. The bulimic first binges on high-calorie food, then seeks to prevent its absorption by inducing vomiting (for example, by taking an emetic drug such as syrup of ipecac), or by using laxatives or other cathartic drugs to cause bowel movements. Sometimes diuretics are also used compulsively to help remove body water. Such purging endeavors can result in severe dehydration, chemical imbalances within the body, and other physical problems.

These eating disorders are serious and potentially life threatening, and they usually require a combination of therapies to change the patient's self-perception and basic belief system. Psychiatric care is often required.

---

considered useful as an appetite suppressant. As the result of an FDA OTC drug review panel's findings, PPA was identified initially as a safe and effective OTC drug for curbing appetite. Consequently, nearly all of the diet aids at one time or another contained this drug, varying only in dosage form (capsules, tablets, or drops), and dosage schedule (25 mg three times a day vs. 75 mg in one time-release capsule).

Some drug authorities, however, disagree about the safety and effectiveness of PPA. Side effects of PPA can include nervousness, restlessness, insomnia, headache, nausea, elevated blood-sugar level, and dangerous increases in blood pressure. Individuals at risk of heart disease, stroke, hypertension, kidney disease, or diabetes have been cautioned to avoid PPA. Increasingly, this drug is being recognized as potentially dangerous to at least 20 percent of the population.[14]

While PPA diet aids might suppress appetite for short periods in some individuals by stimulating the central nervous system, their effect is modest at best.

Benzocaine, a topical anesthetic often used to relieve sore throats and the pain associated with minor cuts, scrapes, burns, and hemorrhoids, is the only other active ingredient approved by the FDA for weight-control products. Contained in lozenges, candies, and gums, the benzocaine is said to numb the tongue and taste buds mildly and temporarily. This numbing effect supposedly reduces one's ability to taste and results in a decreased appetite. However, the anesthetic effect of benzocaine-based candies and gums may interfere with the swallowing process. If these products are sucked or chewed on a continuous basis, hypersensitivity reactions can occur.

Other so-called diet aids are *bulk-formers, laxatives, diuretics,* and *food supplements* containing methyl-cellulose compounds and fiber from grains and fruits. Sometimes, in combination with PPA, the bulk-producers absorb liquid in the stomach, produce a feeling of fullness, and thus reduce the desire to eat. Bulk-forming laxatives are also used inappropriately to control weight by "purging" the body (see box 12.3). Such laxatives relieve constipation and promote elimination by providing fiber (bulk) to the diet. Diuretics, or "water pills," aid in the relief of water retention or bloating. These diuretic drugs cause a temporary weight loss by reducing body fluid, evidenced by increased urination. None of these products is considered safe and effective in promoting a permanent loss of weight.

Many *diet foods, meal replacements,* and *food supplements* are available to help people maintain or slowly lose body weight. Most such products are accompanied by detailed plans for dieting, which can help some individuals lose weight. Basic ingredients usually include proteins (peanuts, whey, calcium caseinate, egg whites, and soy), and vitamins and minerals. Other products may contain artificial sweeteners to provide a sweet taste without sugar's calories, while glucose preparations raise blood-sugar levels and make individuals feel as if they do not need as much to eat.

None of these products has to be proved as safe or effective, because the United States Congress classified OTC vitamins, minerals, and herbs as food supplements. By this action, these products were excluded from control of the FDA.

According to the 1994 Dietary Supplement Health and Education Act, manufacturers of food supplements cannot make direct health claims for their products. Nevertheless, they may promote various mixtures of herbs, chromium pi- colinate and other minerals, bee pollen, leaves, vitamins—literally hundreds of other mysterious and unproven ingredients—for their known effects on the body's structure and function. Americans can purchase fat burners, energy busters, love formulas, blood purifiers, colon helpers, liver detoxifiers, male power builders, and muscle protectants, in addition to the more conventional weight control products.

Though there is no magic wand or "no-work" way to lose weight, many consumers have gladly accepted numerous spurious concoctions that, according to the Consumers Union, are worthless and dangerous fat-melting pills and potions.[15] Among these allegedly fraudulent products are:

1. *Starch blockers* popular in the early 1980s and derived from legumes, effectively prevented the digestion of starch, but resulted in nausea, vomiting, and stomach pains that often required hospitalization. These products were eventually banned by the FDA, but stayed on the market for a number of years due to the ineffectiveness of enforcement procedures.
2. *Growth-hormone releasers* containing various amino acids were supposed to cause overnight weight loss. Taking these products on an empty stomach supposedly caused the pituitary gland to secrete growth hormone, which in turn would burn fat and cause weight loss during sleep. As a result of government enforcement actions, most of the growth-hormone-releasing preparations have been removed from the marketplace.
3. *Sugar blockers,* derived from an Indian plant, were sold to help prevent the body from absorbing the sugar in various foods. Such an action could never be proved.
4. *Calories-ban,* made from guar gum, was advertised as a product that prevented the absorption of a major portion of calories, thus assuring automatic weight loss. Guar gum, a soluble fiber that thickens foods, has only minimal value as a bulk laxative, and the substance has never been proven effective. It has remained available in several states because the FDA is conducting a lengthy OTC drug review process on the product.

Despite the popularity and appeal of weight-control products and the often sensational advertising claims for such items, no OTC drug can cause a weight loss. At most, even PPA and benzocaine can only help reduce a dieter's appetite. Ideally, drugs ought to be considered only as temporary, short-term measures in conjunction with a well-planned weight reduction program.

In addition, reducing diets should be undertaken only with the supervision of a physician. In the final analysis, only a reduction in calories consumed or an increase in exercise to burn off excess calories can cause a loss of weight. This effort will likely involve significant, long-term changes in lifestyle.

Cold Remedies

One of the most common causes of human misery and disability is the "common cold," a viral infection of the upper respiratory tract. The infection usually localizes in the head, throat, or chest. Fortunately, colds tend to be a **self-limiting condition;** that is, they run their course to recovery without treatment.

However, the various signs and symptoms of a cold can be discomforting: sneezing, watery eyes, chills, fever, sore throat, stopped up nose, runny nose, post-nasal drip, sore chest, coughing, and the tired, ache-all-over feeling. Although none of these symptoms in itself indicates a cold, together this group of complaints forms the "cold syndrome."

The treatment of a common cold is aimed at the relief of symptoms because antibiotics such as penicillin have no effect against viruses. The drug companies have responded to this human desire for relief with thousands of cold remedies. While some of these drugs will relieve several of the cold symptoms, none of these products will prevent, cure, or even shorten the course of the common cold.

Certain single-ingredient cold products can provide symptomatic relief of a cold's discomforts; nearly all cold and cough remedies contain a combination of two or more drug ingredients intended to relieve a number of different symptoms. Ordinarily, these combination drug preparations appear to be logical drug mixtures for treating multiple symptoms. However, these OTC **fixed-ratio combination products** are considered undesirable for the following reasons:[16]

1. Combination remedies treat a cold with a "shotgun" approach; that is, the multidrug often contains ingredients not needed by the cold sufferer. Those who undertake self-medication, therefore, expose themselves to unnecessary drugs.
2. It is not possible to formulate multidrugs for individual needs, body weight, and metabolism. Certain fixed-ratio combinations might not be appropriate for some individuals.
3. Cold remedies might contain effective ingredients in less-than-therapeutic doses. Consequently, these drugs often have little or no effect.
4. Consumers expose themselves to more risks and side effects of drugs, often due to the interaction of various ingredients in the multidrug preparation. In addition, the combination remedy might interfere with the healing process. For instance, many cold preparations contain an analgesic. Whether the cold sufferer has a headache, the individual is dosed with the drug.

   Moreover, the analgesic also tends to lower fever that in most instances runs its course without harm. While high body temperatures can be extremely dangerous, a lower fever may stimulate the body's immune system into operation. Therefore, drugs taken to lower temperature might also interfere with the body's own healing strategy. Fever reducers might also reduce the effectiveness of *interferon,* a natural antiviral agent within the body.
5. These combination products invariably cost more money than the single-ingredient medications usually recommended and preferred by medical authorities in treating symptoms of the "common cold."

Some precautions should be observed when using any combination- or single-ingredient cold remedy. Cold medications are intended for temporary use only. They should never be taken on a persistent or continuous basis, even if the drugs produce a beneficial effect. People with asthma, emphysema, or smoker's cough should only use these OTC medicines with their physicians' approval. In addition, individuals with diabetes, high blood pressure, heart disease, and thyroid problems should carefully read package labels and inserts that may indicate special warnings pertaining to those ailments.

Lacing oral cold remedies with alcohol is a widespread practice, although there is little evidence that ethyl alcohol relieves the symptoms of either colds or coughs. When the combination medication contains an antihistamine, the alcohol heightens the antihistamine's effect and often produces drowsiness. Such an effect presents a real danger when persons must drive an automobile or operate machinery.

The numerous cold remedies, such as Actifed, Benadryl, Comtrex, Contac, Coricidin, Dimetapp, Nyquil, Sudafed, Triaminic, and Vicks 440, might be marketed as combinations of the following major drug ingredients:

Antihistamines block the effects of the allergy chemical (histamine) in the body and relieve sneezing, watery eyes, runny nose, and itching of the nose or throat. While effective in controlling allergic reactions, antihistamines do not relieve sinus or nasal congestion and have no direct action on colds. They continue to be one of the most common ingredients of cold preparations, primarily because of antihistamine's side effects—drowsiness and a slight drying of nasal secretions.

Decongestants, such as pseudoephedrine, phenylpropanolamine, oxymetazoline, and xylometazoline, unclog blocked nasal passages and sinuses, and prevent postnasal drip into the throat. Marketed as either oral (taken by mouth) or topical (applied in the form of nose drops or sprays) preparations, these decongestants usually cause a *vasoconstriction* (narrowing) of the blood vessels in the nasal passages and thus help clear up stuffy noses.

Although the decongestants are effective, those applied in the form of nose drops and nasal sprays present a potential problem. Initially, the active ingredient causes the swollen blood vessels in the nose to shrink. When the nose drops or sprays are used too long or too frequently, a phenomenon known as the "rebound effect" is likely to occur.

After excessive use of the decongestant, the blood vessels become fatigued and undergo a swelling or dilation when the effect of the drug wears off. The swollen blood vessels contribute to greater congestion and nasal stuffiness. In response to this rebound swelling or vasodilation, the cold sufferer uses more of the nasal decongestant, resulting in a vicious cycle of drug dependency.[17]

Analgesics and *antipyretics* are drugs that relieve pain and reduce fever, respectively. As indicated earlier in this chapter, the major analgesics and antipyretics present in most OTC cold remedies are aspirin, acetaminophen, and ibuprofen. Acetaminophen is a common ingredient because it does not irritate the stomach lining and cause bleeding.

Antitussives or *cough suppressants,* such as dextromethorphan, diphenhydramine hydrochloride, and codeine (a prescription-only drug in some states), are useful in controlling coughs that cause chest pain or interfere with sleep or breathing. (A cough that brings up phlegm—a "productive cough"—should not be suppressed. Such a cough helps clear the respiratory passages.)

Expectorants are drugs that tend to thin and loosen the thick mucus that often accumulates in the respiratory airways of a cold sufferer. Although this drug action may be desirable, an FDA OTC drug review panel concluded that expectorants, including *guaifenesin* (the most widely used), are of limited therapeutic effectiveness. Perhaps in a somewhat irrational combination, some cold preparations contain both an expectorant and a cough suppressant. Such a mixture has a drug intended to make phlegm easier to cough up and another drug intended to suppress coughing.

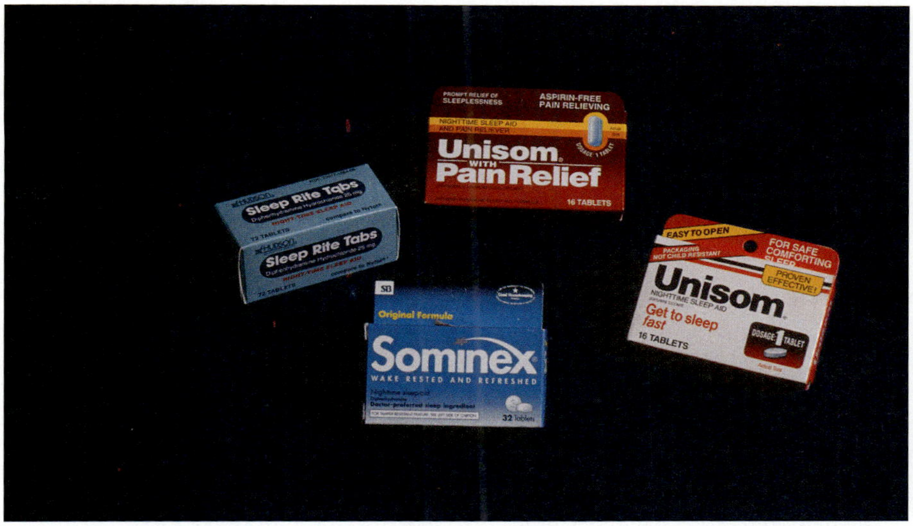

Nearly all OTC sleep aids contain an antihistamine that produces a degree of drowsiness or mild sedation in many users.

© James L. Shaffer

Sleep Aids

Several OTC preparations are marketed exclusively as **sleep aids.** Some popular ones are Compoz, Nervine, Nytol, Sleepeze-3, Sleepinal and Scminex—all of which contain the same active ingredient, diphenhydramine hydrochloride, a common antihistamine. Other sleep aids, such as Doxysom, Ultra Sleep, and Unisom, contain another antihistamine, doxylamine succinate, while Excedrin PM contains both an antihistamine and an analgesic.

The antihistamine drugs reverse the action of a naturally occurring substance, histamine, which causes allergic reactions like runny nose, itching, tearing of the eyes, and sneezing. In addition to relieving allergy symptoms, antihistamines tend to act on the central nervous system and produce a mild form of drowsiness or sedation in some individuals.

However, many physicians and pharmacologists oppose the use of antihistamines as sleep aids because they expose users to several other possible side effects. Frequently reported problems include dizziness, incoordination, fatigue, nervousness, blurred vision, double vision, loss of appetite, dryness of the mouth, throat and respiratory passages, nausea, vomiting, increased urination, constipation, and diarrhea.

For those considering the use of OTC sleep aids, the following advice is offered.

1. Sleeping pills are for short-term use only. If insomnia persists for more than two weeks, even after taking sleeping pills, consult a physician without delay. Persistent insomnia may be a symptom of some serious underlying medical problem.
2. Take sleep aids with extreme caution if alcohol is also being consumed. Drinking an alcoholic beverage while taking an antihistamine, another CNS depressant, can lead to excessive drowsiness and confusion, and, in extreme cases, coma and death.
3. Unless discomfort from minor pain is causing sleeplessness, avoid those sleep aids that also contain a pain and fever reducer.
4. Never give OTC sleep aids to children under twelve years of age. Such medication is for adults only.
5. Do not use these products if you are presently taking another prescribed or OTC medicine without medical consultation; or if you are pregnant or nursing an infant; or if you are suffering from asthma, glaucoma, or enlargement of the prostate gland.
6. Be careful not to exceed the recommended dosage. When the standard dose does not seem to be effective, there is the temptation to take more pills. Overdose then becomes a danger.

Millions of people rely on OTC sleeping pills to purchase elusive sleep, though a variety of nondrug alternatives exist that can promote sleep, including these: modification of eating, drinking, exercise, and relaxation habits; establishing regular times for retiring at night; elimination of caffeine or other stimulants; resolution of personal crises; synchronization of lifestyle with natural body rhythm; biofeedback; and relaxation techniques. Specific recommendations for relieving insomnia are detailed in chapter 7.

Stimulants

When improved mental alertness or motor performance is desired, OTC *stimulants* are used to cover up conditions of fatigue, and thus permit the successful completion of a required task. Common nonprescription stimulants include Caffedrine, Dexitac, NoDoz, Quick Pep, Tirend, and Vivarin. While these drugs might help individuals stay awake, they might not be sufficient to promote the alertness or efficiency needed to drive an automobile skillfully and safely.

The only approved effective ingredient of OTC stimulants is caffeine. This drug can help restore mental alertness or wakefulness in people experiencing fatigue or drowsiness. Each stimulant tablet or capsule contains from 100 to 325 milligrams of caffeine. Usually, the recommended dose ranges from 100 to 200 milligrams of caffeine every three to four hours. Some products, until restricted by the FDA, also contained phenylpropanolamine hydrochloride and ephedrine sulfate mild stimulants. A variety of vitamins and small amounts of sugar have also been added to some OTC stimulants. Vitamins have no stimulating effect, so they do not help people stay awake.

Use of an OTC stimulant may be considered reasonable on an occasional basis, especially when used to reduce fatigue or tedium associated with long, boring, and repetitive tasks. However, self-treatment with a stimulant should not last more than a week. There is no drug substitute for adequate sleep. Although an OTC stimulant may relieve the feeling of tiredness, the body is still fatigued.

Caffeine is a natural component of various plants that are sources of coffee, tea, kola nut extracts, cocoa, and chocolate. Present in many prescription drugs, caffeine is also an ingredient in nearly two thousand OTC medicines, such as analgesics and cold remedies. Used typically in dilute forms, caffeine is a relatively safe drug. However, excessive intake—whether in coffee, tea, cola drinks, OTC stimulants, or OTC analgesics—can contribute to sleep disturbances, nervousness, and irritability.

Caffeine overdoses can result in mood changes, anxiety, insomnia, headache, and restlessness; these are characteristics of *caffeinism,* described in chapter 9. When caffeine doses exceed 5 to l0 grams, convulsions may occur and, on rare occasions, death.

OTC stimulants are concentrated doses of caffeine, so enough coffee, tea, or caffeine-containing cola drinks should be as effective and probably much less expensive.

Herbal Remedies

More Americans are beginning to use natural remedies or herbal products to relieve discomfort and improve their health. Products once sold only in health food stores are now appearing in drugstores and supermarkets and creating a billion dollar market. These products are usually not tested or controlled by the FDA. The only government restriction is that products sold as dietary aids cannot make explicit health claims.[18]

Many of these products have been used for centuries and may relieve or prevent health problems. Others may be worthless or dangerous. As with all health remedies, buyers should use these products cautiously. Be sure you know what you are taking, how much you are taking, and the possible side effects. Talk to your doctor or pharmicist about potential side effects or other problems, especially if you are taking other medications (see box 12.4).

Box 12.4 Some Selected Natural Products Used as Herbal Remedies

Product	Commonly Used For
Bilberry	Cardiovascular and gastrointestinal problems, cancer prevention
Cat's Claw	Allergies, gastrointestinal problems
Chromium	Weight loss, increased energy
Co-Q10	Anti-aging, increased energy, improved cardiovascular and gastrointestinal health
DHEA	Increased energy, antiaging
Echinacea	Prevention of flu and colds
Garlic	Lowering cholesterol and blood pressure, antiaging
Ginkgo Bilboba	Improving circulatory system, antiaging
Ginseng	Stimulating the immune system, increasing stamina
Kava Kava	Promoting relaxation, reducing anxiety
Ma Huang	Weight control, increasing energy
Melatonin	Promoting sleep, cancer prevention
St. John's Wort	Mild depression
Saw Palmetto	Urinary problems

Although popular, most of these products have not been rigorously tested for safety or effectiveness. To protect your health and your pocketbook, check with a health professional before using.

Self-Medication

Many human ailments are distressing only temporarily and produce no lasting changes in the human body. When used with care and discrimination on a temporary basis, over-the-counter drugs can provide a significant degree of relief from various minor discomforts.

The OTC drugs serve yet another function in overall health care. In programs of **self medication,** nonprescription drug use allows medical doctors to concentrate their efforts on more serious health problems of treatment, rehabilitation, and prevention. Without the wise and responsible use of nonprescription medications, and the application of home remedies (rest, sleep, hot water bottles, and ice caps), physicians would be so overwhelmed with patients complaining of minor illnesses that their services would be severely limited. The practice of treating oneself with nonprescription medications has some important advantages, which will likely increase as the cost of health care continues to rise.

Guidelines for Self-Medication

In the interest of avoiding medicine mishaps, getting the best value out of OTC medications, and using self-selected drugs to relieve minor symptoms of illness, this section includes several guidelines for safer self-medication.[19]

Before purchasing any OTC drug for self-medication, *read the label* carefully to make sure the drug is the right one for your symptoms. Federal law requires that OTC drug labels provide sufficient directions for use needed by the average person. Then, *follow the directions for use.* If symptoms persist, stop taking the OTC drug and seek professional advice from a physician. Additional guidelines for self-medication follow.

1. *Do not expect a "miracle cure."* At best, OTC drugs can only relieve symptoms of illness. Though regulated by the Federal Trade Commission, advertising for OTC drugs tends to exaggerate the need for a particular drug, creates health problems that do not exist, or promises more results than one can reasonably expect. In all likelihood, the analgesic promoted as the one remedy to end all headaches will not prevent the next one from occurring.
2. *Never use old medicines.* Leftover drugs often become stale, harmful, or ineffective over long periods. At regular intervals, clear your medicine cabinet of OTC and prescription drugs that have been on hand for a long time. Many OTC medications either lose or increase their strength as time goes by, so the large economy size may not be economical if it will remain unused for several months. Check the medicine's expiration date, often listed on the label or elsewhere on the container.

   Old, outdated drugs should be discarded, preferably by flushing them down a toilet. When no expiration date is listed, one year from the date of purchase should be the maximum time to keep any medication.
3. *Store medicines properly to prolong their effectiveness.* OTC and prescription drugs should be stored away from bright lights in a cool, dry place that cannot be reached by children. Kitchen cabinets and bedrooms are preferred to bathrooms as storage places, because bathrooms tend to be too warm and humid. Unless directed to do so, do not store medicines in the refrigerator. In addition, keep drugs in their original containers, capped tightly when not being used.
4. *Consult your physician and/or pharmacist for information on OTC drug effectiveness and selection of appropriate medications.* While a

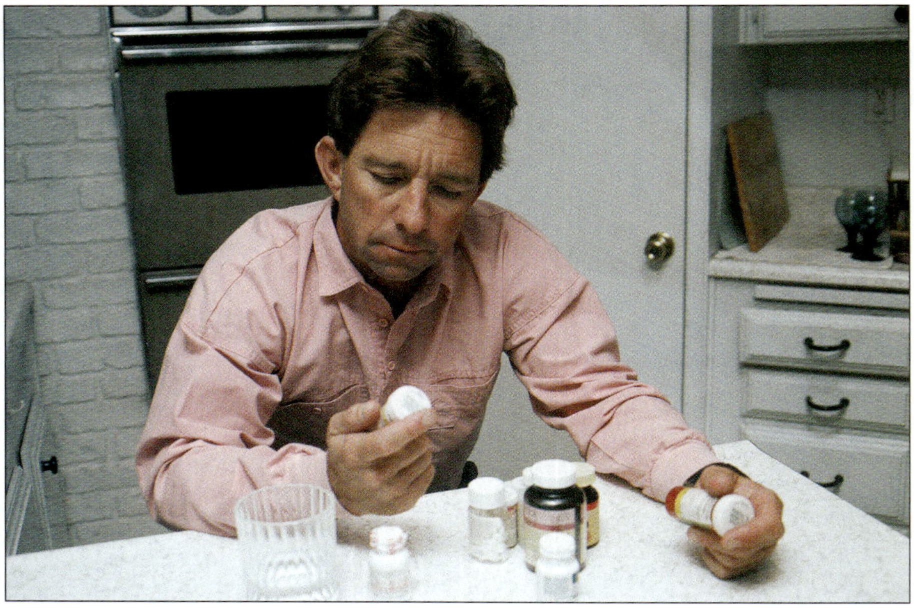

Always check the medicine's expiration date, and discard outdated drugs.

© Felicia Martinez/PhotoEdit

pharmacist may be more readily available, both professionals can assist consumers in selecting OTC products that suit their needs. In particular, a pharmacist may help consumers make informed choices on drug purchases by providing information on comparative drug effectiveness and by advising individuals on the appropriate use of drugs and proper storage of various medicines.

5. *Avoid identical medicines.* Many OTC drugs contain exactly the same ingredients and differ from one another only in brand name, container, and the amount of each ingredient. The major difference is often in the advertised claims, especially for the multidrug combinations. Unknowingly, consumers often purchase these "identical" medications and take them concurrently, and consequently become victims of drug overdose and adverse reactions. By comparing drug labels for lists of ingredients and their specific amounts, you may be able to guard against overdose and adverse reactions and save money.
6. *Save money on the purchase of OTC drugs.* Shop around at discount drugstores and take advantage of special sales and bargains. Undertake a price comparison survey to determine where specific medicines can be bought more economically. Be sure to check the expiration date on the drug container or label before you make your purchase. If a large quantity of drugs must be procured for long-term use, buying the large or king-size container of drugs may result in significant savings, if it has a sufficiently distant expiration date.

   If you have reservations about low-priced drugs, look for the abbreviation *N.F.* or *U.S.P.* on certain OTC drug labels. These symbols stand for the *National Formulary* and the *United States Pharmacopcia,* reference books containing standards for identity, strength, and purity of various drugs and for the inactive ingredients in drug dosage forms. When a drug label lists one of these abbreviations, the drug was made according to official standards and can therefore be purchased with confidence and assurance of the highest quality.
7. *Consider generic OTC drug substitution.* As a potential moneysaving technique, the substitution of **generic drugs** for **brand-name drugs** has received much publicity regarding prescription medicine purchases. However, this practice can also apply to buying OTC drugs. Generics (chemical equivalents of brand-name drugs) or store brands provide identical medications found in their brand-name counterparts. For instance, *aspirin* is the generic name for a leading analgesic. *Bayer* and *St. Joseph* are brand names for different manufacturers' aspirin. Whether you purchase the house or store brand, a generic aspirin, or one of the nationally advertised brands, there should be no differences in the painkilling quality of the aspirin products.

   More than fifteen years ago, tests of Bayer, Norwich, Squibb, and several store (house) brands of aspirin revealed that no one brand performed significantly better than any of the other brands.[20] The tests, conducted by Consumers Union, evaluated the aspirin and salicylic acid content, and the dissolution speed of nine competing brands. Such tests are often used to indicate therapeutic effectiveness and superiority. Despite the various advertising claims of the 400-plus brands of aspirin in the United States, all aspirin is essentially the same according to these tests. As Consumers Union advises, buy the cheapest! Such advice is still valid.
8. *If an adverse reaction occurs, stop taking the OTC drug.* On occasion, any drug will produce some effect other than the intended or anticipated one—the so-called drug **side effect.** When this side effect is unusual, undesirable, discomforting, or life threatening, the side effect is described as an **adverse drug reaction.** If you experience an adverse reaction, stop taking the OTC drug immediately and consult with a physician or pharmacist. These individuals know what actions a drug should have and what adverse effects may be expected. Follow their advice before using the drug again.
9. *Beware of the drug overdose danger.* Although OTC drugs are relatively safe when used in recommended

doses, large overdoses and persistent overuse of such products can prove to be dangerous. This is especially true with large doses of aspirin, which can result in accidental poisoning. Overuse of certain analgesics can cause kidney damage, and antacids can produce an imbalance in the body's secretion of enzymes. Prolonged use of laxatives to relieve constipation can lead to constipation.

To avoid such dangers, never use any OTC drug on a regular, continuous basis or in large quantities, except on the advice of a physician. Additionally, never mix different medicines in one container. Such a practice may be confusing and lead to taking the wrong medication. To avoid another drug-taking error, never take any medicine in the dark.

10. *Exercise extreme caution and consult your physician or pharmacist when using several medications at the same time.* Each drug acts on the body in a characteristic way. However, each drug is also capable of altering the effect of any other drug a person may be taking. On occasion, the combination of drugs can be harmful and fatal. For instance, aspirin increases the blood-thinning effect of some medicines prescribed for heart attack patients. Individuals taking such medicines risk hemorrhage if they use aspirin to relieve headaches. Some combination nasal decongestant-antihistamine cold and allergy remedies should not ordinarily be used with prescription antihypertensive or antidepressant drugs containing a monoamine oxidase inhibitor. Therefore, before using any combination of drugs (prescription with OTC drugs or several OTC drugs taken at the same time), consult your physician or pharmacist.
11. *Never combine OTC sleeping pills or antihistamines with alcohol.* Ethyl alcohol can increase the CNS depressant effect of such drugs, therefore the combination can produce extreme drowsiness, accident, or injury. Whenever taking either prescription or OTC drugs, ask your physician whether drinking beverage alcohol could be hazardous in combination with the medication.

Safety and Effectiveness of OTC Drugs

Each day millions of Americans engage in self-medication. They rely on the purity, safety, and effectiveness of various OTC remedies they purchase, and the adequacy of label information to get the benefits they expect. Such reliance and expectations were not always justified, because neither purity and accurate or truthful labeling nor safety and effectiveness of OTC medications had to be assured before enactment of the first national Food and Drug Act. Passed by the U.S. Congress in 1906, the law forbade interstate commerce in *misbranded* and *adulterated* (impure) drugs.

It was not until 1938, when the federal Food, Drug, and Cosmetic Act (FDC Act) was approved, that new drugs were required to be proven *safe* before their distribution. However, drug manufacturers were not required to prove the *effectiveness* of their products until passage of the Kefauver-Harris drug amendments to the FDC Act in 1962. Since then, drugs used as medicines must be proven safe and effective to the FDA/before being sold in the United States. New drug products were affected immediately, but the monumental problem was the thousands of OTC and prescription drugs already on the market that had never been demonstrated to be effective.

In 1972, the FDA began a long-range regulatory program to apply the "drug efficacy" amendments to drugs sold over the counter. The ambitious program was designed to assure consumers that every OTC drug is safe, adequately and truthfully labeled, and that it will do what the manufacturer claims it will do. More than seven hundred basic ingredients of 300,000 drug products were eventually examined.

To carry out this project, seventeen advisory drug review panels composed of nongovernment experts were formed to evaluate eighty basic OTC "drug classes" for safety and effectiveness. These advisory review panels attempted to place the active ingredients in each OTC drug in one of three categories, namely:

> Category I—drugs determined to be safe, effective, and not mislabeled.
>
> Category II—drugs not usually recognized as safe and effective, or mislabeled. Such drugs must be removed from medications within six months after the FDA issues its final regulations.
>
> Category III—drugs for which there are insufficient data to determine general recognition of safety and effectiveness.

Nevertheless, some drugs of doubtful effectiveness remain on the market, because a drug manufacturer can request a hearing on whether its drug should be ruled ineffective. If such a formal hearing is denied or results in an unfavorable ruling, the drug maker may initiate a legal challenge against the FDA. The drug product in question remains on the open market pending the outcome of the court proceedings—a lengthy process often lasting several months or years.

Sometimes budgetary limitations prevent the FDA from acting as rapidly as possible. For instance, several months after "starch blockers" had been banned by the FDA, numerous stores continued to sell the controversial diet aids. Without sufficient personnel and lacking enforcement resources, neither the FDA nor its counterparts at the state level could visit each retail outlet and confiscate the illegal pills. However, during the entire OTC drug review process (1972–88), the FDA did not initiate any enforcement actions against those drugs that its panels of experts had found to be unsafe.

Despite the best—and sometimes worst—intentions of the U.S. Congress, and the cautious efforts of the FDA, and state agencies dealing with drug products and claims, American consumers have been subject to unreasonable and unnecessary risks to their health by purchasing OTC drugs lacking evidence of safety and effectiveness. The FDA's multiyear evaluation of OTC drugs and the issuance of final monographs has not been completed, although the various advisory panels finished the review process in 1988.

Initial results of the OTC drug-review process indicated that only about 31 percent of the ingredients in the 300,000 brands of nonprescription drug products were safe and effective for their intended uses. By contrast, the effectiveness review process of prescription drugs, completed in September 1984, some twenty-two years after the project was begun, found that, of the 3,300 prescribed drugs that were reviewed, 2,208 (66 percent) were effective for their indicated use.

Chapter Summary

1. There is a widespread belief in the effectiveness of drugs to heal discomfort and prevent disease. In some instances, however, drugs can act as poisons, cause undesirable side effects including adverse drug reactions, alter the effects of other medicines, and produce drug dependency.
2. Common use of over-the-counter drugs—those purchased without a physician's prescription—has been accompanied by widespread drug misuse and by the inappropriate use of medicines, resulting in impaired physical, mental, emotional, or social well-being.
3. Used on a temporary basis for illnesses not requiring a physician's supervision, OTC drugs usually do not cure diseases but do relieve symptoms.
4. The hundreds of thousands of OTC drugs are classified generally according to their primary or intended effect, such as relieving acid indigestion; controlling diarrhea; providing vitamin supplements; stopping growth of bacteria; and relieving symptoms of sneezing, watery nose, and itching of the throat.
5. There are two major types of internal analgesics: the salicylate painkillers containing aspirin, and the nonsalicylate painkillers containing acetaminophen, ibuprofen, naproxen sodium, or ketoprofen. Aspirin, ibuprofen, ketoprofen, and naproxen sodium also reduce fever and act to reduce inflammation and are known as nonsteroidal anti-inflammatory drugs (NSAIDs). Acetaminophen does not reduce inflammation.
6. OTC preparations sold as sleeping aids tend to produce drowsiness. This effect is due to an antihistamine, the major ingredient of nonprescribed sleeping pills and many cold remedies.
7. OTC stimulants usually contain caffeine and help some individuals to stay awake. Usually these drugs do not improve mental alertness or motor performance to the level needed to safely operate an automobile.
8. Fixed-ratio combination products (drugs containing two or more ingredients intended to relieve a number of different symptoms), are often sold as OTC cold remedies. Frequently such multidrug mixtures contain ingredients not needed by cold sufferers.
9. Most diet aids or appetite suppressants contain a mild stimulant (PPA) or a topical anesthetic such as benzocaine. Other weight-control products contain bulk-formers that reduce the desire to eat.
10. Self-medication is often advantageous when guidelines for responsible use are followed. Such guides pertain to reading labels; following directions; discarding old medicines; properly storing drugs; consulting with one's physician or pharmacist on the appropriateness of medications or when using more than one OTC drug at the same time; avoiding identical medicines; stopping drug use when an adverse reaction occurs; guarding against drug overdose; and not combining OTC sleeping pills or antihistamines with alcohol.
11. Due to congressional actions, misbranded and adulterated drugs have been outlawed, and since 1962 new drugs have been required to be proven safe and effective. However, OTC dietary supplements including herbal products and vitamins have been excluded from FDA control.
12. Despite the regulations of the federal Food and Drug Administration and its state-level counterparts, many OTC drugs are of doubtful effectiveness and safety.

World Wide Web Sites

Mayo Foundation for Medical Information and Research

www.mayohealth.org

National Institutes of Health's National Center for Complementary and Alternative Medicine

http://altmed.od.nih.gov

Review Questions and Activities

1. In what ways can drugs taken to restore or improve health harm the body and endanger life?
2. How does drug misuse differ from drug abuse?
3. List the OTC drugs you have taken in the past year. Which of these do you feel were beneficial? Do you think that any of the OTC drugs you have taken were a waste of money? Why? Could you have done anything else to remedy the health problem other than take a nonprescribed drug?
4. What sources are available at your college or in your local community to help you evaluate the effectiveness of OTC drugs?
5. Explain the major function or anticipated effect of each of the following OTC drug types: antiemetic, antihistamine, antiseptic,

analgesic, antitussive, and dermatological.

6. Survey a variety of liquid cold remedies and allergy-relief medications at a local drugstore and determine the relative alcohol content of each item surveyed.

7. In what ways do salicylates and nonsalicylates differ as analgesics? Investigate the names of fifteen oral analgesics available at local drugstores and classify them as either salicylate or nonsalicylate painkillers.

8. How do the NSAID analgesics differ from pain relievers that contain acetaminophen?

9. In what ways might the use of aspirin products cause harm to the body or threaten health status?

10. Why is the use of OTC fixed-ratio combination cold remedies considered to be undesirable?

11. List the anticipated effect of each of the following OTC drug ingredients: appetite suppressant, asthma preparation, expectorant, decongestant, and topical antibiotic.

12. What precautions should be observed when using OTC sleep aids and stimulants?

13. Discuss the practice of self-medication in terms of general guidelines to assure reasonable safety and effectiveness in using OTC drugs.

14. Describe the various activities of the FDA to assure the safety and effectiveness of OTC drugs sold in the United States.

References

1. United States Pharmacopeia, *Complete Drug Reference,* 1996 ed. (Yonkers, N.Y.: Consumer Reports Books, 1995), iv.
2. "Drug Ingredients Banned," *FDA Consumer* 25, no. 2 (March 1991): 3.
3. "FDA Bans Ineffective OTC Drug Ingredients and Adds a Warning," *Health Letter* 7, no. 1 (January 1991): 3–4.
4. Marian Segal, "Rx to OTC: The Switch Is On," *FDA Consumer* 25, no. 2 (March 1991): 9–11.
5. Editors of Consumer Reports Books, *The New Medicine Show,* rev. ed. (Mount Vernon, N.Y.: Consumers Union, 1989), 60.
6. Joe Graedon and Teresa Graedon, *Graedons' Best Medicine: From Herbal Remedies to High-Tech Rx Breakthroughs* (New York: Bantam Books, 1991), 40.
7. Joe Graedon and Teresa Graedon, *The People's Pharmacy* (New York: St. Martin's Griffin, 1996), 85–86.
8. Public Health Service and the Food and Drug Administration, *A Message from the Surgeon General about Reye Syndrome,* U.S. DHHS Pub. No. (FDA) 86-3154.
9. "Over-the-Counter Ibuprofen May Be Hazardous to Your Health, Too," *Public Citizen Health Research Group Health Letter* 5, no. 6 (June 1989): 8.
10. Andrew Whelton and others, "Renal Effects of Ibuprofen, Proxicam, and Sulindac in Patients with Asymptomatic Renal Failure," *Annals of Internal Medicine* 112, no. 8 (15 April 1990): 568–76.
11. "Another OTC Pain Reliever," *FDA Consumer* 18, no. 3 (April 1994): 4.
12. "Over-the-Counter Pain Relief," *University of California at Berkeley Wellness Letter* 10, no. 10 (July 1994): 3.
13. "FDA Bans Ineffective OTC Drug Ingredients and Adds a Warning," *Public Citizen Health Research Group Health Letter* 7, no. 1 (January 1991): 3–4.
14. "Do Not Use Phenylpropanolamine-Containing Products," *Public Citizen Health Research Group Health Letter* 7, no. 1 (January 1991): 3.
15. "Tales from the Bazaar: Automatic Weight Loss with Cal-Ban? Send for Your Refund Now!" *Consumer Reports Health Letter* 2, no. 6 (June 1990): 46–47.
16. Neshama Franklin, "Dubious Drugs for Coughs and Colds," *Medical Self-Care* no. 17 (summer 1982): 38; and S. M. Wolfe, M. Coley, and the Health Research Groups, *Pills That Don't Work* (New York: Farrar, Straus & Giroux, 1981), 12.
17. "Decongestants," *Consumer Reports Health Letter* 1, no. 3 (November 1989): 21.
18. "Sex, Lies and Garlic," *Newsweek,* (6 November 1995): 65–68.
19. H. Winter Griffith, *Complete Guide to Prescription & Nonprescription Drugs* (New York: The Body Press/Perigee, 1996), xix–xx; United States Pharmacopeia, *Complete Drug Reference,* 1723–31; Graedon and Graedon, *The People's Pharmacy,* 79–80; and John Fried and Sharon Petska, *The American Druggist's Complete Family Guide to Prescriptions, Pills, and Drugs* (New York: Hearst Books, 1995), 16–20.
20. "Is Bayer Better?" *Consumer Reports* 47, no. 7 (July 1982): 347–49.

Chapter 13

Prescription drugs

KEY TERMS

Additive Drug Reaction
Antagonistic Drug Reaction
Antihypertensive Drug
Anti-infective Drug
Benefit-Risk Equation
Bioavailability
Bioequivalence
Cardiovascular Drug
Chemically Equivalent Drug
Combination Oral Contraceptive Drug
Controlled Drug
Depo-Provera
Diuretic
Drug Classes or Families
Fail-Safe Medicine
Food-Drug Interaction
Generic Drug
Insulin
Methotrexate
Minipill
Morning After Contraception
Norplant
Patient Medication Instructions (PMIs)
Physicians' Desk Reference
Polypharmacy
Prescription
RU-486
Sedative-Hypnotic Drug
Subdermal Implants
Synergistic Drug Reaction

chapter objectives

After you have studied this chapter, you should be able to do the following:

1. Define the key terms.
2. Explain why so-called prescription drugs, unlike OTC drugs, can be obtained only by the direction of a physician.
3. Discuss the concepts of fail-safe medicine and the benefit-risk equation as they apply to the use of prescription drugs.
4. Identify the common elements appearing on (a) a typical prescription and (b) a typical Rx drug label.
5. Compare and contrast the restrictions placed on the prescribing of drugs under the provisions of the Controlled Substances Act.
6. List at least eight questions to be answered or guidelines to be followed to assure the wise use of prescription drugs.
7. Identify the major anticipated effects of the following drug classes or families: anorexics, antiasthmatics, antidepressants, antihypertensives, antispasmodics, and diuretics.
8. Describe the differences between the major and the minor tranquilizers in terms of their psychotherapeutic uses.
9. Explain the similarities and differences between the combination oral contraceptive pill and the minipill.
10. Identify five of the most serious and life-threatening side effects associated with using oral contraceptives.
11. Name several noncontraceptive benefits associated with the use of oral contraceptives.
12. Compare and contrast the actions of estrogen and progestin hormone agents found in combination oral contraceptives.
13. Distinguish among the following drugs used in emergency oral contraception and pregnancy termination: ordinary oral contraceptive pills, methotrexate, and mifepristone.
14. Describe several relatively mild side effects and several adverse reactions associated with the use of prescription drugs.
15. Explain the significance of the therapeutic index.
16. List at least five guidelines for preventing or minimizing adverse drug reactions.
17. Discuss the relationship between polypharmacy and drug interactions in terms of drug absorption, distribution, metabolism, excretion, and drug reactions.
18. Distinguish between additive and synergistic drug interactions.
19. Describe the potential usefulness of the *Physicians' Desk Reference* to the consumer-patient.

Introduction

Although the major concern of this text is psychoactive drugs and their abuse potential, a related American drug problem is the widespread misuse of prescribed drugs—not just those having their primary impact on the human mind. Therefore, a chapter on physician-prescribed medications seems most appropriate.

To counter the widespread belief in "fail-safe" medicines, the "benefit-risk" equation is described, portraying all medications as having the potential for harm as well as for health and cure. After prescriptions and drug labels are examined, several guidelines are offered for the wise use of prescription drugs. Next, there is an investigation of the most frequently prescribed drugs, including psychoactives. Separate drug classes are described briefly.

Many patients apparently fail to comply with directions for using drugs, because they lack information on what can happen if they deviate from instructions, therefore an extensive section explores the potential for side effects and adverse reactions accompanying drug use. A concluding investigation focuses on the issue of generic versus brand-name drugs.

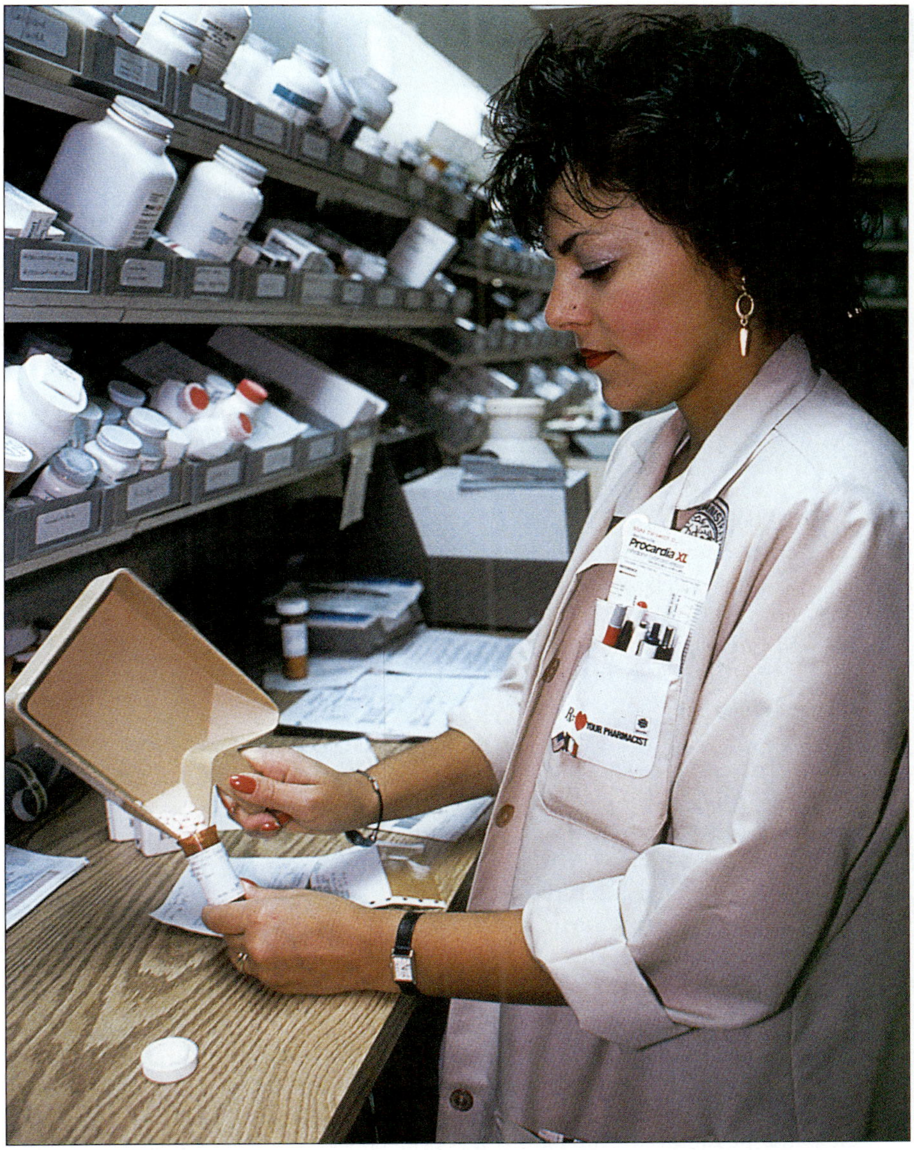

Prescription drugs may be sold only by licensed pharmacists in a variety of drug stores, as well as through pharmacist-supervised mail-order programs.

© Jeff Greenberg/PhotoEdit

Prescribed Drugs: Potent Chemotherapeutic Agents

According to the Food, Drug, and Cosmetic Act, drugs are substances intended for use in the diagnosis, cure, mitigation, treatment, or prevention of disease. Many of these drug substances or medicines are used beneficially in programs of self-medication that relieve minor symptoms. Such drugs that can be purchased over the counter and taken without a physician's supervision have been identified and described in chapter 12.

There are many other drugs that also have a legally recognized therapeutic value, such as Amoxil, Cardizem CD, Premarin, Synthroid, and Xanax. Unlike OTC drugs, these medicines can be obtained only by the direction of a physician and are referred to as *prescription* or *Rx drugs.* Sold only by licensed pharmacists, prescribed drugs are used in treating specific disease conditions of a more serious nature, are usually more powerful than OTC drugs, and are more likely to cause unexpected and adverse side effects.

In comparison with OTC drugs, prescribed medicines have a lower margin of safety when used. They have a greater potential for being habit forming or toxic and an increased likelihood for harmful effects. Moreover, they are produced for treatment of medical conditions that cannot be readily self-diagnosed.[1]

Potent chemotherapeutic agents, prescription drugs require professional supervision in their use because of the complex and powerful actions they can have on human structure and body function. Several nonphysician specialists, such as dentists; podiatrists; and some pharmacists, optometrists, physician assistants, and nurse practitioners—all of whom have been granted limited prescribing privileges in specific states—are qualified to determine the nature of a particular health problem and recommend an appropriate medication.[2] Nevertheless, only physicians are trained professionally to use a broad range of therapeutic drugs safely. Only these professionals can determine how long a specific drug can be taken—and in what amounts—without harm.

The Benefit-Risk Equation

Many people believe in the myth of **fail-safe medicine,** that is, the expectation that all drugs work safely on all people at all times. However, there is a common and not well-publicized reality that exists in medical practice and in many aspects of human endeavor—the so-called **benefit-risk equation.** According to this equation, there is a high probability that absolute safety does not exist. This is particularly true with regard to drugs.

Whether at the conscious or subconscious level, nearly all regulatory judgments are based on a compromise between benefits and risks. This benefit-to-risk judgment applies to crossing a busy street, driving a car, chewing a piece of meat that could cause choking, undergoing surgery, and taking a prescribed medicine. The probability of the good outweighs the possibility of the bad. If a medication poses an unusual or serious risk to the user, then, to justify prescribing it for that person, its benefits must be proportionately high and urgently required.

Indeed, every drug has the potential for causing unanticipated and unintended drug reactions or *side effects.* These side effects may range from relatively minor complaints that are undesirable and discomforting to the more serious effects that can be life threatening, even fatal. The more serious side effects are usually described as *adverse drug reactions.*

It is the competent physician then, together with an informed patient, who must decide if the health-giving or medicinal characteristics of an Rx drug are greater than the drug's potential hazards.

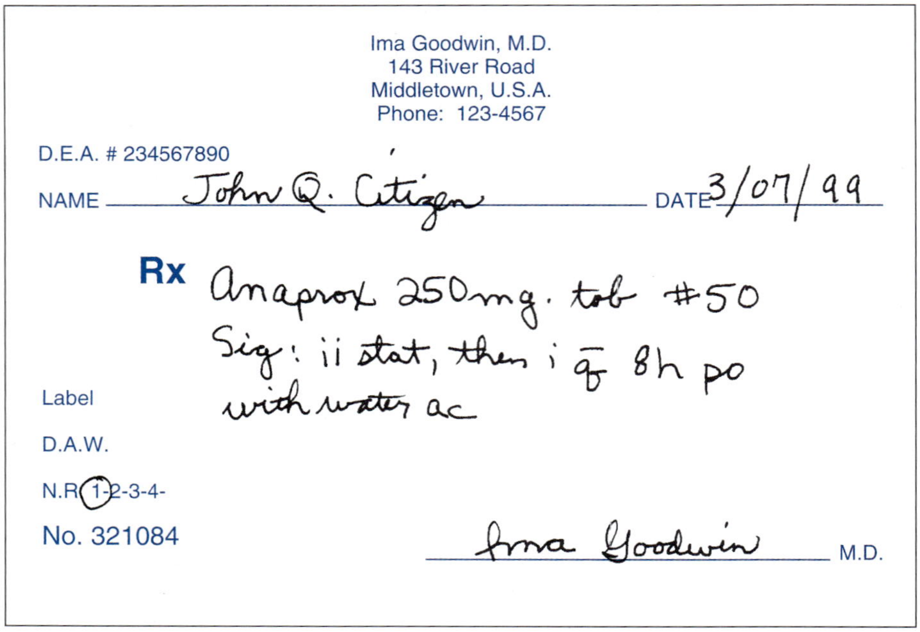
Ima Goodwin, M.D.
143 River Road
Middletown, U.S.A.
Phone: 123-4567

D.E.A. # 234567890

NAME John Q. Citizen DATE 3/07/99

Rx Anaprox 250 mg. tab #50
Sig: ii stat, then i q̄ 8h po
with water ac

Label

D.A.W.

N.R. (1)-2-3-4-

No. 321084 Ima Goodwin M.D.

figure 13.1

This sample prescription is for Anaprox, a brand name for a specific nonsteroidal anti-inflammatory analgesic often used to control pain, swelling, and stiffness accompanying certain types of arthritis. As indicated on the prescription, the pharmacist is directed to give the patient a 250 mg. dose of Anaprox, 50 tablets (#50). The label also states that two tablets should be taken at once as the first dose (ii stat), then the dose should be decreased to one tablet every 8 hours (i q̄ 8h) by mouth (po) with water before meals (ac). The label on the drug container should list the name of the medication ("Label" is not crossed out); the pharmacist must fill the prescription as written and no generic is allowed ("D.A.W." is not crossed out); and the patient may receive one refill.

Consequently, a pharmacist can dispense these powerful drugs only to individuals who have a physician's prescription. But the pharmacist may be the last defense against risky drug interactions. Thus, the assurance of quality and safety in using prescription drugs involves not only the prescribing physician and an informed and cooperative patient, but also the skilled and caring pharmacist.

Prescriptions and Drug Labels

A **prescription** is a physician's order to a pharmacist to dispense a specific drug product to a patient.[3] The prescription may be written or given orally to a pharmacist or nurse, in person or by telephone. According to the Pharmaceutical Manufacturers Association, nearly 70 percent of Rx drugs are dispensed through prescriptions; the remainder are administered directly to patients or provided in hospitals or by physicians.

Reading a Prescription

Although a prescription may appear to be a foreign, garbled handwritten message to a pharmacist, there is no mystery about reading a physician's order if the pharmacists know the special shorthand and can decipher the physician's handwriting. The prescription follows a uniform procedure and includes the elements on a preprinted form as shown in figure 13.1.[4]

Labels on Prescribed Medicines

Though prescription drugs are more powerful and more likely to produce serious side effects than OTC drugs, the labels on prescribed medicine containers

Box 13.1 Know Your Medicines *Common Dosage Forms*

Caplet—a round or elongated tablet with a coated or smooth surface.

Capsule—a thin gelatin case or shell that encloses a medicine.

Inhalant—a breathable mist or fine powder introduced into the body through the lungs.

Injectable—typically, a liquid medication that enters the body by way of a syringe and needle.

Liquid—a solution in which a drug is completely dissolved. A *suspension* is a liquid in which the active drug is only partially dissolved, while an *elixir* or tincture is a solution of a medicinal substance in alcohol. By contrast, a *syrup* is a concentrated solution of sugar that contains the active drug ingredient along with flavoring and stabilizing agents. *Drops* are solutions or suspensions containing a drug introduced behind the eyelid or into the ear. *Nasal sprays* or drops are solutions of a drug in water intended to produce a localized effect in the nostrils.

Suppository—a solid medication inserted into the rectum or vagina, where the drug dissolves.

Tablet—a solid form of medicine made by compressing the powder form of the same drug. Frequently, the term *tablet* is used interchangeably with "pill," although a pill is usually described as a solid form of medicine in a globular or oval mass.

Topical—a drug form such as an ointment, cream, lotion, or liquid applied to an external surface of the body.

Transdermal—a medication absorbed into the body through the skin.

have somewhat limited information in comparison with their OTC counterparts. Prescription drug labels usually carry the following information:

Name, address, and *phone number* of the dispensing pharmacy.

Prescription number, sometimes followed by the initials of the dispensing pharmacist.

Prescribing *physician's name.*

Date when prescription was filled.

Patient's name.

Drug name. In some instances, state laws may require the listing of the originally prescribed drug name and the product's manufacturer, if a generic drug has been substituted.

Directions for use, such as *dosage, frequency of use, when to take the medicine, how to take the medicine, and specific instructions for storage or preparation for use.*

On controlled substances (psychoactive therapeutic drugs having an abuse potential) and noncontrolled medicines, a *special legend* regarding *federal prohibition of the transfer of the drug* to any person other than the patient for whom the medication was prescribed.

Expiration date indicates the month, day, and year after which the medicine's potency is not likely to be maintained and/or the date beyond which the prescription cannot be refilled.

Number of allowable refills, if any.

Labels on prescribed medicines are not required to indicate precisely what the drug will likely do or why the medicine is being prescribed. Common side effects or precautions are not routinely listed. Only a general warning may be provided by the pharmacist, who may attach a small adhesive tag to the drug container or provide a small sheet detailing various precautions to observe, as a service by the dispensing pharmacy. Even the required directions for use might be inadequately stated. For instance, the direction to take a medication "before meals" is not specific enough for most individuals. Adequate instructions would indicate exactly how long before meals the medication should be taken.

This detailed information should come from one's physician. It will not likely be printed on the drug container's label.

The label on an Rx drug will indicate the number of times the medicine can be refilled. Under the provisions of the Controlled Substances Act (see chapters 1 and 15), those therapeutic drugs having a significant potential for producing psychological or physical dependence are restricted according to the following schedule.[5]

1. *Schedule I* drugs, such as heroin, marijuana, and LSD, are used for closely supervised research purposes only, and are not legally available for medicinal use by prescription. According to federal law, drugs in this schedule have a high abuse and dependence potential, and a prescription cannot legally be written for these drugs for medical use. (Although two states have legalized the medical use of marijuana, it still has not been approved by the federal government.)
2. Prescriptions for *Schedule II* medications (those having the highest abuse potential and dependence liability), such as morphine (MS Contin), methadone, Demerol; certain short-acting barbiturates; and specific amphetamines, must be written, not telephoned, to a pharmacy, and they may not be refilled. To obtain more drugs, the patient must return to a physician to obtain another written prescription.
3. Prescriptions for *Schedule III* drugs that have a clear medical use (codeine, hydrocodone, some hypnotics, certain appetite suppressants, and codeine and paregoric in combination with other drugs) may be written or telephoned to a pharmacy by a prescribing physician and may be refilled on the patient's decision up to five times in six months.

4. Prescriptions for *Schedule IV* drugs (propoxyphene, all benzodiazepines, and certain hypnotics) having an abuse and dependence potential somewhat less than drugs in *Schedule III* may also be refilled on the patient's decision up to five times in six months. When a patient requires more medication, rather than issuing a new prescription, a physician may authorize a pharmacist to dispense additional medicine based on the original prescription.
5. *Schedule V* drugs include prescribed and several OTC narcotic preparations of antitussives and antidiarrheals that contain codeine. Schedule V drugs requiring a prescription are processed as any other nonscheduled prescription drug. Some OTC drug preparations can be sold only upon approval by a pharmacist. In addition, the buyer must be at least eighteen years old and is required to sign his or her name in a special record maintained by the pharmacist.

NAME OF DRUG/ DIRECTIONS	SUN	MON	TUE	WED	THU	FRI	SAT

NAME OF DRUG/ DIRECTIONS	SUN	MON	TUE	WED	THU	FRI	SAT
DRUG A— 3 Times a day	8 12 5	8 12 5	8 12 5	8 12 5	8 12 5	8 12 5	8 12 5
DRUG B— once a day in AM	8	8	8	8	8	8	8
DRUG C— 3 Times a day	8 12 5	8 12 5	8 12 5	8 12 5	8 12 5	8 12 5	8 12 5

figure 13.2

Check-off chart for using medicines wisely.

You can make photocopies of the top chart for your use. Write down the times to take your medicines and check them off after you've taken them. You can take it along if you're away from home a lot, or post it at home. The bottom chart example shows the user has taken all doses through 5 P.M. on Tuesday of that week.

Source: National Institute on Drug Abuse and the U.S. Food and Drug Administration

Using Prescribed Drugs Wisely

Labels provide relatively little information about prescribed medicines, and due to the widespread public ignorance regarding drugs and their effects, numerous consumer action groups, along with the Food and Drug Administration, suggest that patients obtain such detailed information from their physicians. But getting the facts, the precautions, the early-warning signs of adverse reactions, and related information on drug effects may involve developing a degree of assertiveness with one's physician. Do not be intimidated by your health care consultant. Remember, your health is at stake!

Ask plenty of questions. Refuse complicated explanations offered in "medical jargon." If you do not understand certain instructions, ask that the physician repeat them slowly so you can write them down. The wise patient is one who has answers to the following questions *before* taking prescribed drugs.[6]

1. *What is the name of the medicine?* Write it down during your visit with a physician; have your physician write it legibly for you; or better yet, ask the physician filling out the prescription to include the drug's name on the label when the medication is dispensed by a pharmacist.
2. *When and how often should the drug be taken?* If your physician tells you to take the drug three times a day, be sure to notice whether it should be taken before or after meals. If "every six hours" is specified, does that mean when you are awake, or should you get up during the night to take the medicine every six hours (see fig. 13.2) To assure proper use of prescribed medicines and to avoid accidental overdosing, keep a record of the names, doses, and frequency of use for each medicine prescribed (see fig. 13.3).
3. *What is the medicine supposed to do?* Will it reduce the pain or get to the cause of the pain, reduce fever, lower blood pressure, or cure infection? Does the drug merely relieve symptoms or eliminate or control an underlying condition? If your state does not require the inclusion of the intended use of the medicine on the prescription, ask your physician to include it. Some states already require this information to appear on drug orders for patients in long-term care facilities.[7]

   You may also want to read the information leaflet that comes with most prescription drugs. Too many of these are often too complicated for most people, so the FDA is proposing to make this information more adequate, useful, and easy to understand. However, it may be 2006 before such revised information is provided to most patients receiving new prescriptions.[8]
4. *Can the new medicine be taken along with others?* If you are taking other

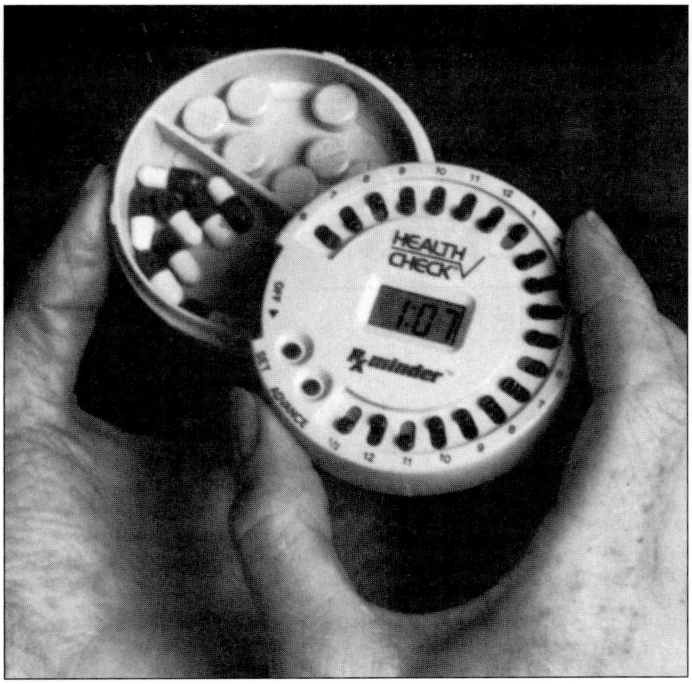

(a)

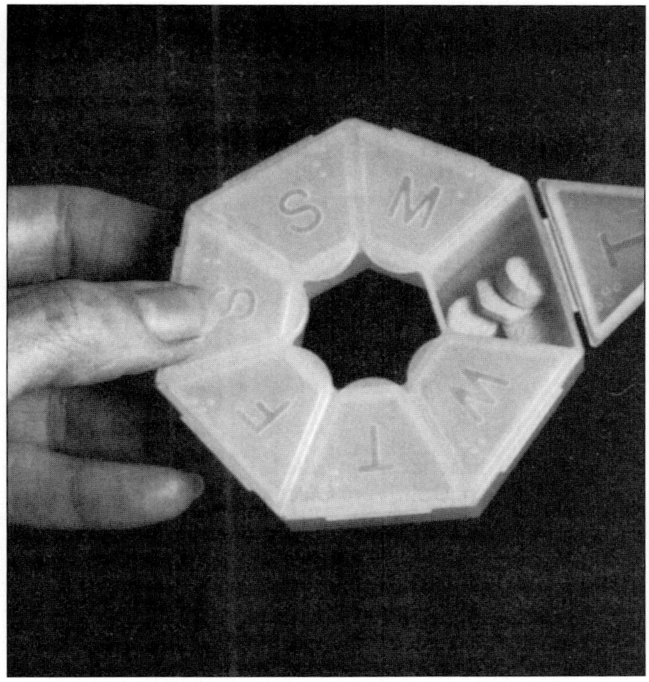

(b)

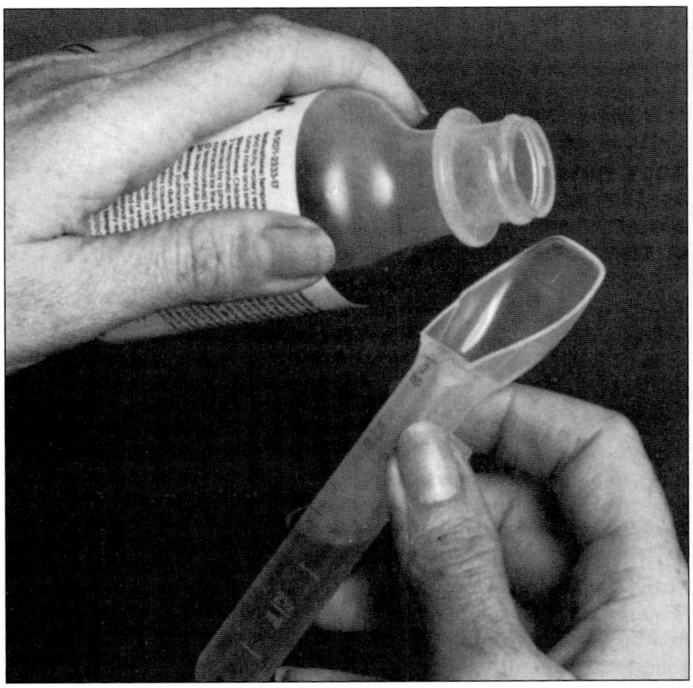

(c)

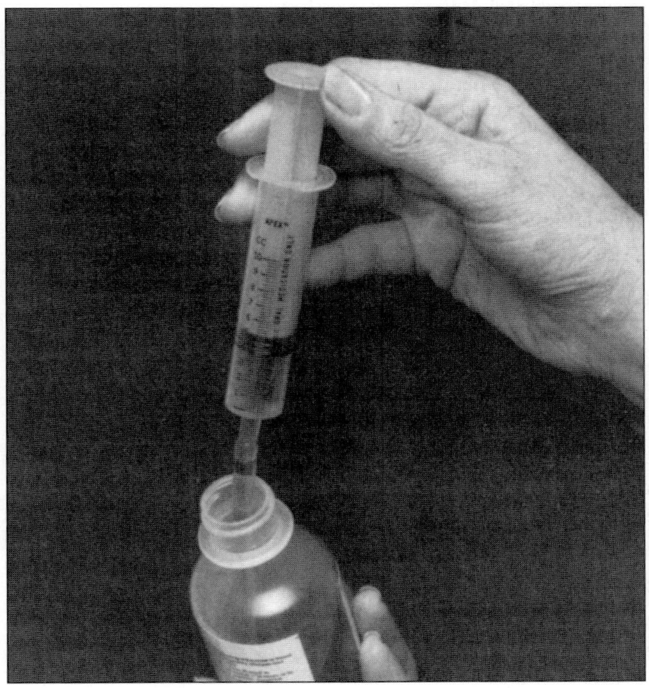

(d)

figure 13.3

Taking the right dose. (a) Several types of aids are available to help people take the right dose of medicine at the right time, like this pill container with a quiet, wristwatch-like alarm that can be set for specific times of day or specific intervals. (b) A pill container with Braille markings that holds a week's worth of pills, divided into the days of the week. (c) A spoon marked with the appropriate dosages for liquid medications. (d) An oral medication syringe, similarly marked.

Source: U.S. Food and Drug Administration.

prescribed or OTC medications, inform your physician and the pharmacist filling your prescription. On occasion, drugs may interact to cause either a decrease or increase in the desired effect or a harmful or life-threatening reaction. The physician and pharmacist may be able to alert you to special precautions in the use of more than one drug at a time.

5. *What unwanted side effects might occur?* In some individuals, medicines might cause drowsiness, nausea, vomiting, dizziness, nervousness, or other reactions. Should an unexpected reaction occur, inform your physician as soon as possible. He or she may want to change your medication.
6. *What precautions should you take?* For example, if the expected reaction to a medicine is drowsiness, dizziness, or unsteadiness, you should not drive or operate machinery.
7. *Are there any particular foods you should avoid while taking the medicine?* Some antibiotics, for example, will not work if you drink milk or eat milk products. Alcoholic beverages should not be used when some drugs are being taken.
8. *Should you take the medicine until it is gone or only until you feel better?* Some medicines must be taken for long periods to cure the disease. If you stop taking the medicine too early, even when you feel better, the symptoms and disease may recur.

Supplied with the answers to the foregoing questions, the consumer-patient may wish to consider several additional guidelines in using prescription medicines.

The following suggestions are designed to safely enhance the effectiveness of a drug.[9]

- *Follow the directions for using a drug* as specified on the label.
- *Inform your physician and pharmacist about any medication problems you may have and all medications you are taking* or have taken during the past few weeks.
- *If you are pregnant, planning to become pregnant, or breast-feeding, consult with your physician* before taking any medicines, including OTC drugs.
- *Before surgery of any kind,* including dental surgery or emergency treatment, *inform your physician, surgeon, or dentist of any medication you are taking.*
- After completing your course of medication, *discard the remaining prescribed drugs.*
- To avoid medication errors, *never take a medicine in the dark or from an unlabeled container.*
- *Store your medication properly* in its original container, away from bright lights, and in a cool, dry place, out of the reach of children.
- *Do not use outdated medications,* because certain drugs lose their effectiveness or potency with age.
- *Never give your prescribed medications to another person,* and never take medicine prescribed for anyone else.

Box 13.2 Know Your Medicines *Types of Drug Effects*

Buccal—general or whole-body effects resulting from the slow absorption of a medicine through the cheek.

Dental—localized effect when a drug is applied to the teeth or gums.

Inhalation—local or even systemic (general) effects when a drug is inhaled into the lungs in breathing.

Mucosal—local drug effect when a medication is applied to mucous membranes, such as the inside of the mouth.

Nasal—local drug effect when a medicine is used in the nose or nostrils.

Ophthalmic—local drug effect when a medication is applied directly to the eyes.

Otic—local drug effect when a medication is introduced into the ear.

Parenteral-local—localized effects in a specific body area, when the drug is injected.

Rectal—local or systemic (general) effect when a drug is used in the rectum.

Sublingual—general or whole-body effects resulting from the slow absorption of a medicine placed under the tongue.

Systemic—general or whole-body effect; descriptive of medicine taken by mouth or by injection.

Topical—local drug effect when a medication is applied directly to the skin.

Vaginal—local or systemic (general) effect when a drug is used in the vagina.

Frequently Used Prescription Drugs

Each year, a nationwide survey, the National Prescription Audit (NPA), indicates which drugs are most often dispensed in chain, independent, food store pharmacies, and long-term care facilities and through mail-order prescription programs in the United States (see table 13.1).[10] The NPA, a continuing study of the movement of prescription drugs from retail outlets to patients, is based on prescriptions dispensed by pharmacists, not on prescriptions written by physicians. Such a procedure reflects the growing importance of retail pharmacists' decision-making authority regarding multiple-source drugs, when **generic drugs** may be substituted for brand-name drugs.

An analysis of the National Prescription Audit reveals that the total number of prescriptions filled each year in the United States is 2.3 billion. This number includes refills (1.02 billion) and new prescriptions (1.29 billion) and brand-name and generic drugs.

table 13.1 Top Twenty Most Prescribed Drugs for 1998

Rank	Drug Name	Generic Name	Therapeutic Use
1	Premarin Oral	conjugate estrogen	Replacement female hormone therapy
2	Synthroid	levothyroxine	Thyroid hormone
3	Trimox	amoxicillin	Antibiotic; anti-infective, penicillin
4	Hydrocodone/APAP	hydrocodone/acetaminophen	Narcotic analgesic with acetaminophen; pain relief
5	Prozac	fluoxetine	Treatment of mental depression
6	Prilosec	omeprazole	Antiulcer drug; supresses gastric secretion
7	Zithromax	azithromycin	Antibiotic
8	Lipitor	atorvastatin	Reduced total and LDL cholesterol
9	Norvasc	amlodipine	Relieves and controls angina (chest pain) and hypertension; calcium channel blocker
10	Claritin	loratidine	Nonsedating antihistamine
11	Lanoxin	digoxin	Improves contraction force of heart muscle
12	Zoloft	sertraline	Treatment of mental depression
13	Albuterol Aerosol	albuterol	Antiasthmatic
14	Paxil	paroxetine	Treatment of mental depression
15	Amoxicillin	amoxicillin	Broad spectrum antibiotic
16	Prempro	estrogens and medroxyprogesterone	Menopausal osteoporosis
17	Zestril	lisinopril	Antihypertensive
18	Vasotec	enalapril	Antihypertensive
19	Augmentin	amoxicillin	Antibiotic
20	Cephalexin	cephalexin	Broad spectrum antibiotic

Source: Dr. Harold Crossley, DDS, Ph.D. Baltimore College of Dental Surgery University of Maryland, Baltimore

By the mid-1990s, the average cost of a prescribed drug had risen to just over $29. While brand name prescription prices rose 3.3 percent in one year, the price of generic drugs fell 11.5 percent for the same year.

Furthermore, the audit confirmed once again the ongoing trend of physicians to prescribe generic drugs when writing new prescriptions. At least 15 percent of new prescription drugs are generic.

Of all prescribed drugs, other than those administered to hospitalized patients, only a small proportion (5 percent or less) are **controlled drugs,** scheduled medications that have a significant potential for abuse and addiction. These psychoactive drugs are under the regulatory control of the Drug Enforcement Administration (DEA), an agency of the U.S. Department of Justice. Most of these controlled medicines are antianxiety drugs, minor tranquilizers (benzodiazepines), narcotic analgesics, sedatives, and hypnotics.

Prescription Drug Classes

The huge numbers of prescription medications are often subdivided into major groups. These **drug classes or families** share important characteristics in terms of their chemical composition or in their actions within the human body. Typically, the several drugs within a class or family behave in particular and somewhat similar ways. There are, to be sure, some important exceptions.

Careful analysis of the various drug classes reveals that within each class or category there may be several medications containing the same or similar basic drug ingredients marketed under different brand names. Identified here are several of the major drug classes or drug families, together with representative brand-name medications.

Analgesics relieve pain and produce insensibility to pain without loss of consciousness. Mild analgesics include Darvocet, Darvon, Percodan, Talwin, and Valadol. Some stronger analgesics are Demerol, Dolophine (methadone), and Leritine.

Anorexics, many of which are amphetaminelike central nervous system stimulants, are occasionally prescribed for weight loss because they tend to reduce one's appetite. Commonly prescribed diet pills are Desoxyn, Didrex, Ionamin, Meridia, Preludin, and Tenuate.

Antialcohol preparations produce a sensitivity to ethyl alcohol resulting in an unpleasant reaction when the patient takes even small amounts of alcohol. Antabuse is a brand name of disulfiram frequently used to deter drinking of ethanol in the management of alcoholism.

Antiarthritics are used to treat joint diseases, specifically rheumatoid arthritis, osteoarthritis, and related arthritic conditions. The anti-inflammatory action of these drugs reduces joint swelling, pain, and duration of morning stiffness and improves functional ability of arthritic patients. Nonsteroidal (Ansaid, Feldene,

Indocin, Motrin, Naprosyn, and Voltaren) and corticosteroidal (Decadron and Prednisone) medications are examples of antiarthritic drugs.

Antihistamines block the action of a specific chemical, histamine, and are used in the treatment as well as prevention of various allergic reactions, especially the prevention of allergic rhinitis. This condition is the inflammation of the nose and upper airways, resulting from a reaction to an allergen, such as pollen, dust, or animal fur. These antihistamine drugs are used to relieve itching, swelling, and redness characteristic of allergic reaction involving the skin. Among the frequently prescribed antihistamines are Actidil, Atarax, Claritin, Hismanal, and Seldane.

Antiasthmatics, or bronchodilators, by dilating bronchial tubes (airways) that are in sustained constriction, relieve difficult breathing associated with acute attacks of bronchial asthma and with other disorders characterized by spasm of the bronchial tubes. Albuterol Aerosol, Bronkodyl, Bronkosol, Choledyl, Intal, Isuprel, Neothylline, TheoDur, and Theolair are antiasthmatics.

Anti-infective drugs, or antimicrobials, such as antibiotics, sulfonamides (sulfa drugs), antifungal preparations, and antiseptics are pharmaceutical agents that inactivate and eliminate invading, disease-causing microbes. Drugs in this family destroy bacteria or inhibit the growth and multiplication of infecting microorganisms. Among the most frequently prescribed drugs are the antibiotics, represented by cephalosporins (Ceclor), erythromycins (E.E.S.), penicillins (Amoxil, Augmentin, Trimox), and tetracyclines (Achromycin). Gantrisin is a commonly used sulfa drug.

Antidepressants are prescribed for the relief of emotional depression, dejection, and withdrawal. Sometimes these drugs also reduce feelings of anxiety and produce a sedative effect. The foremost antidepressant is *Prozac,* a somewhat controversial psychopharmacological medication. Another prescription antidepressant is *Zoloft.*

The *tricyclic antidepressants* include Aventyl, Elavil, Surmontil, and Tofranil. Another group of antidepressants, the *monoamine oxidase* (MAO) *inhibitors,* are represented by Marplan, Nardil and Parnate. These drugs have amphetamine-like actions, inhibit a particular brain enzyme, and produce neurotransmitters that tend to maintain normal mood and emotional stability.

Antidiabetic agents, taken by mouth and by injected forms of **insulin,** help to maintain the diabetic patient's blood sugar at a nearly normal level and keep the urine as free of sugar as possible. Prescribed oral antidiabetics help the body to release its own insulin and are represented by Diabinese, Dymelor, Micronase, and Orinase. Injected insulin, for which a prescription is not required, is used to restore the body's ability to use sugar normally in the condition of diabetes. Examples of injected insulin preparations are Iletin, Lente Insulin, Regular Insulin, and Ultralente Insulin.

Antidiarrheals are used in the management and control of diarrhea (increased frequency and fluid content of fecal discharge). Antidiarrheals containing narcotics or narcotic derivatives tend to reduce intestinal movements. Other drugs in this family relax the smooth musculature of the intestinal tract or destroy specific bacteria causing the diarrhea. Donnagel-PG, Lomotil, Paregoric, and Parepectolin are frequently prescribed to control diarrhea.

Antihypertensive drugs are special types of cardiovascular (heart and blood vessel) drugs used to reduce high blood

Box 13.3 The Drug Approval Process

Before any new over-the-counter or prescription drug can be marketed in the United States, an enormous amount of research and testing must be accomplished. Such an extensive undertaking involves many people and a great deal of money and can often last from 5 to 10 years. The drug approval process consists of two major stages:

Preclinical Stage:

- test drug to determine effects/side effects (usually done in a lab on animal subjects)
- determine most effective method of administering drug
- ask FDA for approval to test drug on humans

Clinical Stage:

- Phase 1—test drug on small number of healthy humans to determine safety
- Phase 2—test drug on small number of patients with the disease the drug is supposed to help to determine effectiveness
- Phase 3—administer drug to more patients (several hundred to several thousand) to establish effectiveness, safety, and dosage levels

Test data compiled in the earlier portion of the clinical phase are submitted to the FDA on a New Drug Application (NDA). These data must prove that the new drug is safe and effective. The FDA review of the NDA may require two or more years. Once the FDA grants its approval for marketing the new drug, the manufacturer then begins a period of postmarketing surveillance to collect information about side effects and other possible uses of the drug other than the one for which it was originally developed and approved. According to the FDA, only one in five drugs tested is eventually approved, and some FDA-approved drugs have been removed from the market due to the occurrence of adverse reactions that did not surface in either preclinical or clinical testing.

The FDA has implemented procedures to speed up access to new drugs and improve the drug review process as described. Under the accelerated approval initiative, so-called breakthrough drugs will be approved at the earliest time at which safety and effectiveness can reasonably be established.

Sources: Modified from "Updates: Initiatives Speed Access to Drugs", in *FDA Consumer,* vol.26, no. 6, pages 2–3, July–August 1992; and Ken Flieger, "Testing Drugs in People" in *FDA Consumer,* vol. 28, no. 6, pages 16–19, July–August, 1994.

pressure. Some of these drugs act directly on the heart to lower heart rate and blood pressure (the alpha- and beta-blockers), while others—the diuretics—help rid the body of excess water and salt and thus produce an antihypertensive effect. Aldomet, Capoten, Inderal, Loniten, Lopressor, Minipress, Tenormin, Vasotec, and Zestril are common antihypertensive drugs.

Antineoplastics are used in treating specific cancerous conditions. These drugs are often prescribed to reduce the pain and other symptoms of cancer and include various pharmaceutical agents, such as antibiotic derivatives, antimetabolites, hormones, steroids, and derivatives of nitrogen mustard. Among prescribed antineoplastics are Adrucil, Cytoxan, Fluorouracil, Leukeran Megace, and Mexate.

Antispasmodics and antiulcer agents are prescribed for the control of various disorders of the stomach and intestinal tract. These drugs tend to reduce the muscular contractions or spasms of the gastrointestinal tract or reduce acid secretion in the stomach. Examples of these drug families are Anaspaz, Bentyl, Darbid, Donnatal containing phenobarbital, Prilosec, Robinul, Tagamet, and Zantac.

However, medical research has revealed that almost all duodenal ulcers are due to a spiral-shaped bacterium, *Helicobacter pylori,* as are nearly 80 percent of gastric ulcers.[11] As a consequence, treatment of ulcers—the open sores in the lining of the stomach or the upper part of the small intestine—will involve more use of an antibiotic in combination with another drug that eases severe heartburn.

Cardiovascular drugs affect the function of the heart and blood vessels of the body. In addition to the widely used antihypertensives that control high blood pressure, cardiovascular drugs include (1) calcium channel-blocking *antianginal preparations* (Calan, Cardizem, and Procardia), which dilate blood vessels supplying the heart and thus relieve pain; (2) *antiarrhythmics* (Inderal, Norpace, Tonocard), which help restore normal rhythm to one's heartbeat—Inderal also has other positive effects on heart function; (3) *digitalis* (Digoxin, Lanoxin), which increases the strength of the heart's contraction; (4) *coronary vasodilators,* such as nitroglycerin (Arlidin, Nitro-Bid, Vasodilan), which increase the blood flow to heart muscle; and (5) *vasopressors* (Aramine), which increase systolic and diastolic blood pressure and are thus used in treating low blood pressure.

Cholesterol-lowering drugs tend to reduce the amount of damaging blood fats that contribute to the build-up of fatty deposits in the arteries of the body. Some of these (Colestid, Questran) block the reabsorption of cholesterol-carrying bile salts, while others (Atromid-S, Lopid and Lorelco) prevent the conversion of fatty acids to lipids in the liver.

Diuretics help the body to pass excess water and salt and cause a sudden and copious flow of urine. Drugs such as Aldactone, Diuril, Dyazide, Lasix and Losol are frequently prescribed to lower blood pressure and to manage symptoms of liver and kidney diseases and congestive heart failure.

Sedative-hypnotic drugs are prescribed to induce sleep or to produce a reduction in tension and anxiety. Noludar and Placidyl are hypnotics used to counter insomnia on a short-term basis. Another nonbarbiturate sedative is Phenergan, an antihistamine with sedative action.

Dalmane, Halcion, and Restoril (representing the benzodiazepine antianxiety drug family) are used frequently as bedtime sedatives to induce sleep. The barbiturates, Amytal, Nembutal, Phenobarbital, Seconal, and Tuinal, may be prescribed as sleeping drugs due to their depressant effect on the central nervous system.

Stimulants are drugs that speed up the function of the central nervous system. Biphetamine and Dexedrine may be used to treat children with attention deficit disorders and narcolepsy (uncontrollable desire for sleep or sudden attacks of deep sleep). Cylert, another CNS stimulant structurally different from the amphetamines, is used as part of a management program for children with attention deficit disorders and hyperkinetic syndrome.

Tranquilizers include two different types of psychotherapeutic drugs used in the management of various physical or psychological disorders.

Major tranquilizers, such as Haldol, Mellaril, Prolixin, and Thorazine, are prescribed to relieve symptoms of a psychotic nature. One drug, Clozapine, has been most effective in relieving chronic schizophrenia.

By contrast, the *minor tranquilizers* or benzodiazepines are used in treating anxiety and reducing tension. These antianxiety drugs function somewhat like the sedative-hypnotics in restoring emotional calm. Minor tranquilizers include Atarax, Ativan, Librium, Serax, Tranxene, Valium, and Xanax. When these drugs are used in large doses for an extended time, they often produce a psychological or physical dependence, or both, along with tolerance and withdrawal symptoms when the drug is discontinued (see chapter 7). Some of these antianxiety agents also control vomiting in stressful situations, relieve muscle or skeletal disorders, prevent convulsions, and prevent withdrawal reactions in drug-dependent individuals.

There are, of course, many other drug classes or families, including *anticoagulants* (which reduce blood clotting), *anesthetics* (which produce a loss of sensation), *eye and ear preparations, hormones* (which regulate various body processes), *muscle relaxants, narcotic antagonists,* and *narcotic detoxification agents.* However, from the consumer-patient's viewpoint, knowing what drug has been prescribed, to which drug class or family the prescribed medicine belongs, and the other members of the same drug class, may prove useful in

1. preventing any interactions that could reduce the effectiveness of drug actions; and
2. lessening the chance of experiencing unanticipated and sometimes hazardous, adverse drug effects.[12]

Oral Contraceptives

Prescription drugs that prevent pregnancy by keeping the ovaries from developing and releasing mature ova or eggs are referred to as oral contraceptives. Formulated in the late 1950s by Dr. John Rock and his associates, oral contraceptives are among the most effective ways of

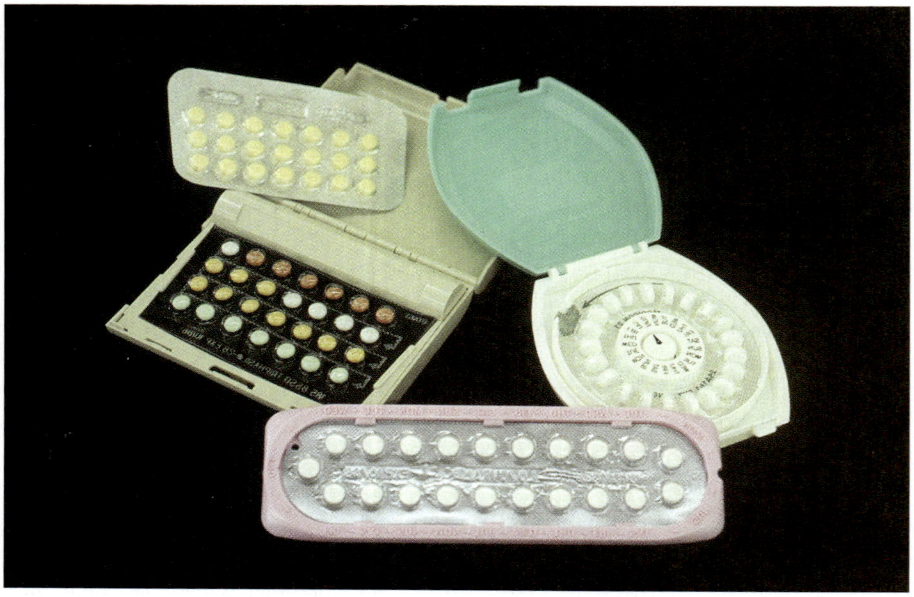

Oral contraceptive pills are frequently prescribed birth control drugs because they are effective despite their potential for adverse and harmful effects.

©James L. Shaffer

preventing conception. (The only known method that is more effective is sterilization.) Although these drugs are convenient and relatively free of major side effects for most women, they are still available only by prescription. Moreover, the use of these drugs cannot guarantee absolute safety or effectiveness. When used alone, birth control pills offer no protection against the transmission of HIV (the AIDS-causing virus) or other sexually transmitted diseases.

Combination OCs

Two major types of oral contraceptives (OCs) are on the market.[13] By far, the most widely used is the **combination oral contraceptive drug**—a combination of two synthetic female hormones, estrogen and progestin. It is this combination OC that is usually referred to as "birth control pills" or "the Pill." It is also this same, combined oral contraceptive, but in much higher doses, that is occasionally prescribed as a "morning-after pill." Such use of OCs will be described later in this chapter.

More than forty-five different formulations of oral contraceptives are listed in the *Physicians' Desk Reference,* reflecting numerous brand names with varying dosage levels of hormonal ingredients. Therefore, any reference to the oral contraceptive must consider the many different pills and their unique characteristics.

The combination drug or pill has proven to be more effective (approaching 99 percent) than the minipill, although the combined OC is associated with the more serious side effects and health risks. The estrogen component appears to be responsible for the greater effectiveness and the greater potential dangers of the Pill.

The present brands of OCs contain far less estrogen and progestin than the combined products first available almost thirty-seven years ago. Extensive research has allowed doctors and their patients to choose from "highest dose" combined pills (more frequently related to serious complications), "lowest dose" pills (associated with "spotting" and "missed menses"), and the "intermediate dose" variety. Most physicians prescribe the lowest dose for new patients.

The Minipill

By contrast, the progestin-only **minipill** is somewhat less effective (only about 97 percent) than the combination OC. However, the minipill apparently has fewer undesirable side effects, particularly headaches, high blood pressure, and leg pain.

Certain physical conditions, such as irregular genital bleeding, indicate a potentially dangerous consequence of using minipills, so the absolute contraindications to the use of estrogen-containing combination pills also apply to the minipill.

Estrogen Hormone Agents

From a contraceptive point of view, estrogen has several major actions.[14] The first action is the blocking or inhibition of the process of ovulation, the release of an egg from the ovary.

Second, the implantation or "nesting" of the fertilized egg in the uterine lining is inhibited by the presence of relatively high blood levels of estrogen. This action is especially effective when the estrogen is given after an unprotected act of intercourse during the middle of the menstrual cycle. Estrogen brings about certain changes in the lining of the uterus and makes the lining inhospitable so that the attachment of a fertilized egg is not likely to occur. High-dose oral estrogens have been given in emergency situations as a "morning-after pill," consisting of a substance known as diethylstilbestrol (DES).

Other actions of estrogen include changing the rate of passage of the ovum within the oviduct and the degeneration of the corpus luteum. This latter effect results in a decline in blood levels of progestin and thereby prevents normal implantation of a fertilized egg or placental attachment.

Progestin Hormone Agents

Whether occurring in the combination pill or in the minipill, progestins also have major contraceptive effects. The progestin changes the cervical mucus so that it becomes thicker and forms a plug that makes sperm movement through the cervix more difficult.

Implantation of the fertilized egg may also be blocked when progestins are given before ovulation. It is probable that progestins interfere with the process of capacitation, a complex action occurring in the uterus and oviducts that enhances the sperm's ability to penetrate the egg. Normal transport of the ovum may also be slowed when progestins are taken before fertilization.

Side Effects of Oral Contraceptives

While the majority of women can take oral contraceptive pills safely, there are some who are at increased risk of developing serious conditions that can threaten life or cause temporary or permanent disability or even death. Such risk is typically associated with those who smoke tobacco cigarettes; have high blood pressure, diabetes, high blood cholesterol levels, past or present blood clotting problems; or have had a heart attack, a stroke, cancer of the breast or sex organs, or malignant or benign liver tumors.

Although oral contraceptives are highly effective in preventing pregnancy, many women do not use the Pill because of their concerns about safety and side effects. The following are among the most serious of these problems:

1. *Cardiovascular* (heart and blood vessel) *diseases* have been associated with the use of combined oral contraceptives, especially those containing more estrogen than is usually used today. Three major cardiovascular effects have been identified:

   Heart attack. The relative risk for having a heart attack (myocardial infarction) is between 2 and 6 times greater in Pill users, but is confined primarily to those who smoke, have high blood pressure and high blood cholesterol, and are obese. However, the risk is low in women under the age of thirty.

   Abnormal blood clotting in the veins of the legs. A blood clot may break off from the clot-site in the veins of the legs or pelvis and then travel to the lungs where a pulmonary embolism (blockage of a blood vessel) may occur and result in death. Such a risk is between 1.5 and 6 times greater for women with predisposing conditions for blood clotting problems, but the risk disappears after pill use has stopped.

   Stroke. When a blood vessel in the brain becomes blocked or ruptures, the result is a stroke. Part of the brain is thus deprived of oxygen and dies. Early studies of women revealed the increased risk of stroke was greatest in women older than thirty-five years and in those who smoked and had high blood pressure. Research on women using only low-estrogen oral contraceptives indicates no stroke risk.[15] The risk of stroke is rare among women of childbearing age.

Standard for *PDR* Warning for Prescribers of Oral Contraceptives*

Cigarette smoking increases the risk of serious cardiovascular side effects on the heart and blood vessels from oral contraceptive use. This risk increases with age and with heavy smoking (15 or more cigarettes per day) and is quite marked in women over 35 years of age. Women who use oral contraceptives should not smoke.

2. *Benign* (nonmalignant) *tumor of the liver.* While such unwanted tumors or growths do not spread, they may result in the rupture of the liver's outer capsule, with extensive bleeding that could be fatal.
3. *Primary liver cancer.* Though an exceptionally rare disease in most developed countries, hepatocellular carcinoma (malignant tumors of liver cells that may infiltrate surrounding tissues and give rise to metastases) in noncirrhotic livers has been attributed to long-term oral contraceptive use.
4. *Gallbladder disease.* Associated with the liver, the gallbladder is a small saclike organ that stores and concentrates bile. Oral contraceptive use is not an important risk factor for development of gallbladder disease, but may speed up the development and appearance of gallbladder problems in women who are susceptible to such conditions.
5. *Hypertension.* Although hypertension (high blood pressure) resulting from the use of oral contraceptives is usually reversible, it can lead to permanent complications unless closely monitored by a physician. However, this condition is rare in women using low-dose pills and is more likely to occur in older users and with prolonged intake.

One side effect formerly associated with use of oral contraception—dangers to a developing fetus—is no longer considered as significant. The risk of having a baby with birth defects does not seem to be increased in Pill users who become pregnant.[16]

Other side effects sometimes experienced by users of the Pill, but are not likely to be life threatening, include nausea, vomiting, breast tenderness, weight gain or loss, swelling of the ankles, spotty darkening of the skin (especially on the face), and unexpected vaginal bleeding (spotting) between periods. More serious side effects observed are worsening of migraine headaches, asthma, epilepsy, kidney or heart disease due to edema (retention of water in the body), and mental depression.[17] The vast majority of pill users have only minor difficulties.

Noncontraceptive Benefits

Though the scientific literature details many potential side effects of oral contraceptives, millions of women in the United States and throughout the world have continued to use these pregnancy-prevention drugs with relative safety and a minimum of adverse reactions. In comparison with the possible risks and discomforts associated with conception, pregnancy, and childbirth, the risks from oral contraceptive side effects are almost negligible. Effectiveness, convenience of use, and the lack of interference with the act of intercourse have combined to make the Pill popular.

* Source: *Physicians' Desk Reference,* 50th. ed. (Montvale, NJ: Medical Economics Company, 1996), 1872, 1876–1877, 2088, 2091, 2093, 2747, 2749, 2756.

There are also a number of noncontraceptive benefits associated with oral contraceptive use. The Pill appears to provide a "protective effect" against pelvic inflammatory disease. Oral contraceptives tend to relieve a variety of unwanted menstrual symptoms, particularly menstrual cramping. The number of days of bleeding is shortened and the amount of blood loss is reduced. Premenstrual tension is often milder.

Most studies in the past demonstrated no increased risk of breast cancer in users of OCs. Research now suggests that OCs might have a breast-cancer-promoting effect on a specific subgroup of women. Some studies have also shown an increased risk for cervical cancer among Pill users. Nevertheless, use of oral contraceptives lowers the risk of ovarian cysts, ovarian and endometrial cancers, and benign breast disease.[18] Use of oral contraceptives may also improve acne conditions and enhance the enjoyment of sexual relations for both females and males, presumably by reducing the fear of pregnancy.

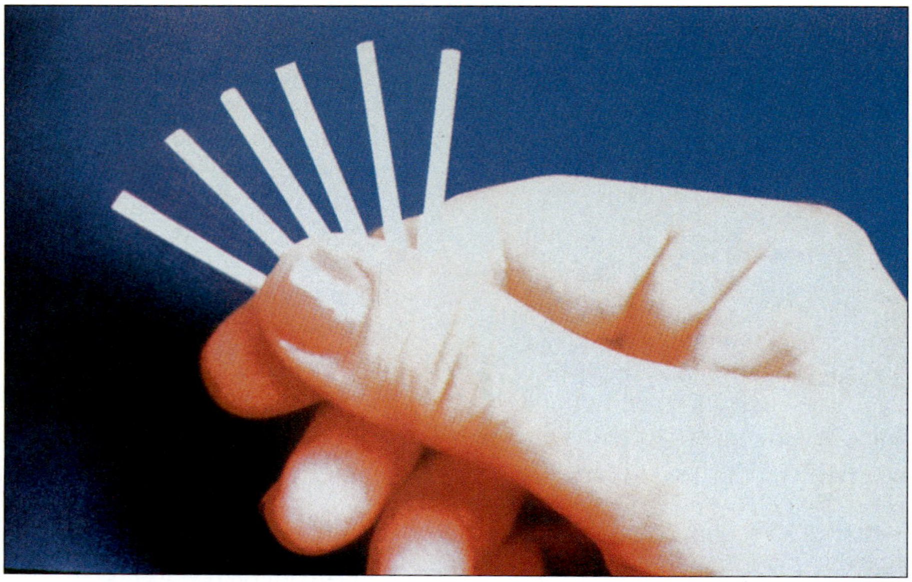

Norplant, the subdermal contraceptive consists of six small capsules surgically implanted just beneath the skin on a woman's upper arm. Each capsule contains a progestin-only substance that is released slowly and provides a long-acting contraceptive effect.
Courtesy Wyeth-Ayers Laboratories.

The Future of Drug-Based Contraception

It is likely there will never be an absolutely safe and perfectly effective oral contraceptive for either the female or the male. However, techniques being researched and developed may enable many people to select what is appropriate and reasonably safe.

Long-acting injectable progestin, known as **Depo-Provera** (depomedroxyprogesterone acetate, or DMPA) is approved for use in the United States. A single intramuscular injection of DMPA, given every three months, blocks ovulation by suppressing FSH and LH blood levels. The development of an "inhospitable endometrium"—one that does not allow implantation of a fertilized egg—and a thickening of cervical mucus that decreases sperm penetration, are additional contraceptive actions. Some common side effects of this drug include menstrual irregularities and weight gain. Depo-Provera should not be taken by women who have liver disease, unusual vaginal bleeding, breast cancer, or blood clots. Pregnancy should be ruled out before the drug is taken.

Subdermal implants consisting of Silastic capsules are inserted beneath the surface of the skin, where a slow-release, progestin-only chemical, levonorgestrel, exerts a contraceptive effect for as long as five years. The FDA approved this **Norplant** subdermal implant as an implantable contraceptive in 1990. The implant is a fanlike arrangement of six match-size, silicon rubber rods, each containing a progestin-only hormone. Surgically inserted just beneath the skin at the inner arm just above the elbow, the rods slowly release the hormone into the bloodstream. While not visible, the rods can be felt under the skin.

According to the FDA, Norplant is more than 99 percent effective in women weighing less than 150 pounds, but its effectiveness may decrease in heavier women.[19] If a woman wants to become pregnant or experiences undesirable effects, including irregular menstrual bleeding, headaches, nausea, nervousness, and mood changes, the patient can have the implants removed by outpatient surgery.

One drug product being tested makes use of a chemical substance, LHRH, originating in the hypothalamus of the brain. This chemical influences the pituitary gland and thus affects the ovulatory cycle. It is hoped that this new drug will not have the potentially serious side effects associated with oral contraceptives.

The future of drug-based contraception may include an antipregnancy vaccine for women, an antifertility vaccine for men, and an injectable hormone preparation of testosterone that suppresses sperm production. An extract from cotton plants, known as *Gossypol,* is being used experimentally on a limited basis in the People's Republic of China to suppress sperm production and to change the structure and transport of sperm cells.

Emergency "Morning After" Oral Contraception

In a controversial action, the FDA declared that ordinary oral contraceptive pills—already available on the market—can be used safely as a form of emergency, **morning after contraception.** Six brands have been proved as effective 75 percent of the time in preventing conception, if taken within seventy-two hours of unprotected intercourse. A second dose is then taken twelve hours after the first.[20]

In higher doses than used in ordinary oral contraception, these "emergency use" pills stop pregnancy in one of four ways:

1. prevention of ovulation;
2. prevention of fertilization;
3. interference with the movement of either the ovum or fertilized egg within the oviduct; and
4. blocking the implantation of a fertilized egg into the uterus.

Women's advocates, The Population Council, and the Planned Parenthood Federation of America have applauded the FDA's action, because physicians may now legally prescribe oral contraceptives for emergency use. However, right-to-life advocates insist that such use of oral contraceptives amounts to approval of abortion. According to their belief, these "emergency pills" likely prevent the fertilized egg—a new human life—from undergoing the normal implantation process.

Despite the FDA's decision, the major United States manufacturer of oral contraceptives has no plans to market its existing products for emergency contraception. The company is fearful of costly product-liability lawsuits.

Chemically Induced Abortion

For many years, birth control scientists have sought to perfect a relatively safe and effective medical alternative to surgical abortion. Esoteric potions, rare herbal preparations, and strange concoctions of chemicals have been tried with varying degrees of success and much failure. But, until recently, no drug has been discovered or formulated with the reliability and safety determined as essentials in any method of drug-induced pregnancy termination.

Two drugs—**methotrexate** and *mifepristone*—have become available to accomplish chemically-induced abortion with relative effectiveness, safety to the mother, and convenience.

Methotrexate

In 1996, the FDA endorsed a Planned Parenthood Federation of America study of a two-drug abortion method. Approved years ago only for the treatment of specific diseases and abnormal conditions, the two prescribed drugs in this first medical procedure are:

> *Methotrexate*—used to treat certain cancerous diseases, severe psoriasis (a skin disease with sores), and adult rheumatoid arthritis, and
>
> *Misoprostol*—used to prevent gastric ulcers in patients who take nonsteroidal anti-inflammatory drugs (NSAIDs).

Research studies have revealed that methotrexate, when injected into a woman no more than seven weeks pregnant, stops development of the placenta and embryo. Several days later, misoprostol tablets are inserted into the woman's vagina. This second drug causes the uterus to contract. Eventually, the embryo is expelled. So far, the only reported adverse side effects of this "methotrexate method" include vaginal bleeding, nausea, vomiting, and diarrhea.[21]

Although the prescribed use of these drugs is legal, some physicians will be hesitant to use them until they are also approved by the FDA for terminating pregnancies. Others will object to using this combination of drugs because of moral objection to abortion and general concern for professional liability.

RU-486

More than fifteen years ago, extensive studies in France determined that the drug, *mifepristone* or **RU-486,** is highly successful in causing menstruation in a woman whose menstrual period is up to six weeks late.[22] A single dose of RU 486 is given by mouth and is then followed 36 to 48 hours later by the administration of *prostaglandin,* another drug.

Known as the "abortion pill," RU-486 is an antiprogesterone chemical first used in 1982 to end human pregnancies. This drug can be used only during the first forty-nine days of pregnancy and produces a menstrual flow, the menses, when given late in the menstrual cycle.

Mifepristone prevents the implantation process or causes a sloughing or shedding of the innermost lining of the uterus along with the implanted fertilized egg, when administered within several days after ovulation. Prostaglandin then produces strong uterine contractions that expel the uterine lining and the implanted fertilized egg or embryo.

Although pain and bleeding often result from this abortion procedure, RU-486 has been determined by the FDA to be safe and effective when used under the close supervision of a physician. Nevertheless, an estimated 5 percent of women who undergo the RU-486 abortion will have to have a surgical abortion anyway.[23] Although mifepristone has been used in the United States only in clinical trials, it is expected to be approved by the FDA for widespread use.

Despite the introduction of RU-486, the debate over the abortion pill continues. Those in support of abortion rights, such as The Population Council, view this drug as a desirable medical option to surgical abortion, a form of postcoital contraception, menses induction, or voluntary pregnancy termination. Opponents of abortion see RU-486 as an abortifacient (a substance that causes abortion), an agent of murder, and a "chemical coat hanger" used to destroy unborn children.

Other New Drugs of Interest

In March of 1998 the FDA approved the first oral pill to treat impotence or erectile dysfunction in males. *Viagra* (sildenafil citrate) does not cause penile erections but increases the muscle relaxant effects of the chemical nitric oxide, which allows blood to flow into the penis, causing an erection. Side effects of this drug may include headache, flushing, and indigestion. Men with cardiac problems need to discuss the risks of this drug with their doctors, as it may cause sudden drops in systemic blood pressure. Men taking organic nitrates in any form should not take this drug.

Premarin is a brand of conjugated estrogens for use in menopausal and postmenopausal women. It is used to treat symptoms of menopause, such as hot flashes and vaginal dryness. It is also used to prevent osteoporosis, a bone-thinning condition. The side effects of estrogen replacement therapy may include mild acne, stomach bloating, and migraine headaches. Women should discuss the risks of taking this medication with their doctor if they have a personal or family history of bone disease; cancer (especially breast cancer); endometriosis; epilepsy; gallbladder, heart, kidney, or liver disease; or circulatory problems. Women who smoke should not take estrogens as the combination may increase the risk of blood clots.

Evista (raloxifene) is one of a class of new drugs called selective estrogen receptor modulators (SERMs) prescribed for postmenopausal women to help prevent bone thinning from osteoporosis. Evista increases bone density, lowers blood lipids, but does not negatively affect breast and uterine tissue, which may be a side effect of other estrogen replacement therapies. Women who smoke or may be pregnant should not use it because the most serious risk associated with this drug is the threat of blood clots.

A new antiobesity drug called *Meridia* (sibutramine) was approved by the FDA in 1997. This drug is used in conjunction with a low-calorie diet to help control obesity. Meridia works by inhibiting the reuptake of the neurotransmitters norepinephrine and serotonin. This drug does not seem to cause the serious side effects of pulmonary hypertension or heart valve disease reported with two diet drugs taken off the market—fen-phen and Redux (fenfluramine and dexfenfluramine).

Side Effects and Adverse Reactions of Prescribed Drugs

Earlier in this chapter it was emphasized that all medicines ought to be considered as having the potential for both helping and harming an individual. All medicines are double-edged swords.

Secondary Side Effects of Medicines

Drugs can reduce symptoms and cure disease—the primary, intended, and expected functions of medicine. Nevertheless, the same medicine can also produce secondary side effects that are sometimes unintended, unexpected, and often undesirable or fatal (adverse drug reactions). Such side effects can result from the use of both Rx and OTC medicines, and they are related to variations in individual responses to drugs, such as sensitivities, allergies, and changes in body chemistry. Every person reacts somewhat differently to medicine; some will sustain undesired effects, while most will have beneficial results.

Relatively minor side effects of certain medicines may include skin rash, mild headache, nausea, and drowsiness. More severe adverse reactions appear as prolonged vomiting, bleeding, extreme weakness, or impaired vision or hearing. Such symptoms are the body's way of telling an individual that the medicine is acting in an unfavorable, adverse way. Prolonged use of some drugs may even result in a variety of nutritional deficiencies. For instance, aspirin can decrease the body's ability to absorb and use vitamin C, folic acid, and vitamin K; tetracycline antibiotics can reduce the body's uptake of vitamin C; and anticonvulsants used in treating epilepsy can lower the level of folic acid and vitamin D, and thus contribute to anemia and rickets (or bone-softening disease). Unless appropriate nutrient supplements are prescribed, these side effects can lead to drug-caused malnutrition.

Therapeutic Index

Pharmacologists, because of the potential for side effects and adverse reactions, have established an index for assessing the relative safety of drugs for use in large populations. This index is known as the *therapeutic ratio*, or *therapeutic index*. The therapeutic index is a measure that relates the dose of a drug required to produce a desired effect to that which produces an undesired effect.[24]

The therapeutic index is expressed as the ratio between the median lethal dose (LD_{50}) and the median effective dose (ED_{50}) of a particular drug used for a specific effect (see chapter 3). Those drugs with a low ratio have a relatively small margin of safety between an effective (therapeutic) dose and an overdose effect, whereas drugs having a high therapeutic ratio possess a relatively greater margin of safety. For instance, a therapeutic index of 3 indicates that the 50 percent lethal dose is only three times the 50 percent effective dose. Accordingly, 1 milligram of a drug will produce the desired effect in half of the test population, but 3 milligrams of the same drug will kill half of the test population.[25] The higher the ratio, the safer the drug; that is, the drug can be taken safely by most individuals, and even if the recommended dose were slightly exceeded, adverse effects would not likely occur. Nevertheless, for thousands of individuals, even the therapeutic dose causes harm.

Although a sizable proportion of adverse drug effects is somewhat predictable, the exact percentage of life-threatening reactions has not been determined.[26] Many such reactions, however, are preventable. Therefore, renewed emphasis should be placed on safeguarding one's health from potentially dangerous drug injuries.

Preventive Measures

Preventive measures involve the prescribing physician, the dispensing pharmacist, and the consumer-patient, and focus on

- informing one's physician of previous adverse reactions to a drug;
- reporting of general and specific allergic conditions to one's physician, dentist, and pharmacist;
- respecting known contraindications (situations that would prohibit the use of a drug) regarding any particular drug;
- exercising precautions in using drugs, such as intermingling of two or more drugs without consulting a physician, and avoiding alcoholic beverages when using depressant drugs;
- following prescribed dose recommendations;
- recognizing and reporting early warning signals of adverse reactions to one's physician;

- having your physician monitor the drug's effects through periodic exams, if necessary; and
- having your physician submit to the U.S. FDA an "Adverse Reaction Report" or file one yourself.

There are two special areas of concern in preventing adverse drug reactions. One deals with polypharmacy; the other involves food and drug interactions. Both areas require the active involvement and cooperation of the consumer-patient.

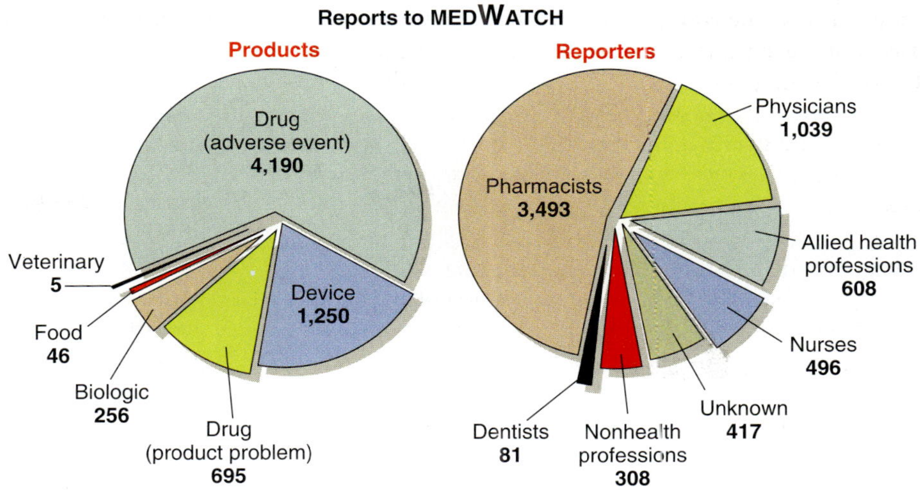

figure 13.4

In one recent eight-month period, MedWatch, the U.S. Food and Drug Administration's medical product reporting program, received reports of 6,442 events or other problems. The chart on the left shows reports according to type of product; the chart on the right depicts reports by profession of the reporters.

As a partner in the MedWatch program, the independent, nonprofit organization of medical and pharmaceutical professionals and consumers, known as the United States Pharmacopeia, has established a Practitioners' Reporting Network (PRN) that consolidates concerns and suggestions involving drugs, radiopharmaceuticals, medical devices, animal drugs, actual or potential medication errors, and adverse events so that product manufacturers and regulatory agencies are kept informed of the problems observed. The reporting network and consequent actions of the Food and Drug Administration (FDA) have resulted in product improvements, corrections, and recalls in support of federal and state government efforts to protect the public health by helping to identify serious adverse effects.

Source: U.S. Food and Drug Administration

Polypharmacy: Drug-Drug Interactions

The use of two or more drugs at the same time during the course of treatment for a particular illness is known as **polypharmacy.** Mixing two different medications can result in unexpected and sometimes dangerous chemical interactions within the body. Such a practice requires your physician's close supervision and knowledge of other drugs you may be taking, including those prescribed by another physician.

In general, the occurrence of adverse reactions increases in proportion to the number of drugs being taken. Sometimes the drug interactions influence the treatment outcome. Consequently, the best policy is to use the fewest drugs possible at any one time.

Drugs interact in a variety of ways. One medication may make another act faster or slower, or more powerfully or less powerfully than it normally would act. As a consequence, one drug may change the effect another has on the body. Some of these interactions are described in the following paragraphs.

Changes in drug absorption, distribution, and metabolism may take place when one drug interacts with another. For example, if a person having a circulatory problem due to clotting of blood in an artery or vein is prescribed an anticoagulant drug, the prescribed medicine would tend to thin the blood and help dissolve a clot. However, if this individual were to take an antacid, even an OTC drug, the anticoagulant may be absorbed at a much slower rate than required to do its job properly.

Alteration of a drug's excretion can also occur with polypharmacy. One drug can either slow down or speed up the excretion of another drug from the body, thus exaggerating, prolonging, or reducing its effect.

As indicated in chapter 3, when drugs are taken in combination, the drug effects can usually be classified as either *independent, antagonistic, additive,* on *potentiating.* Drugs taken together may work independently of each other; that is, neither one affects the drug action of the other. However, when drugs taken together interact so that the effect of either or both agents is blocked or reduced, the action is described as an **antagonistic drug reaction.** For example, certain antibiotics, barbiturates, and tranquilizers tend to reduce the effectiveness of oral contraceptives.

An **additive drug reaction** may occur when two or more drugs that are similar in their general effects interact in the body. The impact of adding one drug's action to that of another so that a doubling of the drug effect takes place is described as a "cumulative" reaction. The result (effect) is the sum of the parts.

Synergistic drug reactions and *potentiation drug reactions* describe the interactions of two or more drugs that produce an exaggerated effect—one that goes beyond what might be expected from adding the effect of one to another. With such drugs, the result is greater than the sum of the parts. Such a drug reaction, in which the effects of the two drugs are multiplied, can speed up the beneficial effect of a particular medicine, as when the

Box 13.4 Potentially Harmful Food-Drug Interactions

Tetracycline (a commonly prescribed antibiotic) and *dairy products*—calcium in milk, cheese, and yogurt impairs absorption of this drug, thus interfering with its effectiveness in the body.

Drugs in combinations with soda pop or acid fruit or vegetable juices—these beverages can result in excess acidity that may cause some drugs to dissolve quickly in the stomach instead of in the intestine, where they can be more readily absorbed into the bloodstream.

High blood pressure medications in combination with *natural licorice products*—the natural licorice extract, still used in imported products, counteracts the effect of the medicine.

Anticoagulants (drugs that prevent blood clotting) and *liver* and *green leafy vegetables*—excess consumption of foods rich in vitamin K, as are liver and spinach, hinders the effectiveness of anticoagulants.

Monoamine oxidase (MAO) *inhibitors*—drugs used to counter depression and high blood pressure—and *foods containing tyramine*—tyramine is found in foods such as aged cheese; chicken livers; pickled herring; fermented sausages; yogurt; sour cream; beef liver; canned figs; bananas; soy sauce; active yeast; and specific alcoholic beverages, including Chianti wine, sherry, and other wines in large amounts. MAO inhibitors react with tyramine to force the blood pressure to dangerously high levels, thus causing severe headaches, brain hemorrhage, and possibly death. MAO inhibitors also are suspected of reacting adversely with cola beverages, coffee, chocolate, and raisins.

Colchicine (a prescription drug for gout) and *mineral oil* (an ingredient in some OTC laxatives) block the proper absorption of nutrients by the intestines.

Diuretics, or "water pills," used over a long period can lead to severe potassium depletion in the body. Potassium is an important mineral needed for proper body function.

Oral contraceptives tend to deplete the blood's content of folic acid and vitamin B_6. Such vitamin loss is not usually serious among healthy women with good diets, but it can present serious problems in women with poor nutrition, such as impoverished women.

OTC antacids, used persistently without a physician's supervision, can cause phosphate depletion—a body condition producing muscle weakness and vitamin D deficiency.

Source: Modified from the U.S. Food and Drug Administration.

antibiotic trimethoprim may be used to enhance the activity of another drug, sulfamethoxazole, in combating certain infections.

But synergistic reactions can also pose dangers, especially when alcoholic beverages are mixed with sleeping aids, pain relievers, or tranquilizers. Even OTC drugs can have synergistic effects. Aspirin greatly increases the blood-thinning action of oral anticoagulants. People taking such medication may risk hemorrhage if they use aspirin to alleviate a headache. OTC cold remedies containing antihistamines can produce synergistic effects when combined with CNS depressants, including anesthetics, barbiturates, hypnotics, sedatives, and analgesics.

Food-Drug Interactions

When a person is taking a drug, the food that he or she has eaten could make the drug work faster or slower or even prevent it from having any effect. More alarming is the possibility of severe adverse reactions to drugs that can be caused by specific foods or alcoholic beverages. Some of the reactions, if left unchecked, can be life threatening. As indicated in box 13.4, there are several potentially harmful **food-drug interactions.**

To prevent such undesirable food-drug interactions, be certain to follow your physician's directions about when to take drugs and what foods and beverages to avoid while taking medications. Read any patient information materials distributed by your physician or pharmacist. Never be afraid to ask how drugs might interfere with your favorite edibles. While taking medicines, always report to your physician about any unusual complaints or experiences that occur when you consume specific foods and beverages.

Drug Information for Patients

The U.S. Food and Drug Administration, because of increasing public concern about the lack of adequate information on prescription drugs, has endorsed the American Medical Association's voluntary program that makes **Patient Medication Instructions (PMIs)** available to practicing physicians for distribution to their patients. Use of PMIs promotes improved effectiveness of drug therapy, reduces the risk of improper drug use, decreases the occurrence of preventable and serious drug reactions, and helps patients comply with instructions about taking their medication properly.

A growing number of laypersons have sought pertinent facts about drugs from a variety of sources because of a perceived reluctance on the part of many physicians to share basic information on Rx drugs with patients. One of the more popular and authoritative sources of such information on prescription drugs is the ***Physicians' Desk Reference*** (PDR), compiled by representatives of pharmaceutical companies. An annual publication, the PDR has nearly 2,900 pages and includes detailed information on thousands of drug products, accounting for nearly all of the leading prescription drugs.[27]

The *Physicians' Desk Reference* provides "full disclosure" of how a specific drug product works, what it is used for, possible side effects and adverse reactions, contraindications, and other precautions and warnings about potential hazards. In the front of the massive volume are several convenient indexes and sections, the more useful of which are described as follows:

1. *Manufacturers' Index*—a listing of all drug manufacturers who have provided information to the PDR. Addresses and emergency phone numbers of manufacturers are also listed.
2. *Brand and Generic Name Index*—an alphabetical listing of drug products by their brand and generic names. Only those medications currently available from participating drug manufacturers are included.
3. *Product Category Index*—a listing of products according to their appropriate category (classification or drug type), such as analgesics, diuretics, antihistamines, and so on.
4. *Product Identification Guide*—approximately forty pages of full-color photographs that depict tablets and capsules in actual size under company headings. Pictures of tubes and syringes are reduced in their dimensions.
5. *Product Information Section*—a list, in alphabetical order according to the name of the manufacturer, of more than 2,500 pharmaceuticals that are fully described as to brand name, generic or chemical name, indications for usage, dosage, administration, description, clinical pharmacology, supply, warnings, contraindications, adverse reactions, overdosage, and precautions in use.
6. *Diagnostic Product Information Section*—descriptions of and use guidelines for various diagnostic agents, such as tests for tuberculosis screening, cellular hypersensitivity, and pituitary gland function.

The *PDR* also contains a listing of certified poison control centers, a telephone directory for the FDA, and a national directory of drug information centers.

Some libraries also have copies of recent PDRs. The publisher of this reference on prescription drugs has issued a companion pharmaceutical directory, the *PDR for Non-Prescription Drugs.* This latter volume is also proving to be a best-seller.

Generic Drugs

One of the more complex issues pertaining to prescription drugs is the "generic brand name controversy." With the increasing cost of health care, some consumers, physicians, pharmacists, the FDA, and the pharmaceutical companies that make drugs have become concerned about the quality and cost of comparative drugs. The controversy includes the naming of drugs, possible differences in quality between brand-name drug products and their generic counterparts, the cost differential between the two name types of medication, and the substitution of the generics for brand-name drugs.

Drug Names

To better appreciate the nature of this controversy, understand that drugs prescribed for therapy are named in three different ways.

1. The *chemical name* describes the chemical structure of the drug molecule. Typically, such a name is rather long, unwieldy, and written in a complex chemical jargon seldom used by either physicians or pharmacists. For instance, a common antibiotic drug has the following chemical name: *D.-(−)α-amino-p-hydroxybenzyl penicillin trihydrate.*
2. The *generic name* refers to a drug's official or nonproprietary name, that is, a name that is *not* patented, trademarked, or owned by a private individual or company. Assigned to a drug after it has demonstrated some therapeutic usefulness, the generic name is usually a contraction of the more complex chemical name. The antibiotic drug identified in number 1 has the generic name *amoxicillin.* Drugs are frequently referred to by their generic names in academic and scientific situations.
3. The *brand name* or trademark (registered with the U.S. Patent Office) is assigned to a generic-name drug by a particular pharmaceutical company. Usually, the brand name is shorter than the generic name, easier to remember, and often devised to suggest the pharmacological action of the drug. For instance, SmithKline Beecham Laboratories' brand name of amoxicillin is Amoxil; Wyeth-Ayerst's is Wymox; and Squibb's is Trimox.

There are several other brand names and generic versions of amoxicillin marketed in the United States by different drug manufacturers. It is the brand name of a drug, however, that is advertised to the medical profession, although the generic name must also appear in advertising and labeling in letters at least half as big as that of the brand name.

Chemical Equivalence Versus Bioavailability

According to the FDA, all drugs, whether sold under their brand names or their generic names, must meet the same FDA standards for safety, strength, purity, and effectiveness. An extensive sampling and analysis of frequently prescribed generics revealed no significant differences in the quality of the generics compared to the brand-name products.[28]

None of the samples tested posed a health hazard to patients when the drugs were examined for potency, dissolution rate, and content uniformity.[29] Consequently, the FDA believes there is no significant difference in quality between generic and brand-name drugs. Supposedly, generic drugs are equivalent to those sold under their brand names.

While generics contain the same amounts of active ingredients in the same dosages—and are, therefore, **chemically equivalent drugs**—many physicians, pharmacists, and drug manufacturers contend that the quality of the generics varies considerably. This variation is expressed usually as **bioavailability,** a measure of a drug's activity within the body, determined by the quantified levels of that particular drug in the blood.

Considered as trade secrets, various fillers, binders, coloring agents, lubricants, preservatives, drying agents, flavors, disintegrants, coatings, and wetting agents—the inactive ingredients used in formulating and manufacturing a drug product—are what determine how available the active ingredient will be in the body. Sometimes these inactive substances affect the drug's absorption, how much of the active ingredient gets to its desired destination, and how fast it gets there.

This variation can make an important difference between apparently similar drugs. When the bioavailability of brand-name drugs and generics are the same, the drug products are described as having the same **bioequivalence.** This means that the medications produce the same therapeutic effect in the body. But any difference in bioavailability between brand names and generics may alter the clinical or therapeutic effects of the medications. In such a situation, then, the drugs would not share the characteristic of bioequivalence because they might not function similarly at the site of action within the human body.

To be regarded as therapeutically equivalent to an already FDA-approved, brand-name drug, a generic product may differ only in such characteristics as color, taste, tablet shape, packaging, and inert or inactive ingredients.

In comparison with their brand-name counterparts, generics must contain the same active ingredients; be identical in strength, dosage form, and route of administration; be used generally for the same illnesses (with the same precautions, warnings, and instructions); and be bioequivalent, meaning that they must release the same amount of drugs into the body at the same rate and must affect the body in the same way.

Despite the antigeneric position of the pharmaceutical manufacturing industry, a majority of generics are made by the major drug firms in the United States. These drug companies are often the same ones that also research, develop, and market the brand-name drugs. Some of the large firms distribute, under their own brand names, drug products that have been manufactured, packaged, and labeled by firms that make only generic drugs.

Generic Drug Prescription

The consumer-patient will likely find that generic drugs cost less. The savings can be as much as 50 percent. Such a difference can translate into a significant dollar amount, especially if the drug must be taken over a long period of time.

To benefit from such savings, the consumer needs the cooperation of both physician and pharmacist. Ask your physician to write a prescription so that it permits a generic version to be dispensed, and tell your pharmacist you want the least expensive version of the medicine that has been prescribed for you.

In addition, the consumer should compare prices at chain stores and independent pharmacies because some generics have cost more than brand-name drugs, on occasion. Although pharmacists usually pay less at wholesale for generics, they often have a higher markup than their brand-name counterparts. Sometimes, a pharmacy might feature a bargain price on a brand-name drug—lower than the generic price—due to a special order or deal from a pharmaceutical manufacturer.

Generic prescription has increased rapidly, surpassing the smaller annual increase in brand-name perscription. As more patents expire on brand-name drugs, it is anticipated that not less than 80 percent of the top-selling prescribed medications will one day be open to generic competition.

The trend to generic prescription has been promoted now that all fifty states have laws allowing, and in some instances requiring, pharmacists to substitute a generic drug for a brand-name medication, unless the prescribing physician mandates the use of a specific brand-name product.

Additional factors advancing the trend to generics are the many hospitals, military installations, and other government health care facilities that routinely dispense generics whenever possible. Even cost-conscious employers and health insurance companies encourage members to urge their physicians to write prescriptions that can be filled with generic drugs.

The upswing in generic prescribing indicates that more physicians are convinced that generic drugs are good drugs, despite the deluge of pro-brand-name propaganda by the major drug-developing companies. But the trend to generics may also represent the effort by consumer-patients to take some control of their own health care costs.

Chapter Summary

1. Prescription medicines are chemotherapeutic agents, more powerful than OTC drugs, that require a physician's supervision in their use. They are also more likely to cause unexpected side effects and adverse drug reactions.
2. Although many people believe that all drugs work safely on all people at all times (the fail-safe concept), there is no absolute safety regarding the use of prescription drugs. The benefit-risk equation applies in the use of such medications.
3. A prescription typically lists the physician's name, address, phone number, and DEA number; patient's name and address; date; name of drug prescribed; dosage form; strength of dose; amount to be dispensed; directions for use; number of refills allowed; and the physician's signature.
4. The label on an Rx drug container typically lists name, address, and phone number of the dispensing pharmacy; prescription number; prescribing physician's name; date of dispensing; patient's name; drug name; directions for use; federal restriction; expiration date; and number of allowable refills.
5. Dispensing of controlled drug substances is restricted according to major drug schedules, under the provisions of the Controlled Substances Act.
6. Guidelines for the wise use of Rx drugs pertain to knowing

medication's name, directions for use, expected drug effects, possible side effects, precautions in use, avoiding use of other drugs and particular foods, and duration of recommended use.

7. Additional guidelines for responsible use of Rx drugs relate to informing one's physician about medication problems, possibility of pregnancy, and multiple-drug use; discarding old drugs; proper storing of medicines; and avoiding medication errors.

8. According to the National Prescription Audit, new and refill prescriptions total nearly 2 billion per year. Nearly 15 percent of new prescriptions are for generic drugs. Psychotropic drugs (minor tranquilizers, sedatives, hypnotics, antidepressants, major tranquilizers, and antimanics) account for only 5 percent of prescriptions.

9. Rx drug classes or families are composed of drugs that share important chemical characteristics and tend to produce similar effects in the human body. Major drug classes include anti-infectives, antihypertensives, antineoplastics, cardiovascular drugs, diuretics, sedative-hypnotics, and stimulants.

10. The combination pill and the minipill are types of oral contraceptives that prevent pregnancy by keeping the ovaries from developing and releasing mature ova.

11. Highly effective and relatively safe to use, oral contraceptives can produce serious but rare adverse reactions, such as cardiovascular disorders, benign liver tumors, primary liver cancer, and gallbladder disease.

12. New forms of drug-related contraception and pregnancy termination (abortion) have become available, particularly emergency "morning after" oral contraceptives; the methotrexate-based abortion procedure; and RU-486, the so-called abortion pill containing mifepristone.

13. Rx drugs that reduce symptoms of illness and cure disease can also produce unexpected side effects and life-threatening adverse drug reactions.

14. Mixing two or more different medications can result in changes in drug absorption, distribution, and metabolism; alteration of a drug's excretion; and either additive or potentiation drug interactions.

15. Patient Medication Instructions and the *Physicians' Desk Reference* are two important sources of information on Rx drugs.

16. There has been an increase in the prescription of generic drugs that have an official, nonpatented, nontrademarked name. Although generics tend to be chemically equivalent to brand-name Rx drugs, some physicians believe the generics produce variable levels of drug activity in the body. As such, generics may alter the therapeutic effectiveness of a brand-name drug.

World Wide Web Sites

Federal Drug Administration: Information on Prescription Drugs

www.verity.fda.gov or www.fda.gov/medwatch

Internet Medical Site for Clinicians and Consumers

www.medscape.com

Review Questions and Activities

1. In what ways do Rx drugs differ from OTC drugs?
2. How does the benefit-risk equation apply to the use of prescribed drugs?
3. Can you think of any reason why directions for use on a prescription often include a Latin form of medical shorthand?
4. Examine a prescription drug container and determine if the recommended information elements are included on the label.
5. Do you believe the federal government should continue to restrict the prescription of controlled drug substances, under the provisions of the Controlled Substances Act?
6. Develop a "plan of action" to enhance your chances of using a prescription drug safely and responsibly.
7. Investigate how you as a patient might improve your communication skills with a physician, especially regarding the use of prescribed medications.
8. Identify some of the major Rx drug classes or families that are prescribed frequently in America.
9. What are some of the more frequently prescribed psychoactive drugs?
10. How do major tranquilizers differ from the so-called minor tranquilizers?
11. From both a female and male viewpoint, discuss the "pros" and "cons" of using oral contraceptives.
12. Explain in detail precisely how oral contraceptives prevent pregnancy. Distinguish between the effects of estrogen hormone and those of progestin hormone.
13. What are some of the common side effects of using oral contraceptives? What are some adverse reactions associated with these Rx drugs?
14. What are the differences and similarities between methotrexate and mifepristone when used as drugs to induce an abortion?
15. In what ways can the practice of polypharmacy affect drug actions within the human body?
16. What foods can sometimes cause adverse drug reactions?
17. Interview local pharmacists to determine the level of generic drug prescriptions in your community.

18. Survey several pharmacies and compare the prices of various brand-name drugs with their generic counterparts. What conclusions might be reached as a result of your comparative study?

19. Contact a regional or district official of the Federal Food and Drug Administration for information on testing of new drugs, actions taken concerning Rx drugs already in use, and related matters concerning drug safety and effectiveness.

References

1. Tamar Nordenberg, "Now Available Without a Prescription," *FDA Consumer* 30, no. 9 (November 1996): 6–11.
2. Andrew Purvis, "Unlocking the Pill Bottles," *Time,* 17 December 1990, 95.
3. Pharmaceutical Manufacturers Association, *Key Facts about the U.S. Prescription and Medical Device Industries* (Washington, D.C.: Pharmaceutical Manufacturers Association, n.d.), 2.
4. Editors of Consumer Guide, *Prescription Drugs* (Lincolnwood, Ill.: Publications International/Signet Reference, 1995), 6–11.
5. James Rybacki and James Long, *The Essential Guide to Prescription Drugs,* 1996 ed. (New York: Harper Perennial, 1996), 1159.
6. Ibid., 14–16.
7. Dixie Farley, "Making It Easier to Read Prescriptions," *FDA Consumer* 29, no. 6 (July/August 1995): 25–27.
8. Dixie Farley, "FDA's Rx for Better Medication Information," *FDA Consumer* 29, no. 9 (November 1995): 5–10.
9. United States Pharmacopeia, *Complete Drug Reference,* 1996 ed. (Yonkers, N.Y.: Consumer Reports Books, 1995), 1717–31.
10. "Top 200 Drugs of 1995," *Pharmacy Times* 62, no. 4 (April 1996): 27–30, 32–34, 36.
11. Ricki Lewis, "Surprise Cause of Gastritis Revolutionizes Ulcer Treatment," *FDA Consumer* 28, no. 10 (December 1994): 15–18.
12. Rybacki and Long, *The Essential Guide to Prescription Drugs,* 1059.
13. Robert Hatcher and others, *Contraceptive Technology,* 16th rev. ed. (New York: Irvington, 1994), 285–86.
14. Ibid., 224.
15. Diana Petitti and others, "Stroke in Users of Low-Dose Oral Contraceptives," *New England Journal of Medicine* 335, no. 1 (4 July 1996): 8–15.
16. Hatcher and others, *Contraceptive Technology,* 275.
17. Ibid., 227.
18. Ibid., 231.
19. "Implantable Contraceptive Approved," *FDA Consumer* 25, no. 2 (March 1991): 2–3.
20. Leon Jaroff, "Rx: ` Morning After' Pills," *Time* 148, no. 4 15 July 1996, 59.
21. Catherine Crocker, "Clinics OK Abortion by Drugs," *Dayton Daily News,* 12 September 1996, Sec. A, p. 3
22. Louise Silvestre and others, "Voluntary Interruption of Pregnancy with Mifepristone (RU-486) and a Prostaglandin Analogue," *New England Journal of Medicine* 322, no. 10 (8 March 1990): 645–48; and Hatcher and others, *Contraceptive Technology,* 418.
23. John Marks, "The Secret World of the Abortion Pill," *U.S. News & World Report* 121, no. 13 (30 September 1996): 55.
24. Henry Boune and James Roberts, "Drug Receptors and Pharmacodynamics," chap. 2 in *Basic and Clinical Pharmacology,* 4th ed., ed. Bertram Katsung (Norwalk, Conn.: Appleton & Lange, 1989), 24.
25. Tibor Palfai and Henry Jankiewicz, *Drugs and Human Behavior* (Dubuque, Iowa: Brown & Benchmark, 1991), 76.
26. Rybacki and Long, *The Essential Guide to Prescription Drugs,* 16–19.
27. *Physicians' Desk Reference,* 50th ed. (Montvale, N.J.: Medical Economics Company, 1996).
28. Frank Young, "Ensuring the Safety of Generic Drugs," *FDA Consumer* 23, no. 10 (December/January 1989/1990): 5–7.
29. "Generic Drugs: Still Safe and Effective According to New Study," *Public Citizen Health Research Group Health Letter* 6, no. 10 (October 1990): 8–10.

Part Six

New Dimensions of Drugging, Drinking, Medicating, and Prevention

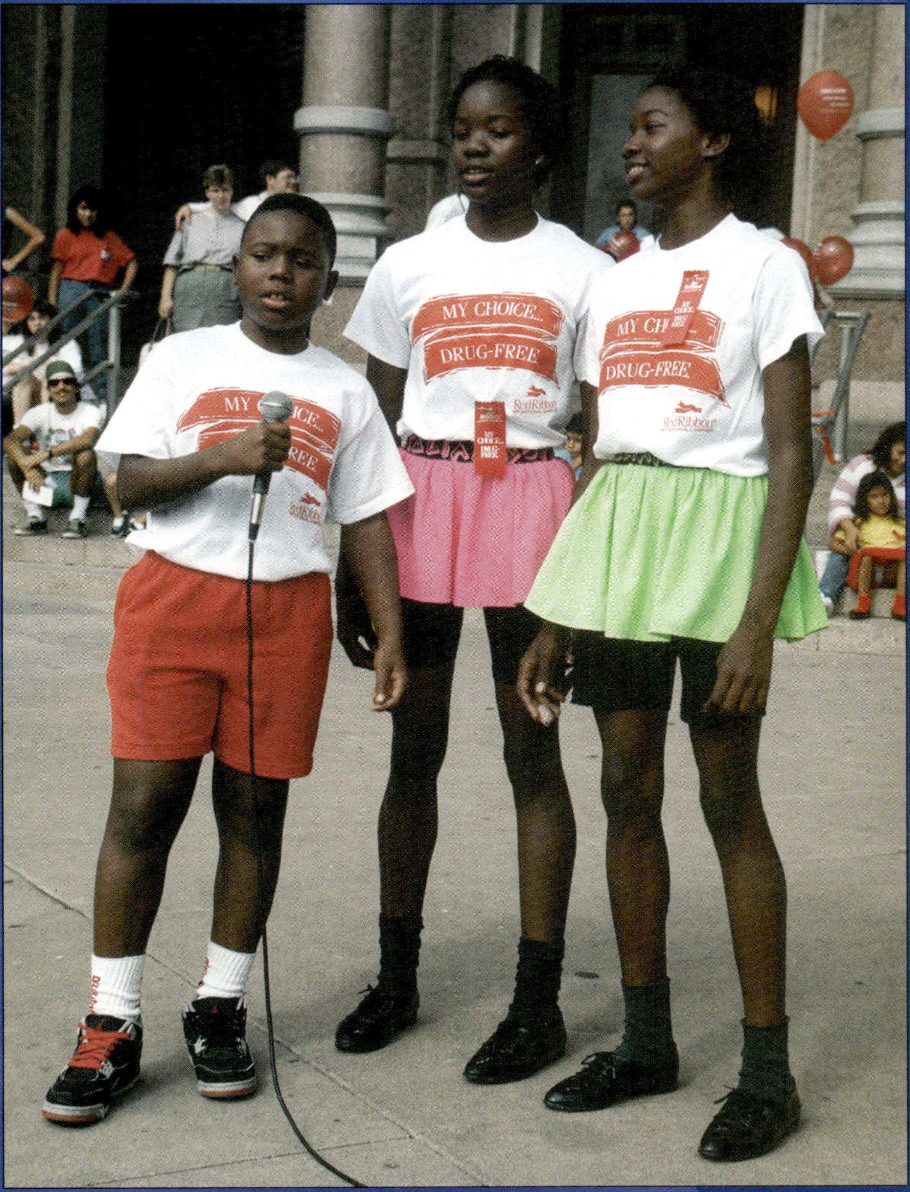

Questions of concern

1. If all members of special populations began to drink and use illegal drugs like white nonminorities, would the current drug scene be different?
2. Why aren't known risk factors for drinking and illegal drug-taking used more often to reduce psychoactive substance abuse problems in special minority groups?
3. If women and the elderly are more likely to visit their physicians more often than men, how could these special populations have so many more drug-related problems?
4. What strategies should communities and schools use to prevent the use of alcohol, tobacco, and other drugs by youth, and to prevent drug and alcohol abuse among adults?
5. Some drug-abuse prevention programs promote only abstinence from illegal drugs. Does this adequately prepare young people for their probable interactions with legal drugs after they leave the school setting?
6. Why are so many prevention programs directed at the illegal drugs, when alcohol and tobacco appear to cause more personal and social problems than the illegal psychoactives?
7. Although legalizing drugs might increase the number of deaths due to drug use and abuse, would it not eliminate the enormous profits of drug dealers, spare users the high costs of drugs, and reduce the cost of crime to society?

Chapter 14

Alcohol and other drugs in special populations

KEY TERMS

Acculturation
Anabolic-Androgenic Steroid
Congenital Abnormality
Early-Onset Alcohol Abuse or Dependence
Ergogenic Agent
Gender Gap
Late-Onset Alcohol Abuse or Dependence
Machismo
Medication Error
Mutagenic Effect
Polydrug Use
Sexual Dysfunction
Therapeutic Agent

chapter objectives

After you have studied this chapter, you should be able to do the following:

1. Define the key terms.
2. Explain how women appear to be closing the gender gap in the use and abuse of psychoactive drugs.
3. Identify several gender-related hazards associated with the use of psychoactive drugs by females.
4. Describe how heavy use of alcohol can become both the cause and consequence of female sexual dysfunction.
5. Explain how substance abuse contributes to sexual violence and exploitation.
6. Distinguish between mutagenic effects and congenital abnormalities in relation to a pregnant woman's use of psychoactive drugs.
7. List ten specific possible effects of psychoactive drugs on the developing fetus.
8. Compare and contrast the extent of alcohol and other drug use and abuse among the major racial and ethnic minorities in the United States.
9. Explain why alcohol and drug abuse affects racial and ethnic minorities to a greater extent than the white population in the United States.
10. Identify the major factors that influence or determine the drinking and other drug-taking practices of African Americans, Hispanic Americans, American Indians and Alaska Natives, and Asian Americans and Pacific Islanders.
11. Describe the flushing reaction and its effects on drinkers of Asian ancestry.
12. Distinguish between the use of therapeutic drugs and the use of ergogenic drugs among athletes.
13. Name at least five major types of ergogenic drugs banned by the NCAA and/or the USOC.
14. Identify at least five potentially adverse side effects associated with the use of AAS by athletes.
15. Describe how the use of alcoholic beverages can interfere with athletic performance.
16. Explain why athletes seem to be psychologically vulnerable to the use and abuse of psychoactive drugs.
17. Describe how some older Americans are mismedicated.
18. Identify four major factors that contribute to the increased potential for drug misuse, drug abuse, and drug interactions among the elderly.
19. List several examples of medication errors often experienced by the elderly.
20. Distinguish between early-onset and late-onset alcohol abuse or dependence.
21. State five factors that seem to place the elderly at increased risk for problem drinking.
22. Explain why older problem drinkers may not be detected and diagnosed as early or treated as effectively as younger problem drinkers.

Introduction

Over the past fifty years, research into drinking and other drug-taking behaviors has provided a good deal of information about psychoactive drug use and drug-related problems. Factors influencing nonuse and low-risk alcohol intake, chronic consumption of narcotics, so-called recreational use of marijuana, and smoking of tobacco cigarettes have all been explored. The onset, development, signs and symptoms, complications, and treatment of various drug dependencies have also been identified.

Much of this valuable, accumulated knowledge, however, has been gathered from studies conducted with mostly white American males. Nevertheless, for many years, the white male dimensions of using and abusing alcohol and other drugs were assumed to apply equally to females and to members of specific minority populations, now distinguished by race, ethnic group, athletic status, and age.

When females and representatives of various minorities were eventually studied, significant differences in drug use patterns and drug-related problems were revealed. Women appear to be influenced more dramatically by alcohol than are men, and alcohol and drug abuse apparently affect racial and ethnic minorities more dramatically and severely than nonminorities. Despite athletes' preoccupation with performance-enhancing drugs and the elderly's frequent interaction with prescribed medications, these groups tend to have major difficulties with alcohol. Such differences in these special populations will also affect treatment and prevention efforts in the future.

Therefore, this chapter will focus on the emerging alcohol and other drug-related problems and their origin that have been recognized among women, four racial and ethnic groups in the United States, athletes, and the elderly.

Alcohol and Drug Use and Abuse Among Women

While there is general agreement that fewer women drink, smoke, and use illicit drugs than do men, the number of American females who use psychoactive substances is significant. At least 21.5 million women smoke tobacco products; 4.5 million are alcoholics or alcohol abusers; 3.1 million regularly use illegal drugs; and 3.5 million also misuse prescription drugs, such as tranquilizers and anti-depressants.

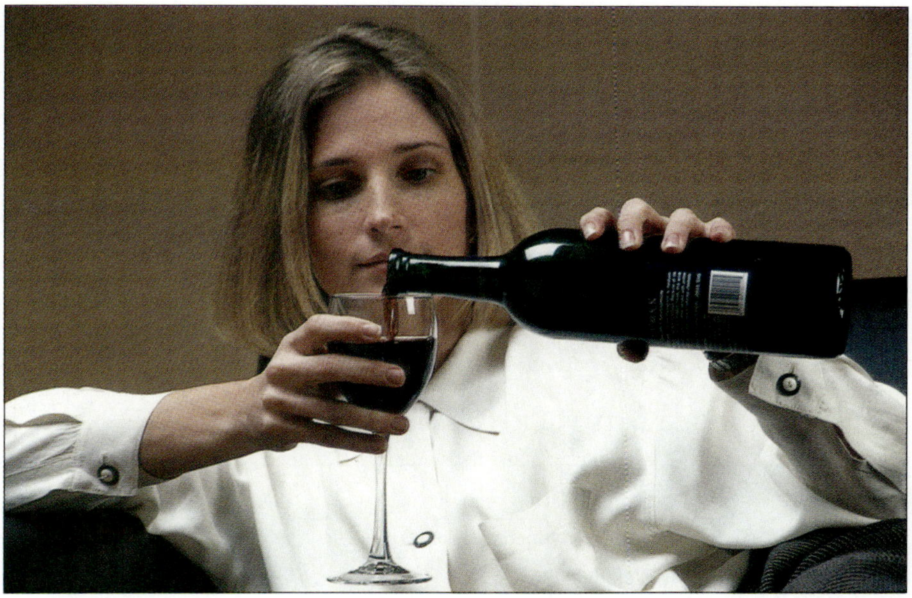

As women seek to close the gender gap in employment and income, they are also closing the gender gap in the use and abuse of alcohol.

Closing the Gender Gap

There are fewer females than males who use and abuse alcohol and other drugs, so many people incorrectly assumed that women didn't have drug-related problems or their abuse was not serious. However, American women have never been safe from such problems and are closing the **gender gap** of using and abusing drugs with men, particularly among teenagers and young adults. In many ways, women are becoming like men in the extent to which they use and abuse psychoactive substances. They are suffering the same adverse consequences of their involvement with drugs as men. The evidence, collected by the National Center on Addiction and Substance Abuse, speaks for itself:[1]

- The percentage of women who quit smoking is less than that of men. If the present trend continues, eventually, the number of women who smoke will equal the number of men who smoke.
- The percentage of drug-addicted women doubled between 1960 and 1980. Today, nearly 40 percent of crack addicts are females.
- The percentage of women and men who abuse prescription drugs is nearly equal.
- Among adolescents, boys and girls are equally likely to drink and to have used illegal drugs, especially marijuana.
- Today's daughters are fifteen times more likely than their mothers to have begun using illegal drugs by the age of fifteen.

Women have come a long way in closing the gender gap in employment, the professions, military service, and earning power. But in substance abuse and drug-related problems, women seem to have come the wrong way. Now that women are beginning to smoke, drink, and "do drugs" like men, they are beginning to get sick and die like men!

Gender-Related Hazards

Encouragement to adopt moderate drinking practices has become an important method of reducing alcohol-related problems. But moderate drinking

Box 14.1 Alcohol Impairment Chart

This chart is intended as a guide, not a guarantee.

Alcohol affects individuals differently. Your blood alcohol level may be affected by your age, gender, physical condition, amount of food consumed and any drugs or medication. In addition, different drinks may contain different amounts of alcohol, so it's important to know how much and the concentration of alcohol you consume.

For purposes of this guide, "one drink" is equal to 1.25 oz. of 80 proof liquor, 12 oz. of regular beer, or 5 oz. of table wine.

A woman drinking an equal amount of alcohol in the same period of time as a man of an equivalent weight may have a higher blood alcohol level than that man. Therefore, **women should refer to the female "Know Your Limits" chart.**

Some stats have set .08 percent Blood Alcohol Concentration (BAC) as the legal limit for Driving Under the Influence. For commercial drivers, a BAC of .04 percent can result in a DUI conviction nationwide.

IMPAIRMENT BEGINS WITH YOUR FIRST DRINK.

Men

Approximate Blood Alcohol Percentage

Drinks	Body Weight in Pounds								
	100	120	140	160	180	200	220	240	
1	.04	.03	.03	.02	.02	.02	.02	.02	Impairment Begins
2	.08	.06	.05	.05	.04	.04	.03	.03	Driving Skills Significantly Affected
3	.11	.09	.08	.07	.06	.06	.05	.05	
4	.15	.12	.11	.09	.08	.08	.07	.06	
5	.19	.16	.13	.12	.11	.09	.09	.08	Possible Criminal Penalties
6	.23	.19	.16	.14	.13	.11	.10	.09	
7	.26	.22	.19	.16	.15	.13	.12	.11	Legally Intoxicated
8	.30	.25	.21	.19	.17	.15	.14	.13	
9	.34	.28	.24	.21	.19	.17	.15	.14	Criminal Penalties
10	.38	.31	.27	.23	.21	.19	.17	.16	

Subtract .01% for each 40 minutes of drinking.
One drink is 1.25 oz. of 80 proof liquor,
12 oz. of beer, or 5 oz. of table wine.

Women

Approximate Blood Alcohol Percentage

Drinks	Body Weight in Pounds									
	90	100	120	140	160	180	200	220	240	
1	.05	.05	.04	.03	.03	.03	.02	.02	.02	Impairment Begins
2	.10	.09	.08	.07	.06	.05	.05	.04	0.4	Driving Skills Significantly Affected
3	.15	.14	.11	.10	.09	.08	.07	.06	0.6	
4	.20	.18	.15	.13	.11	.10	.09	.08	.08	Possible Criminal Penalties
5	.25	.23	.19	.16	.14	.13	.11	.10	.09	
6	.30	.27	.23	.19	.17	.15	.14	.12	.11	Legally Intoxicated
7	.35	.32	.27	.23	.20	.18	.16	.14	.13	
8	.40	.36	.30	.26	.23	.20	.18	.17	.15	
9	.45	.41	.34	.29	.26	.23	.20	.19	.17	Criminal Penalties
10	.51	.45	.38	.32	.28	.25	.23	.21	.19	

Subtract .01% for each 40 minutes of drinking.
One drink is 1.25 oz. of 80 proof liquor,
12 oz. of beer, or 5 oz. of table wine.

Data Supplied by the Pennsylvania Liquor Control Board.

The National Clearinghouse for Alcohol and Drug Information
A Service of The Substance Abuse and Mental Health Services Administration

rules for men cannot be applied to women. Until recently, few people realized that women become intoxicated after drinking much less than men. One alcoholic drink will affect a woman more severely and more rapidly than an identical dose per pound will affect a man. The concepts of moderate drinking for women will have to change (see box 14.1).

Women also experience the undesirable short- and long-term effects of alcohol more quickly than do men.[2] Women metabolize alcohol somewhat differently due to a gender-based enzyme deficiency in their stomachs. More alcohol enters the female bloodstream more rapidly than a male's, therefore a woman tends to get drunk faster than men (as explained in chapter 3); they become addicted to drugs more easily; and develop alcohol-related cirrhosis of the liver more readily.[3]

Women develop alcohol-induced liver disease in a shorter period and at lower levels of consumption than do men. The number of alcoholic women who develop such liver disease is somewhat higher than among alcoholic men.

table 14.1 Risk Factors for Problem Drinking over a Woman's Life Span

A risk factor is some behavior or element of a person's history or genetic makeup that may increase the likelihood of developing a particular condition, in this case, a harmful drinking pattern. The term problem drinking is used here to include all alcohol-related disorders. It is believed that many behaviors or elements of a woman's life occur only at specific periods or phases and may function as risk factors for developing problem drinking only during those periods of the life cycle.

General Factors for Problem Drinking Throughout the Life Span

- family history of problem drinking
- peer and spouse pressure
- psychological depression
- stress, distress, poor coping ability

Risk Factors Among Adolescents

- behavior problems
- school-related difficulties
- family history of alcohol abuse
- marital conflict in parents
- inadequate parenting skills
- early alcohol intoxication and
- marijuana use
- anticipation of the alcohol "high"
- alienation

Risk Factors Among Young Adults

- college enrollment
- nontraditional occupation
- low-status job
- recent layoff and unemployment
- single, divorced, or separated
- in a cohabiting relationship
- spouse or partner's heavy drinking
- reproductive disorders
- miscarriage, hysterectomy
- smoker
- use of prescribed and illegal psychoactive drugs
- public drinking
- driving offenses
- conflict and emotional distress during decade of the thirties

Risk Factors Among Middle-Age

- unlikely to acquire new roles, new job or new friends
- "empty nest" status
- distress, feelings of abandonment
- heavy spousal drinking
- marital disruption
- drinking pattern: at home, alone
- abuse of prescribed psychoactive drugs
- comorbidities: depression, eating disorders, phobias, panic disorders, anxiety state

Risk Factors Among Older Women

- heavy drinking by significant others
- widowhood
- retirement or husband's retirement
- use of prescribed sedatives and tranquilizers

Source: Edith Lisansky Gomberg, "Risk Factors for Drinking Over a Woman's Life Span," *Alcohol Health & Research World*, Vol. 18, No. 3 (1994): 220–27.

Women's use of psychoactive drugs can have other harmful consequences, too. Each year since the mid-1980s, smoking cigarettes has been responsible for more women's deaths due to lung cancer than breast cancer. Thousands of women also die annually of smoking-related heart disease; chronic lung disease; and cancers of the esophagus, larynx, and cervix.

While hormone levels also affect the way women metabolize alcohol, with blood alcohol levels peaking faster just before menstruation, repeated bouts of intoxication may suppress hormonal activity. There is a higher occurrence of menstrual dysfunction and more rapid onset of menopause among alcoholic women.

Even light to moderate alcohol intake may influence the development of certain diseases in women. As few as three drinks per week may increase a women's risk of breast cancer. Alcohol may also make a woman more susceptible to hemorrhagic stroke in which a blood vessel breaks and may interfere with bone calcification. Consequently, some women are at higher risk for osteoporosis, a disease characterized by a loss of bone mass and thinning of the bones.

In so many ways, then, the gender gap seems to be at its widest when considering the use of alcoholic beverages. Although women tend to drink on fewer occasions and consume fewer drinks than men, women appear to suffer far greater harmful consequences from using alcoholic beverages. Perhaps women interact with more risk factors for problem drinking than do men and are therefore more susceptible to alcohol abuse and alcohol dependence (see table 14.1).

Sexual Dysfunction

For many centuries, both men and women have viewed alcohol as an aphrodisiac, a substance that allegedly increases sexual desire and performance. While alcohol may have a disinhibiting or facilitating effect at first, larger amounts inevitably interfere with the human sexual response cycle, resulting in male impotence and various female **sexual dysfunctions,** in other words, difficulties in sexual arousal and reaching orgasm.

In contrast with the positive expectancies associated with alcohol use are the serious consequences of heavy drinking and alcohol dependence. These unexpected and undesirable results surface as sexual dysfunctions, namely, lack of sexual desire, decreased sexual arousal, and inability to achieve orgasm in women. Research suggests that a preexisting sexual dysfunction may motivate a woman to drink in the hope of improving her sexual desire and performance. This self-medication drinking may then develop into problem drinking and alcohol dependence.[4]

These women may become disappointed with their own inadequate performance because of alcohol's harmful effects on sexual function. Now they may drink more alcohol to lessen feelings of inadequacy or failure or in the ongoing hope of improving their sexuality. In time, a self-reinforcing vicious cycle develops in which heavy drinking becomes both the cause and consequence of sexual dysfunction.[5]

Connecting Substance Abuse with Sex and Violence

The association between substance abuse and sex and violence is also a serious threat to the well-being of females. Again, as noted by the National Center on Addiction and Substance Abuse:[6]

- Teenage girls who drink more than five times a month are five times more likely to have sexual relations and a third less likely to engage in "protected" sex than girls who do not drink.
- Women who have been drinking are more likely to become the objects of unwanted sexual advances on the part of men.
- Sixty percent of women who had been drinking report that another drinker had become more sexually aggressively to them.

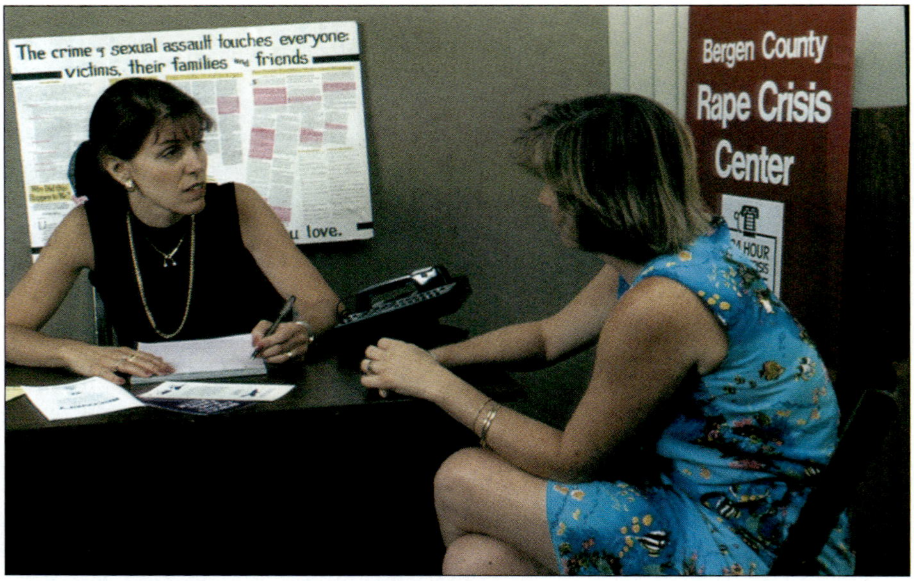

In most rape cases, either the victim or the rapist has been drinking, and drinking by victims is more likely to result in completed rather than attempted rape.

- In 75 percent of rapes and 70 percent of domestic violence cases, either the victim or the assailant has been drinking alcoholic beverages. However, drinking by the victims is more likely to result in a completed rather than an attempted rape, because the disabled females are not able to resist as well as sober individuals or to be clear about their nonconsent.

Although alcohol has a direct pharmacological effect on individuals' abilities to make judgments about sexual assault, even so-called moderate drinking can have some unfortunate results on the perception of the assault situation.[7] For instance, drinking women judged their assailants as having used less force and their assailants' behavior as more acceptable.

Whether drinking or not, many males, along with many females, believe that an intoxicated female thereby gives implied permission to be exploited sexually in a rape situation. Both men and women often assign more responsibility for the sexual assault to an intoxicated rape victim than to a sober one. However, the offender in such cases tends to be blamed less when intoxicated than when sober.

Psychoactive Drugs and Pregnancy

Large numbers of female drug users are women of child-bearing age. Each year, nearly 800,000 women endanger their own health and that of their infants by smoking, drinking, and using drugs during pregnancy. Many infants are born with cocaine, nicotine, alcohol, and heroin in their systems.

A female's offspring will eventually develop from ova that are present in her ovaries from the beginning of her embryonic life. Therefore, the first major concern is the possibility of **mutagenic** (gene toxic) **effects** of drugs on future offspring. Mutagenic effects involve sudden changes from the parent that appear in the offspring, due to some poisonous or undesirable force (such as a drug) on a gene or chromosome. Such mutagenic effects carry a risk of infertility and cancer.

Of equal concern is the effect of various drugs on the embryo and fetus if the mother takes psychoactive substances during pregnancy (see table 14.2). While drug-induced **congenital abnormalities**—physical and mental irregularities originating after conception—occur primarily during early pregnancy, some drugs have the potential to affect growth of the fetus and its postbirth be-

table 14.2 Drug Use During Pregnancy

Drug	Effect on Fetus	Safe Use of Drug
Alcohol	Increased risk of spontaneous abortion, "fetal alcohol syndrome," and infant addiction; low birth weight, mental retardation, physical deformity, and behavioral problems, including hyperactivity, restlessness, and poor attention span. Especially dangerous during first three months of pregnancy.	Should be avoided.
Amphetamines	Possibility of numerous birth defects resulting in damage to the liver, heart, and brain; abnormal bone and organ development; greater risk of miscarriage, stillbirth, and premature birth; poor coordination after birth.	Only under doctor's supervision.
Aspirin	During last three months of pregnancy, frequent use may cause excessive bleeding at delivery and may prolong pregnancy and labor.	Under doctor's supervision.
Barbiturates	Mothers who take large doses may have babies who are addicted. Babies may have tremors, restlessness, irritability, breathing difficulties, poor coordination, and slow reflexes.	Only under doctor's supervision.
Cocaine	Possible neurological damage, diminished motor abilities, smaller body length, lower birth weight, smaller head circumference; higher risk of kidney disorders, heart problems, seizures and strokes; increased risk of sudden infant death syndrome, and greater likelihood of visual problems, lack of coordinated movements, and developmental retardation with disturbed behavior and possible learning difficulties.	Should be avoided.
Inhalants	Possibility of "fetal solvents syndrome" with physical defects and mental retardation similar to fetal alcohol syndrome; increased likelihood of miscarriage or stillbirth.	Should be avoided.
Marijuana	Possibility of low birth weight and premature birth; and increased risk of behavioral problems in newborns.	Should be avoided.
Narcotics	Infant addiction, increased risk of miscarriage, early death, HIV infection; slowed growth, possible learning disabilities.	Should be avoided.
Nicotine	Higher risk of miscarriage, premature birth with low-birth-weight babies; increased risk of infant death, slowed growth, bleeding problems in delivery; increased risk of infant heart and lung disease.	Should be avoided.
Psychedelics	Some psychedelics, such as PCP, are linked with brain and nervous system damage, muscle control problems, deficits in speech and social skills.	Should be avoided.
Tranquilizers	If drug is taken during the first three months of pregnancy, there is the possibility of cleft lip or palate or other congenital malformations; infant addiction, damage to heart and blood vessels, mental retardation.	Avoid if you might become pregnant and during early pregnancy. Use only under doctor's supervision.

Source: Modified from the National Institute on Drug Abuse.

havioral and mental performance when exposure occurs at later stages of pregnancy. Even after birth, maternally consumed drugs can enter the newborn through milk from the mother's breast.

A pregnant woman's use of a psychoactive drug will result in the transfer of that drug to the fetus. The drug, present in the mother's bloodstream, crosses the placenta where it is then distributed into the fetus and sometimes the fetal brain. Such a drug will then accumulate in the fetus to levels that are at least as high as those achieved in the mother. Whether the drug will have toxic or adverse effects on the fetus depends in part on the size and frequency of doses that the mother takes and the ability of the drug to cross the blood-brain barrier.

As detailed in table 14.2, specific effects of various illegal and prescribed drugs recognized as congenital abnormalities, can threaten the health and life of the fetus and the newborn infant.

Of pregnant women who use illegal drugs, slightly more than 50 percent smoke marijuana; 20 percent use cocaine; and 14 percent use heroin, methamphetamine, or other illegal substances.[8] In addition, more than a quarter of pregnant women misuse prescription drugs. More dangerous to the developing fetus is a mother's multi-drug use. Pregnant women who use drugs often tend to use more than one drug, for example, combining smoking and drinking or drinking and marijuana use. Thousands of women who have contracted the AIDS-causing virus run the risk of endangering the lives of their own babies by infecting them with HIV.

It should be clear that nondrug using women are far more likely to give birth to healthy babies. Therefore, drug use of any kind should be avoided or strictly supervised by a physician throughout pregnancy and during the nursing period. It is tragic that so few women are aware of their pregnant state until the developing embryo is well into the vulnerable stage of prenatal growth and development.

Female Athletes and Drugs

Another aspect regarding drug use and abuse among women relates to the growing number of female athletes. As more females increase their participation in sports and intensify their competition, their growing success and heightened aspirations have produced a corresponding increase in performance-enhancing drug usage.

Women's greater commitment to sports training has been accompanied by the use of chemicals to improve athletic performance, the so-called ergogenic drugs described later in this chapter. Some female athletes may use steroids to increase their athletic prowess despite the steroids masculinizing effects on the female body.

Emphasis on "being thin" and striving for a high percentage of lean muscle mass and a low percentage of body fat have also produced chemical problems for some women. Laxatives, diet pills, diuretics, and amphetamines are often used to control weight and lose body fat. These conditions, in turn, have been related to the epidemic of serious eating disorders, such as anorexia nervosa and bulimia, and to alcohol abuse and alcohol dependence among women.

Racial and Ethnic Minorities

In the United States, racial and ethnic diversity reflects a wide range of drug-taking behaviors and drug-related problems among our minority populations.

Alcohol and drug abuse appear to affect racial and ethnic minorities in a disproportionate way. More unfavorable consequences tend to occur in these populations with negative effects on employment, school achievement, family stability, and increased risk of disease and death. Minorities seem to be at greater risk than whites of nonfatal and fatal consequences of alcohol and drug abuse due to their preference for injecting drug use and their choice of more dangerous drugs.[9]

The following analysis by the National Institute on Drug Abuse, and other sources as indicated, will reveal some other major concerns associated with alcohol and other drug use among America's racial and ethnic groups, as defined by the Census Bureau: African Americans, Hispanic Americans, American Indians and Alaska Natives, and Asian Americans and Pacific Islanders.[10]

African Americans

Young African Americans tend to drink less alcohol and have lower levels of illegal and legal drug use than other racial/ethnic groups. Usually, African American high school seniors report lifetime and annual use rates that are much lower than those for white or Hispanic seniors. Nevertheless, illicit drugs are a major problem in the African American community. Those adults who use alcohol and other drugs experience higher rates of drug-related health problems than do users from other ethnic groups. This may be because inner-city minorities have poorer diets and less access to health care. In addition, African Americans appear to be more severely affected by an increase in crime, often resulting from the indirect effects of drug usage and trafficking.

By contrast, African American adult males are most likely of all minorities to be current users of marijuana or cocaine. Along with Hispanic Americans, African Americans are also severely victimized by certain of their drug-taking behaviors. While African Americans and Hispanic Americans together make up about 22 percent of the United States population, these two minority groups account for nearly 50 percent of the reported cases of AIDS. The extremely large numbers of both minority groups among injecting drug users with AIDS is due in part to their preference for *injecting drugs* over other methods of drug administration.

Another variation related to the consequences of drug usage is somewhat surprising. When African Americans go to a hospital emergency room with a drug-related problem, they are more likely than white drug abusers to be treated and then released, whereas whites with similar conditions are more likely to be hospitalized. This situation is probably related to differing abilities to pay for treatment, but also because a greater proportion of whites relate their drug abuse occurrence to a suicide attempt.

Drinking patterns among African Americans had been characterized for many years by a preference for group drinking, weekend and holiday alcohol consumption, and a tendency to either drink heavily or abstain.[11] Yet, research indicates that, overall, black and white men have similar drinking patterns, although black men have higher abstention rates than whites; the same pattern tends to exist for women, with more black women than white abstaining.[12]

Throughout the years, various historical, social, psychological, and economic factors have been offered to explain alcohol use among African Americans. Heavy drinking has been described as a reaction to the isolation of racial segregation, the consequence of accessible liquor stores in black neighborhoods, and a method of coping with the frustrations of racism and lack of employment. However, emphasis has been placed on the concept of *racial consciousness* and pride as a basic attitude influencing drinking behavior. The higher one's racial consciousness as an African American, the less likely the person is involved in alcohol abuse or tolerant of such behavior.

African Americans and whites differ with respect to the age of distribution of drinking and related problems. Frequent heavy drinking among white males is most prevalent between 18 and 29 years of age, whereas, among African American males in that age group, heavy drinking is less frequent. Between 30 and 39 years of age, the rates of heavy consumption continue to be high for white males, but those of African American males rise sharply, surpassing those of whites.

According to the National Institute on Alcohol Abuse and Alcoholism, racial differences in consumption patterns are even more pronounced among women.[13] African American women tend to drink less. Nearly half of African American women are abstainers, compared with only one-third of white women. A much smaller proportion of African American women than white women are heavy drinkers. In the 18–29 age group, African American women are significantly less likely to drink at all or to drink heavily than are white women. Substance abuse among pregnant black women is reported at approximately ten times the rate of white women, although many studies indicate that illicit drug use among pregnant women is similar regardless of race or socioeconomic status. It appears that minority and poor women are more likely to be reported for substance abuse than their white counterparts.[14]

African Americans, especially males, tend to be at high risk for acute and chronic alcohol-related diseases, such as cirrhosis of the liver; alcoholic fatty liver; alcoholic hepatitis; heart disease; and cancers of the mouth, larynx, tongue, esophagus, and lung. High rates of problem drinking and alcoholism in high density, urban African American communities have been associated with assaults, homicides, accidents, trouble with the law, and family problems. Nationally, death rates associated with the alcohol dependence syndrome are highest for blacks, perhaps because of lack of adequate health care, including treatment. The extremely high rates of medical problems seen in blacks thus occur among a smaller percentage of the black population when compared with whites.

Hispanic Americans

Hispanic Americans make up one of the fastest growing and youngest segments of the United States population. The Hispanic American median age is only 25.3 years compared with 32.8 years for the U.S. population. A larger proportion of Hispanic Americans may be at increased risk for drug use because such a large proportion of this population segment is so young. Data reveal that Hispanic Americans have higher drug abuse rates for illegal drugs than non-Hispanic American whites.

As a group, Hispanic American high school seniors have the highest "lifetime" and "annual use" rates for some extremely dangerous classes of psychoactive drugs, namely, cocaine and crack cocaine. It appears that Hispanic Americans are exposed to cocaine somewhat earlier than other population segments. Other drugs of particular concern are inhalants and alcohol, the latter being the first, the most frequent, and the most injurious drug being used.[15] However, when all age groups—both adolescents and nonadolescents—and both females and males are considered together, Hispanic Americans have lower "ever used," "past year" use, and "past month" illegal drug use rates than both whites and African Americans.

As also seen in the African American population segment, large numbers of Hispanic Americans are among those injecting drug users with AIDS. This is related again, in part, to their preference for injecting drugs over other methods of taking psychoactive substances.

Although many variations exist within the Hispanic American population group, alcohol use among Hispanics, is usually marked by heavy consumption in males who tend to have high rates of alcohol-related problems. By contrast, female Hispanic Americans tend to abstain or to be light or infrequent drinkers, usually within a family setting.

Several factors likely determine the problem-producing drinking behavior of young Hispanic American males. Contrary to common belief, there is little indication that lower socioeconomic status and perceived stress related to social disadvantage are necessarily linked to alcohol use among these adolescents. In terms of explanations for using and abusing alcohol, greater emphasis is placed on the role of **acculturation** and the concept of **machismo**—the demonstration of a male's exceptional ability or drinking skill, in other words, the idea that a "real man can hold his liquor." As a consequence, when young Hispanic American males drink, they often engage in "binge drinking," the rapid consumption of large amounts of alcoholic beverages in a short period. Moreover, the alcohol-related problems of these males often continue throughout adulthood, more frequently than among white males.

Acculturation. the adoption of cultural traits or behaviors of another group, especially a dominant one, also appears to be a major factor influencing the drinking behavior of Hispanics, especially Mexican Americans. Male immigrants appear to quickly adopt a drinking pattern that blends the high frequency characteristic of white male drinking with Hispanic high quantity per occasion practices. Among Mexican American females, acculturation appears to be related with increases in the proportion of women who drink and the amount they consume. Such changes tend to occur more often in the first generation born in the United States rather than in the immigrant generation. In both male and female Mexican Americans, acculturation has been associated with a more permissive attitude toward alcohol consumption and a more neutral view of alcohol.

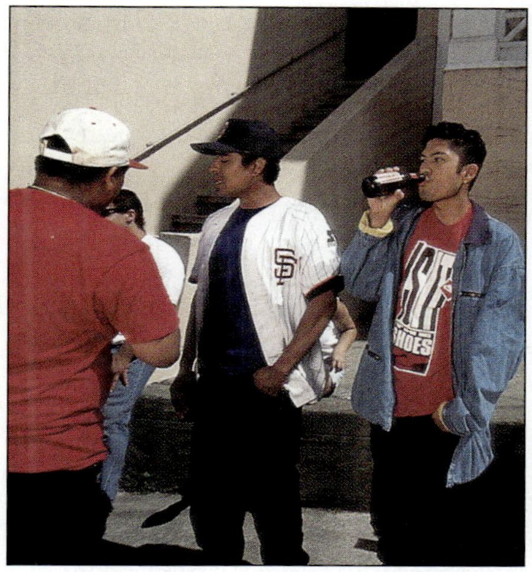

Generally, in the Hispanic American population, alcohol use is marked by heavy consumption by males, while women tend toward abstinence or light and infrequent drinking.

Hispanic American males tend to experience a disproportionate number of problems related to alcohol abuse, including alcohol dependence, when compared with African American and white males in the United States. Hispanic American women, however, are at lower risk for such alcohol-related problems than are white women.

Native Americans and Alaskan Natives

Alcohol and other drug use is a serious concern among American Indian populations. There is more substance use among this minority segment than most, if not all, ethnic minority groups in the United States. Native Americans and Alaskan

Natives report the highest occurrence of "past-month" drug use for marijuana, cocaine, cigarettes, and any illicit drug.

Young Native Americans begin using various psychoactive substances at an earlier age than their white counterparts. They are more likely to try marijuana and begin this experimentation at an earlier age than white youth. Moreover, inhalant use among Native American youth is twice as high as the national average. Toluene-based solvents are frequently the first drugs used by these youths. This form of drug abuse often precedes first-time alcohol use.

This population segment consists of over three hundred distinct tribal and ethnic groupings of Native Americans and Alaskan Natives, each of which has significantly different social, economic, and educational customs and conditions. These variations also extend to alcohol and other drug use patterns, attitudes toward psychoactive substances, and the occurrence of drug-related problems. As a consequence, some tribes are identified as nondrug-using, others report drinking moderately with few problems, while other groups demonstrate high rates of alcohol and drug use and highly visible drug-related problems.

Although alcohol use varies tremendously from one tribe to another and may be influenced by reservation and urban settings, the majority of Native American youth reports experimentation with alcohol. Such alcohol involvement is especially serious because death from alcohol-related causes is most common in younger years.

Two common drinking styles are especially problem-producing among Native American and Alaskan Natives: *recreational* and *anxiety*.[16] The recreational drinkers are typically young males who drink with friends for weekends, parties, and special occasions. As with other groups of young persons, drinking and intoxication are important for social cohesion and are highly valued.

By contrast, the anxiety drinkers tend to be older; drink chronically; are more solitary in the use of alcohol; and are usually dependent on alcohol, in other words they are alcohol addicts.

Heavy recreational and "binge" drinking among certain tribes may account for unusually high rates of alcohol-related arrests and accidental deaths in young Native American and Alaskan Native males. By contrast, Native American women drink considerably less than men, but the occurrence of drinking among these women is growing rapidly in some tribes. This drinking trend may help explain the increase in reported cases of Fetal Alcohol Syndrome.

Available data suggest that alcohol abuse is a contributing factor in five leading causes of death for Native Americans: motor vehicle crashes, alcoholism, cirrhosis, suicide, and homicide. An estimated 75 percent of traumatic deaths and suicides among Native Americans are alcohol-related. Deaths from alcohol-related causes are especially prevalent in the 25 to 44 age group. Many Western tribes have dramatically higher accident mortality rates than the national average, and fatal accidents among Native Americans are at least twice the national average.

A widely held myth suggests that "Indians cannot hold their liquor." Such a misconception persists, despite that science has demonstrated that Indians have no inherited or natural physiological deficit or vulnerabilities that would account for a differential, adverse reaction to alcohol. Researchers now focus on social, cultural, and psychological factors to account for the disproportionately high rates of alcoholism and alcohol-related problems among American Indians. Causes of excessive drinking by Indians are likely rooted in poverty, racial discrimination, and cultural rejection.

Asian Americans and Pacific Islanders

This minority segment of the population consists of more than sixty separate racial/ethnic groups that are different from one another. However, the most consistent finding of the limited research conducted to date reveals that drug use among Asian Americans and Pacific Islanders' drug use is less frequent than that of all non-Asian populations in general. When both males and females and all age groups are combined, Asian Americans and Pacific Islanders report the lowest prevalence of "past-month" drug use for any illicit drug, marijuana, cocaine, alcohol, heavy alcohol use, and cigarettes. Within the Asian American and Pacific Islander group, only native Hawaiians drink alcohol at levels similar to those of whites.

Certain minority groups may possess specific genetic traits that either predispose them to or protect them from adverse effects of using psychoactive drugs. Few such traits have been discovered. However, the so-called flushing reaction found in its greatest influence among people of Asian ancestry, is one example. Flushing has been linked to variants of genes for enzymes involved in alcohol metabolism and biotransformation. The reaction is a physiological response to drinking alcohol and consists of a reddening of the face and neck due to increased blood flow to those areas. In addition, flushing may be accompanied by headaches, nausea, palpitations (abnormally rapid beating of the heart), and dizziness—all of which are perceived as unpleasant sensations. Flushing can occur even when small amounts of alcohol are consumed, although some Asian Americans display a relatively slow response, appearing only after two or more drinks, or no response. Although flushing appears to discourage alcohol use, people with this trait may still consume alcohol.

For many years it was believed that Asian Americans limited their alcohol use to avoid the flushing response. However, such avoidance behavior is only one factor, along with sociocultural and environmental forces, that influences drinking patterns. Contributing to relatively low rates of alcohol abuse and alcoholism are norms or unwritten rules that permit alcohol use, especially at social functions, but discourage drinking to excess, and tight family and community regulation of alcohol use. Despite these genetic and social controls, the progressive assimilation of Asian Americans into American value systems may lead to increases in drinking problems among recent Asian immigrants.

Considerable variations in drinking patterns have been identified by ethnicity, age, and sex. Those most likely to drink are men under the age of forty-five years who have higher social status, whose attitudes toward alcohol use tend to be permissive, and whose friends tolerate drinking. A relatively high proportion of heavy drinkers exists among Japanese American and Filipino American men. By contrast, Chinese American men and women tend to have significantly lower prevalences of alcohol use and abuse. Asian American women usually drink far less than men, and this gender difference tends to hold true across various ethnic groups.

As the percentage of U.S.-born Asian Americans and Pacific Islanders increases, alcohol consumption and alcohol-related problems for these groups are expected to increase. In addition, as the number of Asian Americans and Pacific Islanders has been growing rapidly, they may become a marketing target for the alcoholic beverage industry, just as African Americans have been targeted for sales.[17]

table 14.3 Drug Classes Banned or Restricted by the National Collegiate Athletic Association (NCAA) and the United States Olympic Committee (USOC)

Stimulants, including amphetamines, cocaine, ephedrine, "cat," Ritalin, Anorex, Dexatrim, Sudafed, and certain use levels of caffeine
Beta-blockers
Diuretics
Adrenergic Bronchodilators
Peptide Hormones and Analogs, including Growth Hormone and EPO
Anabolic-Androgenic Steroids
Specific Recreation Drugs:
marijuana and heroin banned by the NCAA, but not by the USOC
cocaine banned as a stimulant and local anesthetic by the NCAA and USOC
LSD, mescaline, and PCP or angel dust use strongly discouraged by both organizations
alcoholic beverages banned for riflery events by the NCAA, but not by the USOC
tobacco products, both smoked and smokeless, banned during NCAA games and practices
Corticosteroids or anti-inflammatory drugs not banned by NCAA, but certain forms are banned by the USOC
Certain types of *local anesthetics*
Note: Blood doping procedures are also banned by the NCAA and USOC.

Source: United States Pharmacopeia, *Complete Drug Reference* (Yonkers, New York: Consumer Reports Books, 1996), 1747–50.

Drug Use and Abuse Among Athletes

There is nothing new about the use of drugs among athletes. Traditionally, chemical compounds have been employed in treating injuries, alleviating anxiety and nervous conditions, and relieving pain and inflammation sustained in sports competition. Drugs used in this manner are referred to as **therapeutic agents,** and include antibacterial medications, muscle relaxants, anti-inflammatory drugs, and analgesics (painkillers).

Ergogenic Drugs

Certain drugs have also been used not to cure disease or restore health but rather to enhance athletic performance. When used to artificially improve athletic skills or competition, drugs are described as **ergogenic agents.**

Occasionally, some ergogenic drugs are effective. Others appear to work because of the "placebo effect"—the user's strong faith in or expectation of benefit from the substance used. This placebo effect is explained in detail in chapter 3.

Many of the psychoactive ergogenics are potentially hazardous, often causing dramatic changes in behavior, heart failure, strokes, and blood vessel disease. Although their use has been universally condemned, ergogenics still appear to be abused widely in many amateur and professional sporting contests. Some observers believe that certain records achieved in national and international sports competition are due to the use of ergogenic drugs.

In reaction to the increasing use of ergogenic drugs, now described as an epidemic of biomedical challenges, the National Collegiate Athletic Association (NCAA) and the United States Olympic Committee (USOC) have forbidden or severely restricted numerous ergogenic substances (see table 14.3):[18]

Stimulants, such as, amphetamines, cocaine, ephedrine, "cat," Ritalin, Anorex, Dexatrim, and Sudafed may be used to quicken reaction times, heighten alertness, reduce feelings of fatigue, enhance confidence and ability to concentrate, and elevate one's mood. These are valuable factors in improving athletic performance. On occasion, amphetamines and cocaine have been used together by athletes engaged in contact sports, but these drugs might also be used to increase the stamina of runners and cyclists.

Some forms of *beta-blockers* (antihypertension drugs) are used in certain sport activities, particularly shooting events, because these drugs tend to lower heart rate, which in turn steadies one's nerves and the trigger finger.

Diuretics are sometimes taken to lose body weight rapidly, because they flush water from the body, and to reduce the concentration of other banned substances in the urine.

Inhaled *adrenergic bronchodilators* (antiasthma drugs) are forbidden by the USOC and oral bronchodilators are banned by the USOC and NCAA, because these drugs can increase muscle mass in much the same way as anabolic steroids.

Peptide hormones and their synthetic *analogs* are often abused by athletes because these drugs cause the release of growth-related chemicals in the body. *Growth hormone* increases strength and muscle mass, stimulates growth, and strengthens tendons and ligaments. *EPO* increases the level of red blood cells in the hope of increasing endurance.

Anabolic-andergenic steroids have been used frequently to increase the growth and development of muscle mass and strength. These substances are discussed at length in the next section of this chapter.

Corticosteroids are anti-inflammatory drugs that are not banned by the NCAA. However, injected, oral, and rectal administration of these substances is banned by the USOC.

Topical *anesthetics,* applied to a small surface of the skin to reduce sensibility to pain, are permitted, but those containing other banned substances are also forbidden by the NCAA and the USOC. Various restrictions are placed on the injected use of anesthetic agents.

Anabolic-Androgenic Steroids

Of these ergogenic substances, the **anabolic-androgenic steroids** (AAS)—originally called anabolic steroids—are the most frequently abused. (*Anabolic* means "building-up of muscle"; *androgenic* means "producing male characteristics"; and steroids are the class of drugs that resemble bodily hormones.)

Commonly known as "roids," AAS drugs are synthetic derivatives of testosterone, the major male sex hormone; they are used by both male and female athletes to build lean muscle mass and to improve the strength and mechanical efficiency of skeletal muscles. Many athletes also believe that these drugs enhance aggressiveness, another desirable characteristic in competitive sports. As a consequence, anabolic steroids are viewed as giving athletes an added advantage in training and in competition.

Restricted originally to world-class power lifters and weight lifters, steroids eventually became available for use in various sports at both the professional and amateur levels. These drugs have become popular among athletes in swimming, track and field, weight lifting, football, basketball, and bodybuilding.

However, other groups are also involved in using these forms of self-medication.[19] These groups include law enforcement officers, firefighters, bar bouncers, and even some construction workers who believe that AAS drugs will give them a competitive edge to "always be on top." The other nonathletes taking steroids are the "aesthetic users" who want to look better and feel better about themselves.

Abuse of Anabolic-Androgenic Steroids

Studies on the prevalence of use and abuse indicate that more than three hundred thousand individuals take AAS drugs each year and that there are more than one million current or former AAS users in this country.[20] Most of the AAS use in the past year has been concentrated among those less than twenty-six years of age. It is apparent that AAS use affects a large number of men and women from various racial and age groups across the nation. Furthermore, use has spread from the Olympic, professional, and college levels of competition to recreational athletes and to young students in high schools, junior highs, and grade schools.

The following items also suggest the extent of consumption and the countermeasures to prevent such use.

- Until recently, at least 70 percent of the steroid production in the United States has not been used for legitimate medical purposes. Although a prescription is needed to get these drugs legally, almost no one has needed a prescription to obtain them.
- An estimated $400 million worth of the drugs are bought and sold annually on the "black market."
- Discouraging the use of AAS has proved to be difficult and frustrating, due to the following sequence of events: junior and senior high school athletes want to take steroids because they want to be college stars and college athletes take them because they want to be professional stars.
- The National Football League includes steroid testing when testing for drug abuse among its players.
- The National Collegiate Athletic Conference tests for both anabolic steroids and chemical "masking agents" sometimes taken in an attempt to cover up steroid use. Under new drug-testing measures, first-time offenders could lose an entire year's playing eligibility. Players testing positive for steroids a second time will be banned for life from NCAA sports.
- In response to the Anabolic Steroids Control Act of the U.S. Congress, the Drug Enforcement Administration (DEA) placed anabolic steroids on Schedule III of the Controlled Substances Act in 1991. As controlled drugs with high abuse potential, anabolic steroids may not be manufactured, distributed, or dispensed without a registration from the DEA. Special record keeping, inventory, and security procedures apply to nearly all of the anabolic steroids. Various penalties apply for violation of the newly established procedures, for instance, any person who gives anabolic steroids to a minor can be sentenced to prison for ten years.

Patterns of Use

The various anabolic-androgenic steroids can be taken either by mouth or by injection; the latter method is preferred by most users. Oral anabolic-androgenic steroids include Android-10 and -25, Anadrol-50, Oxandrin, and Winstrol, while injectables are represented by Deca-Durabolin, Durabolin, and DEPO-Testosterone. Developed originally for patients with muscle problems, these drugs are also used medically to treat certain types of breast cancer, growth problems, arthritis, long-term infections, and anemia.

Frequently, these drugs are used in increasingly higher doses, a practice known as "pyramiding." When several different types of steroids, or a combination of different strengths of pills and injectables, are taken jointly or in cycles, the usage pattern is described as "stacking." For instance, about four or five months before competition, dosage levels will be gradually increased to 10 to 100 times greater than recommended therapeutic amounts. Then, to avoid detection, dosage levels are reduced several weeks before the mandatory drug testing for a particular event. Sometimes these drugs are taken in a cyclical manner, with a six- to twelve-week period of use followed by a drug-free period of one to several months.[21]

Benefits versus Risks

Despite the expected benefits of using AAS drugs—greater endurance, increase in lean muscle mass and aggressiveness, enhanced physical appearance, and a decrease in muscle recovery time—the 1996 edition of the *Physicians' Desk Reference* carries this advisory for such drugs: "Anabolic steroids have not been shown to enhance athletic performance."[22]

However, controlled research on males has confirmed that high doses of anabolic-androgenic steroids, when combined with strength training, can increase fat-free mass and muscle size and strength in normal men. These AAS drugs are variations of testosterone, the male sex hormone that has masculinizing effects in the female, therefore they can probably increase a woman's strength too. There is no evidence of an increased capacity for aerobic work.[23]

Although the use of ergogenic drugs often gives athletes an assumed competitive edge against other contestants, their repeated intake carries the risk of potential threats to the health of the drug users. Amphetamine users often find they must resort to sedatives or tranquilizers to facilitate sleep. And painkillers, by masking the body's messages of injury, can lead to crippling damage of the joints.

Anabolic steroids can also have a variety of life-threatening side effects, including higher blood pressure, less favorable blood-fat ratios, higher cholesterol levels, and increased risk of heart attack and liver cancer, and numerous other serious, potentially dangerous conditions identified in figure 14.4.

Serious psychiatric risks have been associated with steroid use. Users typically display elation; overestimation of their capacities; irritability; and hyperactivity or recklessness in their driving, spending, or sexual habits. These behaviors are common symptoms of mania—an abnormal state of euphoria beyond normal happiness, joy, and pleasure.[24]

Another symptom sometimes reported is heightened, inappropriate aggressiveness, the so-called "roid rage." Displayed not only during use, but also as part of the withdrawal process, roid rage may also include major psychological depression, irritability, and antisocial behavior. New research, however, has found no evidence of or scientific basis for this rage of anger and aggression.[25] No significant changes in mood or behavior were reported during a ten-week period of AAS use by adult males subjects, their spouses, or their partners.

Evidence suggests that many long-term steroid users develop a steroid addiction or dependence. Loss of control over the amount of steroids used, preoccupation with continued use, development of tolerance, and the use of steroids to avoid or control withdrawal symptoms are part of AAS dependence.[26]

Sport fans may also be encouraging this type of drug abuse by expecting perfection of athletes. Many fans tend to value winning—often at any cost—more than honest competition. They will frequently "boo" the loser and cheer loudly when a player "draws blood" from a competitor.

There is also an ethical viewpoint regarding the use of ergogenic agents. When athletes use performance-enhancing drugs, they break the code of conduct that governs most sport activities. Involving cheating and lying, this form of drug use violates the spirit of competition by rewarding willingness to cheat or take health risks. These characteristics and attitudes oppose natural ability, skill, and willingness to train intensively—the qualities a sport is intended to reward.

Dangerous Alternatives to Anabolic-Androgenic Steroids

A number of equally dangerous alternatives to using AAS have been devised to achieve performance-enhancing effects for competitive athletes. First is "blood doping," the injection of blood, one's own or another's, in an attempt to enhance performance and increase endurance by increasing the number of red blood cells available for oxygenation. This procedure involves blood transfusion, therefore infections and even fatal reactions due to error may occur.

Lately, a synthetic form of the human hormone erythropoietin or EPO (Epoetin and Epogen) has been used by some athletes to increase red blood cell production in the human body. Unlike typical blood doping, this synthesized product can be self-injected. This drug can lead to increased blood clotting, so its use is vigorously discouraged by medical authorities.

Gamma hydroxybutyrate (GHB) and clenbuterol are two additional steroid alternatives. GHB, a common ingredient in many so-called performance enhancers, is a deadly, illegal drug that can cause headaches, nausea, vomiting, diarrhea, seizures, and nervous system disorders. Contrary to popular belief, GHB does not produce a "high" in its users. Clenbuterol, an extremely popular item on the black market, can unexpectedly produce muscle tremors, fast heart rates, headaches, nausea, and chills.[27]

More recently, a synthetic form of human growth hormone (HGH) has been used by some athletes to increase tendon and ligament strength and to avoid bone damage that sometimes occurs with the use of anabolic-androgenic steroids. Potentially adverse effects of this relatively new ergogenic drug include hypothyroidism, heart disease, increased incidence of leukemia, and impaired metabolism of various body chemicals.

Creatine

Probably the most popular natural supplement marketed to athletes for ergogenic benefits is creatine. This amino acid occurs naturally in the body and seems to work by drawing fluid into the muscle cells, thus providing more nutrients. This results in better muscle recovery and strength. While some studies indicate that creatine may be a safe nutritional supplement, long-term side effects are not known.

Recreational Drugs

Increasing attention has been focused on drug abuse in sports, since college and especially professional athletes have been

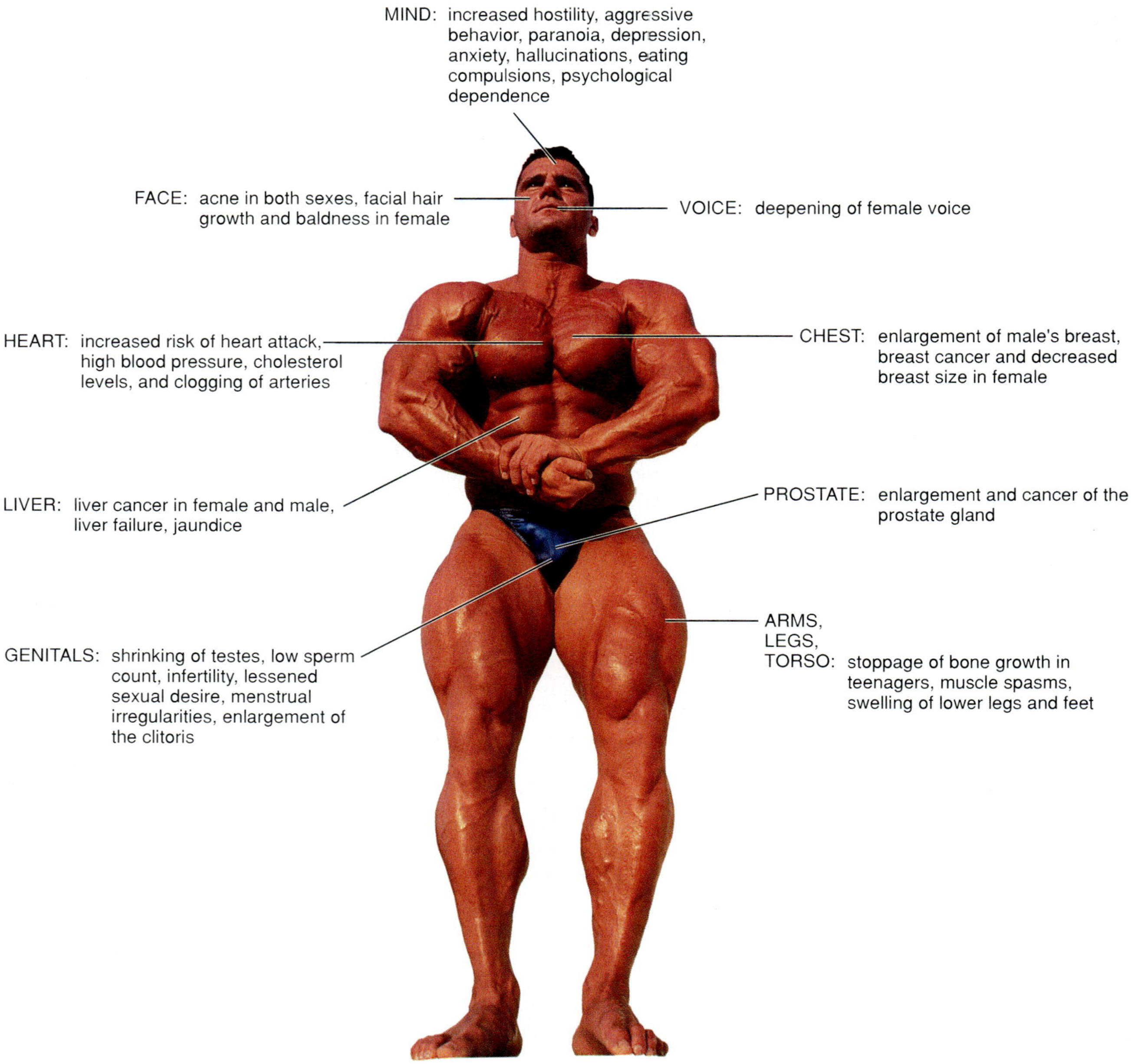

figure 14.4

Adverse side effects of anabolic-androgenic steroids. Developed originally for patients with muscle problems, these drugs are also used medically to treat certain types of breast cancer, growth problems, arthritis, long-term infections, and anemia. But anabolic steroids can have many undesirable side effects, some of which can be life-threatening, especially with long-term, high-dose use without close medical supervision.

Photo © Uniphoto Picture Agency

charged with possession or use of illegal recreational drugs or found to be addicted to some psychoactive substance. In response to charges of scandal and in an effort to prove their athletes were "clean" or not using social drugs, many colleges began NCAA-sponsored drug testing to reduce and, perhaps, eliminate drug use among students participating in college sports (see table 14.4).

Most colleges and universities, and many high schools, have rather comprehensive drug-testing programs, often in combination with drug education and counseling. Testing is typically accomplished by obtaining urine samples from athletes. After the samples are frozen and divided, they are tested for separate drug categories and specific drug substances.

In addition to the performance-enhancement use of anabolic-androgenic steroids and amphetamines, the most frequently abused psychoactive drugs

table 14.4 Selected Drugs for Which College Athletes Are Frequently Tested

Anabolic-Androgenic Steroids	Benzodiazepines (Dalmane, Librium, Valium)
Stimulant Drugs	Phenothiazine, chlorpromazine
Amphetamines	**Narcotic Drugs**
Methamphetamine	Heroin
Phenmetrazine (Preludin)	Morphine
Cocaine	Codeine
Depressant Drugs	Meperidine (Demerol)
Barbiturates	Hydromorphone (Dilaudid)
Phenobarbital	Methadone
Short-acting barbiturates (Amytal, Nembutal, Seconal)	**THC or Its Metabolites**
Methaqualone	Marijuana
Tranquilizers	Hashish
	Phencyclidine (PCP)

by athletes are alcohol, marijuana, and cocaine.

Marijuana has no ergogenic value, so its use is primarily related to producing feelings of relaxation after the excessive pressures of competition. Using marijuana prior to sport activities tends to lower blood pressure, blocks normal sweating, and interferes with the ability to follow a moving object from one point to another, a function referred to as tracking ability.

Cocaine, which has performance-enhancing properties, is a rather expensive and dangerous way of reexperiencing the euphoria of competition or reinforcing one's self-image as an invincible, conquering hero. As a central nervous system stimulant, however, cocaine can also remove the psychological sting of defeat.

Alcohol Use and Abuse

Alcohol is, by far, the number one drug of abuse at the collegiate and the professional level of athletics. Moreover, it is no secret that brewers sponsor a wide variety of sporting events on radio and television. Indeed, beer makers promote their products as the perfect, necessary adjunct to athletic events. Despite the frequent association between former professional athletes and the beers they endorse, drinking any alcoholic beverage is one of the surest ways to interfere with athletic performance.[28]

1. Even small amounts consumed just before or during sports activities will slow down one's physical performance, due to alcohol's depressant effect on the central nervous system. Reaction time, hand-eye coordination, accuracy, balance, and gross motor skills are adversely affected. With higher blood alcohol levels, voluntary motor actions become increasingly clumsy.
2. Although alcohol is a concentrated source of calories, it provides little energy. Alcohol cannot be used directly by the muscles because it must first be processed by the liver. Thus, alcohol is an inefficient source of fuel.
3. Even at low to moderate doses, alcohol causes blood vessels within muscles to constrict, while the blood vessels at the surface of the skin dilate. Performance tends to deteriorate because blood cannot easily reach the working muscles where it is needed.
4. The pancreas tends to produce an excessive amount of insulin in the presence of alcohol. When this occurs, a condition known as temporary hypoglycemia (low blood sugar) can develop, which results in fatigue during exercise.
5. Moderate to heavy drinking blocks the release from the pituitary gland of ADH, a hormone that regulates the amount of water retained by the kidneys. This action can cause dehydration, marked by extreme thirst and physical weakness.

Psychological Factors

To be certain, athletes are influenced by the same influences that determine the use and abuse of recreational drugs in the general population. Yet, a number of psychological forces seem to have special significance for athletes and their interaction with psychoactive substances.[29]

Sensation seeking reflects a particular type of personality in relation to a person's toleration of various levels of sensory and neurological stimulation. Higher risk individuals (those who play football, basketball, and hockey) tend to be more sensation seeking and are more likely to use stimulant drugs, such as amphetamines and cocaine. By contrast, lower sensation seekers are more likely to choose depressant drugs, such as barbiturates.

The sport world, supposedly based on health and drug-free competition, has gradually adopted the use of performance-enhancing substances, pain reducers, and muscle builders over the past thirty years. The encouragement to use these drugs, including alcohol, suggests that the use of all drugs is acceptable and even expected.

The macho role or machismo, the concept of exaggerated male skills or abilities has been linked with alcohol use and abuse for many years. According to society, real men can drink a lot and drink often. Presumably, since athletes are perceived as supermen, they should be able to drink even more and more frequently. This common myth is taught to young people and young athletes by adult athletes; sport celebrities; and nonathletic, adult spectators who consume alcoholic beverages at sporting events. The underlying message is that drinking and sports mix well. The influence of advertising and the sponsorship of various sporting events by beer manufacturers can also be impressionable on the young and the vulnerable.

Stress reduction is a common motivating factor for using alcohol and other recreational drugs. However, athletes at all levels of competition appear to face unique stressors, often to a greater extent than nonathletes. The constancy of practice, travel, preparation for peak performance in competition, and time constraints often add to the stress they would normally experience in nonathletic endeavors. Consequently, taking recreational drugs may be a way of reducing the perceived stress, loneliness, and isolation that may accompany athletic ability. Use of psychoactive drugs is also a way of trying to cope with the reality of career termination or a disruption of athletic competition due to injury or replacement by a another athlete.

In these special ways, athletes, because of their talents and abilities, seem to be vulnerable to some important risk factors for using and abusing mind-changing drugs.

Box 14.2 Inappropriate Drug Prescribing for the Elderly

This study was based on a survey of 6,000 people over sixty five years of age who were not hospitalized or confined to a nursing home. Inappropriateness of prescriptions was determined by the availability of safer alternative medications, because the drugs prescribed by physicians were not needed by patients, were ineffective, or were addictive or otherwise harmful or debilitating. These drugs, however, are still among the more frequently prescribed medicines for the elderly.

Prescribed Drug Class with Specific Examples of Brand Name Drugs Considered Inappropriate

Antianxiety medications (minor tranquilizers), sedative or hypnotic agents: Valium, Librium, Librax, Dalmane, Miltown, Equagesic, Equanil, Nembutal, Seconal.

Antidepressants: Elavil, Endep, Etrafon, Limbitrol, Triavil

Arthritis drugs: Butazolidin Indocin

Diabetes drugs: Diabinese

Analgesics or pain relievers: Darvocet, Darvon Compound, Wygesic, Talwin

Dementia treatments: generic Cyclandelate, generic Isoxsuprine

Blood thinners: Persantine

Muscle relaxants, spasm relievers: Flexeril, Norflex, Norgesic, Robaxin, Soma

Antinausea, antivomiting drugs: Tigan

Antihypertensives: Inderal, Aldoril, Aldomet, Regroton, Hydropres

Source: Sharon Wilcox, David Himmelstein, and Steffie Woolhandler, "Inappropriate Drug Prescribing for the Community-Dwelling Elderly," *Journal of the American Medical Association,* Vol. 272, No.4 (July 27, 1994): 292–96.

Alcohol and Drug Use and Abuse Among the Elderly

If you want evidence of senior citizens' drug use, inspect the medicine cabinet or bedside table in the homes of your parents and grandparents. If you have an aged relative confined in a nursing home, inquire about the number of prescribed medications being taken by that individual. You will likely be shocked at the sheer volume of drugs, both prescribed and nonprescribed, taken by the elderly.

Americans over the age of sixty comprise just over 18 percent of the population. Yet, each year, senior citizens use approximately 30 percent of prescription drugs and 40 percent of sleeping pills.

Today, the average American senior citizen gets fifteen prescriptions each year. About four in ten seniors also use five or more of these prescriptions at the same time. Even more alarmingly, these older Americans account for 30 percent of hospitalizations and 51 percent of deaths from adverse drug reactions.[30]

With the number of senior citizens increasing rapidly, the amount of medicine used by this segment of the population will likely become phenomenal. The improper use of drugs, misdiagnoses by physicians, and inappropriate dosage levels—already major problems—will also become phenomenal. Already one in five Americans over the age of sixty has had at least one adverse reaction to prescription drugs. Many of these unanticipated and undesirable responses are the result of interactions between different drugs.

Emerging from a national conspiracy of silence and neglect is an epidemic of inappropriate drug prescribing for the elderly.[31] Research has revealed that nearly a quarter of Americans aged sixty five or older are routinely given prescriptions for drugs that they should almost never take and often do not even need (see box 14.2).

Prescribing errors among noninstitutionalized patients and those in health care facilities have become extremely high, resulting in almost a quarter million older Americans being hospitalized each year due to the side effects of their medicines. Seniors often see a variety of medical specialists for their ailments, therefore these patients are the ones most likely to experience harmful drug interactions.[32] For example, it is not unlikely for one person to be prescribed arthritis medication from an internist or rheumatologist; high blood pressure pills and aspirin to prevent blood clots from a cardiologist; heartburn and antiulcer medication from a gastroenterologist; and still more drugs from a urologist or dermatologist.

Some physicians and drug companies have used elderly patients as test subjects for drug experiments without obtaining informed consent from the affected individuals. In addition, adverse drug interactions are routinely seen in hospitals and in nonsupervised settings.[33] These situations are part of the "mismedication" of older Americans.

While the wise use of medications can be beneficial for older people, a number of factors related particularly to the elderly contribute to the increased potential for drug misuse, abuse, and numerous drug interactions with serious and undesirable side effects.[34]

1. *Aging is accompanied by normal changes in the body that make adverse drug reactions more likely.* Older adults typically weigh less and have a

smaller amount of water and a larger proportion of fat than younger adults. These changes affect the amount of a drug needed per pound of body weight or body water to be safe and effective, the dilution of a drug after it enters the body, and the duration of drug action. In addition, many older adults experience an increased sensitivity to many drugs and decreased abilities to maintain blood pressure and compensate for changes in temperature.

Other common changes include impaired kidney and liver function, which reduces the ability to metabolize and clear drugs or their by-products from the bloodstream; a weakened heart; lowered effectiveness of the immune system; and loss of intestinal flexibility. These body changes make the elderly more likely to need drug therapy. At the same time, these changes combine to reduce the effectiveness and efficiency of drugs and to increase the risk of side effects due to the buildup of chemical substances in the body.

2. *The occurrence of the pharmaceutical revolution in conjunction with the decline of the extended family.* Without family support or consolation, the elderly are increasingly placed on chemical tranquilizers; antidepressants; and sedatives to combat their depression, loneliness, and isolation.
3. *Changes in sleep patterns that often lead to drug dependency.* Confronted with the inability to sleep as well as when they were young, many older people are prescribed sleeping pills containing depressant drugs, hypnotics, and tranquilizers. If such medication is stopped, these people often experience increased wakefulness and nightmares, which are sufficient to motivate continued use of the drugs.
4. *Many physicians overprescribe psychoactive drugs for the elderly.* Encouraged by the promotional practices of pharmaceutical companies, physicians have tended to increase their reliance on drugs as their primary method of treatment. This is especially true regarding the emotional life and sleeping pattern of older patients. This situation allegedly has occurred without a similar increase in the pharmacological training of physicians regarding geriatric patients.
5. *Mismanagement of medicines is a common problem among the aged.* It is not unusual for older people to be taking three or more drugs—often prescribed by two or more physicians—at the same time. This pattern of taking multiple drugs concurrently is **polydrug use.** Because of self-medication, any number of drugs purchased over the counter may also be used simultaneously. Multiple drug use makes it difficult for many people to remember whether they have taken a particular drug. Inability to distinguish between colored medicines, impaired vision that prevents reading label instructions, and decreased ability to hear or understand directions all combine to precipitate numerous **medication errors.** Unintentional, inappropriate uses of medicines, these medication errors include decreasing or increasing recommended dosage, improper timing of taking the medicine, sharing prescribed drugs with relatives and friends, forgetting to take a dose as directed, or stopping the use of the medicine because of lack of funds or because they are feeling better (see table 14.5).

table 14.5 Common Medication Errors Experienced by the Elderly

- Failure to take medicines at the right time
- Difficulty in remembering to take medicines
- Trouble opening the bottle, jar, or container
- Difficulty separating or breaking tablets
- Problems encountered with mixing or preparing medication
- Inability to maintain an adequate supply of medicine
- Difficulty reading the label and understanding directions
- Taking a greater or smaller dosage than specified in the directions
- Inability to distinguish between medicines that look alike

There is a greater need for drug education for the elderly and their physicians. There appears to be an equal need to become aware of nondrug alternatives to the health problems of the aged, especially problems solved by sleeping pills and tranquilizers. Until the overmedication syndrome is reversed in treating and caring for the elderly, one might conclude logically that older Americans are more abused than are their drugs.

While the misuse of pain-relieving medicines, minor tranquilizers, barbiturates and other sleep-inducing drugs, and numerous over-the-counter medications is common and a growing problem for the elderly, most senior citizens have little involvement with illegal psychoactive substances. Although this situation may change, the major drug problems of the elderly center around legal prescription drugs and alcohol, often used in combination.

Alcohol Abuse and Alcoholism or Alcohol Dependence Among the elderly, these are usually classified on the basis of age of onset. **Early-onset alcohol abuse or dependence** represents the continuation of lifelong drinking problems, and represents nearly two-thirds of elderly problem drinkers. Such problematic use is more likely to be associated with a family history of alcoholism or psychological disorders. By contrast, **late-onset alcohol abuse or dependence** usually develops after many years during which no alcohol problems were experienced and is typical of about one-third of older problem drinkers.

This late-onset form is sometimes triggered by a life crisis or major life change usually involving a series of losses—loss of employment, retirement, decreased income, death of a spouse, diminished mobility due to illness, loss of familiar environment and longtime friends when forced to move to smaller homes, and increased isolation from former support groups or individuals.

As a group, older Americans have unique concerns and risk factors associated with drinking:[35]

- Older persons can experience the physical and mental effects of alcohol while drinking less, in other words, a smaller dose, because of changes in body function as a person ages, including a loss of lean body mass in which to distribute water-soluble alcohol.
- The effect of a given blood alcohol on the brain tends to increase with age. This effect may also be more severe because of the use of prescribed medicine that interacts with alcohol.
- Family, friends, and physicians may sometimes mistakenly confuse the physical effects of alcohol with the natural aging process or the side effects of medication. Consequently, alcohol problems may be discovered or diagnosed only with difficulty.
- Alcohol problems may be worsened by combining certain prescription and over-the-counter drugs with alcohol, resulting in dangerous and life-threatening drug interactions. This risk is especially evident when alcohol is combined with sleeping medications, antianxiety drugs (tranquilizers), antidepressants, antihistamines, certain blood pressure medicines, antiarthritic medications, blood thinners, and antidiabetic medicines.
- Alcohol tends to slow brain activity and impairs mental alertness, judgment, physical coordination, and reaction time, so the chances of falling or being injured are increased.
- Drinking may mask pain and disguise the warning signs of heart attack or some other health problem because of alcohol's analgesic (pain-relieving) effect.
- Heavy drinking can produce symptoms similar to dementia (general mental deterioration). Incorrect diagnosis can result in unnecessary institutionalization.

The reality of drinking and alcohol abuse and dependence among older Americans suggests that alcohol problems do not necessarily decrease with age. The identification of older alcoholics is challenging and elusive, with many individuals being first diagnosed by emergency department physicians. Fortunately, older alcoholics tend to achieve the same treatment success rates as younger alcoholics.

Unlike alcohol abuse in younger age groups, several conditions tend to complicate the early detection, formal diagnosis, and effective treatment of alcohol problems in the elderly. These include the following:[36]

1. The elderly are more able to hide or deny their drinking problems. This situation applies especially to the 8 to 9 million Americans over age sixty-five who live alone, and thereby escape the social controls placed on those who work outside the home. Those who live isolated lives and have few friends may never be confronted with the consequences of their otherwise problem-producing use of alcohol.
2. The elderly are frequently unaware they have a drinking problem, particularly if they are affected by chronic aches, pains, and other physical and psychological complaints. The elderly often suffer from symptoms that they and their physicians do not associate with their use of alcoholic beverages. Many indications of physical, psychological, and social deterioration associated with alcoholism are attributed falsely to the "natural aging process" or to Alzheimer's disease.
3. Families and physicians are unable or unwilling to recognize alcohol abuse among the elderly. In some instances, children encourage their aging parents to use alcohol to promote sleep and alleviate aches and pains, while physicians mistakenly assume their elderly patients are too old to have a drinking problem.
4. In too many instances, physicians are unsure about how to handle alcohol problems in the elderly and are usually pessimistic about the effectiveness of treatment.

Chapter Summary

1. Special populations, including women, racial and ethnic minorities, athletes, and the elderly, often have significant differences in drug use patterns and drug-related problems from white males.
2. American women are closing the gender gap with men in terms of use and abuse of psychoactive substances and drug-related problems.
3. Gender-related drug hazards for women include the tendency to get drunk faster than men; to develop alcohol-related cirrhosis more readily; and to experience menstrual dysfunction, more rapid onset of menopause, and sexual dysfunction.
4. Use of psychoactive drugs by mothers-to-be may contribute to undesirable mutagenic effects in the offspring. Use of any drug, including alcohol, during pregnancy may contribute to various congenital birth defects that could affect the health and growth of the fetus and its postbirth behavioral and mental performance.
5. Alcohol and drug abuse appear to affect racial and ethnic minorities in disproportionate ways with more negative effects on employment, school achievement, family stability, and increased risk of disease and death. Serious consequences of drug abuse are often related to some minorities' preference for injecting drug use and their choice of more dangerous psychoactive substances.
6. African American males have high rates of marijuana and cocaine use, although their drinking patterns are similar to white males. Alcohol abuse

in this population has been related to various factors: isolation of racial segregation; accessibility to alcohol outlets in black neighborhoods; and coping with racism, lack of employment, and the level of racial consciousness.

7. Young Hispanic Americans have extremely high use rates for cocaine and crack cocaine, though when all age groups and both males and females are combined, this minority population has lower use rates of illegal drugs than whites and African Americans. Alcohol use among Hispanics is marked by heavy consumption in males—influenced by machismo and acculturation, and by abstinence or light drinking among females.
8. American Indians and Alaska Natives display high rates of psychoactive drug use, especially alcohol, marijuana, and inhalants. While some tribes have relatively few drug-related problems, others display many adverse consequences of alcohol abuse, especially motor vehicle crashes, alcohol-related traumatic deaths and suicide, alcoholism, and cirrhosis.
9. Asian Americans and Pacific Islanders usually have much less drug use than any other non-Asian population. The so-called flushing response or reaction is one factor likely contributing to relatively lower rates of alcohol abuse and alcoholism. Asian American women usually drink far less than men. This gender difference holds true across most ethnic groups.
10. Ergogenic aids, drugs used to artificially improve athletes' performance in competition, include stimulants, beta-blockers, bronchodilators, hormones, anabolic-androgenic steroids (AAS), and various anesthetics.
11. Continued use of various anabolic-androgenic steroids—now Schedule III controlled substances—can result in numerous life-threatening conditions, such as high blood pressure and elevated blood cholesterol levels, increased risk of heart attack and cancer of the prostate and the female breast. These drugs can also result in various growth and developmental problems, including baldness and deepening of the female voice, shrinking of the testes, menstrual irregularities, and enlargement of the clitoris.
12. Use of alcoholic beverages tends to impair athletic performance due to alcohol's CNS depressant effect, its function as an inefficient source of fuel, the tendency of alcohol to constrict blood vessels within muscles, and its potential for causing dehydration.
13. Some athletes seem to have unique risk factors for using psychoactive drugs, namely, high levels of sensation seeking; involvement in the sport world, which has a strong pro-use message; the influence of the macho role; and alcohol's function as a perceived stress reducer.
14. Prescribing errors among elderly patients have been extremely high, allegedly, because of prescriptions for drugs that patients ought not to have and often do not need. In addition, several factors contribute to increased potential for drug misuse, abuse, and adverse interactions among the elderly, including normal body changes with aging, greater prescription of psychoactive drugs for the institutionalized and the noninstitutionalized, changes in sleep patterns, and mismanagement of medicines by patients who engage in polydrug use and unintentionally make medication errors.
15. Among the elderly, alcohol problems develop as either early-onset alcohol abuse/alcoholism or as late-onset alcohol abuse/alcoholism, triggered by a life crisis involving losses. Alcohol problems are often overlooked in this population group because senior citizens frequently hide or deny their drinking problems, they are unaware of their own alcohol abuse and confuse their difficulties with normal aging, physicians typically fail to diagnose such abuse, and children encourage their elderly parents to drink to promote sleep or to lessen common aches and pains.

World Wide Web Sites

Gatorade Sports Science Institute

www.gssiweb.com

Higher Education Center for Alcohol and Other Drug Prevention

www.edc.org/hec

National Association for Children of Alcoholics

www.health.org/nacoa

Review Questions and Activities

1. What is the so-called "gender gap" in relation to psychoactive drug use by men and women in the United States?
2. Survey class members or several friends or acquaintances to determine their definitions of moderate alcohol use for men and women. Can you detect any gender differences in these descriptions?
3. Identify several distinct ways in which women experience undesirable short- and long-term effects of using various psychoactive drugs.
4. How can heavy use of alcoholic beverages become both a cause and consequence of sexual dysfunction?
5. In your opinion, why is psychoactive substance abuse so often associated with violence and sexual exploitation against women?
6. Name at least one specific adverse effect that ten psychoactive drugs may have on a developing embryo or fetus.
7. Compare and contrast psychoactive substance use and abuse among African Americans, Hispanic

Americans, American Indians/Alaska Natives, and Asian Americans and Pacific Islanders.

8. Relate the following terms to the use and abuse of psychoactive drugs by racial/ethnic minorities in the United States: injecting drug use, racial consciousness, machismo, acculturation, binge drinking, and the flushing reaction.
9. What is the difference between therapeutic drugs and erogenic drugs?
10. For what specific reason or outcome do some athletes use each of the following: stimulants, diuretics, human growth hormone, blood doping, and anabolic-androgenic steroids?
11. Explain why the use of anabolic-androgenic steroids can be potentially harmful and life-threatening to users.
12. In what ways might sport fans be contributing to the use of ergogenic agents among athletes?
13. Describe how drinking alcoholic beverages can interfere with athletic performance.
14. Relate each of the following risk factors to athletes' psychological vulnerability to using and abusing psychoactive drugs: sensation seeking, the environment of the sport world, the macho role, and stress reduction.
15. Explain what is meant by the "mismedication of older Americans."
16. Survey your older relatives or friends to determine how many different over-the-counter and prescription drugs they take in one year. Compare the results of this study in class. What factors likely influenced the outcome of your findings?
17. What normal changes in the aging human body contribute to adverse drug reactions in the elderly?
18. Distinguish among the following paired terms: medication error and polydrug use; and early on-set alcohol abuse/alcoholism and late-onset alcohol abuse/alcoholism.
19. Why is the use of alcoholic beverages among the elderly more likely to be problem-producing than among younger drinkers?
20. How do some older drinkers, their families or friends, and their physicians sometimes complicate the early detection, diagnosis, and treatment of alcohol problems?

References

1. The National Center on Addiction and Substance Abuse at Columbia University, *Substance Abuse and The American Woman* (New York: The National Center on Addiction and Substance Abuse, 1996), 4.
2. National Institute on Alcohol Abuse and Alcoholism, *Alcohol Alert: Alcohol and Women* (Rockville, Md.: Public Health Service, Alcohol Drug Abuse and Mental Health Administration, 1990), 1–4; Jacqueline Horton, ed., "Addictive Behaviors," chap. 5 in *The Women's Health Data Book* (Washington, D.C.: Elsevier and The Jacob's Institute of Women's Health, 1992), 75–87; and "Wine, Women and Health," *Harvard Women's Health Watch* 1, no. 9 (May 1994): 2–3.
3. Stephen Deal and Judith Gavaler, "Are Women More Susceptible Than Men to Alcohol-Induced Cirrhosis?" *Alcohol Health & Research World* 18, no. 3 (1994): 189–91.
4. Jeanette Norris, "Alcohol and Female Sexuality: A Look at Expectancies and Risks," *Alcohol Health & Research World* 18, no. 3 (1994): 197–201.
5. Sharon Wilsnack and others, "Predictive Onset and Chronicity of Women's Problem Drinking," *American Journal of Public Health* 81, no. 3 (1991): 305–18.
6. The National Center on Addiction and Substance Abuse at Columbia University, *Substance Abuse and The American Woman*, 6.
7. Jeanette Norris, "Alcohol and Female Sexuality," 200.
8. The National Center on Addiction and Substance Abuse at Columbia University, *Substance Abuse and The American Woman*, 8–9.
9. National Institute on Drug Abuse, *Drug Use Among Racial/Ethnic Minorities*, NIH Pub. No. 95-3888 (Rockville, Md.: Public Health Service, National Institutes of Health, 1995), 93.
10. Ibid., 2–4.
11. Frederick Harper and Elaheh Saifnoorian, "Drinking Patterns Among Black Americans," in *Society, Culture, and Drinking Patterns Reexamined* (New Brunswick, N.J.: Rutgers Center of Alcohol Studies, 1991), 327–38.
12. National Institute on Alcohol Abuse and Alcoholism, *Alcohol and Health, the Eighth Special Report to the U.S. Congress* (Rockville, Md.: Public Health Service, National Institutes of Health, 1994), 25.
13. National Institute on Alcohol Abuse and Alcoholism, *Preventing Alcohol-Related Problems Among Ethnic Minorities*, Program Announcement PA-93-47 (Rockville, Md.: Public Health Service, National Institutes of Health, 1993), 3.
14. I. Chasnoff, H. Landress, and M. Barrett, "The Prevalence of illicit-drug or Alcohol use during Pregnancy and Discrepancies in Mandatory Reporting in Pinellas County, Florida," *New England Journal of Medicine* 322, no. 17 (28 April 1990): 1202–6.
15. Jose Szapocznik and Steve Fein, "Issues in Preventing Alcohol and Other Drug Abuse Among Hispanic/Latino Families," in *A Hispanic/Latino Family Approach to Substance Abuse Prevention*, Center for Substance Abuse Prevention Cultural Competence Series 2 DHHS Pub. No. (SMA) 95-3034 (Washington, D.C.: GPO, 1995), 10.
16. Philip May, "The Prevention of Alcohol and Other Drug Abuse Among American Indians: A Review and Analysis of the Literature," in *The Challenge of Participatory Research: Preventing Alcohol-Related Problems in Ethnic Communities*, Center for Substance Abuse Prevention Cultural Competence Series 3 (Washington, D.C.: GPO, 1995), 189–90.
17. Kiyoko Parrish, "Alcohol Abuse Prevention Research in Asian American and Pacific Islander Communities," in *The Challenge of Participatory Research: Preventing Alcohol-Related Problems in Ethnic Communities*, Center for Substance Abuse Prevention Cultural Competence Series 3 (Washington, D.C.: GPO, 1995), 407.
18. United States Pharmacopeia, *Complete Drug Reference* (Yonkers, N.Y.: Consumer Reports Books, 1996), 1747–50.
19. Corinne Groark, "When Pumping Up Can Lead to Serious Health Problems and Side Effects," *Employee Assistance: Solutions to the Problems* 4, no. 4 (November 1991): 8.
20. Charles Yesalis and others, "Anabolic-Androgenic Steroid Use in the United States," *Journal of the American Medical Association* 270, no. 10 (8 September 1993): 1217–21.
21. Barry Stimmel and the editors of Consumer Reports Books, *The Facts About Drug Use* (New York: The Haworth Medical Press, 1993), 293.
22. *Physicians' Desk Reference*, 50th ed. (Montvale, N.J.: Medical Economics Company, 1996), 2338.
23. Stimmel and others, *The Facts About Drug Use*, 295.
24. Harrison Pope and David Katz, "What Are the Psychiatric Risks of Anabolic Steroids?" *Harvard Mental Health Letter* 7, no. 10 (April 1991): 8.
25. Shalender Bhasin and others, "The Effects of Supraphysiologic Doses of Testosterone on Muscle Size and Strength in Normal Men," *The New England Journal of Medicine* 335, no. 1 (4 July 1996): 1–7.

26. Harold Doweiko, *Concepts of Chemical Dependency,* 2d ed. (Pacific Grove, Calif.: Brooks/Cole Publishing Company, 1993), 171–72.

27. Raja Mishra, "Steroids and Sports Are a Losing Proposition," *FDA Consumer* 25, no. 7 (September 1991): 25–27.

28. U.S. Department of Health and Human Services, Office for Substance Abuse Prevention, *The Performance Edge* (Washington, D.C.: GPO, 1989), 2–3.

29. Steven Heyman, "Psychological Factors in Athletes' Substance Use," *The Prevention Researcher* 3, no. 2 (spring 1996): 3–5.

30. Hank Tweed, *Drugs and Alcohol: What Older People Should Know* (Tempe, Ariz.: D.I.N. Publications, 1994): 1–2.

31. Sharon Willcox, David Himmelstein, and Steffie Woodhandler, "Inappropriate Drug Prescribing for the Community-Dwelling Elderly," *Journal of the American Medical Association* 272, no. 4 (27 July 1994): 292–96.

32. Joe Graedon and Teresa Graedon, *The People's Guide to Deadly Drug Interactions* (New York: St. Martin's Press, 1995), 139.

33. David Schneider, "The Pharmacology of Aging," in *Frontiers in Therapeutic Drug Monitoring and Clinical Toxicology* [Special issue], *Clinical Chemistry News* (June 1992): 22–26.

34. John Fried and Sharon Petska, *The American Druggist's Complete Family Guide to Prescriptions, Pills, and Drugs* (New York: Hearst Books, 1995), 43–44; and "Nine Reasons Why Older Adults Are More Likely to Get Adverse Drug Reactions Than Younger Adults," *Public Citizen Health Research Group Health Letter* 6, no. 11 (November 1990): 5–6.

35. Nan Robertson, "The Intimate Enemy: Will That Friendly Drink Betray You?" *Modern Maturity* 35, no. 1 (February–March 1992): 26–30, 65; and "Elderly At Risk for Alcohol Problems," *The Prevention Pipeline* 7, No. 2 (March/April, 1994): 32–34.

36. Council on Scientific Affairs, American Medical Association, "Alcoholism in the Elderly," *Journal of the American Medical Association* 275, no. 10 (13 March 1996): 797–801; and National Institute on Alcohol Abuse and Alcoholism, *Alcohol and Health,* Eighth Special Report to the U.S. Congress (Rockville, Md.: Public Health Service, National Institutes of Health, 1994), 29–30.

Chapter 15

Drug-abuse prevention

KEY TERMS

Alternatives Approach
Antiparaphernalia Movement
Controlled Substances Act (CSA)
Demand Reduction
Detection
Distribution of Consumption Theory
Drug Enforcement Administration (DEA)
Drug Testing
Enforcement Techniques
Inoculation Strategy
Interdiction
Intervention Process
Macroapproach
Primary Prevention
Referral Process
Responsible Drug Use
Secondary Prevention
Supply Reduction
Surveillance
Tertiary Prevention
Trafficking

chapter objectives

After you have studied this chapter, you should be able to do the following:

1. Define the key terms.
2. List two examples that reflect the application of each general strategy in a drug-abuse prevention program.
3. Discuss the significance of the macroapproach to preventing drug abuse.
4. List two examples of each intervention level (primary, secondary, and tertiary) that might be applied in a drug-abuse prevention program.
5. Identify at least five routine law-enforcement techniques used by law-enforcement agents in their drug-abuse prevention activities.
6. Describe the nature and objectives of the federal government's strategy in combating drug abuse.
7. Name at least four federal law-enforcement agencies concerned directly with drug-abuse prevention activities.
8. Compare the advantages and disadvantages of using a "summons" rather than making an "arrest" of an underaged person caught using alcoholic beverages.
9. Compare, in general terms, the drug laws of other nations with those of the United States.
10. Explain the meaning of the "alternative behaviors" approach as a drug-abuse prevention measure.
11. Name some alternative behaviors to using drugs that are appropriate to various levels of experience or types of satisfaction desired.
12. Discuss in detail the concept of "responsible drug use" as a drug-abuse prevention measure.
13. Describe "responsible drug use" in terms of situational responsibilities, health responsibilities, and safety responsibilities.
14. Explain why drug abuse is often seen as a family affair.
15. Identify several common signals or indicators of drug use among young people and adults.
16. List at least five guidelines parents could use to help their children overcome a drug problem.
17. Describe the major stages frequently seen in adolescent chemical use.
18. Explain how the family can function in the primary prevention of drug abuse.

Introduction

Prevention activities are undertaken to avoid, reduce, or eliminate the adverse consequences of using, misusing, and abusing psychoactive drugs. Various prevention strategies of reducing the drug supply, lessening the demand for drugs, and protecting users from the more negative consequences of drug abuse are explained.

Primary, secondary, and tertiary prevention efforts are identified as levels of program intervention or application. Various therapies for drug dependencies have already been described in earlier chapters, therefore the major emphasis here is on substance-abuse prevention in the workplace, drug law enforcement,

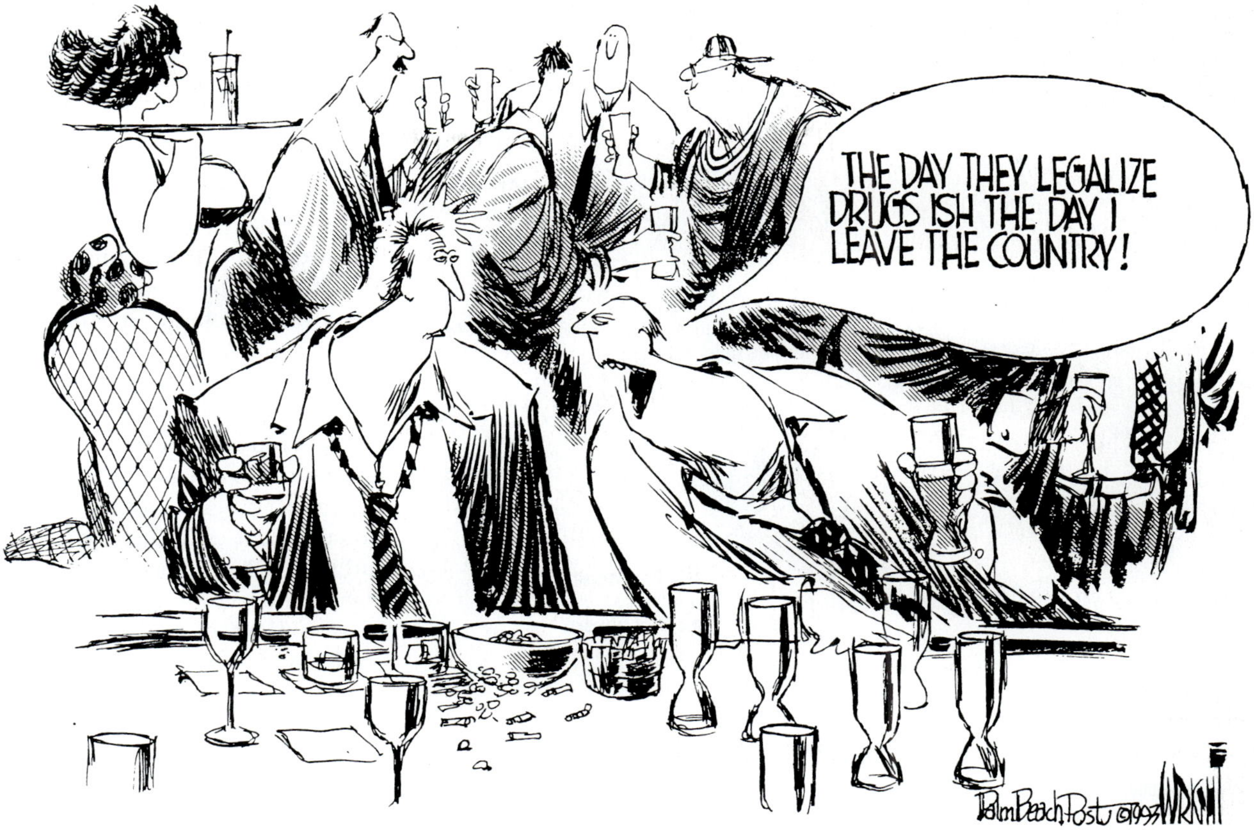
THE DAY THEY LEGALIZE DRUGS ISH THE DAY I LEAVE THE COUNTRY!

figure 15.1

Although the debate over legalizing certain psychoactive drugs continues, prevention of alcohol, tobacco, and other drug-related problems is often hampered by commonly held misconceptions, as noted in this cartoon. Does the "war on drugs" overlook certain mind-changing chemicals by focusing so narrowly on illegal psychoactives?

Reprinted by permission: Tribune Media Services.

the promotion of alternative behaviors as a substitute for taking drugs, and the consideration of responsible drug use, a somewhat controversial proposal.

Although prevention activities take place at school, in the workplace, and in the community at large, the final section of this chapter focuses on the role of the family in preventing drug problems. It is within the family unit that primary and secondary interventions are likely to have their greatest potential effect.

Prevention: The War on Drugs

What can be done to prevent alcohol, tobacco, and other drug problems? From time to time, a coordinated national effort—a so-called war on drugs, or the National Drug Control Strategy—is declared or renewed by the president. Such a "war" or strategy has many dimensions. For instance, officials at the federal, state, and local levels pledge their best efforts to reduce, if not entirely eliminate, the many personal and social difficulties related to the use and abuse of mind-changing substances. Often reflecting the political and economic expediency of the federal government's legislative branch, the U.S. Congress enacts tougher antidrug laws, threatens or suspends foreign aid to drug-producing countries, and slashes prevention programs considered too expensive, ineffective, or not punitive enough. Meanwhile, the U.S. military services, and businesses and industries, continue programs of drug testing to deter drug use and chemical dependency in the interest of national security and worker productivity, respectively.

The foregoing activities demonstrate this nation's ongoing anxiety and frustration about a serious and potentially life-threatening issue. There is a persistent concern, because of the wide-spread use of both legal and illegal psychoactives (fig. 15.1), about stopping or reducing the tragic consequences and mounting expenses associated with the use, misuse, and abuse of these drugs. The need for counter measures seems obvious, because we pay a staggering price for our national drug problem. A huge part of the cost of national health care is related directly to alcohol, tobacco, and other drug-related

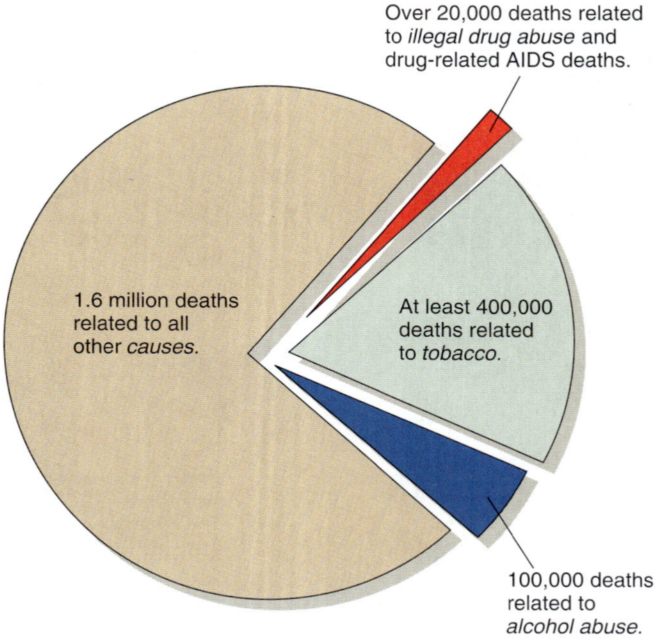

figure 15.2

Of the 2.1 million deaths per year in the United States, about one in four—between 520,000 and 575,000—is now related to alcohol, tobacco, and other illegal drugs.

medical expenses, and amounts to over $5 million every hour—money some believe could be better used in reducing the national debt or funding health care reform.

However, our continuing preoccupation with drug-related problems is also due to increasing interest in health promotion and the growing awareness that alcohol, tobacco, and other drug abuse often results in serious problems for family life, school performance, and worker efficiency. There is another factor responsible for the need to act against these drugs—the growing awareness that using alcohol, tobacco, and other drugs often contributes to crime, violence, homelessness, urban decay, and preventable illnesses and injuries. At least half a million Americans die each year from alcohol, tobacco, and illicit drugs, thus making substance abuse the single largest preventable cause of death in this country (see fig. 15.2).[1]

Health, social welfare, educational, and law enforcement agencies, among others, have placed greater emphasis on efforts to block, avert, forestall, or eliminate those unfavorable results of using, misusing, and abusing psychoactive chemicals. Such efforts are particularly evident in the rapid growth of parent groups alarmed by their children's drug usage.

Realistically, can the war on drugs be won? Has the nation already lost such a war? Despite billions of dollars spent and more than a million arrests each year, the war on drugs has turned into a war on drug users, and drug-related violence, crime, ill health, social tension, and compromised civil liberties have increased.[2] Reasonable answers to such questions can be given only when and if the "enemy" in this war is better understood and recognized for what it is. The war will not likely be won soon because of the country's continuing demand for psychoactive drugs—both legal and illegal. There can be no significant victory until there is a basic change in the national acceptance of and reliance upon mind-altering substances. People have yet to learn that taking pills is not the best way to handle indigestion, stress, or emotional conflict, and that drinking alcoholic beverages is not necessary for a successful party or essential for gracious living.

As long as the demand for drugs is great, the supply will be there, despite the antidrug wars on the local and national levels. Illegal drugs, and the legal ones too, are "big business," and a profitable one at that! The inhabitants of the earth are estimated to spend more on illegal drugs than on food, housing, clothes, education, medical care, or any other product or service. In the United States, consumers of illegal drugs spend an estimated $140 billion annually on illicit drugs.[3] In this instance, the enemy in the war against drugs is a formidable international narcotics industry described as ruthless, rich, and largely unseen. This menacing operation consists of criminals in an underground empire in which crime and governments embrace in the promotion of drug trafficking.

But the enemy is also a nation in which the annual advertising budget for one brand name of "light beer" is more than twenty times greater than the annual prevention budget for the National Institute of Alcohol Abuse and Alcoholism. While urging other nations to destroy their major cash crops of cocaine, heroin, and marijuana, Americans continue to subsidize the number one drug killer in our country—tobacco. In these ways, we are the enemy too!

The war on drugs will not likely be won for a long time, if ever. But we cannot afford to stop fighting; we cannot retreat; we cannot lose. The stakes are too high, and defeat would be too costly in terms of human lives. In theory, the battle plan in this war consists of various countermeasures, referred to as *prevention activities,* to combat alcohol, tobacco, and other drug abuse. These activities are aimed at ensuring healthy, safe, and productive lives for Americans. In general, prevention includes those efforts that keep alcohol, tobacco, and other drug (ATOD) problems from occurring by reducing risk factors and by increasing protective factors.[4] Prevention also occurs when people do not use certain substances in conjunction with other behaviors, such as drinking alcoholic beverages

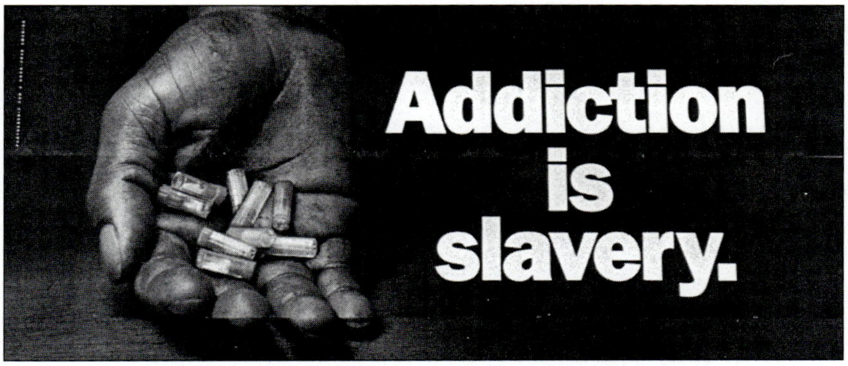

Public awareness campaigns that communicate the adverse effects of psychoactive drugs are important parts of any overall effort to promote a drug-free environment.

© Toni Michaels/The Image Works

and then driving, and when those who have already developed an ATOD problem stop using these substances.

Prevention activities are usually based on general strategies or plans in terms of desired outcome, and they are applied at three different yet related levels of intervention, described in the following sections.

General Strategies of Preventing Drug Abuse

Though alcohol and other drug abuse is hardly a new phenomenon, it was not considered a major problem in the United States until the "youth rebellion" of the 1960s. When middle-class teenagers and young adults suddenly adopted a wide range of unconventional behaviors, including the recreational use of illicit psychoactive chemicals, the nation realized that something had to be done.

Initial efforts at combating drug abuse were aimed at scaring youths into nonuse through information-only school programs and at finding and treating drug abusers for their illness or penalizing them for their criminal behavior. Evaluation of early school-based drug education programs revealed that such efforts had little or no effect on drug-using behavior. In some instances, students seemed to increase their recreational drug usage after exposure to drug education programs.[5] It was also recognized that there would never be sufficient treatment facilities or caregivers to "cure" the mounting numbers of "addicts," and the jails were not big enough to accommodate a whole generation. Countermeasures were eventually devised that focused on preventing the problem before it developed. Today, effective programs of alcohol, tobacco, and other drug abuse prevention combine a variety of activities that reflect the following general plans or strategies.

Supply Reduction Strategy

This concept of drug-abuse prevention is not new. The Harrison Narcotic Act of 1914 and the Eighteenth (Prohibition) Amendment to the U.S. Constitution—later to be repealed by the Twenty-First Amendment—represented early attempts at drug-abuse prevention (see fig. 15.3). Both were based on the idea that enforcement of laws controlling the manufacture and distribution of certain drugs would stop people from using those drugs. These and similar laws reflect a plan of **supply reduction**—one that intends to lower, restrict, or eliminate the availability of a drug. With less use, eventually there will be no use. Without use, there can be no misuse or abuse.

Reducing the supply of illegal drugs and limiting the availability of therapeutic drugs with abuse potential are important parts of the current abuse prevention policy in the United States.[6] Other aspects of supply reduction include disrupting major drug-trafficking organizations, eradicating American and foreign marijuana crops, driving drug prices higher by limiting availability and discouraging use, interdicting foreign-manufactured drugs at the nation's borders and ports of entry, heavy taxation of ethyl alcohol, criminal penalties for trafficking in drugs, and limiting the number of retail beverage alcohol outlets and their hours of operation. The implementation of supply reduction techniques has not always produced the desired effect, however. Some people believe that laws curtailing the supply of drugs have almost no impact on drug-taking behavior.

The relationship between the average level of consumption in a population and the percentage of heavy consumers has been debated and extended to the phenomenon of alcohol and drug abuse. According to this **distribution of consumption theory,** there is a relationship between the per capita consumption of drugs used in a society and the prevalence of heavy drug use and abuse. Therefore, highly restrictive controls on accessibility to drugs will lead to lower consumption which in turn, will result in fewer drug abuse problems. Although the theory supporting supply reduction has some validity, the social, economic, and political costs of implementation are often perceived as outweighing their potential benefits. Moreover, the severity of restrictions—often known in the alcohol-abuse prevention field as "neoprohibition" tactics—would likely be found unconstitutional.

Demand Reduction Strategy

Another major plan for preventing drug abuse is to reduce the demand for drugs. Techniques based on **demand reduction** include a wide range of activities that help individuals (primarily youth) create positive mental attitudes, values, behaviors, skills, and lifestyles that will enable them to mature as adjusted and competent citizens who will not need to resort to the use of drugs. Demand reduction also involves medical or other therapy for current drug abusers and drug dependent

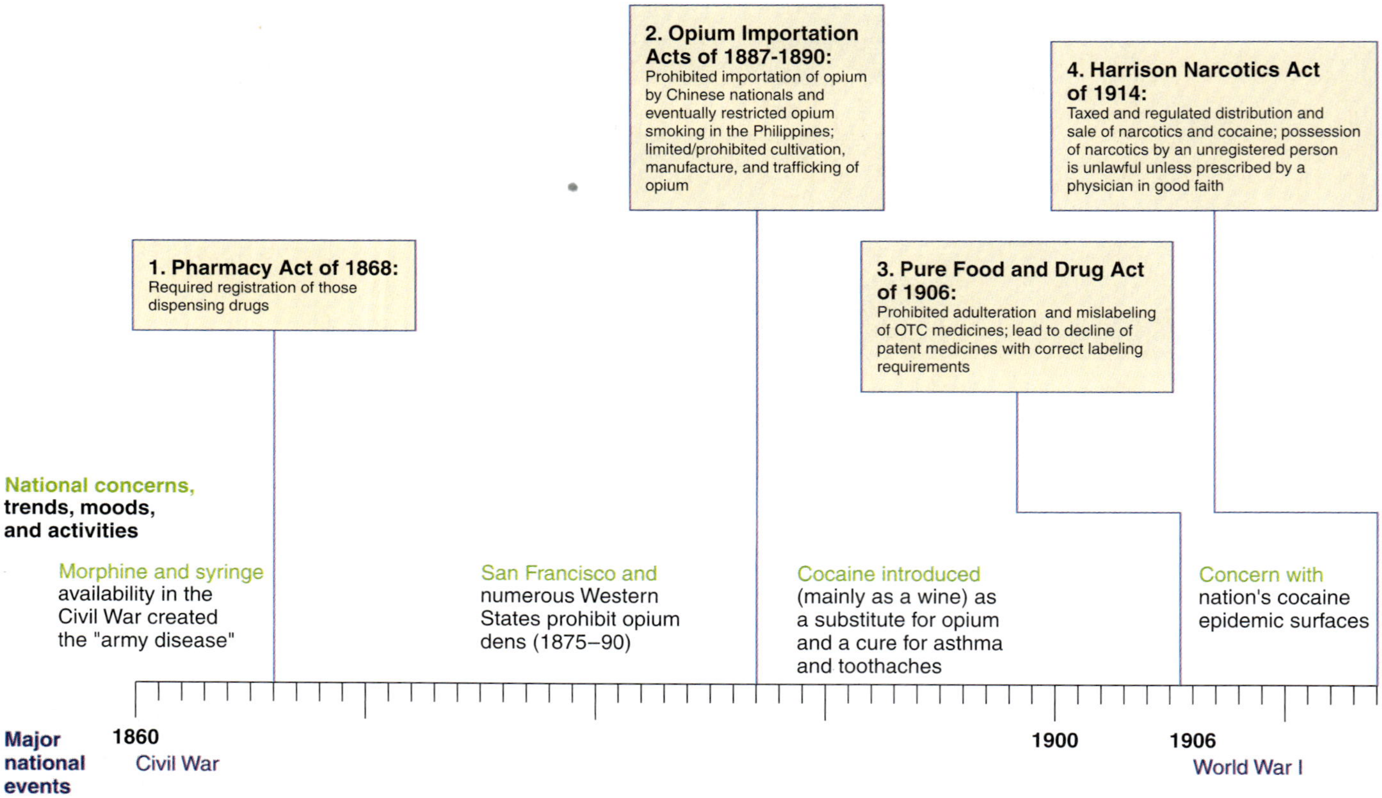

figure 15.3

Major federal legislation in early United States drug control efforts.

Source: Office of Justice Programs. Bureau of Justice Statistics. U.S. Department of Justice, modified.

individuals who will no longer be in the drug-using population.

Information programs conducted via various media can provide accurate and objective information about all types of drugs and their effects on the body. This effort is often referred to as information dissemination and aims at increasing awareness of the effects of drugs on families, communities, and individuals. Such a program also attempts to increase perceptions of the risks associated with alcohol, tobacco, and other drug use.

Educational experiences can be designed to help individuals develop skills in decision making, coping with stress, problem solving, and interpersonal communication. These activities can prove valuable for young people who are not using drugs or for those having only initial or experimental contact with psychoactives.

Though drugs may be available "on the street," the hope is that the demand, desire, or need for their use and anticipated benefits are reduced or eliminated altogether by this strategy. The outcome of such demand reduction is the lessening, delay, or absence of drug-abuse behavior that is not within the bounds of medical therapy and that disrupts normal human development and functioning.

Too often, substance-abuse specialists view supply reduction and demand reduction strategies as conflicting approaches to the prevention of alcohol and other drug problems. However, reciprocal relationships that exist between these strategies should not be overlooked. For instance, while overseas crop eradication and border interdiction activities work primarily to reduce the supply of drugs, they often make the purchase of certain imported drugs more difficult, and therefore, less likely. Similarly, drug education and treatment work primarily to reduce demand, but in doing so they may force suppliers to cut back on production and distribution in an effort to sustain consistent profits in the illegal drug marketplace.

Inoculation Strategy

Abuse prevention based on the **inoculation strategy** attempts to immunize or protect drug users against unhealthy, irresponsible drug taking behavior and thus reduce the harmful and negative consequences so often associated with drug abuse. Rather than reduce either the supply of or demand for psychoactive drugs, inoculation activities seek to increase the proportion of individuals practicing certain styles of moderate and responsible drug use. Emphasis is placed on responsible decision making, that is, decisions involving obligations, accountability, rational limits on use,

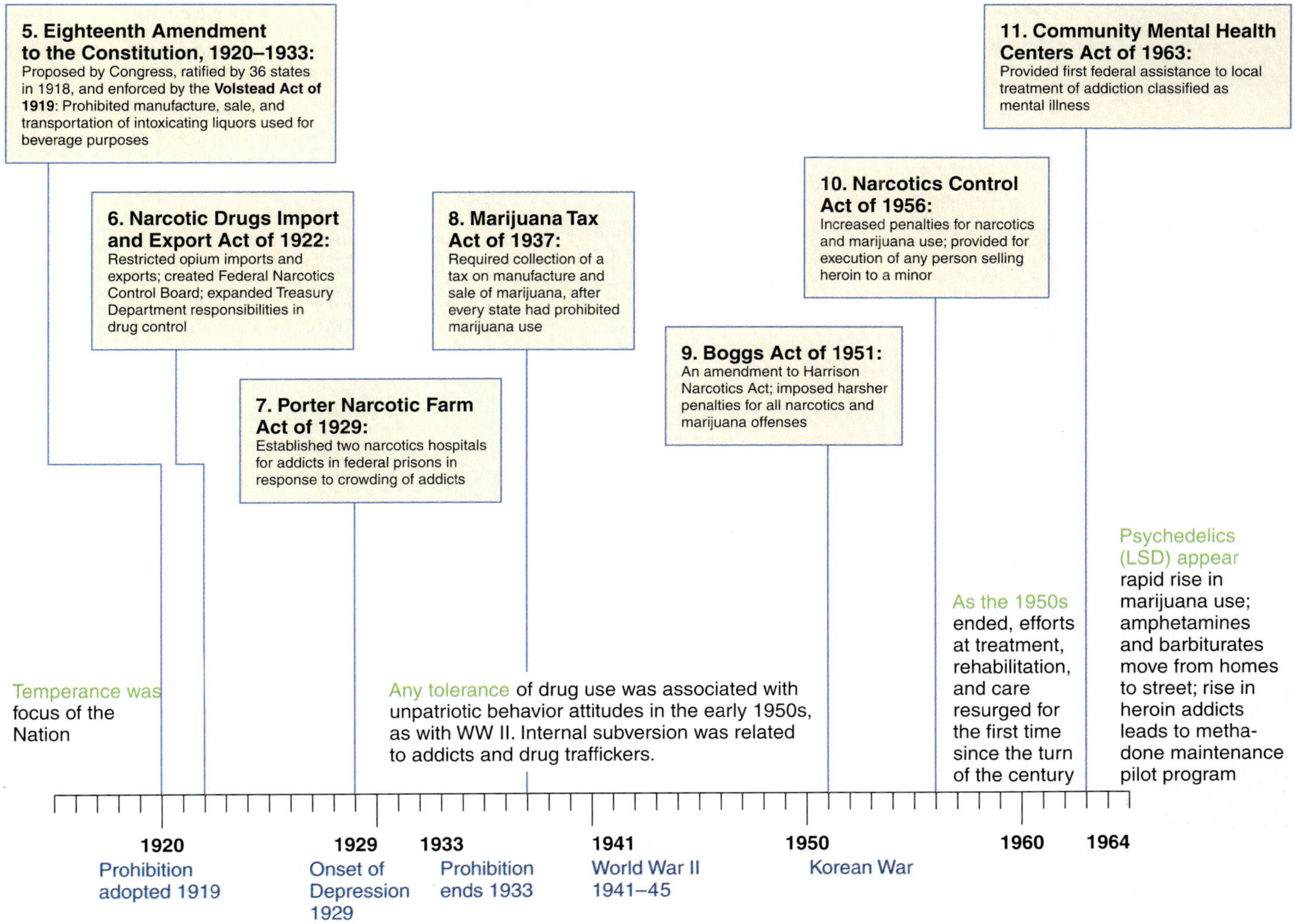

figure 15.3—*continued*

and the exercise of various precautions as individuals interact with specific drugs.

An example of the inoculation strategy is the development of a drinking etiquette for those who use alcoholic beverages. Such an etiquette refers to manners and behaviors that meet standards accepted by a particular social group of drinkers. When practiced, the basic rules of etiquette tend to lessen the number and severity of adverse consequences resulting from drug use or abuse. While inoculation activities may make the drug user resistant to harm, they can never guarantee absolute protection from negative effects. There is some risk associated with use of all drugs, including alcohol.

The Macroapproach

Among drug-abuse prevention specialists, focusing prevention efforts on the entire environment in which any individual lives is called the **macroapproach.** (The word *macro* means large, great, or all-inclusive.) Such a prevention approach involves a number of coordinated activities designed to create a community climate of nondrug use or a reduction in severe ATOD problems.

To accomplish these broad-based goals, several major activities or methods have been identified as keys to effective prevention and treatment services. As described in box 15.2, these prevention activities include information dissemination, education, alternatives, problem identification and referral, community-based process, and environmental changes.

By using these activities, a communitywide effort can be undertaken to prevent or reduce ATOD problems. Such desirable outcomes, however, will depend on committed individuals, activated citizen advocacy groups, and the often reinforcing effects of government policy. In an application of the macroapproach, comprehensive prevention activities can be most successfully undertaken within the community-at-large, the family setting, the school and other educational organizations, and the workplace (see box 15.1).[7]

The Community-At-Large

Developing comprehensive *community-at-large projects* to prevent or reduce drug

Box 15.1 What Communities Can Do About Drug and Alcohol Abuse

Community Projects

Youth Organizations
Social Policies, Laws, and Regulations
Community-based Counseling
Assessment of Community Needs
Health Promotion
Media Impact
Networking Resources
Community Coalitions

School Programs

School Policies
Positive Peer Programs
Peer Resistance to "Gateway Drugs"
Drug and Alcohol Information Programs
Comprehensive Health Education Curriculum
Student Assistance Programs
Alternative Programs

Parent/Family Activities

Parent Support Groups
Parent Action Groups
Family Life Skills Development
Parent Drug and Alcohol Education
Training for Service Providers and the Elderly

Workplace Initiatives

Drug and Alcohol Policies
Employee Assistance Programs
Family Assistance Programs
Health Promotion
Drug and Alcohol Information Programs
Encouragement of Social Responsibility

Source: National Institute on Drug Abuse and Center for Substance Abuse Prevention.

and alcohol abuse involves many segments of the community, including civic, youth, and voluntary organizations; professional and medical associations; industry; law enforcement and other government agencies; and the mass media. A community-based task force might consider the following.

1. Establishing youth programs that emphasize drug- and alcohol-free behavior and provide positive peer influence to prevent drinking/drug-taking and driving fatalities.
2. Developing social policies, norms, laws, and regulations that provide consistent messages about drugs and alcohol. Restricting "happy hours," banning drug paraphernalia sales, and not allowing youths to leave school during the day can all help prevent chemical abuse problems.
3. Providing community-based counseling that would refer clients to other programs, and providing resources that might better prevent or reduce problems of substance abuse.
4. Assessing community needs and involving youth in constructive community service projects.
5. Highlighting and supporting health promotion techniques that advocate healthy lifestyles and alternatives to drug-taking activities.
6. Encouraging local newspapers and radio and television stations to deglamorize drug and alcohol use, and to provide current and accurate information regarding drug use and abuse.
7. Promoting "networking" (working together through developing interrelationships) among public and private groups to assure consistent and comprehensive solutions to drug-related problems.
8. Forming coalitions of concerned people to provide a public forum for the sharing of ideas and perceptions about issues related to alcohol and other drugs in the local community.

Parents and Families

Parents and families are often affected the most by drug and alcohol problems in the community. However, they are often the most dedicated antidrug abuse activists on the local level. Some actions to consider include

1. forming parent support groups through which parents help one another as they cope with drug and alcohol problems in their homes and neighborhoods;
2. establishing parent action groups that work with state and local governments, schools, law enforcement agencies, and businesses to influence social policies regarding alcohol and drug use;
3. enabling parents and children to communicate more effectively and learn personal and interpersonal skills through family life skills development programs;
4. encouraging parent drug and alcohol education programs emphasizing pharmacology of abusable substances and the impact of such drugs on personal health status; and
5. training service providers and informing the elderly about the proper use of medicines and effective communication skills with physicians and pharmacists.

School-Based Programs

Today's *school-based programs* to prevent alcohol and drug abuse consist of more than information sessions to discourage the use of psychoactive drugs. Working together, students, teachers, parents, school administrators, school counselors and nursing personnel, community officials, local professionals, and other concerned citizens have made a significant impact on young people's use of mind-altering chemicals. Some effective school strategies include the following.

1. Adopting and enforcing fair and clear school policies regarding use and possession of drugs and alcohol both on and off school property.
2. Establishing positive peer programs that use student peers as role models, facilitators, helpers, and leaders for

other school-age children. Such programs can help young people who are having problems, undergoing normal adolescent stresses, wanting to confide in someone, and who want to take part in school and community service activities.

3. Developing peer resistance programs relating to use of cigarettes, marijuana, cocaine, and alcohol. These programs usually help students learn that the use of such drugs is not as common as they perceive, that not "everybody" is doing it, and that there are clear ways to say no to the use of drugs.
4. Offering school team training for teachers, administrators, support staff, and other interested community people who can then implement action plans in schools that will improve the school's emotional climate and address alcohol and other drug-related issues.
5. Introducing comprehensive health education and other curricula that increase students' knowledge about their own health and help them assess their feelings and values. Sometimes these curricular offerings focus on specific chemicals of abuse, whereas others seek to enhance healthy, constructive lifestyles.
6. Initiating student assistance programs for those who may be at high risk for developing drug, alcohol, and other problems. Such programs, modeled after the Employee Assistance Programs in business and industry, can also serve as an intervention tool with students who have already developed problems.
7. Offering alternative programs that provide specific activities and involvements that are healthy, positive options to drug use (see table 15.2). Some alternatives already being promoted for youths include helping the elderly, preventing crime and vandalism, finding jobs and learning job skills, restoring historic sites, and building community parks and playgrounds.

Business and Industry

Substance abuse continues to pose a major problem to *business and industry* in terms of worker health and productivity. Listed are some of the strategies being used to prevent alcohol and drug abuse in the workplace.

1. Adopting appropriate, clear, and fair policies relating to drug and alcohol use and abuse, and their consistent enforcement.
2. Implementing employee assistance programs (EAPs) that help troubled employees, including those with drug and alcohol problems, through referral to counseling, treatment, and rehabilitation agencies.
3. Establishing family programs that provide counseling and referral services to workers' family members when employee problems originate from nonwork issues. Flexible work schedules and maternity leaves have been used to help families in periods of stress.
4. Developing health-promotion endeavors that inform employees about general health issues and provide them with opportunities to improve their fitness, nutrition, and other health-related behaviors.
5. Offering drug and alcohol education programs that provide information about the negative health effects of drug and alcohol use and positive reinforcement for nonuse of drugs and alcohol.
6. Encouraging social responsibility by offering training programs about use of safety belts and the hazards of drinking and driving. A corporation may also exercise crowd control procedures and offer nonalcoholic alternatives to consumption of alcoholic beverages at holiday parties and company picnics, in the interest of promoting more responsible behavior of its employees.

Risk Factors and the Macroapproach

Another version of the macroapproach interprets alcohol, tobacco, and other drug use as a major health problem influenced by various risk factors in five life areas of young people—individual, family, school, peer group, and community. In each of these five risk areas, specific risk factors are identified and then appropriate intervention strategies are proposed (see box 15.2).[8] While no single initiative can ever address all such risk factors, various "high-risk" youth demonstration programs have been implemented to develop and field test innovative approaches aimed at preventing ATOD use and helping young people make healthy, productive, and self-affirming life decisions.

This rather detailed description of two macroapproaches to drug abuse prevention reveals the many interrelated efforts that can be used to influence the host, agent, and environment in solving a communitywide problem. It is essential that all parts of the community work together to address the various factors and causes underlying alcohol, tobacco, and other drug use and abuse. Slowly, many communities are discovering the great power they have to solve their own drug-related predicaments.

Intervention Levels of Abuse Prevention

Activities undertaken to prevent the occurrence of some disease or disabling condition are often described on three levels of intervention or application. Each intervention level is intended to reduce the number of individuals who suffer from a disease or are afflicted by some impairment. According to public health practices, these levels refer to the timing when intervention (prevention) activities are begun. Identified as **primary, secondary,** and **tertiary prevention,** the three levels are described here.

Primary Prevention Level

The first level of intervention pertains to activities begun before drug abuse occurs. Primary prevention takes place "before the fact" and prevents an individual

Box 15.2 Risk Factors for Alcohol, Tobacco, and Other Drug Problems and Promising Countermeasures

Individual-Based Risk Factors	Promising Countermeasures
Individual life skills	Social and life skills training in problem solving, decision making, controlling anger and aggression
Lack of self-control, assertiveness, peer-refusal skills	
Low self-esteem and self-confidence	Alternative activities to build self-esteem and self-confidence
Emotional and psychological problems	
Favorable attitudes toward ATOD use	Individual and group counseling
Rejection of commonly held values and religion	
School failure	Tutoring and homework support
Lack of school bonding (commitment)	Mentoring (intergenerational) and surrogate nurturers
Early antisocial behavior (lying, stealing, aggression)	

Family-Based Risk Factors	Promising Countermeasures
Family conflict and domestic violence	Family therapy
Family disorganization and lack of family rituals	Family skills training in effective parenting
Lack of family cohesion	
Social isolation of family	
Heightened family stress	
Family attitudes favorable to drug use	Play therapy, especially for young children of ATOD-abusing parents
Ambiguous or inconsistent rules regarding ATOD use	Parent training
Poor child supervision and discipline	
Unrealistic expectations for development	Parent involvement in youth activities

School-Based Risk Factors	Promising Countermeasures
Ambiguous or inconsistent rules regarding drug use and student conduct	Teaching reform that involves youths as active learners; educational planning
Favorable staff and student attitudes toward ATOD use	School alcohol and drug policy that is clear and consistently enforced
Poor student management practices	Availability of ombudsperson or advocate for parents and students
Availability of ATOD on the school premises	Availability of prevention services to youths and professionals in contact with the youths
Lack of school bonding (commitment, lack of motivation)	

Peer-Based Risk Factors	Promising Countermeasures
Association with delinquent, ATOD-using peers	Membership in positive peer clubs or groups
Association with peers having favorable attitudes toward ATOD use	Correcting perceptions of norms concerning ATOD use in peer and general population
Susceptibility to peer pressure	Peer resistance training to develop skills of saying no
Strong sense of external focus (locus) of control, that is, the belief that oneself is controlled by outside pressures, family, friends, chance, or luck	Positive peer/youth models who do not use ATOD
	Peer leadership and counseling interventions

Community-Based Risk Factors	Promising Countermeasures
Community disorganization with few potential leaders	Cultural enhancement via learning of group's history, traditions, values, identity, and pride
Lack of community bonding (no identification)	
Lack of cultural pride	Orientation to community services
Lack of bicultural competence	Rites of passage to become responsible, mature members of society
Community attitudes favorable to ATOD use	
Ready availability of alcohol, tobacco, and other drugs	Positive drug-free youth groups
	Community service and media education activities
Inadequate youth services and opportunities for prosocial involvement	Provision of "safe havens" that provide secure areas for those wishing to avoid gangs and drug dealers
	Community advocacy for changes in social policy that glamorize ATOD use
	Involvement of the faith community that links ATOD use with the moral authority of a church institution

Source: Modified from the Center for Substance Abuse Prevention.

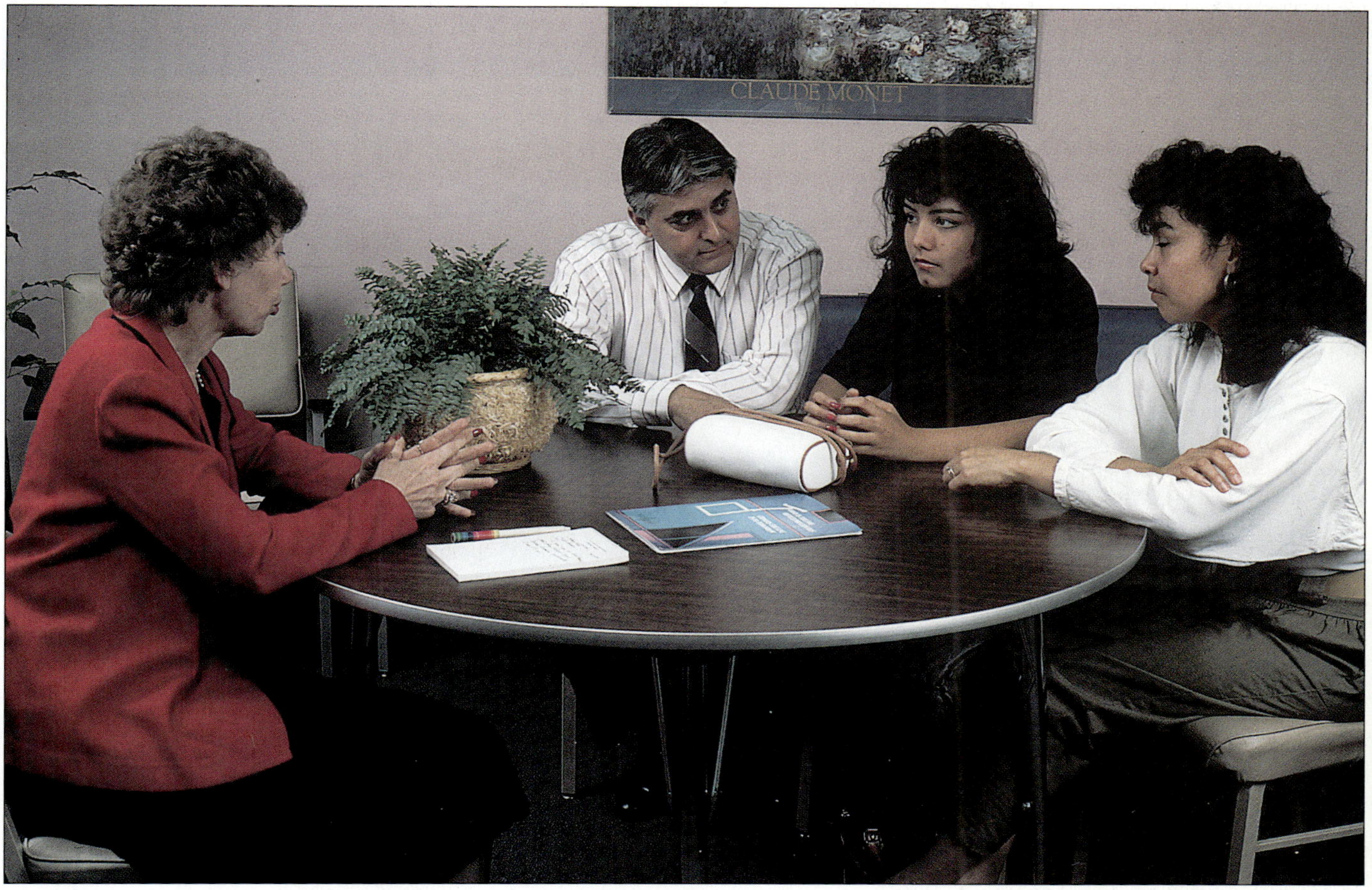

The typical intervention process includes a planned, rehearsed, and supervised confrontation between family members and the drug dependent individual. This effort is an attempt to motivate or persuade the drug abuser to seek help for his or her drug problem.

© Bob Daemmrich/The Image Works

from becoming diseased or impaired in the first place. As a consequence, no new cases of drug abuse develop. Common primary prevention techniques include legislation and law enforcement, information programs, education for responsible decision making, knowledge of risk factors, and the development of non-drug-related alternative behaviors.

One example of primary prevention aimed at the host is motivating young people to say no to alcohol and drugs. Also a demand reduction procedure, the task has been formalized into a ten-step program to be used by parents and others who work with preteens—those in the 9- to 12-year-old age group (see box 15.3). During these "in-between" years, young people are old enough to understand various adult subjects but still young enough to accept guidance from parents and other family members.

The ten-step program is based on proven communication techniques that can lead to strengthened parent-child relationships. Furthermore, each of the specific steps can be implemented independently. Whether one or all of the steps are used, they can provide young people with the solid foundation needed for the confusing adolescent years.

Secondary Prevention Level

On the second level of intervention are those prevention activities applied during the early stages of drug abuse. Through crisis intervention, early diagnosis, crisis monitoring, and referral for treatment, efforts are made to detect the problem as soon as possible and to get it treated effectively so that the condition does not progress. Secondary prevention attempts to restore to health those who have been drug abusers, and thus reduces the number of existing drug-problem cases.

Many initial activities of the war on drugs have been secondary prevention endeavors. Two of these—early **detection** and *referral* and *family intervention*—are described here in some detail because of their potential for success and their widespread application in the general population.

Early Detection and Referral

It is important to recognize the outward indicators of chemical abuse because

Box 15.3 Ten Steps to Help Young People Say No to Alcohol and Other Drugs

1. *Talk with your child about alcohol and other drugs.* Parents can intervene to help change mistaken ideas their children may have obtained from peers and the media, such as "everybody drinks."

   Challenge the common myths; clearly explain why young people should not drink or take drugs.

2. *Learn to really listen to your child.* Children are more likely to communicate when they receive positive verbal and nonverbal cues that show their parents are listening.

   Rephrase your child's comments to show you understand; watch your child's face and body language; give nonverbal support and encouragement; use the right tone of voice for the answer you are giving; use encouraging phrases to show your interest and to keep the conversation going.

3. *Help your child feel good about himself or herself.* Self-regard is enhanced when parents praise efforts, as well as accomplishments, and when they correct by criticizing the action rather than the child. Give lots of praise; help children set realistic goals; don't compare your child's efforts with others; use "I messages" to take responsibility for your negative feelings; give your children real responsibility.

4. *Help your child develop strong values.* A strong value system can give children the courage to make decisions based on facts rather than pressure from friends.

5. *Be a good role model or example.* Parental drinking and drug-taking habits may strongly influence children's perceptions about alcohol and other drugs, including medicines.

6. *Help your preteen deal with peer pressure.* Children who have been taught to be gentle and loving may need parental "permission" to assertively say no to negative peer pressure. Teach your child to value individuality; explore the meaning of friendship with your child; encourage your child to practice saying no.

7. *Make family policies that help your child say no.* It's helpful when parents verbalize specific family rules against alcohol and other drug use by minors, and the consequences of breaking those rules.

8. *Encourage healthy, creative activities.* Hobbies, school events, and other activities may prevent children from experimenting with alcohol, tobacco, or other drugs out of boredom.

9. *Team up with other parents.* When parents join support groups, they can take steps that will reinforce the guidance they provide at home.

10. *Know what to do if you suspect a problem.* Parents can learn to recognize the telltale signs of alcohol and drug abuse and even experimentation.

Source: Modified from the National Institute on Alcohol Abuse and Alcoholism.

many drug abusers tend to conceal their drug-taking behavior (see box 15.4).

Though one should be alert to both general and specific signs of possible drug abuse, it is necessary to realize that even drug experts have difficulty on occasion in early identification of chemical abuse. Therefore, it is recommended that concerned individuals not act solely on their own, because such an undertaking could lead to falsely accusing an innocent person. After identifying an indicator of possible drug abuse, seek professional advice and help from the "experts"—physicians and the agencies specializing in drug problems.[9]

After early detection and the willingness to break the silence of denial, the next task involves getting the drug abuser into some form of treatment so that chemical dependence does not progress to its more serious and devastating phases. This sometimes frustrating and complex procedure is the **referral process**—directing, convincing, and encouraging the drug abuser to contact some drug and alcohol treatment program for assistance.

Just as difficult may be the location of appropriate information and treatment centers, and other agencies that support either the drug abuser or members of the drug abuser's family. Consulting the local telephone directory for such valuable knowledge is a recommended first step. Look on the inside front cover, and in the white and yellow pages, for numerous listings of information and referral centers, treatment and rehabilitation programs, and self-help groups. Examining one telephone directory from a medium-size city revealed the multiple sources of assistance listed in box 15.5. Self-help organizations for family members of a drug abuser may also be available, including Al-Anon Family Groups, Nar-Anon Family Groups, Families Anonymous, and TOUGHLOVE.

The Intervention Process

One example of secondary prevention that focuses on the host or drug abuser is the **intervention process.** Sometimes this process or procedure is referred to as a form of crisis intervention because the family and friends of the drug-dependent individual attempt to create a crisis that will motivate or persuade the drug abuser to seek help.[10] In practice, the process of intervention is a technique used in helping drug abusers overcome their psychological denial and accept that a problem exists.

Planned and implemented under the supervision of a trained counselor or family therapist, the intervention process is structured to help drug-dependent

Box 15.4 Indications of Possible Chemical Abuse

Common Signs

Changes in attendance patterns at work or school.
Change from typical capabilities, such as work habits, efficiency, self-discipline, mood or attitude expression.
Poor physical appearance, including lack of attention to dress and personal hygiene.
Unusual effort to cover arms to hide needle marks.
Association with known drug users.
Increased borrowing of money from friends or family members; stealing from employer, home, or school.
Heightened secrecy about actions and possessions.

Specific Indications

Narcotics:
Appearance of scars ("tracks") on the arms or back of hands, caused by injecting drugs.
Constricted pupils.
Frequent scratching of various parts of the body.
Loss of normal appetite.
Immediately after a "fix," user may be lethargic, drowsy, i.e., "on the nod," an alternating cycle of dozing and awakening.
Restlessness, sniffles, and red, watery eyes and yawning, which disappear soon after drug is administered.
Users often have syringes or medicine droppers, bent spoons or metal bottle caps, small glassine bags or tinfoil packets.

Depressants:
Behavior like that of alcohol intoxication, with or without the odor of alcohol on the breath.
Sluggishness, difficulty in thinking and concentrating.
Slurred speech.
Faulty judgment, moody.
Impaired motor skills.
Falls asleep while at work.
Anxiety, weakness, tremors, sweating, insomnia relieved by another dose.

Stimulants:
Excessively active, irritable, nervous ("wired") or impulsive.
Abnormally long periods without eating or sleeping, with the likelihood of being or becoming emaciated.
Repetitive, nonpurposeful behavior.
Dilated pupils.
Chronically runny nose, respiratory problems related to snorting cocaine.

Users may have straws, small spoons, mirrors, and razor blades.

Psychedelics (Hallucinogens):
Behavior and mood vary widely. The user may sit or recline quietly in a trancelike state or may appear fearful or terrified.
Difficulty in communicating.
Profound changes in perception, mood, and thinking.
May experience nausea, chills, flushing, irregular breathing, sweating, and trembling of hands after consuming the drug.

Phencyclidine (PCP) and Related Drugs:
User is likely to be noncommunicative and exhibit a blank, staring appearance with eyes repeatedly flicking from side to side.
High-stepping, exaggerated gait.
Increased insensitivity to pain.
Amnesia.
Profound changes in perception, mood, and thinking, which can include self-destructive behavior and mimic an acute schizophrenic disorder.

Marijuana:
Shreds of plant material in pockets, bobby pins, or other small clips used to hold end of cigarette (joint), cigarette papers, pipes.
Intoxicated behavior.
Lethargy, inability to concentrate.
Impaired motor skills.
Distorted sense of time and distance that would make driving hazardous.

Source: Modified from the U.S. Drug Enforcement Administration.

individuals become aware of and desire recovery from their dependency. Such intervention can assist drug abusers to achieve the first steps in recovery—identification of the need to make significant lifestyle changes and recognition of the need for help in the recovery process. The intervention process is not always successful and may further alienate the drug user.

Tertiary Prevention Level

As the third level of prevention, tertiary intervention is initiated during the later or advanced stages of drug abuse. To avoid the relapse of recovering drug abusers and to maintain their health status after therapy, the following techniques are used: various physical, mental, social, and spiritual treatment procedures; detoxification of chemically dependent individuals; and institutionalization or drug-maintenance programs (see box 15.6). Tertiary efforts are intended to prevent the reactivation of the drug abuse phenomenon. In this text, tertiary prevention techniques are described more fully in chapters pertaining to specific psychoactive drugs.

Though treatment is the major feature of tertiary prevention, it is essential that common barriers to treatment be removed or reduced. Emotional support must be available for continuing recovery and rehabilitation of the drug-dependent individual. Financial support, often inadequate, must be assured through job counseling, job training, and eventual employment. Special treatment needs of recovering addicts and drug abusers may require support groups, child care, and various medical therapies. If these treatment enhancers are not present, tertiary prevention often fails.

Box 15.5 Sources of Help Frequently Listed in Telephone Directories for Drug-Related Problems

Al-Anon and Alateen Family Groups

Alcoholics Anonymous Information

Alcoholism and Drug Treatment Programs

Alcoholism Information and Treatment Centers
- Inpatient and outpatient family programs
- Aftercare programs
- Specialized hospitals
- Chemical Dependency Clinics

Cocaine: 1-800-COCAINE Hotline

Counseling Associates

County/City Crisis Service

Drug Abuse and Addiction Information and Treatment

Drug Abuse Helpline

Drug Education and Information Programs

Emergency Information and Referral Service of the United Way

Families of Alcoholics

Family Helpline

Mental Health Services (Mental Health Resources Corporation)

Narcotics Anonymous

Outpatient Recovery Program

Turn-in a Drug Pusher Hotline

Box 15.6 Alcohol and Drug-Abuse Treatments

Many health authorities view dependence on alcohol or other drugs as a chronic relapsing disease. As such, drug dependence is often marked by the return of disease symptoms after their apparent cessation. Therefore, to measure the effectiveness of treatment, it is necessary to use graded measures of change. It is more reasonable to think in terms of remissions (lessening or reduction of symptoms) rather than cures.

There are so many different types of drug-dependent people, with so many variables—presence or absence of psychiatric disorders, educational or occupational achievements, family/social support system, family history, and genetics—therefore a wide range of treatments are available after appropriate diagnoses have been made.

A partial listing of drug-abuse treatments includes:

Drug-Free Treatments

- Therapeutic community
- Self-help groups such as Alcoholics Anonymous, Narcotics Anonymous, and others
- Psychotherapy of various types, including supportive-expressive, cognitive/behavioral, family therapy, and others
- Behavioral therapy specifically aimed at prevention of relapse

Drug-Based Treatments

- Methadone maintenance
- Naltrexone (nonaddicting narcotic antagonist, also used in treating alcoholism)
- Antabuse (blocks alcohol metabolism)
- Psychoactive medication when indicated

Source: National Institute on Drug Abuse.

Substance Abuse in the Workplace

Though there is no precise measure of the extent of drug use in American businesses and industries, there is a consensus that illegal drugs have become pervasive in the workplace among both blue- and white-collar workers. Indeed, people who use drugs regularly are likely to use them at work on occasion and sometimes arrive at work already "high" or intoxicated. Consequently, one of the major battlefields in the war on drugs is the workplace, where both new and old procedures are being used to assure a drug-free place of employment for labor and management.

Effects on Business and Industry

While cocaine often replaces marijuana as the most common workplace drug, the misuse of prescription and OTC drugs has also become an extensive problem for industry and business. Alcohol, America's number one drug problem, continues to contribute to absenteeism, expensive medical bills, and reduced employee productivity.

Available statistics suggest that substance abuse in the workplace and drug usage affecting the workplace present a staggering problem.[11]

- Approximately 70 percent of users of illegal drugs are employed.
- An estimated 1 out of 5 workers 18 to 25 years of age, and 1 out of 8 workers 26 to 34 years of age, abuse drugs on the job.
- Workplace ATOD problems cost U.S. companies over $100 billion each year. The costs to individual companies usually exceeds 2.5 percent of payroll.
- Drug-abusing employees acquire 300 percent higher medical costs and benefits, which consequently increases health insurance rates.

- Illicit-drug users are five times more likely to file a workers' compensation claim.
- Employees using drugs are 3 times more likely to be late for work and 2.5 times more likely to have absences of eight or more days. Absenteeism among problem drinkers or alcoholics is 3.8 to 8.3 times greater than normal. Statistics also show that drug users ask for early dismissal or additional time off 2.2 times more often than nonusers do.
- Drug use in the workplace breeds drug dealers in the workplace. Of workers surveyed, nearly one-third know of drug use by fellow employees on the job, and 10 percent have been offered drugs while at work.
- Drug users in the workforce are 3.6 times more likely to have workplace accidents. They also are 9 times more likely to have a domestic altercation or accident away from work. And according to the Employee Assistance Society of North America, up to 40 percent of industrial fatalities and 47 percent of industrial injuries are associated with alcohol abuse and alcoholism.

One study that measured the association between the presence of marijuana and/or cocaine in a preemployment drug screen and employment outcomes confirmed that drug-using behavior was linked with adverse results.[12] However, the risk was much less than previously estimated. Those with marijuana-positive urine samples had 55 percent more on-the-job accidents, 85 percent more injuries, and a 78 percent increase in absenteeism. For those with cocaine-positive urine samples, there was a 145 percent increase in absenteeism and an 85 percent increase in injuries.

In terms of the economic burden on society, the annual cost of alcohol and other drug abuse in the United States is estimated to range from $200 to $400 billion. This amount reflects expenses associated with treatment, research, prevention programs, treatment of related health problems, crime, motor vehicle accidents, reduced productivity, and lost employment. In addition, businesses and industries are also concerned with increased on-the-job accidents and injuries, inappropriate decisions and actions that endanger human lives, and on-site thefts to finance employee addiction.

Workplace Countermeasures

To reduce alcohol and other drug abuse on the job, the American business community, in compliance with the *Comprehensive Drug Free Workplace Act of 1988,* has developed a variety of countermeasures to lower the enormous costs associated with drug-impaired worker performance. These procedures and programs apply to employers with federal contracts and all federal grantees, and are described as follows.

> *Development of clear, drug-free workplace policies* that state expectations of behavior, employee rights and responsibilities, and actions to be taken in response to employees found to be using illegal drugs.
>
> *Establishment of a comprehensive and continuing drug education and awareness program* covering the elements of the drug-free workplace program, the signs and symptoms of drug use, and the services available to help users.
>
> *Introduction of a detection program* to help supervisors recognize and address alcohol and other drug use by employees, and to deter and discover the use of alcohol and other drugs through drug testing.
>
> *Implementation of employee assistance programs or other appropriate mechanisms* that will enable those in violation of established policies to be evaluated prior to proper treatment and/or rehabilitation.
>
> *Reporting to the federal government any convictions* stemming from drug crimes committed in the workplace.

Although neither testing nor treatment is required by the federal act, many businesses, agencies, and the private sector (in response to executive order, not law) have added several supplements to the federal initiative. In an attempt to demonstrate "good-faith effort" in maintaining a drug-free workplace, some companies use random drug testing of employees' urine specimens to detect or screen for substance use and abuse in the workforce. Other supplemental measures involve observation of telltale signs of drug abuse, use of undercover agents and surveillance videocameras to detect drug trafficking operations on company property, and searches of employees and their possessions to locate illegal drugs and to discourage the use of drugs during work.

Drug Testing in the Workplace

Drug testing has become one of the most effective techniques in promoting a drug-free workplace in America. The procedure has also become controversial because drug testing has evolved into a major civil rights issue, complicated by numerous grievances, complaints, and lawsuits.

The detection of drug use and abuse through random screening of urine specimens is required for specific employees of the federal government, such as the executive branch, the Nuclear Regulatory Commission, the military services, and millions of workers in safety-related jobs with the Department of Transportation, as well as railroad employees, airline pilots, flight attendants, and mechanics. In addition, many Fortune 500 companies—major corporations, manufacturers, public utilities, and transportation services—conduct drug screening by urinalysis during preemployment physicals. And random

At Issue

Is drug testing in the workplace an appropriate weapon in the "war on drugs"?

Point: Absolutely not! Except in certain occupations that directly influence public safety or national security, drug testing is a violation of a worker's rights. Requiring individuals to urinate in the presence of supervising observers to get a job or keep a job is a gross invasion of privacy and a human indignity. Moreover, such a requirement often reflects a class and/or racial bias as it rarely affects management personnel, especially those who make or enforce such a regulation. However, there are important legal questions that have not been resolved. The Fourth Amendment to the U.S. Constitution guarantees individual freedom from unreasonable searches and seizures. Without probable cause for the test, it is difficult to describe drug testing as legal or constitutional. Furthermore, because drug testing is expensive, not reliable, often produces false results, and is frequently applied without relationship to job impairment, the testing procedures appear to violate the Constitution's Fifth Amendment, which assures due process and freedom from self-incrimination.

Counterpoint: There is a consensus that drug problems threaten the nation's well-being, so drug testing in the workplace, military, and schools and colleges is justified, even at the expense of reduced personal freedom. We do not live in utopia! Drug testing is not a constitutional issue; it is a public safety, management, and education issue. We need to deter illegal drug use, and drug testing is the best available weapon in the "war on drugs." In some instances, drug testing may be the last line of defense in combating the epidemic of drug abuse. Whether the person is an airline pilot, a production worker, or a professional or collegiate athlete, a drug-abusing employee or player costs money, threatens productivity, and endangers good business management. We cannot tolerate the expenses associated with drug abuse in the workplace.

testing of college athletes is mandated by the National Collegiate Athletic Association.

Types of Drug-Testing Programs

Several types of drug-testing programs are available in the United States.[13]

- Random and comprehensive testing of employees in sensitive positions
- Voluntary testing of any employee or appointee who wishes to participate in the drug-testing program
- Reasonable suspicion testing (based on specific and particular facts and reasonable inferences from those facts)
- Special condition testing (as part of an examination following an accident or unsafe practice)
- Follow-up testing (administered by an agency or company during or after counseling or rehabilitation through an employee assistance program)
- Testing applicants for any position or appointment

In American businesses regulated by the U.S. Department of Transportation, five types of testing are usually required, including, preemployment, periodic as part of required medical examinations, random, reasonable suspicion, and postaccident. However, most private companies with drug-testing programs use only the following three options:

1. *Reasonable suspicion testing.* Employers may require urinalysis in "for cause" testing of a particular employee identified by observation, absenteeism, health problems, accidents, or any other means as having job-related problems possibly associated with substance abuse. With positive urine results, employees may either receive disciplinary action or be referred to an employee assistance program for counseling, referral, and treatment.
2. *Random testing.* Most effective in early detection and in its deterrent effect on drug usage, random testing requires all employees to submit to urine tests routinely, every six months or on an annual basis.
3. *Applicant testing.* Employers might use a urine test to screen all new job applicants. Those who test positive for drug usage might be refused employment, cautioned that the positive test will limit their eligibility for certain positions, or referred for evaluation and possibly treatment.

Large-scale drug testing is conducted on urine samples as a first test or screening technique for chemical substances such as marijuana and cocaine. Most frequently, the tests also check for heroin and other opioids, amphetamines, phencyclidine (PCP), barbiturates, methaqualone, methadone, and certain minor tranquilizers. Urine is used as a test specimen because it is a normal product of the body, is readily available, and is easily collected in a relatively nonintrusive manner, although the use of urine as the test medium imposes practical limitations on the frequency of collection.

Urinalysis Testing

Two common urine-testing procedures used for initial screening are:[14]

- *Immunoassay tests,* specifically the *enzyme multiplier immunoassay test* (EMIT), used most often in industry, and the *radioactivity immunoassay* (RIA) favored by the military. Both procedures use drug-specific antibodies to distinguish positive and negative samples. These tests are relatively fast, inexpensive, and sensitive for most drugs.

- *Thin-layer chromatography* (TLC) identifies drugs by color retention, distance of travel over a coated glass plate or plastic film, and appearance under ultraviolet light. This particular test is somewhat less sensitive than EMIT.

If a urine specimen tests positive, then a *confirmatory test* will be performed using the *gas chromatography/mass spectrometry* (GC/MS) *technique*. More complicated, more time-consuming, and much more expensive than other tests, GC/MS is the most accurate, sensitive, and reliable method of urine testing. This procedure detects specific drug classes and drug metabolites based on molecular structure following separation with a GC absorbent material.

Urine testing for psychoactive drugs merely differentiates between people who have exposed themselves to the drugs being tested and those who have not. Thus, results of such testing give no indication of the pattern of drug use, whether the user abuses or is dependent upon a drug, or whether an individual is impaired physically or mentally by the drug at the time the sample is taken. (An exception to this general limitation is testing for urinary ethyl alcohol, whose concentration can be correlated with blood-alcohol content, from which degrees of impairment can be determined. But ethyl alcohol is not frequently checked for in urinalysis because it is oxidized within a relatively short time after consumption. Thus, even chronic alcoholics could pass a urine test if they refrained from alcohol for twelve hours prior to the test.)

Drugs other than ethyl alcohol tend to leave the body more slowly (see box 15.7).

Box 15.7 The Length of Time Drugs Can Be Detected in Urine Varies by Drug

Type of Drug	Average Time Detectable After Ingestion*
Cocaine (metabolite)	2–3 days
Cannabinoids (marijuana)	
Single use	3 days
Moderate use (4 times per week)	5 days
Heavy use (daily smoking)	10 days
Chronic heavy use	21–27 days
Opiates (including codeine, heroin, morphine)	48 hours
Phencyclidine (PCP)	About 8 days
Amphetamines & methamphetamines	48 hours
Benzodiazepines (including Librium, Valium)	
Therapeutic dose	3 days
Barbiturates	
Short-acting (including secobarbital)	24 hours
Intermediate-acting	48–72 hours
Long-acting (including phenobarbital)	7 days or more
Propoxyphene (including Darvon)	
Unchanged	6 hours
Metabolite	6–48 hours

*Interpretation of the time detectable must take into account many variables such as drug metabolism and half-life, subject's physical condition, fluid balance and state of hydration, route and frequency of ingestion, and testing technique and cutoff level used. These are general guidelines only.

Source: Office of Justice Programs, Bureau of Justice Statistics, U.S. Department of Justice.

Common Concerns with Urine Testing

Though drug testing by urinalysis is used increasingly by federal, state, and local governments, and by businesses and industries, many social and legal questions have arisen. For instance, to maintain the integrity of specimen collection, a supervisor should watch the testee urinate to prevent substitution of another's urine, contamination, or dilution of the specimen. The collection procedure may violate the individual's right of privacy. But, is not the assurance of public safety more important than maintaining one's privacy?

Despite claims of high rates of accuracy and reliability, initial urine tests are somewhat fallible, with demonstrated error ranges of 0 to 100 percent. Laboratory and testing errors can contribute to *false positive results* (erroneous indications that at least one drug is present) and *false negatives* (inaccurate indications that a drug is absent from the urine specimen). Therefore, a confirmatory test is always necessary when the initial screening test is positive.

False positive results are sometimes related to other substances in the urine.[15]

For instance, ibuprofen preparations (Advil, Medipren, Motrin IB, Nuprin, and Rufen) can cause a false positive when a specimen is being tested for marijuana; drinking certain herbal teas can produce a false positive when testing for cocaine; and nonprescription stimulants (phenylpropanolamine and ephedrine) may test positive for amphetamine.

There are also several ways of producing false negative results, such as accidental or intentional switching of specimens, using diuretics, changing urine acidity/alkalinity chemically, and adding large amounts of salt to the specimen. Specimen switching has become a major enterprise generating a profitable black market for drug-free urine. To reduce such manipulation and contamination, most test subjects are observed during collection of specimens.

While urine screening is good at identifying most drug users, the procedure does so only at the cost of falsely implicating at least some nonusers. The tests show only drug use and not necessarily abuse, therefore many workers are opposed on the grounds that this may lead to further invasion of one's privacy while not at the worksite. Some management opposition has also developed regarding the relatively high cost of drug testing for large numbers of employees and because of the likelihood of prolonged challenges to the tests in courts of law.

Alternatives to Urine Testing

Urine testing is the most common form of drug testing. It is the most revealing test of drug use at the time the sample is obtained. It is probable, however, that with the development of more effective and donor-friendly techniques, alternatives to urine testing will eventually come into regular use. These new testing procedures may be used either as a substitute for or a supplement to existing urine tests.

Hair Analysis Some of the objections to urine tests may be resolved when hair analysis is approved as a means of drug testing.[16] With a radioimmunoassay process, strands of hair can be tested for cocaine, heroin, marijuana, methaqualone, and phencyclidine. Human hair gives a history of drug use, therefore hair samples can differentiate between recreational and chronic use and can reveal what drug was in the body in what amount, how often, and at what time. However, the use of radioimmunoassay hair analysis to detect illegal drugs is not yet scientifically supported by forensic toxicologists.

Nevertheless, hair has several advantages over urine testing for drugs of abuse:

> Hair analysis expands the "time window" for the detection of an illicit drug up to several months or more, depending on the length of the hair.
>
> Brief periods of abstinence from drugs will not significantly change the outcome of hair analysis.
>
> Hair is relatively inert and easy to handle, and it requires no special storage facilities or conditions. Compared with urine samples, hair presents fewer risks of disease transmission.
>
> Having some hair snipped from the head is less invasive and embarrassing for most people than supplying a monitored urine specimen.
>
> Collecting comparable samples for repeat testing is easier with hair than with urine.
>
> Contaminating or altering a sample to distort or manipulate test results is much more difficult with hair than with urine.

In comparison with urine testing, hair testing does reveal more "positives" for illegal drug use, due to the longer "window-of-detection"—months as against days or hours when testing urine.[17] Additional comparative studies concluded that:[18]

1. Hair analysis is a better indicator of cocaine use over an extended time and can more accurately identify a long-term drug user. But, urine analysis is better able to measure short-term exposure to cocaine.
2. Urine analysis seems to be a better way to detect opioids, particularly codeine. Hair testing is designed to detect morphine-based compounds.
3. Both tests appear to have an equal capability in detecting the presence of marijuana.
4. Hair and urine testing can complement one another because of their capacity to expose different patterns of drug use.

Sweat Test The first sweat patch system for detecting amphetamines, cocaine, and opioids has received the FDA's marketing clearance. However, this procedure is for use by trained drug abuse testing personnel in clinical and rehabilitation centers.

According to the FDA, the test system consists of a patch applied to the skin to collect sweat and an analysis to detect drugs.[19] The patch is a waterproof, adhesive pad approximately the size of a playing card.

Applied to the back, upper arm, or lower chest, the patch can be worn for a period of up to seven days. During this time, the patch collects skin perspiration containing small amounts of detectable drugs. A tamper-proof feature restricts the patch to a single application, so it cannot be removed and then reapplied.

Additional Techniques

Another method of drug testing that is difficult to subvert is FACTOR 1000, a computer-based test that measures hand-eye coordination and reaction time. This method will also measure other nondrug related impairments such as fatigue and failure to concentrate.

Yet another potential alternative to urine testing may evolve with the hoped-for perfection of brain scan equipment that will check for drug effects—brain waves called drug-evoked potentials that correlate specific brain-wave patterns with specific chemicals.

Employee Assistance Programs

Employee assistance programs (EAPs) are formal employer-financed programs administered by a company or through an outside contractor.[20] An EAP is designed to help in the identification and resolution of productivity problems associated with employees impaired by personal concerns, which might include health, marital, family, financial, alcohol and other drugs, or stress.

There are more than 300,000 EAPs in the United States. Originating as a special resource for employees, they attempt to maintain and improve the health of a company's workers while minimizing the negative impact of problematic behavior, such as alcohol and other drug abuse, on worker productivity and employers' profits. In countering ATOD users, EAPs have concentrated on detection, counseling, and referral to treatment programs. Several interrelated functions are emphasized, including identification of impaired employee performance due to alcohol and other drug abuse; confrontation of the employee by a supervisor; referral for treatment; restoration of job productivity through the rehabilitation process; and follow-up procedures to assure continued worker effectiveness in the workplace. Such efforts are an example of secondary prevention activities.

More recently, EAPs have been expanded to combat employee abuse of prescription and OTC drugs and illicit psychoactive substances. Other areas of concern are also considered, including marital and family crises, money management and financial difficulties, and health problems other than alcohol and drug abuse, all of which can have unfavorable consequences on the well-being of workers and managers.

Usually, the stated purpose of most EAPs has been to reduce problems associated with impaired job performance. However, helping employees to achieve personal, social, and professional growth on the job is becoming an important secondary and concurrent goal of such programs. Model programs of health promotion that not only help prevent or postpone disease but also enhance wellness are being implemented in large companies and small businesses.

An essential component of many EAPs are various *health-promotion activities* that promote employee wellness and contribute to worker productivity, increased self-esteem, and reduction of stress generated in certain jobs. Health-promotion activities include

1. *environmental reform:* efforts to improve the mental health of employees through better working conditions, such as less stressful management styles and work-area restructuring;
2. *dissemination of health information:* use of posters, mailings, and presentations on various health-promotion and disease-prevention activities related to therapeutic and recreational drugs, nutrition, mental health, family living, communicable and noncommunicable diseases, and personal health status;
3. *voluntary lifestyle changes:* company-sponsored projects that bring about smoking cessation, stress management, improved physical fitness, and weight reduction among employees;
4. *risk identification:* use of health-screening laboratory tests, risk appraisal, and physical examinations to identify potential physical and mental problems before symptoms appear and referral to treatment and rehabilitation are needed; and
5. *high-risk intervention:* detection, intervention, and referral options associated with the secondary level of prevention. Individuals identified with various health problems—such as diabetes, hypertension, or substance abuse—are referred for treatment, rehabilitation, and eventual return to the workplace.

Alcohol-, tobacco-, and other drug-free workplace policies and procedures; employee assistance programs; employee and family education; worksite wellness programs; and changes in workplace culture and norms effectively reduce costs to the employer. According to the Center for Substance Abuse Prevention,

- For every dollar employers invest in EAPs, they can save $5 to $16.
- Workplaces free of alcohol, tobacco, and other drugs have a competitive edge in maintaining productivity and quality, improving employee health, and reducing medical claims and absenteeism.[21]

Drug Law Enforcement

A major part of society's response to drug abuse is expressed in the numerous laws and governmental programs intended to reduce the availability of illegal drugs to the general public and to penalize the promoters of such drugs. Sometimes, the victims of drug abuse have been punished for their social offenses. Drug laws and their enforcement are considered important parts of any drug-abuse prevention program. The many laws are intended to reduce drug supplies and deter consumption, and though their enforcement is sometimes imperfect, they are nevertheless an example of primary prevention activities (see fig. 15.4).

Efforts to control illegal drug sales and use are conducted by federal, state, and local agencies. Increasingly, these different levels of government join forces in a coordinated system and work together smoothly. On occasion, however, they still act independently, jealously guarding resources and sources from one another.

Routine Enforcement Techniques

Local, state, and federal agents use a variety of **enforcement techniques** in their prevention activities against illicit drug use.[22] The following are among those frequently employed.

Informants—using a second party, sometimes a paid "underworld" figure, who becomes the eyes and ears of the drug enforcement officer, develops contacts, and obtains information that otherwise would be inaccessible to the investigating officer.

Surveillance—secret and usually continuous watching of suspected individuals, vehicles, places, or objects to obtain information about criminal activities.

Undercover operations—investigations conducted by a law officer who uses various identities, disguises, or pretexts to gain the confidence of criminal suspects. This technique is

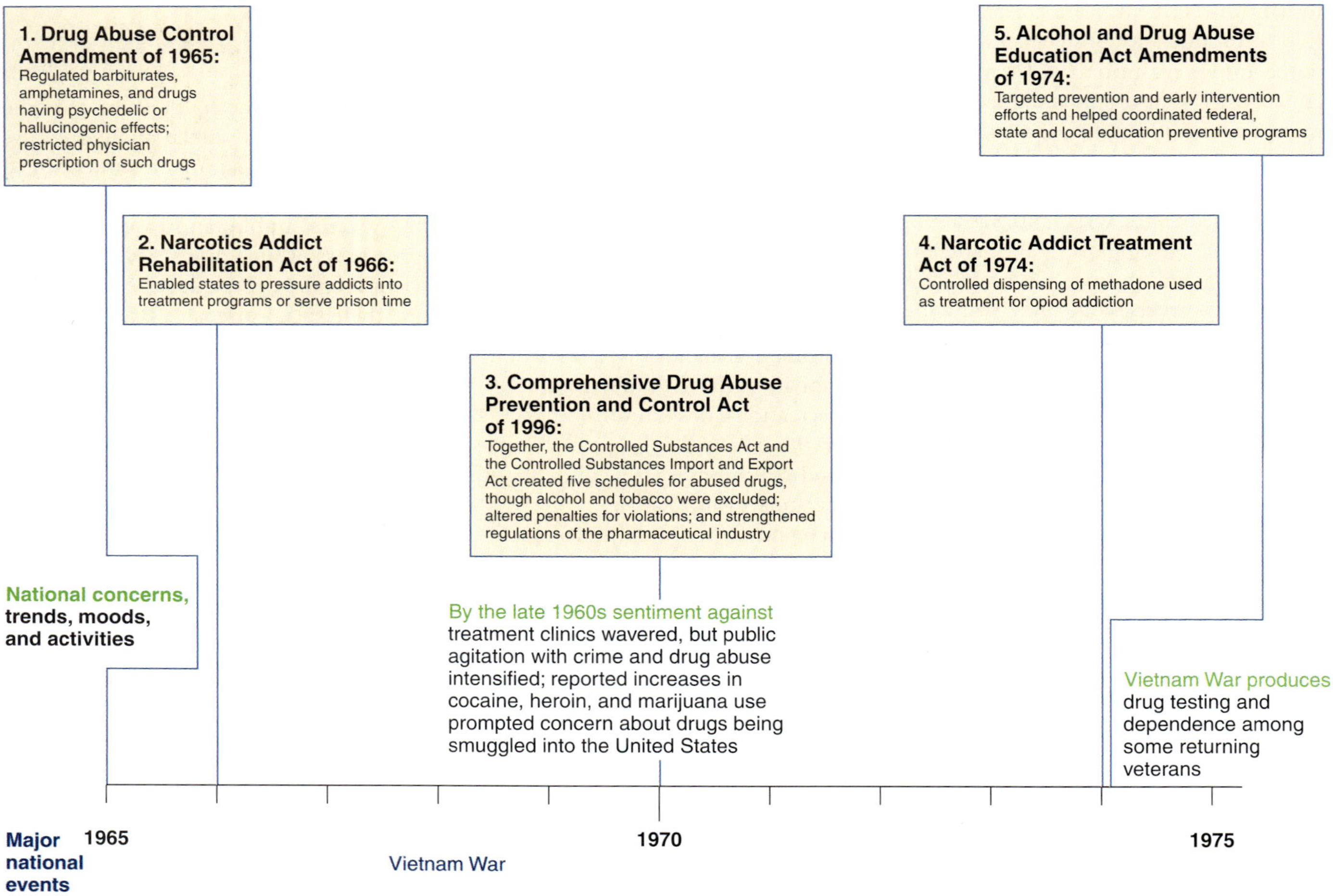

figure 15.4

Over the past thirty-five years, the U.S. Congress has sought to control the supply of and demand for drugs.

Source: Office of Justice Programs. Bureau of Justice Statistics. U.S. Department of Justice, modified.

especially hazardous and time consuming, and it is undertaken to determine the nature and extent of any criminal action in which the suspects may be involved.

Drug raids—searches of specific places, based upon "probable cause," that is, the reasonable belief that a criminal offense is being committed and that evidence of illegal drugs can be found in a particular location.

Interdiction—confiscating illicit drugs at national borders or ports of entry or seizing contraband at sea to prevent them from entering the United States.

Intelligence gathering—acquiring and organizing information in a systematic way that would lead to better enforcement of laws.

In addition, there is the process of "carding," with which many college students are familiar. Carding is a technique in which local or state-level police officials inspect the identification cards of young-looking individuals who are present in a tavern. Such on-the-spot checking of IDs is an attempt to prevent underage individuals from buying and/or drinking alcoholic beverages in a public place.

Federal Law Enforcement Agencies

To implement the goals and objectives of the National Drug Control Strategy, as detailed in box 15.8, numerous cabinet departments, departmental agencies, and special action organizations at the federal level have been assigned various responsibilities for drug-abuse prevention. The principal agency for drug law enforcement, including drug trafficking, investigation, drug intelligence, and regulatory control, is the **Drug Enforcement Administration (DEA).** However, the Federal Bureau of Investigation (FBI) has been assigned concurrent jurisdiction with the DEA to investigate drug offenses. This expansion in the war on drugs has improved greatly the resources and personnel available for drug enforcement activities. The DEA and the FBI are administered within the Department of Justice.

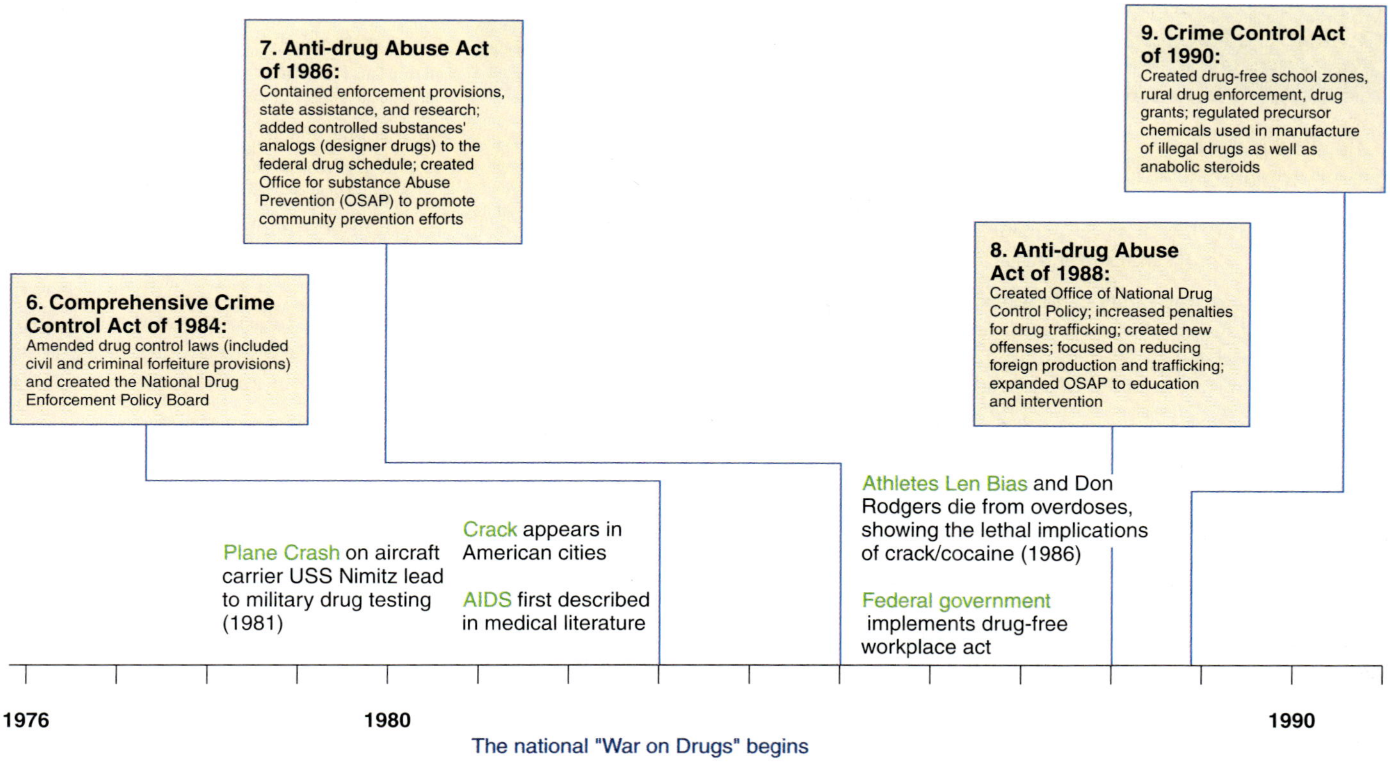

figure 15.4—*continued*

In addition to setting standards for quality and content in alcoholic beverages and establishing and collecting taxes on the production of beverage alcohol, the Bureau of Alcohol, Tobacco, and Firearms (BATF) pursues major drug violators who use or traffic in firearms to support and protect illegal drug activities. Established together with the BATF under the Department of the Treasury are two other agencies that contribute to the drug-abuse control efforts of the federal government: (1) the Internal Revenue Service (IRS), which gathers intelligence and conducts investigations dealing with the tremendous untaxed profits generated by the illegal drug traffic industry; and (2) the U.S. Customs Service, which conducts financial investigations directed at drug-smuggling organizations, border-control measures, and air interdiction of illicit drugs. Within the Justice Department, the Immigration and Naturalization Service conducts advanced investigations of drug trafficking when focusing on other criminal activity associated with its regularly assigned functions.

Reversing a 100-year ban that had prohibited military intervention in civilian affairs, Congress passed legislation allowing the use of available military resources in providing information and equipment support to civilian law-enforcement agencies. This action has the potential for significantly improving the federal attack on drug smuggling and enhancing the effectiveness of the U.S. Coast Guard, the U.S. Customs Service, and the U.S. Border Patrol. At-sea interdictions by the U.S. Navy will also help implement the federal war against drugs.

Federal Control Mechanisms

The legal foundation for federal efforts in reducing the consumption of illicit drugs is the Comprehensive Drug Abuse Prevention and Control Act of 1970 and its amendments, including the Anti-Drug Abuse Acts of 1986 and 1988. The major control mechanisms imposed on the manufacture, purchase, and distribution of controlled substances, as specified in the **Controlled Substances Act** (CSA), are summarized in table 15.1.[23]

Criminal penalties for trafficking are the most common and well-known control mechanisms. **Trafficking** is the unauthorized manufacture, distribution (delivery whether by sale, gift, or otherwise), or possession with intent to distribute any controlled substance. The stiffer sanctions imposed by the Anti-Drug Abuse Act of 1986 (Narcotics Penalties and Enforcement Act) vary according to the CSA schedule, the weight of a mixture or substance containing a detectable amount of a CSA Schedule I or II controlled drug, whether the penalty is for a first or subsequent trafficking offense, and whether the defendant is an individual, a company, or a business association. In the latter instance, the fine imposed for "other than an individual" is usually two and one-half times greater than for an individual offender.

Box 15.8 The 1998 National Drug Control Strategy

Strategic Goals and Long-Term Objectives

Goal 1: Educate and enable America's youth to reject illegal drugs, alcohol, and tobacco. (Children must be nurtured and protected from drug use and other forms of risky behavior to ensure that they grow up as healthy, productive members of society.)

Long-Term Objective: 50 percent reduction in current drug use and an increase of thirty-six months in the average age of first use by 2007.

Goal 2: Increase the safety of America's citizens by substantially reducing drug-related crime and violence. (A large percentage of the 12 million property crimes committed each year is drug-related as is a significant proportion of nearly 2 million violent crimes. Drug-related crime can be reduced through community-oriented policing and other law-enforcement tactics.)

Long-Term Objective: 30 percent reduction by 2007.

Goal 3: Reduce health and social costs to the public of illegal drug use. (Drug dependence is a chronic, relapsing disorder that exacts enormous costs on individuals, families, businesses, communities, and nations. Providing treatment for America's chronic drug users is compassionate public policy and a sound investment.)

Long-Term Objective: 25 percent reduction in consequences by the year 2007.

Goal 4: Shield America's air, land, and sea frontiers from the drug threat. (The United States is obligated to protect its citizens from the threats posed by illegal drugs crossing our borders. Interdiction in the transit and arrival zones disrupts drug flow, increases risks to traffickers, drives them to less efficient routes and methods, and prevents significant amounts of drugs from reaching the United States.)

Long-Term Objective: 20 percent reduction in the rate at which illegal drugs successfully enter the United States by 2007.

Goal 5: Break foreign and domestic drug sources of supply. (International supply-reduction programs not only decrease the volume of illegal drugs reaching our shores, they also attack international criminal organizations, strengthen democratic institutions, and honor our international drug-control commitments.)

Long-Term Objectives: 30 percent reduction in the flow of drugs from source countries and a 50 percent reduction in domestic marijuana cultivation and methamphetamine production by 2007.

Source: Office of National Drug Control Policy, *The National Drug Control Strategy: 1998*

The penalties for a *trafficking offense* can be complex, and most severe. For instance, in a first-time violation of trafficking in 5 kilograms or more of a substance containing a detectable amount of cocaine (its salts, optical and geometric isomers, and salts of isomers), an individual shall be sentenced to a term of imprisonment that may not be less than ten years or more than life. However, if death or serious bodily injury results from the use of such substance, the sentence shall be not less than twenty years imprisonment or more than life. A fine not to exceed $4 million if the defendant is an individual, or $10 million if the defendant is other than an individual, will be imposed. In addition, a term of supervised release of at least five years of probation, in addition to any imprisonment, shall be imposed.

Simple possession of any illegal, non-prescribed controlled substance in any of the CSA schedules for one's own use is a violation of law punishable on the first offense by a maximum of one year imprisonment, a fine of not less than $1,000 but not more than $5,000, or both. Second-time offenders shall be sentenced to a minimum of fifteen days imprisonment with a maximum of up to two years, and a fine of not more than $10,000.

If a person is found guilty of a first-time violation of simple possession after trial or upon a plea of guilty, the court may, without entering a judgment of guilty, defer further proceedings and place such person on probation up to one year. After the probation period, the court may discharge the individual without court adjudication and dismiss proceedings against him or her. If the offender was not over twenty-one years of age at the time of the offense, he or she may apply to the court for a complete removal of pertinent official records.

In addition to the general federal statutes that make it a crime to deal in and illegally possess a controlled substance, there are special laws designed to protect children and schools from illegal drugs, as noted.[24]

> Selling drugs within 1,000 feet of a public or private elementary or secondary school is punishable by up to double the sentence that would apply if the sale occurred elsewhere. More severe mandatory penalties apply for repeat offenders.
>
> When anyone over 21 years of age sells drugs to anyone under 18 years of age, the seller runs the risk of receiving up to double the sentence that would ordinarily apply to a sale to an adult. And if any person knowingly provides or distributes a controlled substance or controlled substance analogue to any person under 18 years of age, or if the individual employed, hired, or used in drug trafficking is 14 years of age or younger, the offender is subject to a term of imprisonment for not more than 5 years or a fine of not more than $50,000 or both.

State Legal Control Mechanisms

Along with the federal statutes dealing with trafficking and possession of controlled substances, there are numerous laws enacted by cities and states restricting the use or availability of certain drugs. For instance, at the state level, departments of alcohol beverage control (ABCs) or liquor control boards regulate alcoholic beverages, usually by controlling production, distribution, marketing, hours of sale, and by taxation.

All states have also established a minimum legal drinking age. At the urging of Mothers Against Drunk Driving (MADD) and with the support of the president, the U.S. Congress passed legislation that would persuade individual states to raise their minimum drinking age to twenty-one years. Under provisions of this law, if states did not adopt the twenty-one-years

table 15.1 Regulatory Requirements

Controlled Substances	Schedule I	Schedule II	Schedule III	Schedule IV	Schedule V
Registration	required	required	required	required	required
Recordkeeping	separate	separate	readily retrievable	readily retrievable	readily retrievable
Distribution Restrictions	order forms	order forms	records required	records required	records required
Dispensing Limits	research use only	Rx: written; no refills	Rx: written or oral; refills[a]	Rx: written or oral; refills[a]	OTC (Rx: drugs limited to M.D.'s order
Manufacturing Security	vault/safe	vault/safe	secure storage area	secure storage area	secure storage area
Manufacturing Quotas	yes	yes	NO but some drugs limited by Schedule II	NO but some drugs limited by Schedule II	NO but some drugs limited by Schedule II
Import/Export *Narcotic*	permit	permit	permit	permit	permit to import; declaration to export
Import/Export *Nonnarcotic*	permit	permit	[b]	declaration	declaration
Reports to DEA by Manufacturer/ Distributor *Narcotic*	yes	yes	yes	manufacturer only	manufacturer only
Reports to DEA by Manufacturer/ Distributor *Nonnarcotic*	yes	yes	[c]	[c]	no

[a]With medical authorization, refills up to five in six months
[b]Permit for some drugs, declaration for others
[c]Manufacturer reports required for specific drugs
Source: U. S. Drug Enforcement Administration.

standard, they risked losing a certain percent of federal highway funds. This congressional action represented a federal inducement to the states to act against alcohol-impaired driving.

Such legislation was eventually found to be constitutional by the U.S. Supreme Court, after several states challenged the law. Whether the imposition of a nationwide minimum drinking age will have the desired effects and anticipated benefits remains to be seen, though total yearly deaths related to alcohol-impaired operation of motor vehicles have been declining.

Another moderate approach to drug law enforcement pertains to people having reached the age of eighteen years but who are still underage in terms of the minimum legal drinking age. Where such individuals are found in violation of the state's alcoholic beverage laws, police officers in some states may issue a summons or warning instead of making an arrest.

The summons is similar to a traffic ticket. It permits the underaged person to avoid arrest, jail, and the embarrassment of a criminal record and a court appearance with parents. (A court appearance, however, is still necessary.) As a substitute for arrest, the summons is used typically when drinking is the only charge. Possession of other drugs, disorderly conduct, and driving under the influence of an intoxicating drug would still result in arrest. While perceived as a lenient approach to underage alcohol users, the summons procedure enables police officers to catch more underage drinkers.

States also have numerous laws restricting the possession, sale, cultivation, and manufacture of illegal psychoactive drugs and furnishing such substances to minors. Sometimes the penalties are harsher than those for corresponding federal offenses. The penalties tend to vary from state to state and with the specific drug or class of drugs (marijuana, hashish, hash oil, heroin and cocaine, LSD, amphetamines and barbiturates, and peyote, mescaline, and psilocybin), the relative amount of drug possessed, and the relative amount of the drug intended for sale.

The Antiparaphernalia Movement

The rapid growth of illicit drug use in the nation has prompted many community groups to seek legislation at the state and municipal levels of government to control the availability of drug-related paraphernalia. (This is known as the **antiparaphernalia movement.**)

The term *paraphernalia* refers to those articles used in administering, preparing, packaging, and storing drugs. Though it can refer to equipment for legal or illegal administration of legal or illegal substances, the term *paraphernalia* has been used more often with products intended for use with recreational drugs, especially marijuana and cocaine.

Some common paraphernalia items sold at retail outlets include smoking papers, rolling machines, roach clips, lighters and matches, pipe/bowl screens, bowl loaders, bongs and water pipes, stash cleaners and containers, isomerizers, spoons, straws, snorters, screens, adulterants, drying devices, conversion/purification kits, nasal irrigators, cultivation kits, crack kits, freebasing kits, and diluents and adulterants designed for use in "cutting" controlled substances.

Nearly all states and the District of Columbia attempt to control the sale of drug paraphernalia under state law or local ordinances. In most cases, such legislation is based on a model act proposed by the Drug Enforcement Administration.[25] Various legal options are used in controlling paraphernalia sales, including

- Forbidding the use of U.S. Postal Service, or any other interstate conveyance, as part of a scheme to sell drug paraphernalia.
- Prohibiting the importation and exportation of drug paraphernalia.
- Zoning and licensing regulations barring sales of paraphernalia to minors, limiting the type of advertising and display of such items, and controlling where "head shops" (retail outlets) can be located.
- Advertising restrictions banning the printed advertisement of the sale of paraphernalia.
- Prohibiting sales, including the gift or delivery of drug paraphernalia to minors, or permitting sales to minors only when they are accompanied by a parent or legal guardian.
- Banning drug paraphernalia, that is, a full-scale prohibition on the manufacture, sale, and possession of drug paraphernalia.
- Civil forfeiture, a legal procedure that permits the seizure and destruction of paraphernalia items without arresting the retailer or the person possessing the paraphernalia object.

The effectiveness of such legal measures has not been established, though their constitutionality has been upheld by the U.S. Supreme Court.

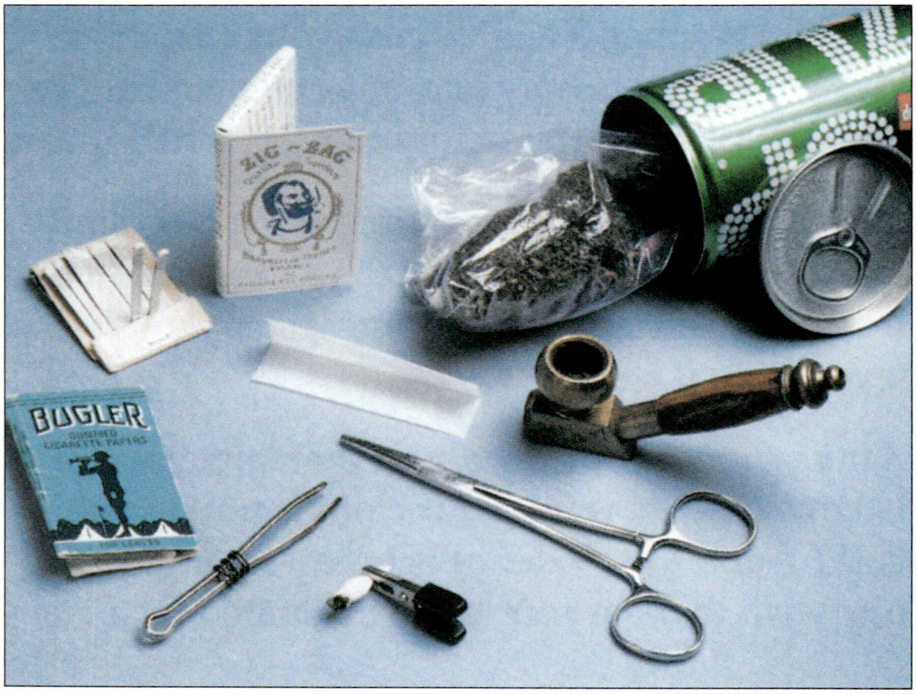

(a)

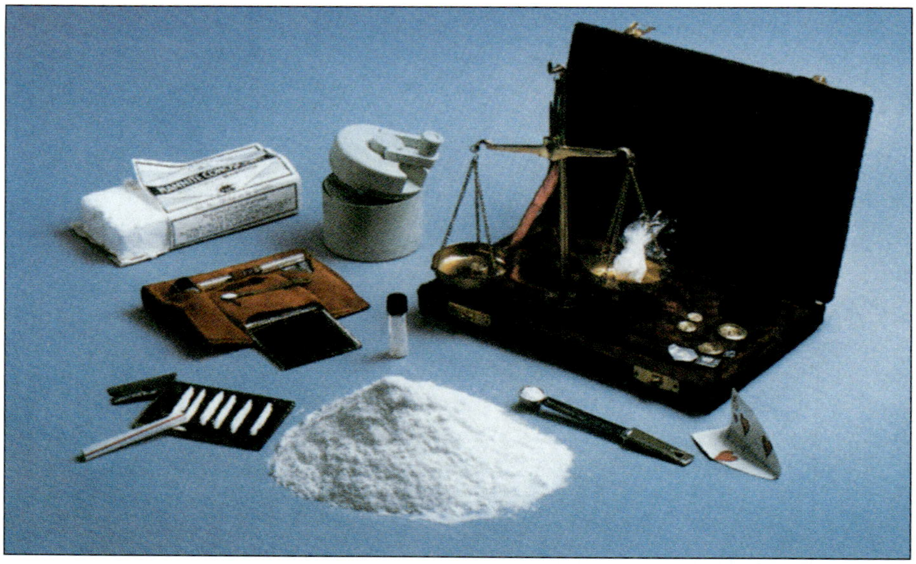

(b)

(a) Marijuana paraphernalia includes rolling papers, clips, and pipes. (b) Cocaine paraphernalia includes mirrors, razor blades, and scales used by drug dealers.

Source of photos: Office of the Attorney General, State of California and the U.S. Drug Enforcement Administration.

Drug Laws of Other Nations

Penalties for violating drug laws vary considerably from one state to another within the United States. However, in comparison with drug laws of certain other nations, the United States is typically viewed as being easy on users of illicit psychoactives. "Draconian" is the best description for the drug laws of some countries in the Near East, Far East, Africa, and South America. Many nations impose long prison sentences—even life imprisonment—heavy fines, and permanent expulsion from the country for what Americans would probably consider relatively minor offenses. In some instances, illegal drug possession and drug use carry the death penalty.

Most Americans are uninformed about other nations' systems of justice. Many months of pretrial confinement can pose hardships of hunger, intimidation, torture, beatings from fellow prisoners, and extortion. In some countries, entrapment of foreigners in purchasing or smuggling illegal drugs is a national pastime. Neither the American ambassador nor the consul can get an American civilian out of a foreign jail. Consequently, travelers are encouraged to check out the drug laws of those nations to be visited. By leaving illegal drugs at home and by not purchasing them when abroad, Americans can avoid the degradation and pain of being imprisoned in another country.

Alternative Behaviors as Alcohol and Other Drug-Abuse Prevention

A practical technique of abuse prevention, the **alternatives approach** is a way of helping young people respond to their real needs without using alcohol and other drugs. Emphasis is placed on expanding the individual's interests outward into life. Characterized as easy to implement yet requiring a long-term commitment, the alternatives program seeks to provide youths with attractive optional substitutes, not just to drugs but to drug-using lifestyles.

The alternatives approach to drug-abuse prevention is based on several principles of drug-using behavior:[26]

- People use drugs voluntarily—that is, because they want to.
- People are taught by example of others and by the media that drugs are an effective way to feel better.
- People take drugs to feel better, get high, or experience adventure. They also use drugs to deal with negative feelings and stressful situations.
- People do not usually stop using drugs until they discover something better.
- The same effects produced by drugs can usually be achieved through alternative means that are more personally and socially constructive.
- Drug abuse can be prevented by helping people experience satisfying nonchemical behaviors.

Involvement in an alternative behavior should not be regarded merely as a substitute for using a drug, as in the case of a natural "high." Rather, an alternative to drug use should lead to a long-term constructive activity, and not just a short-term gratification.

Possible nondrug alternatives have been proposed, as seen in the examples in table 15.2.

Though there is considerable value in offering accurate information about the effects of drugs in a drug education program, education about the nonchemical alternatives on each level of experience is frequently viewed as the best method of drug abuse prevention.

Responsible Use as Alcohol and Other Drug-Abuse Prevention

One of the more controversial aspects of drug-abuse prevention is the precise definition of what is to be prevented. This controversy is equaled in the prevention area by the complex definition of what is to be encouraged. Problems of preventing drug abuse, misuse, and use are as perplexing and debatable as is the goal of encouraging responsible drug use.

The various meanings associated with "abuse of drugs" and "responsible use of drugs" contribute to the competition and even contradictions found among prevention efforts. For instance, law enforcement officials typically view drug abuse as the use of any illicit drug. By contrast, medical authorities tend to define drug abuse as the failure of the patient to comply with directions for using prescribed medicines (drug misuse), engaging in dangerous self-medication, or the recreational use of psychoactive drugs. Except for Rx drugs used for therapeutic purposes, legal and medical groups appear to foster abstinence, or nonuse of illegal drugs, as the ultimate goal of drug abuse prevention.

This drug-free, zero-tolerance approach to prevention is precisely the stance taken by the federal government. According to the federal Center for Substance Abuse Prevention, "responsible use" efforts are not compatible with its philosophy that regards the use of alcohol or other drugs, in any amount, as unacceptable behavior for youth. Moreover, the term *responsible use* is not appropriate for adults either, because there is some risk for harm associated with all drug use.

By contrast, another definition offered by some social scientists may be more comprehensive, more acceptable for planning purposes, and more realistic in terms of the drug-using population. This group of professionals defines drug abuse as the use of any drug, including alcohol, that is harmful to the individual or to society. According to this definition, a new element of abuse prevention would have to be recognized: the reduction of negative consequences due to using drugs. Among the negative or adverse consequences to be lessened are illness and death, acute behavioral effects (e.g., paranoia), chronic behavioral impairment (e.g., apathy), intellectual impairment, injury, or death associated with conditions of use (e.g., malnutrition and AIDS—acquired immune deficiency syndrome), developmental difficulties (e.g., adolescent crises), barriers to social acceptance, and

table 15.2 Nondrug Alternatives for Various Levels of Experience

Levels of Experience: Type of Gratification	Corresponding Motives, Needs, Aspirations	Alternative Behaviors
Example 1		
Physical: pertaining to physical well-being and experience of the body	1. Physical relaxation 2. Relief from pain or anticipated illness 3. Increased physical energy, avoidance of fatigue	1. Relaxation exercises, hatha-yoga 2. Dance and movement training 3. Training in positive health habits 4. Dietary and nutritional training 5. Physical recreation, fun sports, and individual activities
Example 2		
Social-Political: pertaining to identification or involvement with social causes or political movements and reaction to social and political inertia or change	1. Identification with antiestablishment forces 2. Rebellions against disliked laws 3. Overcoming discouragement or desperation with social-political future 4. Induced change in mass consciousness	1. Partisan political action, e.g., helping candidate campaigns 2. Nonpartisan lobbying fieldwork with politicians and public officials 3. Involvement in social service 4. Participation in Peace Corps, VISTA, etc.

Nondrug alternatives for other levels of experience include:

Sensory level: developing increased awareness of body position, balance, coordination, and small muscle control; massage; responsible expression of one's sexuality.

Emotional level: competent and empathetic individual counseling; instruction in the psychology of personal development; emotional awareness exercises, such as learning body language and the improvement of honest self-awareness.

Interpersonal level: competently managed peer and group discussion; sensitivity and encounter group activities; experiences in trusting and respecting others; participation in goal-directed groups, such as the Scouts, 4-H groups, church organizations, school clubs, and Big Brother and Big Sister programs.

Intellectual level: hobbies, games, puzzles, reading, and memory training.

Creative level: nongraded experiences in music, art, drama, crafts, sewing, and photography; development of communication skills, including writing, public speaking, and conversation.

Philosophical level: courses on values and ethics; counseling oriented toward meaning and values clarification; association with individuals committed to various personal philosophies; strengthening of ethnic, racial, and minority pride.

Spiritual-mystical level: study of spiritual literature; investigation of different belief systems; meditation; contemplation; prayer; spiritual dance and song.

Sources: Henry, S. Resnik, "It Starts With People: Experiences in Drug Abuse Prevention," National Institute on Drug Abuse, DHEW Publication No. (ADM) 78-590, 1978; Allen Y. Cohen, "The Journey Beyond Trips: Alternatives to Drugs" in *Journal of Psychedelic Drugs,* vol. 3, no. 2, page 19, Spring 1971; Allen Y. Cohen, "Matching Alternatives to Specific Drug Behaviors, in Positive Alternatives: Perspectives and Directions" in *Alternative Pursuits for America's 3rd Century, A Resource Book on New Perceptions, Processes, and Programs,* pages 39–43, National Institute on Drug Abuse, 1975; and Dario McDarby, *Drug Abuse: A Realistic Primer for Parents,* page 7, Do It Now Foundation, Phoeniz, Ariz., 1980.

unfavorable social conditions (e.g., dissolution of marriages and families, unemployment, criminal behavior).

Prevention of such abuse, the negative or adverse consequences identified, is a major shift in thinking and planning efforts away from earlier attempts at imposing nonuse. This emphasis on personal and social aspects of abuse prevention:

- includes *all drugs*—legal and illicit and therapeutic and recreational;
- acknowledges a *distinction* between the occasional or social use of a drug and the use of a substance that constitutes chemical dependency or significant personal and social impairment; and
- fosters *responsible* choices regarding the use of drugs, that is, the choice to use only medically prescribed drugs or the choice to use readily available drugs, even those that are potentially more harmful.

The focus of such prevention activities would be **responsible drug use,** or "responsible decision making" that would eliminate, reduce, lessen, or minimize negative consequences from the use of any drug. Helping people of all ages in making responsible decisions about drug use and nonuse is not beyond criticism, however. In many instances, there are no safe procedures for using a particular drug. Only less-harmful procedures may be offered for consideration.

Certain "responsible use" actions might only reduce the negative consequences to the individual drug user and to society, but not eliminate them. As such, this non-abstinence approach that allows for responsible use as a viable option would meet strong opposition on ethical, religious, political, philosophical, legal, and medical grounds. Indeed, advocating responsible use of illicit recreational drugs appears to be contradictory to many prevention efforts. Moreover, such advocacy tends to encourage breaking drug laws for those who choose to engage in recreational use of illegal psychoactive substances. It is not likely that in the near future the "prevention of harm" will be substituted for the "prevention of use" as the explicitly stated goal of drug abuse prevention.

Yet, a similar prevention approach has been conducted for many years with regard to smoking cigarettes and drinking alcoholic beverages—drug-taking behaviors associated with dangerous, potentially lethal though legal mind-altering chemicals. For example, to reduce the intake of harmful tars in smoke, the smoker is advised to smoke only halfway down on the cigarette; to avoid or minimize the effects of rapid intoxication, the drinker is cautioned never to consume ethyl alcohol on an empty stomach. In each case, the suggested action is part of a drug-abuse prevention program intended to lessen the adverse consequences of using a drug.

Applied to the social-recreational use of other psychoactive substances, primary prevention would stress responsible decision making, and the promotion of specific drug-taking skills that could contribute to nonproblem-producing use of such drugs. The following lists of responsibilities to be considered *before* using psychoactive drugs have been modified from the *Final Report of the Task Force on Responsible Decisions About Alcohol.*[27] Recommendations of this task force (a creation of the Education Commission of the States) are presented here in three distinct, yet related, areas: situational responsibilities, health responsibilities, and safety responsibilities.

Situational Responsibilities

If recreational use of drugs is one of the acceptable behavioral options, it should not be the main purpose of the gathering.

If drug use is socially acceptable within the group, then nonuse should also be an acceptable option.

Recognize that the recreational use of psychoactive drugs need not be an essential ingredient of every social occasion.

Recognize that drug overdose or drug-induced intoxication is neither healthy, humorous, nor safe.

Never urge another person under the influence of a psychoactive drug to continue using more of that drug or to take yet another drug.

Realize that group norms influence drug-taking behavior and ought to include a reasonable time limit and a consumption limit.

Avoid severe drug-related intoxication and help others to do the same.

Make contingency plans for those who might overdose and become severely intoxicated, including accompanying them home, applying appropriate first-aid measures, or calling for medical assistance when needed.

Use recreational drugs only in settings that are conducive to pleasant and relaxing behavior.

Realize that it is usually preferred to use recreational drugs in a group, rather than alone, because the limitations and concern of group members are more likely to reduce the potential for harm.

Health Responsibilities

Remember that there are occasions on which using any recreational drug would be contraindicated, for example pregnancy, the existence of some particular health problem, and upon the advice of a physician.

Set a limit on the amount of any drug consumed in a recreational setting.

Exercise extreme caution about using one psychoactive drug in combination with any other drug.

Recognize that any of the so-called recreational drugs is a drug substance having specific effects on the body, brain, and thought processes of the drug user.

Follow the advice of a physician concerning the use or nonuse of any recreational drug.

Understand that using mind-altering drugs for purposes of coping with life's problems is an extremely high-risk behavior.

Recognize that one need not use drugs in a recreational setting to be liked or accepted by others.

Avoid injecting drugs into a blood vessel (vein) with borrowed or shared needles, because of the possibility of infection and of the transmission of the AIDS-causing virus.

Set definite limits on the amount of drugs used to avoid overdosing.

Safety Responsibilities

Avoid performing complex tasks, such as operating machinery, driving a car, or engaging in other physical activities with obvious safety hazards while using psychoactive drugs.

Refuse to ride with a driver using psychoactive drugs, and discourage such an individual from operating a motor vehicle.

Recognize that the changed behaviors and attitudes resulting from using drugs may affect and influence others through the power of example, especially children.

Confine the use of recreational drugs to those social situations that are relaxing, noncompetitive, and conducive to limited consumption.

Use recreational drugs in moderation, that is, limited to the smallest amount of a drug needed to produce the desired effects.

Be extremely cautious when experimenting with drugs from unknown sources.

The Role of the Family

Increasing interest has been given to the importance of the family in the origin, maintenance, and prevention of alcohol and other drug-related problems. Though experimental drug use by young people appears to be a social phenomenon of adolescence, more serious drug abuse is predominantly a family problem.[28] As indicated in chapter 2, the changing nature of the family—its mobility, loss of traditions, instability due to divorce, and blending of families following remarriage—is often related to the incidence of drug misuse and abuse.

Drug Abuse: A Family Affair

Despite the pro-alcohol and pro-drug influences of peers and the mass media, role modeling by parents is considered the foremost factor in the development of young people's attitudes toward drugs and the likelihood of abusing drugs. There appears to be a strong relationship between parents' use of alcohol and other drugs and the occurrence of drug use and abuse in their children. Thus the family can be considered as the origin or genesis of alcohol and other drug abuse in many instances.

Family dynamics (psychological forces and interactions), especially marked by poor communications, overinvolvement and overindulgence by parents, and punitive and psychologically distant relationships between parents and child, are also identified as supporting the continuation of a drug-abuse problem within the family. Frequently, family members unwittingly or intentionally enable the drug abuser to continue as a chemically dependent individual whose treatment is often delayed or sabotaged.

Identification of Drug Use and Abuse

Detecting a drug problem in its earliest phase is considered the first line of defense parents have against their child's drug use and abuse. Unfortunately, parents often fail to do so, and typically, problems of serious abuse are often denied, even when a son or daughter overdoses or attempts suicide in front of the parents.

Parents need help in determining when drug involvement exists. Though there is no single criterion that would apply in all cases, there are several common signals or indicators of drug use. Box 15.9 lists twenty of these *warning signals* in the form of questions for parents. Taken as a whole, the questions represent the signs and symptoms of a drug problem.

Guidelines for Parental Intervention

When a young person becomes involved with drugs, the parents often panic, become angry, and invariably assume that their faulty rearing practices caused the drug use. Parents often fail to recognize that their only responsibility is to assist their child in overcoming the drug problem. To accomplish such a goal, parents might consider the following guidelines for early drug-abuse intervention.[29]

Try Not to Panic

Drug experimentation is occurring at increasingly early age levels. Many young Americans try at least one drug before the age of seventeen. Remember that most experimentation does not progress to chemical dependence and that your child still loves you.

Attempt to Talk with Your Child

Ask your child about his or her knowledge of drugs. Find out as much as possible about the situation, and then bring any evidence to the child's attention, but do so without nagging or an outburst of anger. Try to understand why your child is taking drugs. Then tell your child that you still love him or her and want to maintain open communication.

Help Your Child Understand that Being Drug-Free Has Its Rewards

Although doing drugs is often seen as a form of peer acceptance, you will have to convince your child that a drug-free lifestyle is the key to many opportunities now and in the future. Relate abstinence from illegal drugs with learning; fulfilling goals; loving oneself and others; making rational decisions; increased energy and strength; feeling of physical, mental, and spiritual wholeness; competition in sports and other activities; and clearer thinking processes. In effect, you will have to demonstrate to your child that having fun is possible without drugs.

Indicate to Your Child that You Do Not Consider Drug Use as an Acceptable Behavior in the Family

State firmly and clearly the family rules on using drugs. Explain the difference between drugs that can cure illness and those that can make a person sick. Also distinguish between legal and illegal drugs, but emphasize that for young people, all so-called "recreational drugs" are illegal, including alcohol and tobacco products. If you choose, establish some code or agreement between you and your child about using drugs in the home and away from home. Specify what your child is expected to do when confronted with a drug-using situation and when offered a ride with a drug-using driver. Make an agreement about informing the parent of the child's whereabouts, complying with special curfew times, and associating with friends who are to be introduced to the parent. Whatever the rules may be, make sure they are clear and consistent and enforced with objective fairness.

Consider the Model You Provide to Your Child Regarding Recreational and Therapeutic Drug Use

Parental misuse often sets a "double standard" for children who see mom and dad popping unneeded tranquilizers, drinking heavily, or using other mind-changing drugs more often than their peers.

Be Prepared to Enforce the Rules of the House Regarding Drug Use and Its Behavioral Consequences

Assure your child that in the future he or she will be punished if caught breaking a rule.

Become Informed About the Drug Scene

Become informed about the drug scene, the pressures to use drugs as experienced by children, the consequences of using drugs, aspects of drug safety, and the adventure and excitement of drugs as perceived by kids. Realize, however, that the majority of young people are drug-free, and that not everyone is doing drugs Then make sure your child gets this powerful message from you.

Box 15.9 Questions for Parents

You may suspect that your child or teenager is having trouble with alcohol and other drugs, but short of smelling liquor on the breath or discovering pills in pockets, how do you tell? While symptoms vary, there are some common tip-offs. Your answers to the following questions will help you determine if a problem exists.

1. Has your youngster's personality changed dramatically? __________ Does he or she seem giddy, depressed, extremely irritable, hostile without reason? __________________ Do his or her moods change suddenly, intensely, and without provocation? __________________
2. Is your supply of liquor, mood or diet drugs dwindling? __________________(Unless you keep a close inventory, you may not detect diminished amounts for months.)
3. Is your youngster less responsible about doing chores? ______ About getting home on time? __________________ About following instructions and household rules? ______________
4. Has he or she lost interest in school? __________________ In extracurricular activities, especially sports? ______________ Are grades dropping? __________________ Has the teacher complained that your youngster is sleeping or inattentive in class? __________________ Is your youngster skipping school? __________________ (Problems at school are frequent warning signs.)
5. Has your youngster changed friends and started hanging out with a drinking and drug-taking group? __________ Are there weekend-long parties?__________________ (A youngster having problems with alcohol or other drugs will abandon old friends and seek out those with similar attitudes and behavior.)
6. Are you missing money or objects that are easily convertible into cash? __________ (A young abuser's need for alcohol or other drugs increases and becomes more expensive. Eventually, the need for drugs overcomes any guilt about stealing from family members or others.)
7. Have neighbors, friends, or others talked to you about your youngster's behavior or drug taking? __________________ (These reports may have substance.)
8. Has your youngster been arrested for drunkenness? ________ Driving under the influence of alcohol or other drugs? __________ Disorderly conduct? __________ Delinquent acts? (Encounters with the legal system often indicate underlying problems with alcohol and other drugs. There is a strong correlation between alcohol and/or other drug abuse and delinquency.)
9. Does your youngster strongly defend his or her right to use alcohol and other drugs? __________________ (People defend that which is most important to them.)
10. Does your youngster "turn off" to talks about alcohol and other drug addictions? __________________ (Abusers would rather not hear anything that might interfere with their behavior, whereas the nonabuser will listen without becoming defensive.)
11. Does your youngster get into fights with other youngsters? ___________ With other family members? ___________ (More than 70% of all beatings, stabbings, and assaults have occurred when one or both participants have been drinking or abusing other drugs.)
12. Are there medical or emotional problems? __________ (Check for ulcers, bronchitis, high blood pressure, acute indigestion, liver and kidney ailments, hepatitis, nosebleeds, malnutrition, weight loss, depression, memory lapses, talk of suicide. Alcohol and other drugs take their toll. Youngsters on "uppers" or "downers" usually lose their appetite. The taking of PCP, "angel dust," leads to paranoia and hallucinations. Long-term marijuana users often develop bronchitis. Heavy drinkers experience problems with digestion, malnutrition, and depression.)
13. Do you detect physical signs—alcohol on the breath, change in pupil size in the eyes, hyperactivity, sluggishness, slurred or incoherent speech? __________________________ (These are all strong clues.)
14. Does your youngster lie to you and others often? _________ (For young abusers, lying becomes automatic. They fib without reason. There is a saying: "Young alcoholics and other drug abusers have two things in common—they have a terminal attack of the 'cool' and are stuck in 'sneak' gear.")
15. Does your youngster volunteer to clean up after adult cocktail parties? __________ (Draining half-empty glasses is a cheap high.)
16. Do you find bottles or drugs in the bedroom, garage, van? __________ (Parents of abusers are amazed to find stashes of alcohol or drugs under mattresses, in stereo speakers, behind insulation in garages.)
17. Is your youngster irresponsible in using the family car—taking it without permission, making excuses for not getting it home on time? __________ (Many teenagers drink in cars and then drive. They frequently cause motor vehicle accidents.)
18. Does your youngster stay alone in his or her bedroom most of the time, bursting forth only occasionally? ___________ Does he or she resent questions about activities and destinations? __________ (Some secrecy, aloofness, and resentment on the part of teenagers is normal. But when carried to extremes, these may signal problems with alcohol or other drugs.)
19. Have your youngster's relationships with other family members deteriorated? __________________ Does he or she avoid family gatherings that were once enjoyed? __________ (An abuser's ability to relate to others suffers. The primary family relationships are affected first.)
20. Has your youngster been caught dealing in drugs or giving them to friends? __________________

Alcohol and other drug abuse can create "Mr. Hydes" out of once happy youngsters and isolate them from those who love them. The youngsters become strangers and sources of frustration, irritation, and disruption to the family.

Develop Life Experiences with Your Child

Work hard at developing life experiences with your child—experiences that are fun, meaningful, and constructive alternatives to drug and alcohol use. Use the supervised activities of other parents, churches, and youth groups, and make certain these individuals and organizations also know what is going on in the community about drug use.

Consult with Other Parents

Within the parent group, work out a common code of basic behavior rules—on drugs, drinking, dating, curfews, chaperoning, and so on. Then present a unified parental front, a community set of standards. Acting together, a group of parents can break up the peer pressure that often fosters experimentation and regular drug use.

Now a nationwide movement, thousands of such parent groups have been formed to combat drug use among teens and preteens.

Decide if Professional Treatment Is Needed When Regular or Frequent Drug Use Persists

Such intervention is usually advised if recommended by a school counselor or law enforcement officer, when the drug use causes other problems, such as truancy, poor school performance, or strained family relations, or when the parents doubt their own ability to cope with the child's drug use.[30]

But the most essential aspect of intervention is for the parents to stop enabling the drug abuser's involvement with mind-changing substances. This step begins with learning "ignoring skills"—the series of disengagement activities that must be accomplished before successful intervention can occur. Several disengagement skills have been identified and often prove helpful:[31]

Do Not

take your drug-abusing child's anger personally;

nag your child or constantly remind him or her of the harmful effects of alcohol and other drug use, because nagging equals provoking, and provoking constitutes enabling; or

make excuses to other family members or friends about your child's drug abuse.

Never

confront your drug-abusing child when you are angry;

use physical or verbal violence toward your child; or

clean up your teenager's messes, such as paying fines, covering bad checks, or financing repair bills.

Avoid

saying things and making idle threats you do not mean or cannot enforce.

Always

remind yourself, over and over, that chemical dependence is a disease. Your son or daughter is sick, and you are not at fault!

Understanding the Stages in Adolescent Chemical Use

Many people fail to recognize that involvement with recreational drugs usually occurs in phases and may be progressive or level off at an early developmental stage.

The four stages frequently seen in adolescent chemical use are described here.[32]

1. *Experimental use*—Late grade school or junior high age students, especially boys, are great experimenters with various mood-altering substances. The majority of these users, however never go beyond the experimental stage.
2. *More regular use*—Simply using more does not, by itself, indicate dependency. But a pattern of regular use, coupled with some adverse behavioral changes, can show a definite move toward possible dependency. . . . This may begin in late junior high or early senior high years.
3. *Daily preoccupation*—Although the user may accept preoccupation with [alcohol or other] drugs as normal, such behavior is one of the major indicators of a chemical problem. More and more of a student's time, energy, and money are spent on thinking about being high, and ensuring that a steady supply of drugs is available. . . . Questioning users at this stage reveals that very few of their daily activities do not include drug use. Although abusers may be able to cut down or quit using drugs altogether for a few weeks, these periods of abstinence generally will not last.
4. *Dependency*—In this stage, negative personal feelings have been building steadily until they require daily, even hourly medication with drugs. In this stage, abusers are unable to distinguish between normal and intoxicated behavior. To them, being high is normal, and no rationale or moral argument can break through their chemically maintained delusion. This delusion persists even in the face of overwhelming evidence that his or her abuse is out of control and is physically, mentally, and emotionally strangling him or her.

The Family and Primary Prevention

Although parents can engage effectively in secondary prevention by identifying chemical use in children and making appropriate interventions, the primary prevention of drug abuse demands a more positive and even more prolonged parental effort.

Admittedly, there is no single method of preventing young people's involvement with drugs. However, there is considerable agreement that children who develop certain life skills or attributes within a healthy family will have little need of drug use, as they learn to manage their own lives effectively in a drug-using society. Characterized by the wholeness of each member, the healthy family is one that can develop in children clear ideas about themselves, about others, and about family boundaries or limits, and the recognition of and respect for differences as well as sameness.[33]

Children who grow up with love and security, who can express themselves freely, who can make sound decisions, and who are realistic, yet optimistic about their own abilities, will likely not become dependent on drugs.

At Issue

How should we fight the drug war?

Point: Let there be no mistake Despite encouraging news about the overall decline in illegal drug use among adult Americans, the level of alcohol and other drug abuse among all age groups remains unacceptably high. Data indicate that the use of marijuana and tobacco products is increasing among our youth. However, the epidemic of illegal-drug abuse is becoming endemic—a permanent condition often concentrating in young and older adults and in inner-city minorities. To fight a war on drugs, we must increase our efforts to limit the supply of drugs and penalize more harshly the drug pushers and users in our communities. We must interdict illegal drugs coming into this country, and stamp out the domestic drug crop and illegally manufactured drug substances here in America. Use the United States military in such a war. If we can fight and win wars halfway around the world, why can't our armed forces involved in restoring law and order in our neighborhoods? Additionally, we should punish more harshly those who traffic in drugs and use drugs to deter use in the future. Jailing the "drug scum" will, at the least, keep them from returning to their lifestyle of addiction!

Counterpoint: Reducing the supply of drugs will never result in more than temporary victories on the battlefield of the drug war. We need to place more emphasis on reducing the demand for drugs. This is no small task, because it involves changing the minds and hearts of our people. Such a war strategy involves awareness and educational programs that encourage people to refuse drug use, as well as nondrug diversionary activities that substitute for the pleasure obtained from drugs. More importantly, drug users and abusers, especially those addicted to cocaine and heroin, need treatment and rehabilitation, not imprisonment. Perhaps the ultimate victory will not be found in a war on drugs, but rather in a "drug peace" that would legalize mind-changing drugs, control drug production, enable police to concentrate on real crime, empty our overcrowded jails and prisons, and deprive organized crime of its most profitable commodity.

Among the life skills or tools needed so desperately by children are these.[34]

The *ability to exercise self-discipline and self-control*—necessary to resist peer pressure and to say no regarding drug use.

Feelings of love and affection—demonstrated by parental attitudes and actions of concern, support, appreciation, consideration, and assigning value and significance.

Clearly defined limits—establishing an acceptable and expected framework of behavior that imparts a sense of dependability in the environment, which is maintained through fair and consistent discipline.

Open channels of communication—enhancing the mutual expression of needs, feelings, problems, and exchange of information through listening, hearing, understanding, and responding by both parents and children.

It is increasingly apparent that to prevent drug abuse, nothing can be more important than for parents to spend "quality" time and "quantity" time with their children. Moreover, drug-abuse prevention within the family is based upon strengthening the personal and social skills of youths—skills of personal competency in clarifying values, making responsible decisions in relation to interrelationships and career choices, processing feelings, establishing positive behaviors, maintaining and enhancing mood via natural "highs," and refusing the allure of chemical "highs."

Strong relationships, therefore, serve as the best though often underused ammunition in the war on alcohol and other drug abuse.[35]

Chapter Summary

1. The prevention of drug abuse involves activities undertaken to avoid, reduce, or eliminate the adverse consequences of misusing and abusing drugs, especially those identified as psychoactive.
2. General drug-abuse prevention strategies include (a) reducing the supply of drugs; (b) reducing the demand for drugs; and (c) inoculating drug users against unhealthy, irresponsible drug-taking behavior.
3. The macroapproach to drug-abuse prevention involves the promotion of a drug-free atmosphere and a communitywide effort to reduce substance abuse and chemical dependency.
4. There are primary, secondary, and tertiary intervention levels of abuse prevention activities. Primary prevention takes place before drug use or abuse occurs; secondary prevention efforts are applied during the early stages of drug use or abuse; and tertiary prevention activities are begun during the later or advanced stages of drug abuse.
5. Among various countermeasures to substance abuse in the workplace are drug testing by urinalysis and the implementation of employee assistance programs.
6. Drug law enforcement techniques include use of informants, surveillance, undercover operations, drug raids, interdiction, and intelligence gathering.
7. The federal strategy of drug law enforcement reflects a major supply

reduction effort, although demand reduction activities are also emphasized.

8. The Drug Enforcement Administration is the principal federal agency responsible for drug law enforcement. Related enforcement activities are also conducted by the Federal Bureau of Investigation; the Bureau of Alcohol, Tobacco and Firearms; the Internal Revenue Service; the U.S. Customs Service; the U.S. Coast Guard; and the U.S. Border Patrol.
9. State, county, and city law enforcement agencies also make important contributions in restricting and/or penalizing possession, use, trafficking, manufacture, distribution, and sale of legal and illegal psychoactive drugs.
10. The legal basis of federal efforts to reduce the consumption of illicit drugs is the Comprehensive Drug Abuse Prevention and Control Act of 1970, Title II of which is known as the Controlled Substances Act.
11. Attempts to control and/or restrict the availability of articles used in administering, preparing, packaging, and storing psychoactive drugs intended for personal use are focused in the antiparaphernalia movement.
12. The alternative behaviors technique is a drug abuse prevention approach designed to provide individuals with attractive, optional substitutes to using drugs and to drug-using lifestyles. Alternative behaviors may be found in various levels of experience, ranging from the physical to the spiritual-mystical.
13. Drug-abuse prevention may also be described in terms of responsible drug use that considers situational, health, and safety responsibilities.
14. The family often plays a significant role in the origin, maintenance, and prevention of drug-related problems among family members, especially youth.
15. There are numerous common indicators of drug use and drug abuse among young people.
16. Frequently seen stages in adolescent chemical use are (a) experimental; (b) more regular use; (c) daily preoccupation; and (d) chemical dependency.
17. By using a variety of techniques, parents can assist children in overcoming drug problems.
18. Parents can function in the primary prevention of drug use and abuse by helping children develop basic life-skills, such as self-discipline, decision making, and benefiting from mistakes, and by providing models of strong and thoughtful adults, a sense of belongingness, feelings of love and affection, and open channels of communication.

World Wide Web Sites

Drug Enforcement Administration (DEA)

www.usdoj.gov/dea/index.htm

National Institute on Drug Abuse, Prevention Branch

www.nida.nih.gov

Prevention Research Letter

www.integres.org/prevres

Review Questions and Activities

1. Explain why there is a growing interest in drug-abuse prevention activities.
2. Compare and contrast the following general strategies of preventing drug abuse: supply reduction, demand reduction, and inoculation.
3. Survey your local community to determine the various components of a drug-abuse prevention program. Then determine whether each component or activity reflects a supply reduction, demand reduction, or inoculation strategy.
4. What efforts, organizations, and procedures would have to be coordinated in a macroapproach to drug-abuse prevention?
5. How do the following intervention levels of drug-abuse prevention differ from one another: primary, secondary, and tertiary?
6. List several activities or procedures that could be used to reduce substance abuse in the workplace.
7. In addition to making "drug raids" or "drug busts," what are some other routine enforcement techniques used by law enforcement agents?
8. Describe the various components of the federal strategy to reduce drug abuse through drug law enforcement.
9. Describe the roles of the following federal agencies in drug law enforcement: Drug Enforcement Administration; Federal Bureau of Investigation; Bureau of Alcohol, Tobacco and Firearms; Internal Revenue Service; U.S. Customs Service; and the U.S. Border Patrol.
10. Identify several federal control mechanisms imposed on the manufacture, purchase, and distribution of controlled substances as authorized by the Controlled Substances Act.
11. Determine the various laws of your state that restrict the use or availability of both legal and illegal drugs. Do you think the minimum drinking age of twenty-one years is effective in reducing alcohol-impaired accidents in your community?
12. Do you believe the issuance of a summons instead of making an arrest is a better way of preventing drug abuse? Give two reasons to support your stand.

13. Explain why you would support or oppose the antiparaphernalia movement in your community.
14. Describe in detail the alternative behaviors approach as a drug abuse prevention technique. List at least ten individual or group activities that might replace, reduce, or prevent drug abuse.
15. Define the concept of "responsible use" as a drug-abuse prevention technique.
16. What types of responsibilities should be contemplated in any consideration of responsible drug use?
17. Do you believe that responsible drug use is an appropriate technique to prevent drug abuse? On what do you base your response?
18. In what ways might a family contribute to originating, maintaining, and preventing drug-related problems?
19. What are some common warning signals of drug use and abuse among young people?
20. If you were a parent, how might you assist your child if she or he were to have a drug problem?
21. What are some of the common indicators that describe the four stages in adolescent chemical use?
22. In what precise ways might a family function on the primary intervention level to prevent drug abuse? In your opinion, what is the most important thing a family can do to prevent drug or chemical abuse?

References

1. Institute for Health Policy, Brandeis University, *Substance Abuse: The Nation's Number One Health Problem* (Princeton, N.J.: Robert Wood Johnson Foundation, 1993), 31.
2. Lester Grinspoon and James Bakalar, "The War on Drugs—A Peace Proposal," *New England Journal of Medicine* 330, no. 5 (3 February 1994): 356–60.
3. Office of Justice Programs, Bureau of Justice Statistics, *Drugs, Crime, and the Justice System* (Washington, D.C.: GPO, 1992), 36.
4. Center for Substance Abuse Prevention, Substance Abuse and Mental Health Services Administration, *Prevention Works: A Discussion Paper on Preventing Alcohol, Tobacco, and Other Drug Problems,* DHHS Pub. No. (SAM) 93-2046 (Washington, D.C.: GPO, 1993), 9.
5. Jack Durell and William Bukoski, "Preventing Substance Abuse: The State of the Art," *Public Health Reports* 99, no. 1 (January–February 1984): 23–31.
6. Office of Justice Programs, *Drugs, Crime, and the Justice System,* 74–75; and Office of National Drug Control Policy, *National Drug Control Strategy: Reclaiming Our Communities from Drugs and Violence* (Washington, D.C.: Executive Office of the President, 1994).
7. Center for Substance Abuse Prevention, Substance Abuse and Mental Health Services Administration, *Prevention Plus II: Tools for Creating and Sustaining Drug-Free Communities,* DHHS Pub. No. (ADM) 89-1649 (Washington, D.C.: GPO, 1993), 181–84.
8. Center for Substance Abuse Prevention, Substance Abuse and Mental Health Services Administration, *Signs of Effectiveness II—Preventing Alcohol, Tobacco, and Other Drug Use: A Risk Factor/Resiliency-Based Approach,* DHHS Pub. No. (SAM) 94-2098 (Washington, D.C.: GPO, 1993).
9. This section is based, in part, on a publication of the Drug Enforcement Administration, *Controlled Substances: Use, Abuse, and Effects* (Washington, D.C.: Department of Justice, n.d.), 1, 4.
10. Ed Storti and Janet Keller, *Crisis Intervention: Acting against Addiction* (New York: Crown, 1988), 5.
11. Governor's Commission for a Drug-Free Indiana, *Putting Drugs Out of Work* (Indianapolis: Governor's Commission for a Drug-Free Indiana, 1993), section 1; and Center for Substance Abuse Prevention, *Making the Link: Alcohol, Tobacco, and Other Drugs in the Workplace,* CSAP Publication No. ML006 (Rockville, Md.: Center for Substance Abuse Prevention, 1994).
12. Craig Zwerling, James Ryan, and Endel Orva, "The Efficacy of Preemployment Drug Screening for Marijuana and Cocaine in Predicting Employment Outcome," *Journal of the American Medical Association* 264, no. 20 (28 November 1990): 2639–43.
13. Office of Justice Programs, *Drugs, Crime, and the Justice System,* 118.
14. Barry Stimmel and the editors of Consumer Reports Books, *The Facts about Drug Use* (New York: Haworth Medical Press, 1993), 324–25; and Norman Miller, *The Pharmacology of Alcohol and Drugs of Abuse and Addiction* (New York: Springer-Verlag, 1991), 301–3.
15. Stimmel and others, *The Facts about Drug Use,* 329.
16. Tom Mieczkowski and others, "Testing Hair for Illicit Drug Use," *National Institute of Justice Research in Brief* (January 1993): 1–5.
17. "Lab Survey Shows Hair Testing Gets More Positive Results Than Urine," *Substance Abuse Report* XXVII, no. 23 (1 December 1996): 8.
18. Tom Mieczkowski, "Hair Analysis As a Drug Detector," *National Institute of Justice Research Brief* (October 1995): 1–4.
19. Sweat Test for Drugs of Abuse," *FDA Consumer* 29, no. 8 (October 1995): 5.
20. Governor's Commission for a Drug-Free Indiana, *Putting Drugs Out of Work,* section 5.
21. Center for Substance Abuse Prevention, *Making the Link.*
22. Office of Justice Programs, *Drugs, Crime, and the Justice System,* 144–53.
23. Drug Enforcement Administration, U.S. Department of Justice, *Drugs of Abuse* (Washington, D.C.: GPO, 1989), 6–8.
24. Modified from the U.S. Department of Education, *What Works: Schools without Drugs* (Washington, D.C.: U.S. Department of Education, 1986), 49.
25. Kerry Healey, *State and Local Experience with Drug Paraphernalia Laws* (Washington, D.C.: GPO, 1988), 69–73.
26. Allan Y. Cohen, "The Journey beyond Trips: Alternatives to Drugs," *Journal of Psychedelic Drugs* 3, no. 2 (spring 1971): 7.
27. Task Force on Responsible Decisions about Alcohol, Education Commission of the States, *Final Report: Booklet 2* (Denver: Education Commission of the States, 1975), 8–9 (summary). The task force project was supported by the National Institute on Alcohol Abuse and Alcoholism.
28. M. Duncan Staton, "Some Overlooked Aspects of the Family and Drug Abuse," in *Drug Abuse from the Family Perspective,* DHHS Pub. No. (ADM) 80-910, ed. Barbara Gray Ellis (Washington, D.C.: GPO, 1980), 3.
29. National Institute on Drug Abuse, *Drug-Abuse Prevention for Your Family,* DHHS Pub. No. (ADM) 81-584 (Washington, D.C.: GPO, 1980), 4–5; Marsha K. Schuchard, "Celebrating Parent Power in Georgia," *NIDA Prevention Resources* 2, nos. 3–4 (winter 1978): 3–4; and Gary Somdahl, *Drugs and Kids: How Parents Can Keep Them Apart* (Salem, Oreg. Dimi Press, 1996), 174–97.
30. Dorothy Cretcher, *Steering Clear: Helping Your Child through the High-Risk Drug Years* (Minneapolis: Winston Press, 1982), 95.
31. Dick Schaefer, *Choices and Consequences: What to Do when a Teenager Uses Alcohol/Drugs* (Minneapolis: Johnson Institute Books, 1987), 82–84.

32. Dennis D. Nelson, *Frequently-Seen Stages in Adolescent Chemical Use* (Minneapolis: CompCare, 1978).
33. Barbara Gray Ellis, "Report of a Workshop on Reinforcing the Family System As the Major Resource in the Primary Prevention of Drug Abuse," chap. 12 in *Drug Abuse from the Family Perspective,* 135.
34. Based in part on National Institute on Drug Abuse, *Drug-Abuse Prevention for Your Family,* 4–5.
35. David Wilmes, *Parenting for Prevention: How to Raise a Child to Say No to Alcohol/Drugs* (Minneapolis: Johnson Institute Books, 1988), 95–160.

Chapter 16

Alcohol, tobacco, and other drug prevention education

KEY TERMS

Comprehensive Approaches to Drug Prevention Education
Comprehensive Policy Against Alcohol and Other Drug Use
Decision Making
Evaluation
Goals
Instructional Objectives
Life Skills
Methods
Normative Beliefs
Personal Commitment
Resistance Skills
Resources
Strategies
Student Assistance Program
Subject Matter
Systematic Planning Process
Values Clarification

chapter objectives

After you have studied this chapter, you should be able to do the following:

1. Define the key terms.
2. Compare the more traditional approach to school-based alcohol and other drug prevention education programs with an expanded, modern, comprehensive approach.
3. State at least three major goals of school-based alcohol, tobacco, and other drug prevention education.
4. List at least three *Healthy People 2010* objectives for each of the following substance areas: substance use and/or abuse and tobacco use.
5. Identify the basic steps in the recommended systematic planning process that can be used in alcohol, tobacco, and other drug education programs.
6. Distinguish among the several program or curricular strategies often used separately or in some combination in school-based alcohol and drug education.
7. Identify several general principles or "key elements" that can be used in guiding the design and implementation of school-based alcohol and drug prevention programs.
8. Name three federal government sources of alcohol and other drug-related information.
9. Describe the basic elements of a comprehensive school policy against the use of alcohol and other drugs.
10. Discuss the several functions of a student assistance program.

Introduction

Most people think that alcohol, tobacco, and other drug prevention education—the major concern of this chapter—is an educational experience targeted largely to young people in school. However, an expanded view of this process involves several communitywide endeavors and a variety of nonclassroom school activities focused on students, parents, and school personnel offering pupil-support services.

National and local goals of alcohol, tobacco, and other drug education are directly related to the prevention of the use of illegal mind-changing drugs by underage individuals. Such goals are also concerned with the prevention of the potentially harmful and life-threatening consequences of using alcohol, tobacco, and other drugs among the general population.

For effective psychoactive drug prevention education in the school, a systematic planning process is described for designing and implementing an appropriate curriculum—all the formal, structured learning experiences provided by the school regarding alcohol, tobacco, and other drug use and abuse. Several curricular strategies for use in schools are also identified, including those involving normative beliefs, personal commitment, resistance skills, alternatives, goal-setting, decision making, self-esteem enhancement, stress skills, and life skills.

A major portion of this chapter lists numerous resources for alcohol, tobacco, and other drug education programs, specifically prepackaged curricula, government agencies, the RADAR Network, private and voluntary agencies and companies, self-help groups, local community organizations and individuals, and periodicals related to alcohol and other

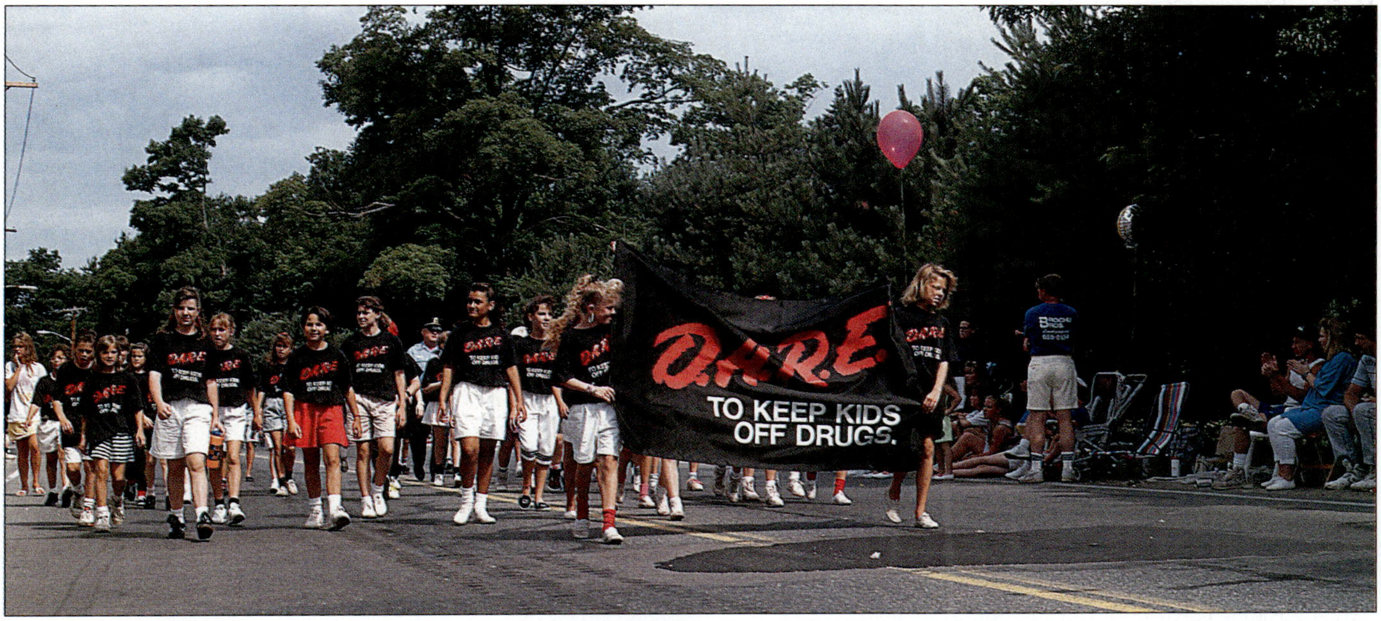

School-based programs to prevent ATOD use and abuse often involve students in out-of-classroom activities. Here youths in Natick, Massachusetts, march through city streets as part of a DARE program to keep kids off drugs.

© Rick Berkowitz/The Picture Cube, Inc.

drugs. The chapter concludes with a section on a comprehensive school policy against alcohol and other drug use, and a description of student assistance programs—a common mechanism for intervention and prevention activities reflecting school policies.

Basic Considerations: The What and Why of Alcohol, Tobacco, and Other Drug Prevention Education

Alcohol, tobacco, and other drug education takes place in many locations and situations other than the classroom. Though school-age youth are the traditional target for alcohol, tobacco, and other drug (ATOD) education, various prevention programs dealing with these mind-changing substances also reach both general and specific populations through other nonschool educational approaches, including these:

- Mass-media campaigns (such as public service announcements emphasizing that "Friends don't let friends drive drunk").
- Publicized communitywide strategies to reduce the supply of or demand for alcoholic beverages and illegal drugs (for instance, strict enforcement of the minimum drinking age and tobacco purchasing age).
- Worksite employee efforts (such as alcohol and other drug awareness projects and employee assistance programs).
- Policy and legislative initiatives (such as laws and regulations that reflect society's attitudes and values about availability, purchase, taxation, and use of alcoholic beverages, tobacco products, and illegal drugs of abuse).
- Training health care professionals and community leaders about alcohol- and other drug-related problems.

Such communitywide **comprehensive approaches to alcohol and other drug prevention education** are essential, because research indicates that individual-directed school-based programs are not as effective in preventing or reducing alcohol and other drug problems when used independently from these more comprehensive techniques.[1] As a consequence, in addition to providing information about alcohol, tobacco, and other drugs, and the consequences of their use, elementary and secondary schools are urged to consider the following elements of an expanded alcohol and drug prevention program:

- Raise awareness and involvement in the local community (e.g., "red ribbon day").
- Increase the knowledge base of teachers, parents, and students.
- Change students' norms and expectations about alcohol and drinking, about tobacco, smoking, and smokeless tobacco products, and about the actual number of those who use marijuana, cocaine, and other illegal drugs.
- Enhance parenting and positive family influences.
- Improve student coping, peer resistance, and decision-making skills.

- Increase involvement in school by parents and students.
- Expand student participation in healthy and legal alternatives to using alcohol and other drugs.
- Implement support services (such as peer counseling and student assistance programs).
- Deter use through regulatory and legal actions (e.g., strict enforcement of school policy on alcohol and other drug use, increased security near schools and other gathering places, strict enforcement of the minimum drinking age, and penalties for bringing other illegal drugs to school).

Now, that is some recipe for potential effectiveness! But all of these primary educational interventions are needed, in addition to a school curriculum about alcohol and other drug use. Each of the efforts will affect youth alcohol and other drug use indirectly by changing one or more of the factors that appear to be related to the use of psychoactive drugs.[2]

At Issue

In ATOD education programs, should the concept of "responsible drug use" be included as part of the goals and objectives?

Point: In terms of school-based ATOD education programs, there should be no reference to the concept of "responsible drug use." Considering responsible use implies that some types of drug use are condoned or even encouraged, when drug substances—even alcohol and tobacco—are illegal for school-age children, and their use is prohibited in most instances. If an educational program is to be preventive in nature, emphasis should be placed on abstinence or nonuse. Postponing the onset of drug use reduces the likelihood of drug use in the future and the probability of developing drug problems. These are proven facts! Saying no to drugs is not just the best policy; it is the only responsible policy.

Counterpoint: It is important for young people to know that most youths do not use drugs, except for alcohol, and that relatively few abuse illegal drugs. However, it is unrealistic to assume that all young people will remain abstinent from alcohol—a legal drug—in a society in which most individuals drink as adults. Should our schools prepare abstaining children to be responsible alcohol users as most adults are? Perhaps abstaining from drug use might be viewed as either a lifelong choice or a temporary restraint until reaching the legal drinking age or applied to specific situations that have a high risk for developing problems. Then, the concept of responsible drug use could appropriately help people of all ages make informed, mature, and personally accountable decisions about drug use. As part of a prevention program, responsible drug use could encourage those people who use drugs to do so in ways that minimize overdosing, intoxication, transmission of the HIV-virus, and other conditions that could threaten health and safety. In reality, as Dr. Jean Mayer suggests, there are no toxic substances, only toxic concentrations of drug substances.

Goals of ATOD Education in the Schools

As stated by the federal Center for Substance Abuse Prevention, ATOD education programs in schools are designed to reduce the extent of alcohol, tobacco, and other drug use and to prevent alcohol-, tobacco- and other drug-related problems from occurring in the future.[3] Such primary prevention is an attempt to lower the number of new users of psychoactive drugs; to delay an individual's first use of alcohol and tobacco products until at least the age of majority; and to improve individual (personal) strengths as an inoculant against using alcohol, tobacco, and other drugs.

Additional goals of ATOD education include the promotion of healthy ways in choosing *not* to use these substances, and offering young people alternative social events free of alcohol and other drugs. On occasion, some ATOD education programs also seek to reduce the number of drinkers, smokers, and other drug users among those youth who have already begun using these substances, by limiting either the duration or the scope of their drug use. (Such efforts may be labeled as targeted prevention, in some instances.) These goals, expressed by alcohol and drug prevention experts, say nothing about promoting "responsible use of alcohol" or low-risk drug-using behaviors, because all underage use is considered unacceptable and illegal behavior.

Healthy People 2010 Objectives

The term *objectives* is often used in educational planning for specific statements of how students are supposed to be changed after a learning experience. The U.S. Public Health Service formulated several specific ATOD-related objectives that served as measurable targets to be achieved by the year 2010. These objectives, part of an extensive national strategy to promote health and prevent disease among Americans, can also serve as general goals of all ATOD prevention efforts. Listed here are modified objectives that pertain directly or indirectly to ATOD education in the schools:[4]

Objectives to reduce substance abuse:

1. Reduce deaths and injuries caused by alcohol and drug-related motor vehicle crashes.
2. Increase the percentage of youth who remain alcohol and drug free.

3. Reduce past month use of illicit substances among 12- to 17-year-old youth.
4. Reduce by one-third the estimated proportion of persons engaging in binge drinking of alcoholic beverages during the past two weeks. (Reduce to 13 percent the proportion of high school seniors reporting binge drinking during the past two weeks).
5. Reduce to 30 percent the number of young people in grades 9 through 12, who reported that they rode, during the previous 30 days, with a driver who had been drinking alcohol.
6. Reduce to one percent the estimated proportion of high school seniors who report use of steroids during the past year.
7. Reduce to 0.7 percent the proportion of youth 12- to 17-years-old who used inhalants during the past year.
8. Increase the percentage of 8, 10, and 12 graders who perceive peer disapproval of substance abuse.
9. Increase the percentage of 12- to 17-year-olds who perceive great risk associated with substance abuse.
10. Increase the number of primary and secondary school-age children with substance abuse problems or who live in substance-abusing households who receive screening, prevention, referral, or treatment of these problems as needed.

Objectives to reduce tobacco use:

1. Reduce the proportion of young people in grades 9 to 12 who have used tobacco products.
2. Increase by at least one year the average age of first use of tobacco products by adolescents.
3. Increase by 40 percent the proportion of young people in grades 9 to 12 who have never smoked.
4. Increase to 100 percent the proportion of schools with tobacco-free environments that include all school facilities, property, vehicles, and school events.
5. Enforce minors' access laws so that the buy rate in compliance checks conducted in all 50 states and the District of Columbia is no higher than five percent.
6. Increase to 95 percent the proportion of 8, 10, and 12 graders, who disapprove of use of one or more packs of cigarettes per day.
7. Increase to 95 percent the proportion of 8 graders who associate harm with tobacco use.
8. Include evidenced-based tobacco use prevention in the curricula in a certain percentage of elementary, middle, and secondary schools, preferably as part of comprehensive school health education.

Source: *Healthy People 2010* Objectives: Draft for Public Comment. U.S. Department of Health and Human Services, Office of Public Health and Science; September 15, 1998.

Planning and Strategies: The How of Alcohol, Tobacco, and Other Drug Education

A major concern of ATOD education is how such a program is developed and introduced in a learning environment. The section focuses on the elements of educational planning, curricular strategies, and principles of curriculum design and implementation.

Educational Planning

An important feature of effective alcohol, tobacco, and other drug (ATOD) education is the process of planning. Whether it describes an entire curriculum or a small teaching unit, a plan usually consists of a written document stating what the learning experiences are designed to do; how the knowledge, attitudes, or skills will be taught; the resources needed for teaching; and the measures used to determine whether the plan achieved its objectives.

The several steps of the **systematic planning process** have been identified as these:[5]

Needs assessment—The process of determining what ATOD problems or concerns need to be included in the plan of instruction. Factors to be considered include surveys of needs, students' interests, district or state requirements, recommendations from authorities and concerned citizens, occurrence of problem behaviors, and society's needs and priorities.

Identification of strategies—Whether a purchased, state- or district-provided, or local curriculum is used, identify and understand its basic philosophy. Several differing educational strategies, as detailed later in this section, are available for selection and provide the basic approaches to curriculum implementation.

Anticipation of instructional problems—Determine the amount of administrative and community support for the curriculum; consider the chances of realistically accomplishing the stated goals and objectives within the limitations of available resources, time, and teacher preparation; plan for possible controversies; and establish the degree to which the curriculum coordinates with other school and community activities relating to ATOD use by young people.

Development of goals—Establish **goals,** broad statements that give direction to instructional efforts and express the nature of change that the educative process will attempt to effect.

Selection of subject matter—Identification of **subject matter** or content areas to be included in the curriculum or teaching plan sets limits to what topics will be considered and at what grade level they will be introduced into learning opportunities. Once appropriate subject matter has been specified, instructional objectives can be formulated. Selected elements of subject matter are detailed in box 16.1.

Formulation of instructional objectives—Developed to guide daily

Box 16.1 Selected Content Elements of Subject Matter Related to ATOD Education

These content items can be used to formulate educational objectives and learning experiences for the grade levels indicated.

Lower Elementary Level

Nature of drugs and medicines
Wide availability of drugs
Difference between drugs and candy
Doctors and parents as sources of drugs
Drugs vs. poisons
Specific mind and behavior modifiers: alcoholic beverages, tobacco products, certain medicines
Activities of drinking, smoking, and drug taking vs. taking medicine
Difficulties in recognizing which substances are safe to eat or touch
Effects of poisons on the body
Occasions for using drugs: meals, family celebrations, communion wine, pain relief, curing illness, adult parties
Effects of smoking on the human body
Family differences in the use of beverage alcohol and tobacco products
Consequences of taking too many drugs at once
Good things about oneself
Social skill of helping others
Appropriateness of asking for help

Intermediate Level

Adult supervision in the use of drugs or medicines
Drug overdoses and poisonings
Hazards of self-medication and experimentation
Difference between over-the-counter drugs and prescription drugs
Variety of substances used to change feelings and behavior: alcohol, tobacco, marijuana, others
Reasons for using various drugs: relieve pain, cure illness, social, dietary, ceremony, pleasure, escape, tradition, curiosity
Reasons for nonuse of drugs, especially psychoactives: personal or family preference, cost, health, legal, religious or moral
Common and uncommon use of psychoactive substances
Saying no to peer pressure
Refusing offers to take drugs from friends and strangers
Legal and illegal use of pyschoactive drugs
Legal controls on purchase, possession, and use
Nature of habits and their development
Importance of rules
Nature of values as guides to behavior
Why it is wrong to take illegal drugs
Importance of helping others
Protective function of laws
Credible sources of information about drugs
Importance of retaining individuality while belonging to a peer group
Elements of healthy friendships

Junior High Level

Formation of attitudes regarding drug use
Influence of peer pressure in relation to using drugs
How drugs work in the human body
Physical and mental changes resulting from use of various psychoactive drugs
Potential benefits vs. possible harmful effects of cigarette smoking
Manufacture and distribution of alcoholic beverages
Differences between beer, wine, and distilled spirits
Consequences of loss of inhibitions, intoxication
Nonuse of alcoholic beverages and cigarettes
Reasons associated with experimental and regular use of marijuana and other controlled substances
Risk taking in relation to living and drug taking

learning opportunities, **instructional objectives** are statements of specific, measurable outcomes and describe patterns of performance to be demonstrated by students upon completion of a particular lesson or series of learning situations.

Method selection—Planned learning procedures and activities that are used to help students accomplish specific objectives are known as **methods.**

Whether they promote individual student responses or student interaction, methods should support the anticipated student behaviors indicated in the educational objectives.

Identification of resources—So-called tools of the trade, **resources** for alcohol education, include personnel and materials that can be used to support the teaching function of the school. Frequently used resources include various instructional media (videocassettes, films, transparencies, etc.) and guest speakers from alcoholism treatment facilities, law enforcement officials, members of voluntary groups of recovering alcohol dependents, representatives of Mothers Against Drunk Drivers, and members and

Box 16.1 Continued

Propaganda appeals commonly used in advertising alcoholic beverages, cigarettes, and over-the-counter drugs
Medicines that cure or heal vs. medicines that control body functions
Development of drug dependencies through the use of psychoactive drugs, laxatives, and nose drops
Dangers of using medicines prescribed for another person
Use of outdated medications
Personal, sociocultural, family, and environmental factors that influence use, nonuse, and abuse of various psychoactive substances
Family drinking problems
Legal drinking age
Drug problems among teenagers, at school, and in society
Student responsibilities in promoting a drug-free school
Policies and laws regarding drug use
Pro-drug messages in music, videos, movies, and TV
Importance of the scientific method in making decisions

Senior High, College, and Adult Levels

Behavioral effects of psychoactive drugs
Recreational drugs vs. therapeutic drugs
Legal vs. illegal psychoactive drugs
Advantages and disadvantages of self-medication
Wise use of medications
Physical effects of cigarette smoking
Cigarette smoking and pregnancy; effects on the newborn
Alcohol's passage through the body
Phenomenon of intoxication
Legal drinking age
Moderate social drinking vs. problem-related drinking
Alcohol abuse and alcoholism
Drinking and driving; driving under the influence of drugs
Women and alcohol
Alcohol and pregnancy; fetal alcohol syndrome
Children of alcoholics and abusers of other drugs
Ways of helping problem drinkers and alcoholics
The appeal and potential for danger in using various psychoactive drugs
Situations in which dangerous drugs might be used socially or as therapeutic agents
Psychological and physical aspects of drug dependency
Drug use vs. drug abuse
Adverse drug reactions and side effects of using any drug; alcohol-drug interactions
Drug overdoses and emergency procedures
Warning signs of substance abuse, including problem drinking
Local, state, and federal laws on controlled substances
Infections related to nonsterile procedures of administering drugs
Treatment and rehabilitation programs for drug-dependent individuals
Stop-smoking programs
Community resources for helping drug-dependent people
Legal consequences of illegal drug use
Physical and mental effects of using steroids
Harmful effects of legal and illegal drugs on fetal development
Myths and stereotypes that seem to encourage drug use
Ways to cope with peers and social pressure to use drugs
Effects of drug use on personal financial resources
Parents' role in prevention of drug abuse
Influence of history and popular media on drug-taking practices
Information about the judicial system, policies, due process, court practices and penalties, and implications of conviction

sponsors of Students Against Driving Drunk.

Development of evaluation procedures—The major concern of **evaluation** is to determine if the curriculum or teaching plan helped students accomplish specific instructional objectives. Various levels and types of evaluation procedures can be used. Process evaluation determines the adequacy of the curriculum design and its implementation in the school setting. Outcome evaluation tries to assess the students' accomplishments of the original objectives. Impact evaluation tries to gauge the effects of an alcohol education prevention program within a certain community or over a specific period.

Revision of the instructional program—Based upon various evaluation procedures, make appropriate changes to either the design or implementation of the curriculum or teaching plan.

Curricular Strategies

In ATOD education activities, several basic **strategies** or underlying

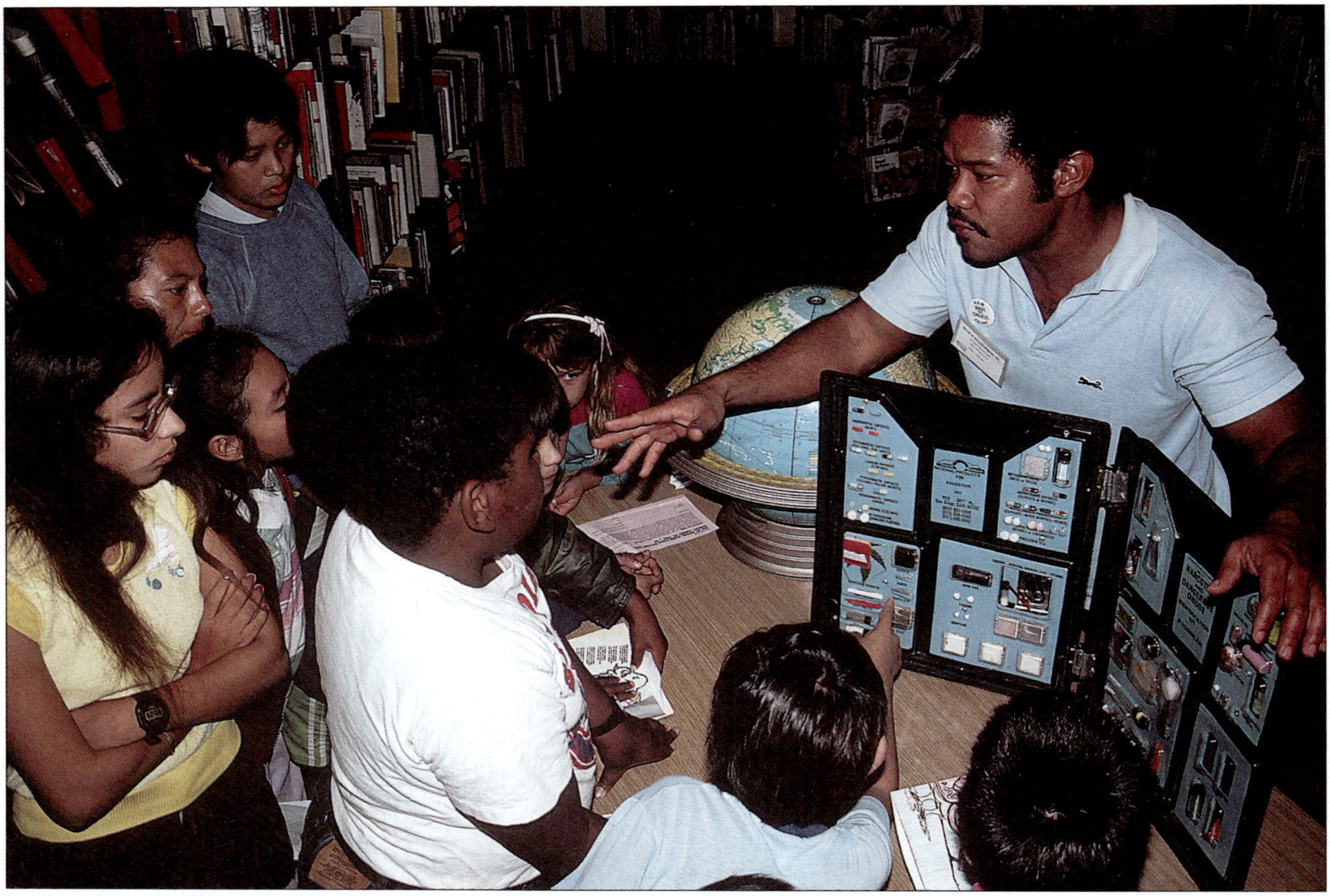

Effective ATOD prevention programs begin in elementary schools where teachers provide information on the "gateway drugs" (alcohol, tobacco, and marijuana), foster development of social skills, and promote a clear "no use" message.

designs of the curriculum have emerged over the years.[6] Early educational efforts relied on scare tactics and moral persuasions that reflected the prohibitionist philosophy of the late nineteenth century, when instruction on the evil and harmful effects of alcohol, tobacco, and narcotics was mandated in many states. Scare tactics, which exaggerate the effects of drug use, usually result in a loss of credibility for the entire antidrug message. Students see that these exaggerated consequences don't usually occur, and they conclude that probably nothing too harmful happens with drug use.

After many years of rather ineffective instruction, the scare strategy of instruction gave way to the "straight facts" approach to alcohol and narcotics education in the 1970s. This information-based strategy assumed that young people would not use drugs or drink when they became informed about the physical and psychological effects of alcohol and other drugs as well as the legal penalty for possession and intoxication.

Then, in the late 1970s, the focus of alcohol and other drug education shifted away from the facts approach to a strategy that concentrated on the personality of the drug user. According to this new theory, young people used alcohol and other drugs because of low self-esteem, poor communication skills, and inadequate decision-making skills. The new curriculum designs featured affective education with strong doses of values clarification exercises, self-esteem building, decision making, and stress management techniques.

During the 1980s, yet another basic curriculum design emerged on the ATOD education scene. This strategy assumed that drinking and resulted drug use from social influences of the environment, and that young people were vulnerable to social pressures to drink or use other illegal mind-changing drugs. Social alternatives to drug use are stressed in this strategy.

Presently, several program strategies are used separately or in some combination in school ATOD education programs.[7] This comprehensive approach is the basis of the many prepackaged and locally developed curricula being used in the hope of preventing alcohol and other drug-related problems. Selected programmatic strategies are described in the following sections.

Normative Beliefs

The **normative beliefs** plan provides information to students about the rates of alcohol and other drug use from surveys, and thereby corrects exaggerations about near-universal drinking, smoking, and other drug use among their peers.

By revealing and comparing personal attitudes and behaviors with others in a group, young people discover that not everyone is drinking, smoking, or taking other drugs, and that use of a psychoactive drug is not necessary to have a good time. Thus, students are freed from the common perception or "normative belief" that they must drink, smoke, or use another drug to be popular or socially acceptable.

Personal Commitment

Based on the theory that young people drink because they have a weak commitment to abstain from alcohol or other drug use, the **personal commitment** strategy encourages students to voluntarily make public or private pledges not to use or abuse alcohol, tobacco, or any other mind-changing drug. The act of pledging increases one's commitment not to engage in drinking, using tobacco, or drug taking.

Values

Use of the values plan assumes that young people who drink, use tobacco products, or take some other drug believe that the psychoactive substance is compatible with their values. Through various **values clarification** exercises, students are challenged to find conflicts between existing personal values and use of such substances. The intent of this approach is to increase the perception that drinking, smoking, or drug taking is inconsistent with one's lifestyle.

Information

The information plan is based on the assumption that drug-taking behavior is the result of one's unawareness of the consequences of alcohol and other drug use and abuse. By providing basic facts about the negative health and social consequences of using and abusing various psychoactive drugs, students increase their feelings of personal vulnerability to the hazards of drinking, smoking, and using other drugs, and thus continue to abstain or delay further use.

Resistance Skills

Peer pressure is thought to be a major reason why young people start using alcohol and other drugs. A curriculum featuring the development of **resistance skills** teaches students how to identify peer and media pressures to drink, smoke, chew tobacco, or use some other drug, and how to cope with pressure situations. By building a cognitive understanding of pro-alcohol influences and developing refusal (resistance) skills regarding the use of various drugs, students will strengthen their belief that they can effectively deal with such pressures.

Alternatives

The alternatives strategy, based on the idea that drug use is the result of a basic unawareness of alternatives to mind-changing drugs for enjoyment, provides young people with information about other, non-drug means for achieving excitement and having fun. Such a plan supposedly decreases the motivation to use alcohol, tobacco products, or other drugs to achieve desired mood states.

Goal Setting

Based on the theory that some young people use drugs because they lack basic goals in life, the goal-setting skills strategy teaches students a system for setting and achieving goals, and motivates them to set and then work on manageable goals and ambitions. In addition to increasing one's goal-setting ability, this strategy also attempts to increase one's feeling of achievement.

Decision Making

Young people sometimes drink or take drugs due to their inability to make reasoned decisions, therefore the **decision-making** curricular plan teaches students a system for organizing information and making choices among alternatives. The strategy's basic intention is to increase the frequency with which reason is used in making choices about using alcohol and other drugs or interacting with those who use these substances, such as deciding to ride (or refusing to ride) in a car with a drinking driver (see box 16.2).

Self-Esteem Enhancement

To increase their feelings of self-worth and better value their personal identity, the self-esteem-enhancement curricular plan encourages students to understand how internal and external events affect self-concept and feelings of self-worth. Students are helped to discover ways to deal with negative feelings toward themselves.

Stress Skills

Drinking and other drug use are sometimes linked with poor coping skills, so students are taught a variety of ways to relax under stress, to cope with pressure, and to resolve problems. With increased ability to cope with anxieties and tension, students can often reduce their stress levels.

Life Skills

The **life-skills** strategy teaches students how to be assertive, how to resolve interpersonal conflicts, and how to communicate more effectively with others. With these newly acquired life skills, students improve their ability to maintain social relations without the use of alcohol, tobacco, or other drugs.

Some Concluding Thoughts

No single curriculum or teaching strategy is adequate to prevent alcohol use and abuse in all school populations. There is no one "magic instructional bullet."

Nevertheless, research reveals that there is a tendency for successful alcohol and drug prevention education programs to include a combination of normative

Box 16.2 Making Decisions About Alcohol and Other Drugs

INTRODUCTION: This activity measures adolescent and preadolescent students' abilities to identify the steps in a systematic decision-making process. Although decision making may be described in many ways, this particular measure views the systematic process as involving five steps:

1. identifying or clarifying the decision to be made;
2. identifying possible decision options;
3. gathering/processing information;
4. making/implementing the decision; and
5. evaluating the decision.

This structured decision-making instrument evaluates this model only and should not be applied in evaluating general decision-making ability.

DIRECTIONS: Read each of the following stories about young people who are trying to make decisions. CIRCLE THE LETTER of the NEXT THING that the person should do to make the best decision. If you are unsure what the person should do, CIRCLE DON'T KNOW.

1. Jane has seen kids smoking in the restrooms at lunch and out on the playground after school. Some of Jane's friends have even tried smoking cigarettes. She figures that her friends may ask her to try a cigarette soon.

   What should Jane do NEXT to make a good decision?
   A. Ask her best friend what she should do.
   B. Decide to try smoking just one cigarette.
   #C. Know that she must decide whether to smoke cigarettes.
   D. Don't know.

2. Mark tried smoking marijuana with some friends a few months ago. Since then he has started smoking more and more. He even smokes before school sometimes. Mark is not doing as well in school as he used to. He is worried that his grades will go down and his parents will get mad. He thinks it may have something to do with smoking marijuana too much. He wants to find a way to stop.

   What should Mark do NEXT to make a good decision?
   A. Decide to find new friends who do not smoke.
   #B. Call a hotline for help about ways to stop smoking marijuana.
   C. Know he must decide on a way to stop smoking marijuana.
   D. Don't know.

3. Donna and her best friend want to go to the school dance Friday night, but they need a ride. Her friend's dad will be able to take them to the dance, but can't pick them up. Donna's older brother is going out with his friend the same night and said he would pick them up. Donna knows her brother likes to drink beer with his friends. She must decide whether to ride home with her brother. Donna and her friend think about what they could do. They could get a ride with Donna's brother or try to find another ride. If they can't find another ride they might not be able to go to the dance. Donna asks some questions in her health class about drinking and driving.

   What should Donna do NEXT to make a good decision?
   A. Know she must decide whether to get a ride from her brother.
   B. Have her friend decide whether they should get a ride with her.
   #C. Decide whether to get a ride home from the dance with her brother.
   D. Don't know.

Source: Modified from *Program Evaluation Handbook: Alcohol Abuse Education*, pages 110–121, Center for Health Promotion and Education, Centers for Disease Control, and Prevention, 1988.

= the most appropriate response

beliefs, personal commitment, information on various mind-changing drugs and their potential effects, resistance skills strategies, and one or two other strategies, such as introducing alternative activities.[8]

Another study indicates that drug-abuse prevention programs conducted in junior high school, with booster sessions in grade 8 and grade 9, can produce meaningful and durable reductions in tobacco, alcohol, and marijuana use, if they (1) teach a combination of social resistance skills and general life skills, (2) are properly implemented, and (3) include at least two years of booster sessions in later school grades.[9]

Based upon an analysis of current educational programs for the prevention of ATOD use and abuse, the following general principles emerge as important components in designing and implementing curricula:[10]

1. Kindergarten through grade 12 ATOD prevention education should be an integral part of a comprehensive school health education program.
2. In dealing with the adverse consequences of ATOD use in young people, concentrate on the immediate effects on the human being and on the use of alcohol and drugs as a major obstacle to responsible behavior, and reduce feelings that the risks of drug taking "cannot happen to me."
3. Provide accurate information on the effects of psychoactive drugs, especially in relation to one's inhibitions and drinking and driving, on laws governing use of alcohol and other drugs, and on the perceived benefits of ATOD use.
4. In elementary and secondary school, provide educational programs on

Box 16.3 Impact Evaluation Indicators

The Department of Education's Regional Centers for Drug-Free Schools and Communities are responsible for assisting state and local agencies, schools, and educators in developing effective prevention programs. They use, and recommend, the following checklist of indicators for evaluating the impact of prevention programs in reducing the use of drugs in schools and in educating students about the dangers of drug use.

Extent to Which Student Body Exhibits Positive Changes in Personal Attitudes, Knowledge, Characteristics, and Behavioral Choices

- demonstrate positive self-esteem*
- demonstrate refusal skills*
- don't use alcohol/drugs
- engage in self-protective behavior* (e.g., use seat belts)
- have networks of nonusing friends*
- know alcohol/drug use is harmful
- know effect of peer influence*
- show change in attitudes toward peer use*
- show change in attitudes toward using alcohol/drugs*

Extent to Which Student Body Participates in Alternative Activities

- access to prevention and intervention programs
- involved in peer leadership programs
- involved in volunteerism
- participate in drug-free activities, events, and parties (e.g., Project Graduation)
- participate in teen clubs
- take part in peer counseling activities

Extent to Which Student Body Exhibits Positive Changes in the Following Education/Schooling Behaviors

- academic achievement
- high school graduation rates
- participation in sports and extracurricular activities at school
- school attendance
- serving as peer tutors

Positive Changes in Youth-Related Statistics

- admissions for detoxification
- alcohol/drug referrals
- alcohol/drug-related hospital admissions
- arrests
- deaths among children and youth
- DUI/DWI
- liquor law violations
- suicides and attempted suicides
- traffic fatalities
- use/abuse of alcohol/drugs*
- use of tobacco products*

Positive Changes in School-Related Statistics

- alcohol/drug related disciplinary referrals
- dropouts
- expulsions
- suspensions
- tardiness
- truancy/school absenteeism

* Typically ascertained via students surveys

Source: Office of Educational Research and Improvement, U.S. Department of Education.

ATOD use with appropriate, planned, and sequential lessons and activities for students at every grade level if possible. Instruction is especially effective when it begins early in life and is continuous.

5. Emphasize that the unlawful possession and use of alcoholic beverages and other drugs is wrong and potentially harmful.
6. In addition to school health education, ATOD education can also be correlated with other subject areas, including sciences, social studies, language arts, psychology, current events, home economics, and driver education.
7. Include information on family and peer norms regarding use, acceptability, and unacceptability. Point out that most youths are not using alcohol or other drugs on a daily basis. Then use peers to make desirable norms more acceptable.
8. Reinforce peer resistance skills, decision making, problem solving, and social (life) competence skills.
9. Include plans and activities that involve parents and community members in supporting ATOD education in the school.
10. Determine if the learning experiences helped students achieve instructional objectives (see box 16.3).

Resources for ATOD Education

Resources are the "teaching tools" used by instructors to enrich and facilitate learning opportunities dealing with ATOD use and abuse prevention efforts in schools and in the community. Books, pamphlets, video tapes, films, projectors, chalkboards, government and private agencies, community groups, and specific individuals who can support an educational program are examples of teaching resources.

Numerous organizations can provide valuable resource materials and information on various aspects of ATOD

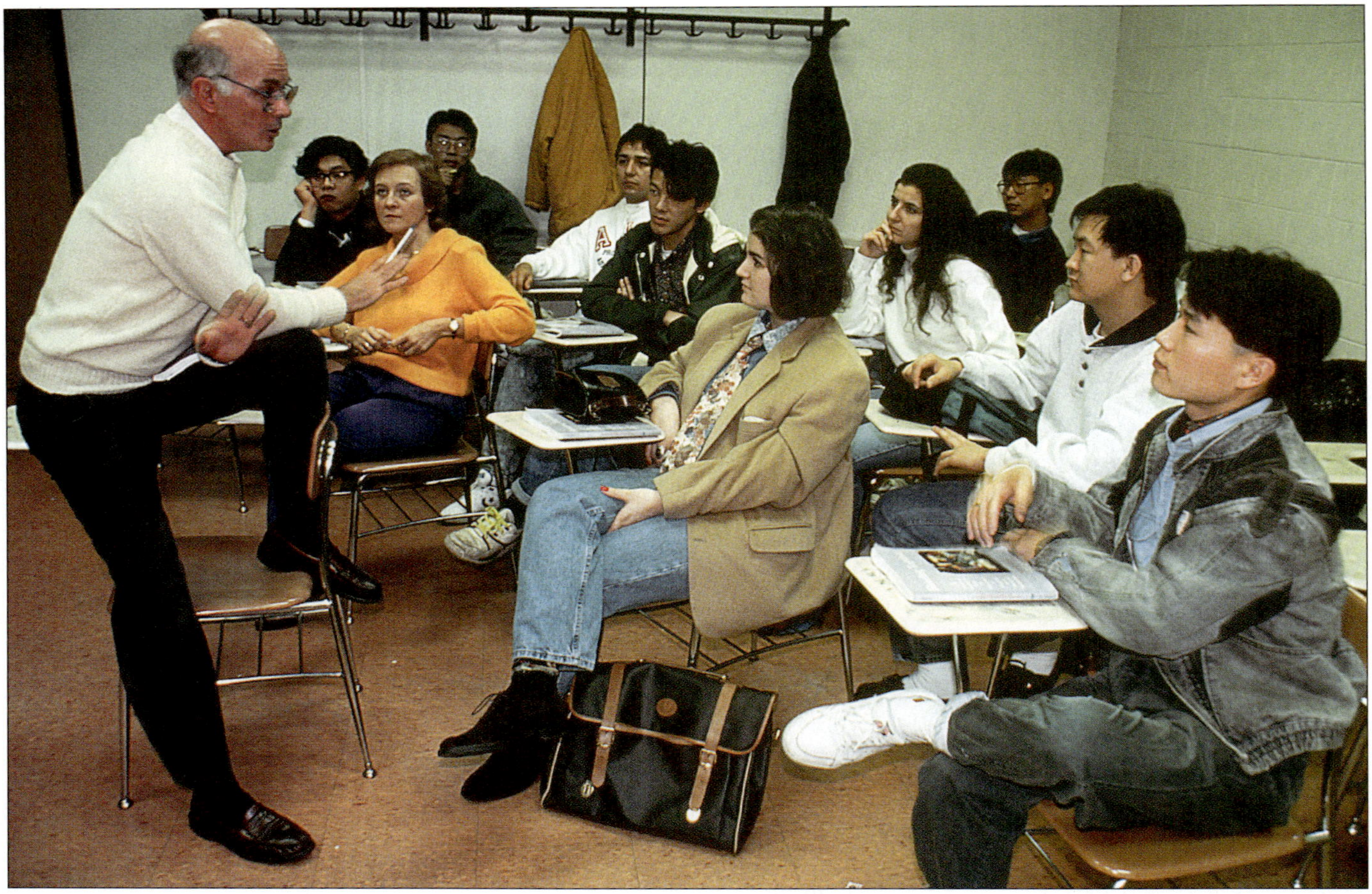

Small group discussions under the guidance of an informed, trained, and empathetic adult are among the most effective ATOD education methods. Here an adult counselor discusses ways for young people to develop refusal skills and to cope with social pressure to use alcohol, tobacco, and other drugs.
© Jeff Greenberg/The Picture Cube, Inc.

use and abuse and on ATOD education. Some materials are free; others are available for loan, rent, or purchase. There is no shortage of instructional media.

Key Elements of Effective Curricula

One resource that is often the most time-consuming in its development and use and possibly the most costly is the curriculum. A guide to classroom teaching-learning activities, the drug prevention curriculum is frequently planned on a local level, typically with the help of a school committee or a city- or countywide task force representing the community.

Some schools prefer to adopt ATOD prevention curricula that have been formulated by private companies or even governmental agencies, including state departments of education. Schools must then choose wisely in selecting a curricular plan that most closely represents the goals and objectives established at the local level. What criteria, then, may be applied to determine which particular plan will be adopted, whether it is purchased or formulated by school personnel and interested parents?

For the past twenty years, in-depth research studies have revealed several elements necessary for successful drug prevention teaching. Some of these "key elements" have been identified in the previous section "Some Concluding Thoughts." However, they are restated here formally along with other related components to assist curriculum planners and evaluators in their respective tasks.

According to an extensive examination and evaluation process, the "key elements" of a successful drug prevention program are:[11]

- help students recognize internal pressures, such as anxiety and stress, and external pressures, such as peer attitudes and pro-drug use advertising, that influence young people to use alcohol, tobacco, and other drugs;
- develop personal, social, and refusal skills to resist the internal and external pressures to use drugs;
- teach students that using alcohol, tobacco and other drugs is not the norm among teenagers, even if students think that "everyone is doing it";

- provide developmentally appropriate materials and activities, including information about the short-term effects and long-term consequences of using alcohol, tobacco, and other drugs;
- use interactive teaching techniques, such as role playing, discussion, brainstorming and cooperative learning, for example, small group assignments or group projects and community service experiences;
- cover necessary prevention elements in at least ten sessions a year, with a minimum of three to five booster sessions in two succeeding years;
- actively involve the family and the community, as described earlier in this chapter;
- include teacher training, availability of resources, and administrative support; and
- include material that is easy for teachers to implement and culturally relevant for students.

Prepackaged ATOD Curricula

Nearly fifty prepackaged drug prevention curricula have been evaluated according to the nine key elements described.[12] No single curriculum emphasized all "key elements" equally. However, as a result of this assessment, some of the most effective school-based drug prevention programs in the United States are:

The Michigan Model—a comprehensive health education program for grades K–8. This curriculum consists of 40 to 60 well-organized lessons per year that address all the elements of prevention. Included is coverage of alcohol, tobacco, and other drugs, while emphasis is also given to resistance skills training within the context of social and personal skills development. Interactive teaching techniques are used effectively.

Alcohol Misuse Prevention Program (Series II)—a middle school drug prevention curriculum for grades 6–8. This clever program, with original activities, focuses on alcohol use prevention. Included are well-developed aspects of normative education, recognition of pro-drug influences, refusal skills, and role playing. The program is recommended for implementation within a two-week period.

Life Skills Training—a state-of-the-art curriculum for grades 6–8 or 7–9. This program focuses on resistance skills training within the context of broader personal and social skills. A core of fifteen sessions is offered in grade 6 or 7, with ten and then eight booster sessions in the two following grades. This well-organized curriculum concentrates on tobacco, alcohol, and marijuana.

Project Alert—a two-year curriculum with eleven sessions in the first year and three in the second for grades 6 and 7 or 7 and 8. This program emphasizes the development of resistance skills to the perceived internal pressures and overt peer pressure to use drugs. In covering alcohol, tobacco, and other drugs, this curriculum also presents good material on normative education.

Project Northland—designed for grades 6–8, this creative program focuses on alcohol use and abuse. In only eight sessions per year, the curriculum places an emphasis on resistance techniques and decision making, and works to set a norm that drinking is not "cool." Special features include family take-home assignments and many opportunities for role playing.

STAR (Students Taught Awareness and Resistance)—a two-year program for grades 5–8. With 10 to 13 sessions in the first year and five in the second, this curriculum focuses primarily on the development of resistance skills along with powerful material on normative education. There is good background information on drugs with an emphasis on short-term effects. Detailed instructions for role play are also offered.

Other selected curricula include:

Comprehensive health education curricula with integrated drug prevention programs:

Actions for Health, grades K–6
Comprehensive Health, grades 5–9
Growing Healthy, grades K–6
Quest: Skills for Action, grades 9–12
Teenage Health Teaching Modules, grades 6–12

K–12 drug Prevention programs:

Here's Looking at You 2000, grades K–12

Elementary and middle school drug prevention programs:

DARE (Drug Abuse Resistance Education), grades 5–6
Growing Up Well, grades K–8
I'm Special, grades 3 or 4
Positive Action, grades K–8
Project Charlie, grades K–6

Middle and high school drug prevention programs

Healthy for Life, grades 6–8
From Peer Pressure to Peer Support, grades 7–12
Ombudsman, grades 5–9
Project All-Stars, grade 6 or 7
Social Competence Promotion Program, grades 5 or 6 or 7
Talking with Your Students About Alcohol, grades 5–12

School Policies on Alcohol and Other Drugs

Instructional planning is an important and necessary step in the successful implementation of an alcohol and other drug use prevention program. However, the planned learning experiences of the curriculum should be seen as only one phase in the school's overall approach to the prevention and management of alcohol and other drug problems.

Before schools can engage in alcohol and other drug education effectively, the community and the professionals involved in working with young people need to establish a **comprehensive policy against alcohol and other drug use** and abuse that is strong, "clearly articulated, consistently enforced, and broadly communicated."[13]

Elements of a Comprehensive Policy

An effective alcohol and drug prevention policy needs to address issues of school security, student access to and distribution and use of illegal substances, use of security police and undercover agents, alcohol and drug seizures by faculty, reporting of suspected alcohol- and other drug-related behavior, alcohol and drug overdoses and emergency actions, in-service training of school staff, due process for student violators, limits on confidentiality, and student involvement in policy development.[14] It is also necessary that such a policy and its implementing procedures addressing the several issues noted be revised regularly and administered fairly.

Additional elements for inclusion in a comprehensive alcohol and other drug prevention policy include the following:[15]

1. A clear statement that alcohol and other drugs and their use are prohibited on the school campus, at school-sponsored functions, and while students are representing the school.
2. A description of the consequences to be expected upon violating the policy and the conditions for reinstatement of students who are disciplined or in treatment programs.
3. Appropriate assistance for students when intervention or follow-up is required within the school due to alcohol and other drug use.
4. Reciprocal communication between school and service agencies that treat alcohol and other drug problems.
5. Lines of communication with the home concerning either suspected or known student alcohol or drug problems.
6. Assurance that school policies on alcohol and other drug use are widely distributed, understood, and made applicable to the needs of the entire school population—school personnel, students, parents, and school board members.
7. A confidential process for referral of identified students and/or their families to qualified human service agencies or treatment programs.
8. Additional resources, such as alternative school programs, for dealing with students who have alcohol and other drug problems.

Student Assistance Programs

School personnel are sometimes reluctant to intervene in cases of student alcohol and other drug use because of the perceived lack of administrative support, feelings of vulnerability to legal sanction, and fear of retaliation by parents and students. Faculty and staff may also be hesitant to get involved with students' drug-related problems unless there is some mechanism for implementing a school's policy on alcohol and other drugs. Such a mechanism has evolved as **student assistance programs.**[16]

Student assistance programs (SAPs) are an approach for intervening in and preventing alcohol and other drug problems among school-age youth. Modeled after the employee assistance programs found in business and industry, student assistance programs focus on behavior and performance at school and use a referral process that includes screening by teachers and other school personnel for alcohol and other drug involvement. Student assistance programs also work with self-referred youth.

As a partnership between community health agencies and the schools, SAPs address a number of important concerns. First, they approach alcohol and other drug use as a problem that affects a student's entire development. Second, they offer a strategy for eliminating alcohol and other drug use both during and after school hours. Third, they give school staff a mechanism for helping youth with a wide range of problems that may contribute to alcohol and other drug use. Last, SAPs can offer assistance to students suffering adverse effects from parental alcohol or other drug use.

Although the components and people responsible for them vary widely, the following activities are found in nearly every school with a student assistance program:

Early detection of student problems

Referrals to designated "helpers" within the school

In-school services (support groups, individual counseling)

Referral to outside agencies (mental health centers or clinics, private physicians, psychologists, family service organizations, Alcoholics Anonymous)

Follow-up monitoring once the student has returned after counseling, treatment, or rehabilitation

Teachers and other school personnel are advised and trained to identify students experiencing problems that interfere with their functioning at school. However, they are not expected to specify the nature of the problem or to intervene personally. Students are referred to appropriate assessment and assistance resources. Regardless of the mix of responsibilities and personnel centered in a student assistance program, the endorsement of the school board, principals, and community leaders is critical to the success of the program.

Chapter Summary

1. Traditionally, school-based ATOD education has been confined to classroom activities in elementary and secondary schools. However, general and specific nonschool populations can now be reached by mass-media campaigns, communitywide supply or demand reduction programs, worksite employee efforts, policy and legislative initiatives, and the training of health care professionals.

2. In addition to providing information about alcohol and other drugs and the consequences of their use, expanded ATOD prevention education programs also try to raise awareness and involvement in the local community, increase the knowledge base of teachers and parents, change students' norms and expectations, enhance parenting and positive family influences, and improve student coping, peer resistance, and decision-making skills. Such programs can also increase parental involvement in schools, expand student participation in legal alternatives to ATOD use, and deter use through regulation and legal actions.
3. The major goals of ATOD education are to reduce the extent of alcohol, tobacco, and other drug use and to prevent alcohol-, tobacco-, and other drug-related problems from occurring in the future.
4. Among the Healthy People 2010 objectives—measurable targets that are to be achieved by the year 2010—are the increase of youth who remain alcohol and drug free, reduction in youthful binge drinking, reduction in steroid and inhalant use by youth 12- to 17-year-old, to increase the proportion of youth who perceive great risk of harm and social disapproval associated with ATODs; and a reduction in the initiation of smoking by young people.
5. A systematic plan for designing and implementing alcohol education consists of the following steps: needs assessment, identification of strategies, anticipation of instructional problems, development of goals, selection of subject matter, formulation of instructional objectives, selection of methods, identification of resources, development of evaluation procedures, and revision of the instructional program.
6. Curriculum strategies used in ATOD education programs include strategies focusing on normative beliefs, personal commitment, values, information, resistance skills, alternatives, goal setting, decision making, self-esteem enhancement, and the development of stress skills and life skills.
7. Key elements of effective drug prevention curricula include: recognizing pressures to use drugs; developing personal, social, and refusal skills; emphasizing normative beliefs, providing information on drugs and their effects; using interactive methods; providing long-term intervention over the school career; involving parents and the community; training of teachers and receiving administrative support; and focusing on materials that are easy to use and culturally relevant for students.
8. Resources, the "teaching tools" of instructors, include various prepackaged curricula; government agencies (especially the National Clearinghouse for Alcohol and Drug Information); state-level prevention resource centers; private, voluntary agencies and companies; self-help groups (including Alcoholics Anonymous); local community organizations; and periodicals related to alcohol and other drugs (see the appendix).
9. In addition to ATOD education, schools need a comprehensive policy against alcohol and other drug use that addresses such issues as school security, student access to and distribution and use of illegal substances, alcohol and drug seizures, reporting of suspected alcohol- and other drug-related behavior, in-service training of school staff, due process for student violators, and limits of confidentiality.
10. An approach for intervening in and preventing alcohol and other drug problems among school-age youth is the student assistance program, modeled after the relatively successful employee assistance programs in business and industry.

World Wide Web Sites

Center for Disease Control

www.cdc.gov

Community Anti-Drug Coalitions of America

www.cadca.org

Parents Resource Institute for Drug Education

www.prideusa.org

Review Questions and Activities

1. Identify examples of "nonschool" alcohol and other education activities in the local community by analyzing newspapers, magazines, and public service announcements on radio and television; by locating businesses and industries that sponsor employee assistance programs and wellness programs; and by interviewing directors of local alcohol and other drug treatment programs. Also determine if there is a local affiliate of the National Council on Alcoholism and Drug Dependence, Inc. How does this organization promote education on alcohol and other drugs?
2. Procure a copy of the laws in your state that pertain to underage drinking; possession of alcoholic beverages, tobacco products, and other illegal drugs; and requirements for alcohol, tobacco, and other drug education in the schools. Share your findings with other class members.
3. Why do the goals of ATOD education in the elementary and secondary schools rarely, if ever, mention responsible use, responsible drinking, or low-risk ways of using marijuana or other illegal drugs as desirable outcomes?
4. Distinguish among teaching strategies based on the following: normative beliefs, personal commitment, values, information, resistance skills,

alternatives, goal setting, decision making, self-esteem enhancement, stress skills, and life skills.

5. After procuring copies of alcohol, tobacco, and other drug education curricula from local schools, determine what major strategies, designs, or methods are used more frequently. If a particular prepackaged curriculum has been adopted, ask the school's ATOD education coordinator or the school principal why such a curriculum was chosen.

6. State several general principles or "key elements" that can be used in guiding the design and implementation of a school-based ATOD education program.

7. What specific advice could you offer to a young person who asks for help in saying no to drinking alcoholic beverages or using a tobacco product or some other illegal drug?

8. Contact your State Prevention Resource Center to determine what types of information and other resources are available for individuals and schools conducting alcohol and other drug education programs.

9. Why do you think schools need a comprehensive policy against alcohol and other drug use?

10. What is the value of a student assistance program?

References

1. Judith Funkhouser, Eric Goplerud, and Rosalyn Bass, "Current Status of Prevention Strategies," chap. 2 in *A Promising Future, Alcohol and Other Drug Problem Prevention Services Improvement,* Office for Substance Abuse Prevention Monograph No. 10, DHHS Pub. No. (ADM) 92-1807, ed. Mary Jansen (Washington, D.C.: GPO, 1992), 42.
2. Jean Linney and Abraham Wandersman, *Prevention Plus III: Assessing Alcohol and Other Drug Prevention Programs at the School and Community Level,* Office for Substance Abuse Prevention DHHS Pub. No. (ADM) 91-1817 (Washington D.C.: GPO, 1991), 20.
3. Ibid., 19.
4. *Healthy People 2010 Objectives: Draft for Public Comment,* U.S. Department of Health and Human Services, Office of Public Health and Science, September 15, 1999.
5. National Institute on Drug Abuse, *Prevention Planning Workbook,* vol. 1 (Washington, D.C.: GPO, 1981), 2–4; and Center for Substance Abuse Prevention, Substance Abuse and Mental Health Services Administration, *Prevention Plus II: Tools for Creating and Sustaining Drug-Free Communities,* DHHS Pub. No. (ADM) 89-1649 (Washington, D.C.: GPO, 1993), 94–164.
6. Mathea Falco, *The Making of a Drug-Free America: Programs That Work* (New York: Times Books, 1992), 33–36; and Phyllis Ellickson, "Schools," chap. 5 in *Handbook on Drug Abuse Prevention,* eds. Robert Coombs and Douglas Ziedonis (Boston: Allyn and Bacon, 1995), 93–120.
7. William B. Hansen, "School-Based Alcohol Prevention Programs," *Alcohol Health & Research World* 17, no. 1 (1993): 54–60.
8. Ibid., 58.
9. Gilbert Botvin and others, "Long-Term Follow-Up Results of a Randomized Drug Abuse Prevention Trial in a White Middle-Class Population," *Journal of the American Medical Association* 273, no. 14 (12 April 1995): 1106–12.
10. Center for Substance Abuse Prevention, *Prevention Plus II,* 40–41; Kevin Volkan and Joyce Fetro, "Substance Use Prevention: Implications of Theory and Practice," *Family Life Educator* 8, no. 4 (Summer 1990): 17–23; U.S. Department of Education, *Success Stories from Drug-Free Schools: A Guide for Educators, Parents, and Policymakers* (Washington, D.C.: U.S. Department of Education, 1992), 30; and Liane M. Summerfield, "Drug and Alcohol Prevention Education," *ERIC Digest* (March 1991): 1–2.
11. Drug Strategies, *Making the Grade: A Guide to School Drug Prevention Programs* (Washington, D.C.: Drug Strategies, 1996), 1–5.
12. Ibid., 6–33.
13. Office of Educational Research and Improvement, *Drug Prevention Curricula: A Guide to Selection and Implementation* (Washington, D.C.: U.S. Department of Education, 1988), 7.
14. John H. Langer, "Problems of Drug Abuse in Schools: The Need for a Consistent Policy" (paper presented to the Coalition of National Health Education Associations at the Center for Disease Control, Emory University Campus, Atlanta, 25 March 1982).
15. Drug Enforcement Administration, *School Drug Abuse Policy Guidelines,* 2d ed. (Washington, D.C.: GPO, and Office of Educational Research and Improvement, 1980), 4–5; and DEA, *Drug Prevention Curricula: A Guide to Selection and Implementation* (Washington, D.C.: U.S. Department of Education, 1988), 3, 7–8.
16. Center for Substance Abuse Prevention, *Prevention Plus II,* 59–61, modified.

Appendix

A Resource Guide for ATOD Information

Government Agencies

National Clearinghouse for Alcohol and Drug Information
P.O. Box 2345
Rockville, MD 20847–2345
(800) 729–6686 or (301) 468–2600
(Sponsored by the federal Center for Substance Abuse Prevention, this clearinghouse is the single best source of free and inexpensive print materials on alcohol, alcohol and drug abuse prevention, and AOD education.)

U.S. Department of Education
Drug Abuse Prevention Oversight Staff
Office of the Secretary
400 Maryland Avenue, SW
Room 4145, MS 6411
Washington, DC 20202

U.S. Department of Justice
Drugs & Crime Data Center & Clearinghouse
Bureau of Justice Statistics
1600 Research Boulevard
Rockville, MD 20850
(800) 666-3332

U.S. Department of Transportation
National Highway Traffic Safety Administration
Office of Traffic Safety Programs
400 Seventh Street, SW, Room 5130
Washington, DC 20590

State Department of Education

State Department of Health

State Drug Abuse Prevention Agency

State Prevention Resource Center
(See box 16.6 for a listing of the Regional Alcohol and Drug Awareness Resource [RADAR] Network, consisting of state clearinghouses.)

Private, Voluntary Agencies, Associations, and Companies

Al-Anon Family Group Headquarters, Inc.
World Service Office
P.O. Box 862, Midtown Station
New York, NY 10018-0862

Alcoholics Anonymous (AA)
World Services
475 Riverside Drive
New York, NY 10115

American Council for Drug Education
c/o Phoenix House
164 W. 74th. St.
New York, NY 10023

American School Health Association
P.O. Box 708
Kent, OH 44240

ARIS (Alcohol Research Information Service)
1106 E. Oakland Avenue
Lansing, MI 48906

ASH (Action on Smoking and Health)
2013 H Street, NW
Washington, D.C. 20006

Association for the Advancement of Health Education
1900 Association Drive
Reston, VA 22091

CompCare Publications
2415 Annapolis Lane
Minneapolis, MN 55441

Do It Now Foundation
P.O. Box 21126
Phoenix, AZ 85036

ETR Associates
P.O. Box 1830
Santa Cruz, CA 95061-1830

Films for the Humanities & Sciences
P.O. Box 2053
Princeton, NJ 08543-2053

Hazelden Foundation
Pleasant Valley Road
P.O. Box 176
Center City, MN 55012

Just Say No Foundation
1777 North California Boulevard
Walnut Creek, CA 94596

Mothers Against Drunk Driving (MADD)
669 Air Port Freeway, Suite 310
Hurst, TX 76053

National Congress of Parents and Teachers
700 North Rush Street
Chicago, Il 60611-2571

National Council on Alcoholism and Drug Dependence, Inc.
12 West 21st Street
New York, NY 10010

Parents' Resource Institute for Drug Education (PRIDE)
10 Park Place S., Suite 540
Atlanta, GA 30303

Rutgers University Center of Alcohol Studies
Publications Division
P.O. Box 969
Piscataway, NJ 08855

Students Against Driving Drunk
P.O. Box 800
277 Main Street
Marlboro, MA 01752

Sunburst Communications
39 Washington Avenue
P.O. Box 40
Pleasantville, NY 10570-0040

Self-Help Groups

Alcoholics Anonymous World Services
475 Riverside Drive
New York, NY 10163 (see local telephone directory)

Al-Anon Family Group Headquarters, Inc.
P.O. Box 862, Midtown Station
New York, NY 10018

Alateen
P.O. Box 862, Midtown Station
New York, NY 10018

Cocaine Anonymous World Services
3740 Overland Avenue, Suite H
Los Angeles, CA 90034

Families Anonymous
P.O. Box 528
Van Nuys, CA 91408

Nar-Anon Family Group Headquarters
P.O. Box 2562
Palos Verdes Peninsula, CA 90274

Narcotics Anonymous World Service Office
P.O. Box 9999
Van Nuys, CA 91409

National Association for Adult Children of Alcoholics
P.O. Box 35623
Los Angeles, CA 90035

National Association for Children of Alcoholics
11426 Rockville Pike
Rockville, MD 20852

Potsmokers Anonymous
208 W. 23rd. St., Apt. 1414
New York, NY 10011

Rational Recovery Systems
P.O. Box 100
Lotus, CA 95651

Secular Organizations for Sobriety
P.O. Box 5
Buffalo, NY 14215-0005

TOUGHLOVE
P.O. Box 1069
Doylestown, PA 18901

Women for Sobriety
P.O. Box 618
Quakertown, PA 18951

Local Community Organizations and Individuals

Alcohol and drug treatment agencies
Community mental health centers
Hospital clinics on chemical dependency
Intervention programs for alcohol-impaired drivers
Members of Alcoholics Anonymous, Al-Anon, Alateen, Narcotics Anonymous
National Council on Alcoholism and Drug Dependence, Inc., local affiliate
Psychologists, social workers, and counselors

ATOD-Related Periodicals

Addiction & Recovery: The Alcohol & Drug Publication
Alcohol, Drugs and Driving
Alcohol Health & Research World
American Journal of Drug and Alcohol Abuse
The Bottom Line on Alcohol in Society
The Drinking and Drug Practices Surveyor
Journal of Adolescent Chemical Dependency
Journal of Alcohol and Drug Education
Journal of Drug Education
Journal of Drug Issues
Journal of Psychoactive Drugs: A Multidisciplinary Forum
Journal of Studies on Alcohol
Journal of Substance Abuse
Prevention File: Alcohol, Tobacco & Other Drugs
Prevention Pipeline: An Alcohol and Drug Awareness Service
Psychology of Addictive Behaviors
Social History of Alcohol Review: The Journal of the Alcohol and Temperance History Group
Substance Abuse: Official Publication of the Association for Medical Education and Research in Substance Abuse
Traffic Safety

glossary

All terms in this glossary have been defined in relation to drug use, drug misuse, drug abuse and chemical dependency, prevention of substance abuse, or education about psychoactive and nonpsychoactive drugs and medicines.

absorption passage of a substance into the bloodstream through the skin, intestinal lining, or other bodily membranes.

abstinence condition of not using a particular substance; refraining from using a drug, such as alcohol.

acculturation adoption by an immigrant group of the cultural traits or behaviors (such as drinking practices) of another group, especially a dominant one.

acetaminophen an over-the-counter nonsalicylate analgesic and antipyretic drug derived from coal tar and marketed as Datril, Tylenol, and Panadol.

acquired immunodeficiency syndrome (AIDS) serious, life-threatening illness (for which there is no present cure), which involves a breakdown of the body's internal defense system.

activation drug action that increases the rate of functional activity in a cell; a stimulating effect.

addiction a pattern of substance abuse characterized by an overwhelming involvement with using a drug and securing its supply, despite adverse consequences associated with use of the drug. A chronic, compulsive, or uncontrollable use of a substance.

additive drug reaction type of drug interaction in which two or more drugs that are similar in their general effects produce a cumulative net effect that is the sum of the effects of the individual substances.

adulteration drug tampering in which cheaper, inferior, or hazardous substances are mixed with a particular drug.

adverse drug reaction a drug effect other than the intended or anticipated one that is unusual, undesirable, discomforting, or life-threatening.

aesthetic experience a psychedelic response related to change in and intensification of sensory input.

agent-related etiology theory that relates drug abuse and drug dependence to a specific psychoactive drug, known as the agent.

alcohol abuse consumption of alcoholic beverages resulting in some degree of physical, mental, or social impairment to either the drinker or someone else; maladaptive pattern of alcohol use leading to significant impairment or distress.

alcohol dependence the diagnosis of alcoholism characterized by tolerance, withdrawal, loss or impairment of control over alcohol intake, and craving.

alcoholics anonymous (AA) voluntary fellowship of problem drinkers who desire help in maintaining sobriety.

alcoholism the disease or condition of alcohol dependence in which an individual cannot consistently exert control over intake of alcohol; pathological pattern of alcohol use marked by impairment in one's social or occupational functioning due to alcohol.

alcohol states of consciousness (ASC) various states of altered consciousness during the duration of alcohol's effects, depending on whether the blood-alcohol concentration is increasing or decreasing.

altered conscious experience a change in your own awareness, typically, to feel better, or different.

alternatives approach technique of drug-abuse prevention that provides individuals with attractive, optional nondrug substitutes not only to drugs, but also to drug-using lifestyles.

ambivalence perception of both positive and negative aspects occurring in the same thing at the same time.

amotivational syndrome pattern of personality changes observed in some frequent users of marijuana and marked by apathy, lack of concern for the future, and loss of motivation, persisting beyond the period of intoxication.

amphetamine synthetic central nervous system stimulant.

anabolic-androgenic steroid formerly called anabolic steroids, these synthetic derivatives of testosterone are used to build lean muscle mass and to improve the strength and mechanical effectiveness of skeletal muscles.

analgesia pain relief.

analgesic drug taken internally to relieve or lessen pain.

anorectic (anorexic) drug that tends to curb the appetite.

antabuse disulfiram, a drug that interferes with alcohol oxidation and prolongs the presence of toxic acetaldehyde in the body, eventually causing severe physical effects. Consequently, Antabuse is used as a deterrent to discourage problem drinkers from resuming alcohol use.

antagonistic drug reaction drug reaction that results when drugs that are taken together interact so that the effect of either or both agents is blocked or reduced.

antianxiety agent a minor tranquilizer that acts somewhat like a sedative-hypnotic and is useful in treating anxiety and neurotic conditions.

antidepressant drug, such as an MAO inhibitor or a tricyclic compound, used to elevate mood and relieve certain types of mental depression.

antihistamine drug that blocks the effects of the allergy chemical, histamine, and relieves sneezing, watery eyes, runny nose, and itching of the nose or throat.

antihypertensive drug drug used to reduce high blood pressure.

anti-infective drug drug that inactivates or eliminates invading, disease-causing microbes; antibiotic, antifungal preparation, sulfonamide, and antiseptic.

antiparaphernalia law law or ordinance restricting or forbidding the sale and/or advertising of items related to use of illegal recreational drugs, such as pipes, bongs, roach clips, and roll-your-own cigarette papers.

antiparaphernalia movement organized community-based attempt, often led by groups of concerned parents, to lobby for legislation or other governmental actions to restrict or prohibit the availability of paraphernalia—articles used in administering, preparing, packaging, and storing drugs.

antitussive drug preparation that relieves coughing.

anxiety/panic reaction mental and emotional effects associated with use of drugs, such as marijuana and the psychedelics, that are perceived as unpleasant or undesirable, including panic, paranoid and/or dependency feelings, hallucinations, nonspecific fears, distortion of body image, and aggressive urges.

aphrodisiac food or drug substance alleged to arouse sexual desire or improve sexual performance or response.

appetite suppressant drug known as a diet aid (anorectic), which helps people curb their appetites, resulting in reduced food intake.

appetite drug use drug-taking behavior motivated by the desire for pleasurable responses and sensations.

aspirin over-the-counter analgesic, antipyretic, and anti-inflammatory drug derived from acetylsalicylic acid and marketed as brand-name aspirin, such as Anacin, Bayer, Bufferin, and Cope.

attention deficit-hyperactivity disorder brain disorder characterized by extreme motor restlessness, poor attention span, and impulsive and sometimes disorderly behavior. In children, this disorder is sometimes treated with amphetamine-like medications.

autonomic nervous system a division of the peripheral nervous system that connects the central nervous system to the organs of the body cavity, such as the heart, stomach, and intestines, and whose nerves function automatically without conscious control.

axon nerve fiber that carries electrical impulses away from the cell body of a neuron.

barbiturate sedative-hypnotic drug derived from barbituric acid and used in medical practice to calm nervous individuals and induce sleep.

beer alcoholic beverage containing 2–6 percent alcohol by volume, derived from cereal grains through the brewing process.

benefit-risk equation principle that in using a drug, the probability of good effects outweighs the possibility of adverse effects, based on the likelihood that absolute safety in drug reactions does not exist.

benzodiazepine antianxiety drug, such as Librium or Valium, used in medical practice to treat anxiety and various neurotic conditions.

binge drinking consuming five or more alcoholic drinks in one sitting for men, or four or more drinks in a row for women.

bioavailability measure of a drug's activity within the body as determined by the quantified levels of that particular drug in the blood.

bioequivalence characteristic or ability of one drug to produce the same therapeutic effect in the body as an apparently similar medication.

biotransformation complex liver functions that change the chemical or pharmacological properties of a drug in the human body to less toxic or nontoxic substances.

blackout early warning sign of alcoholism characterized by alcohol-induced amnesia or memory blank-out, but not loss of consciousness.

blood-alcohol concentration ratio of alcohol present in the blood to the total volume of blood, expressed as a percent; blood-alcohol level.

blood-brain barrier a barrier that restricts the passage of some drugs & molecules from the bloodstream to the brain.

bootlegging secret and unlawful transportation and sale of beverage alcohol.

brand-name drug drug product whose generic name has been assigned a trademarked or patented name by a particular pharmaceutical company for advertising and sale.

breathalyzer one of several instruments used to determine blood-alcohol concentration by measuring the concentration of alcohol in a sample of a drinker's breath.

bromide first drug introduced as a sedative-hypnotic and used initially as a treatment for epileptic convulsions.

bronchogenic carcinoma cancerous growth, malignant neoplasm, that arises in the lining of the bronchial tubes of the lungs.

buspar a prescribed nonbenzodiazepine antianxiety medication that so far has proved effective without causing significant sedation, tolerance, or physical dependence.

caffeine bitter tasting, odorless compound extracted from the fruit of the *Coffea arabica* plant, and one of the most widely used central nervous system stimulants.

caffeinism stimulated condition of chronic poisoning due to overindulgence in caffeine, manifest by mood changes, anxiety, sleep disruption, tremulousness, headache, and ringing in the ears.

cannabinoid chemical compound found only in cannabis products, particularly tetrahydrocannabinol, or THC.

cannabis marijuana or any preparation derived from the hemp plant.

cannabis sativa hemp plant from which marijuana is derived.

carbon monoxide poisonous component of the gas phase of cigarette smoke that combines with the hemoglobin in red blood cells, thus reducing the oxygen-carrying capacity of the blood.

carcinoma *in-situ* noninvasive cancer; cancerous growth remaining at the site of its origin.

cardiovascular disease disease of the heart and blood vessels, including coronary heart disease and atherosclerosis.

cardiovascular drug drug that affects the function of the heart and the blood vessels of the body, including antianginal preparations, antiarrhythmics, digitalis, coronary vasodilators, and vasopressors.

central nervous system that major part of the nervous system composed of the brain and the spinal cord.

cerebellum part of the brain, below the cerebrum and behind the pons and medulla, that serves as a reflex center in coordinating and integrating skeletal muscle movements.

cerebrum largest, most complex part of the brain, which coordinates and interprets internal and external stimuli; site of higher mental functions, for example, memory and reasoning.

chemically equivalent drug drug that contains the same amount of the same active ingredient in the same dosage form as contained in generic or brand-name drugs.

chemotherapy use of drugs to kill or weaken organisms that invade the body or abnormal cells within the body.

chewing tobacco form of "smokeless tobacco" that is chewed.

chronic bronchitis chronic obstructive lung disease marked by recurring inflammation of the bronchial tubes with excessive mucus production, persistent cough, and reduced normal lung function.

chronic obstructive lung disease slow, progressive interruption of the airflow within the lungs due to pulmonary emphysema and chronic bronchitis.

cigarette a roll of finely cut tobacco or marijuana for smoking, usually enclosed in thin paper.

ciliary function sweeping movements of cilia, tiny hairlike projections extending from the surface of the bronchial tubes, which sweep mucus and other debris out of the respiratory system into the mouth.

cocaine powerful central nervous system stimulant of natural origin, extracted from the leaves of the coca plant.

cocaine psychosis severe, relatively rare psychotic reaction characterized by paranoia and hallucinations resulting from prolonged cocaine use.

codeine naturally occurring narcotic widely used in medical practice, particularly as an antitussive, which is closely related to morphine but is less potent.

co-dependence a condition characterized by various maladaptive behaviors that family members often develop in response to a drug-dependent parent, spouse, child, or sibling.

cognitive experience psychedelic experience marked by clearness of thought.

cold turkey process of suddenly quitting the use of a drug, particularly smoking cigarettes.

combination oral contraceptive drug an oral contraceptive containing small amounts of both female sex hormones, estrogen and progestin.

comprehensive approaches to drug prevention education communitywide efforts to prevent ATOD use and/or abuse that involve both schools and nonschool initiatives, including mass-media campaigns, law enforcement actions, worksite drug awareness programs, and policy and legislative restrictions.

comprehensive drug abuse prevention and control act legal foundation for reducing consumption of illicit narcotic and nonnarcotic drugs in the United States, enacted by Congress in 1970, in which most psychoactive drugs were categorized into five schedules according to their presumed potential for abuse and their current acceptability in medical practice.

comprehensive policy against alcohol and other drug use established school policies, in addition to ATOD prevention education, that focus on school security, student access to and distribution and use of illegal substances, use of security police and undercover agents, alcohol and drug seizures by faculty, reporting of suspected alcohol and other drug-related behavior, and in-service training of school staff.

congeners nonalcoholic substances, besides water, present in minute quantities in all alcoholic beverages.

congenital abnormality physical and mental irregularities, including Fetal Alcohol Syndrome, originating after conception during pregnancy, due to some harmful force, such as a drug, acting on the developing embryo and fetus.

controlled drug psychoactive drug or medication having a significant potential for abuse and addiction, and therefore under the regulatory control of the Drug Enforcement Administration.

controlled substances act public law enacted in 1970 that placed most psychoactive substances into one of five schedules according to their abuse potential, likelihood of causing psychic or physical dependence, and current acceptability for medical treatment.

coping process of adjusting or accommodating to the demands of stress and daily living without being overwhelmed so that one's personal and social effectiveness is maintained.

coronary heart disease buildup of cholesterol within the coronary arteries that supply the heart muscle.

crack cocaine a smokable, intensified form of cocaine considered one of the most addictive substances ever known.

crashing disturbing period of mental depression occurring when a person stops taking a central nervous system stimulant after a period of chronic drug use.

craving overwhelming desire to use a drug substance.

cross-dependence condition in which one drug can prevent withdrawal symptoms associated with physical dependence on a different drug.

cross-tolerance condition in which tolerance to one drug, *A*, results in a lessened pharmacological response to another, *B*, of the same drug class, even though the person never used drug *B* before.

dalmane one of the most frequently prescribed benzodiazepines, flurazepam, that is promoted almost exclusively as a hypnotic.

darvon synthetic narcotic (propoxyphene) closely related to methadone, used for relief of mild to moderate pain.

particular human cells known as receptors.

decision making ATOD curriculum strategy that provides students with a system for organizing information about psychoactive drug use and then making choices among alternative behaviors or responses.

decreased awareness condition of escaping from reality, problems, physical and emotional pain.

decriminalization legal process of reducing the penalty for a particular behavior still restricted by law.

delirium tremens severe form of the alcohol abstinence or withdrawal syndrome, characterized by hallucinations, mental disorientation, agitation with continuous motor activity, involuntary body tremors, and convulsions.

demand reduction strategy for preventing drug abuse by reducing or eliminating the demand, desire, or need for various drug substances.

demographics characteristics, such as age, gender, income, education, and occupation, that describe the human population's social and vital statistics.

dendrite nerve fiber that sends electrical impulses toward the cell body of a neuron.

depo-provera long-acting injectable contraceptive drug containing only progestin.

depressant drug that slows down body functions; a sedative that depresses the central nervous system, relaxes, tranquilizes, or produces sleep.

depression reduction in the rate of functional activity; a slowing down effect.

designer drug synthetic substance produced by chemical alteration of an existing drug to make an "act-alike" psychoactive substance that would not be illegal upon its creation.

detection identification of psychoactive substance use or drug abuse through observation of common signs and symptoms of drug-taking behavior or by other measures including drug testing.

detoxification process of making chemical substances nonpoisonous; removal of a toxic substance from the body.

dextroamphetamine synthetic, central nervous system stimulant and one of three major amphetamine drugs.

distilled spirits alcoholic beverages containing 40–50 percent alcohol by volume, made from fermented mixtures of cereal grains or fruits that are heated in a still.

distribution circulation of an absorbed drug to all parts of the body by way of the bloodstream.

distribution of consumption theory an alcohol and other drug-abuse prevention belief that links the prevalence of drug abuse problems with the per capita use of all drugs in a nation or society.

diuretic drug that helps the body excrete excess water and salt, causing a sudden and copious flow of urine.

doping use of ergogenic drugs to artificially improve athletic competition; injecting of extra blood to increase endurance by increasing the number of red blood cells available to carry oxygen.

dose quantity or amount of drug taken at any particular time.

drug any substance that, upon entering a body, can change either the function or structure of the organism.

drug abuse deliberate use of chemical substances for reasons other than their intended medical purposes and that results in physical, mental, emotional, or social impairment of the user.

drug abuse warning network a large-scale drug-abuse data collection system sponsored by the National Institute on Drug Abuse.

drug action the result of a chemical interaction with some part of the human organism.

drug classes see *Drug families.*

drug dependence state of psychological or physical need, or both, for a drug. Usually characterized by compulsive use, tolerance, and physical dependence manifest by withdrawal sickness; chemical dependence; condition often equated with addiction.

drug enforcement administration (DEA) principal federal agency for enforcement of drug laws pertaining to drug trafficking, investigation, drug intelligence, and regulatory control, administered within the U.S. Department of Justice.

drug families major categories or types of drugs that share important characteristics in terms of chemical composition or actions within the body.

drug misuse unintentional or inappropriate use of prescribed or nonprescribed medicine, resulting in impaired physical, mental, emotional, or social well-being of the user.

drug-receptor interaction drug reaction between specific drug molecules and unique, localized portions of or within particular human cells known as receptors.

drug reinforcer any short-term effect of using a drug perceived as beneficial, which increases the likelihood of repeated drug use.

drug testing technique used to detect drug use and abuse through screening or examination of urine, blood, breath, and hair.

early-onset alcohol abuse or dependence a form of alcohol abuse or dependence in the elderly, representing the continuation of lifelong drinking problems, and often associated with a family history of alcoholism or psychological disorders.

ecstasy popular name for a designer drug, MDMA, that has psychedelic qualities and provides a euphoric "rush" of mind-expanding effects.

enabling factors influences that make drug taking behavior and/or substance abuse possible, such as the availability and accessibility of psychoactive drugs, actions of certain relatives or friends or agencies, and existence or lack of personal skills.

endemic drug use continuing presence of a disease condition or behavioral practice (drug use) in a particular population or locality.

endogenous opioid a natural, made-within-the-body substance that resembles morphine and produces opioid-like effects within the body; a booster of one's metabolic rate.

endorphins collective term describing any natural, internal body substance that has opioid-like activity.

enforcement techniques methods used by local, state, and federal law-enforcement agents to prevent illicit drug use, such as use of informants, surveillance, undercover operations, drug raids, interdiction, and intelligence gathering.

enkephalins internal body substance, extracted from the brain and pituitary, identified as having a narcotic effect within the body.

environment one sector or element of the public health model of drug-abuse prevention, specifically relating to the setting or context in which drug use occurs, and the group or community customs, mores, or folkways that influence drug takers.

environmental tobacco smoke mixture of sidestream smoke, smoke from the burning ends of tobacco products, and exhaled mainstream smoke, along with air, in an enclosed space; the mixture of tobacco smoke and air inhaled by a nonsmoker in the process of involuntary or passive smoking.

environment-related etiology theory that relates drug abuse and drug dependence to the sociocultural setting and those external circumstances and interrelational settings (the environment) in which any psychoactive drug is used.

ephedrine natural extract of a shrub that has a central nervous system stimulant effect; an FDA-approved drug for use as a decongestant, but widely advertised as a diet pill.

equivalent amount the quantity of ethyl alcohol, about 0.6 ounce, present in a standard serving of a regular alcoholic beverage.

ergogenic agent a drug, such as a stimulant, narcotic analgesic, or steroid, used for purposes of artificially improving athletic competition.

escape-avoidance drug use drug-taking behavior motivated by the desire for relief from unpleasant sensations, tensions, disturbed interpersonal relationships, fears, and anxieties.

etiology study of the cause or causative factors of a disease condition or behavioral practice.

evaluation process that determines if the curriculum or teaching plan helps students accomplish specific instructional objectives.

exempt narcotic drug preparation containing a small amount of a narcotic substance that can be purchased legally in some states without a physician's written prescription.

fail-safe medicine medicine that supposedly works safely on all people at all times. Though many believe in such a medication, none exists.

federal food and drug act first federal law in the United States, enacted in 1906, that prohibited interstate commerce in misbranded and adulterated drugs sold as medicines.

fentanyl a synthetic narcotic used as an intravenous analgesic-anesthetic.

fetal alcohol effects adverse developmental effects in an embryo or fetus due to prenatal alcohol exposure, but less severe than Fetal Alcohol Syndrome.

fetal alcohol syndrome (FAS) common pattern of birth defects and mental retardation that occurs among some children born of alcoholic or alcohol-consuming mothers, and manifested by central nervous system dysfunction, growth deficiency, facial abnormalities, and other major and minor malformations.

fixed-ratio combination product drug preparation containing a combination of two or more drug ingredients intended to relieve multiple symptoms.

flash short, intense, generalized sensation of total well-being experienced soon after intravenous injection of cocaine or methamphetamine; the "rush" reaction.

flashback undesirable recurrence of a drug's effects with no recent drug consumption to explain changes in consciousness and experience of illusions and hallucinations.

fluoxetine (Prozac) a frequently prescribed antidepressant drug that blocks the reabsorption of the neurotransmitter serotonin, resulting in continued stimulation of brain cells.

food and drug administration (FDA) federal regulatory agency within the U.S. Department of Health and Human Services, with counterparts on the state level, responsible for assuring safety and effectiveness of drugs, protecting consumers against contaminants in food and against falsely represented, worthless, and dangerous drugs, medical devices, and cosmetics.

food-drug interaction interaction between certain foods eaten and drugs being taken, resulting in speeding up or slowing down drug effects, preventing drug effects, adversely affecting the body's use of food, and life-threatening conditions.

formication hallucination associated with stimulant-induced psychosis in which an individual perceives imaginary ants, insects (crank bugs), or snakes crawling on or under his or her skin.

freebasing chemical process of changing common, white cocaine powder into a purer, more potent, smokable form of cocaine "base," which the user then smokes in a glass water pipe that is heated by a butane lighter or small blowtorch.

gender gap variations between males and females who use psychoactive drugs, particularly differences in numbers of those using drugs and the harmful effects of such drugs on users.

generic drug drug product given an official or nonproprietary name, one that is not patented, trademarked, or owned by a private individual or company. The generic name is often a contraction of the drug's more complex chemical name.

genetic predisposition inherited influence that makes some individuals susceptible to certain physical conditions, such as possible increased responsiveness to certain drugs or sensitivity to particular drug effects.

glaucoma disease characterized by increased pressure within the eye, which can damage the optic nerve and eventually lead to blindness.

goals broad, general statements on intent that give direction to a plan, such as an educational program; long-range targets indicating ultimate outcomes of some endeavor.

halcion a frequently prescribed benzodiazepine, triazolam, marketed and promoted for its hypnotic effect.

hallucination groundless false perception having no real external cause.

hallucinogen drug substance that induces or produces hallucinations in a drug user.

hangover temporary, acute physical and psychological distress following excessive consumption of alcoholic beverages or other drugs.

harrison narcotics act federal law enacted in 1914 that established a mechanism of record keeping for the importation, manufacture, distribution, sale, and prescription of narcotic drugs. This act outlawed the nonmedical use of heroin and forbade dispensing of narcotics to known addicts.

hashish cannabis preparation more potent than marijuana and derived from the resinous secretions of the cannabis plant's flowering tops.

hashish oil dark, viscous liquid produced by repeated extraction of cannabis plant materials with a THC concentration greater than that of hashish.

hemp plant leafy plant grown in temperate and tropical areas throughout the world; source of marijuana and other cannabis preparations; *Cannabis sativa.*

heroin a semisynthetic narcotic, one of the more powerful dependency-producing drugs, made by treating morphine with acetic anhydride.

HIV infection invasion of the body by the virus that causes acquired immunodeficiency syndrome (AIDS), the human immunodeficiency virus (HIV).

homeostasis an organism's internal state of constancy or equilibrium necessary for normal functioning.

host one sector or element of the public health model of drug-abuse prevention, specifically relating to individuals and their knowledge about psychoactive drugs, the personal attitudes that influence drug use and patterns of abuse, and drug-taking behavior.

host-related etiology theory that associates drug abuse and drug dependence with some predisposition or unusual condition that makes a person (the host) particularly susceptible to the effects of a psychoactive drug.

hyperkinetic disorder brain disorder characterized by extreme motor restlessness, poor attention span, and impulsive and sometimes disorderly behavior. In children, it is treated by prescribed amphetamines.

hyperplasia precancer change in the lungs characterized by an increase in the number of layers of basal cells that underlie the inner surface of the bronchial tubes.

hypnotic drug that induces sleep, such as a barbiturate, flurazepam, methy prylon, glutethimide, and chloral hydrate.

hypothalamus portion of the brain that is a prime site of action of many psychoactive drugs, which maintains homeostasis by regulating activities of the body cavity, emotions, and behavior.

ibuprofen nonsalicylate analgesic, antipyretic, and anti-inflammatory drug sold originally as a prescription-only painkiller but now available in OTC-strength preparations, marketed as Advil, Medipren, Motrin, and Nuprin.

ice a highly addictive smokable form of methamphetamine that produces a euphoric high that lasts several hours.

idiosyncratic response special sensitivity or unanticipated adverse reaction to a specific chemical substance.

illusion a false or misinterpreted sensory impression of reality; distortion of something that really exists.

immunosuppressive effect decreased effectiveness of the body's structural, cellular, and chemical defense mechanisms that helps protect the human body against assault from disease-causing bacteria, viruses, molds, and toxins.

inactivation drug action that reduces the rate of functional activity in a cell; a depressant effect.

inhalant chemical that evaporates easily and whose vapors, when breathed in, produce mind-altering effects.

inhalation process of breathing in; absorption of volatile chemicals into the blood by passing through the lungs.

injection introduction of a drug into the bloodstream without having to be absorbed through the digestive tract.

inoculation strategy strategy for preventing drug abuse by protecting drug users against unhealthy, irresponsible drug-taking behavior, as promoted through education emphasizing responsible decision making, rational limits on use, and precautions when interacting with psychoactive drugs.

instructional or educational objective curricular component that directs instructional activities on a daily basis; statement of what learners are to be like after they have successfully completed a learning experience.

insulin hormone produced in the body's pancreas that regulates the metabolism of sugar; antidiabetic drug that helps maintain the diabetic's blood sugar at near normal levels and keeps the urine as free of sugar as possible.

interdiction prevention of illicit drugs from entering the United States through confiscation at national borders or ports of entry and through seizure of contraband at sea.

intervention process a structured, confrontational technique used in helping drug abusers overcome their psychological denial and accept the reality of their drug problems.

intoxication temporary state of mental chaos and behavioral dysfunction resulting from the presence of a neurotoxin, such as ethyl alcohol, in the central nervous system.

involuntary smoking form of passive smoking in which the secondhand "sidestream" smoke from the burning tobacco products of others is inhaled by nonsmokers.

ketoprofen an over-the-counter nonsteroidal anti-inflammatory analgesic formerly available by prescription only, but now sold as Actron and Orudis KT.

khat East African shrub containing cathinone, a natural amphetamine-like substance; abbreviated name for methcathinone ("cat").

LAAM synthetic narcotic, chemically related to methadone, that has a duration of action lasting from 48 hours to 72 hours.

late-onset alcohol abuse or dependence a form of alcohol abuse or dependence in the elderly that occurs after many years without alcohol problems and is likely triggered by a life crisis or major life change often involving a series of losses.

legalization legislative declaration approving or authorizing a particular action.

life skills ATOD curriculum strategy that teaches students how to be assertive, how to resolve interpersonal conflicts, and how to communicate more effectively with others to use alcohol, tobacco, and other drugs.

look-alike drug a copy or simulation of a controlled psychoactive drug consisting of one or more legal, uncontrolled nonprescription drugs.

loss of control inability of an alcoholic to predict consistently the length of drinking or the amount consumed once use of the beverage alcohol has begun.

lower-yield cigarette cigarette containing relatively low amounts of nicotine and tar (defined as yielding 15 mg of tar or less per cigarette).

lung cancer uncontrolled cellular growth in the lungs, known specifically as bronchogenic carcinoma.

lysergic acid diethylamide (LSD) one of the most powerful synthetic psychedelics derived from ergot fungus, LSD is the model against which other mind-expanding drugs are compared.

machismo an exaggerated or exhilarating sense of power or strength.

macroapproach all-inclusive, drug-abuse prevention strategy in which the focus of prevention efforts is on the entire environment in promotion of a no-drug climate.

mainlining drug administration method in which a chemical substance is injected directly into a vein; intravenous injection.

mainstream smoke cigarette smoke inhaled by the smoker.

major tranquilizer an antipsychotic drug that relieves symptoms of a psychotic nature, such as schizophrenia and paranoia.

mariani's wine beverage made from the coca leaf and introduced in Europe during the nineteenth century.

MAO inhibitors monoamine oxidase inhibitors, a drug having a central nervous system stimulant effect, which blocks a specific enzyme, thereby increasing a neurotransmitter substance that helps to elevate mood and relieve mental depression; antidepressant drugs.

marijuana any part of the cannabis plant or its extract that produces physical or psychic changes in the human.

marijuana high various mind-altering effects resulting from use of marijuana, including a sense of well-being, feeling of relaxation, and a dreamlike state, perceived as favorable responses to cannabis.

medication error unintentional inappropriate use of a medication (such as decreasing or increasing a recommended dosage).

medicine drug substance used in diagnosis, cure, treatment, or prevention of disease, or in the relief of pain or discomfort.

medulla oblongata direct, upward continuation of the spinal cord within the skull.

mescaline major psychoactive ingredient of the peyote cactus.

metabolism complex chemical changes that alter drugs and convert them to substances that can be eliminated from the body.

methadone synthetic narcotic that produces many of the same effects of heroin and morphine but whose duration of action lasts up to twenty-four hours, thus making the drug useful in the treatment of heroin addiction.

methadone maintenance continuing use of minimal doses of methadone, given orally, to stabilize heroin-dependent patients by reducing their craving for a drug and eliminating the "rush" sensation following heroin injection.

methamphetamine synthetic amphetamine, known as "meth" or "speed," commonly abused by intravenous injection or smoking for the rapid, intense euphoria of the "rush" or "flash" effect.

methcathinone synthetic, powerful stimulant that resembles cocaine and amphetamines, and produces a burst of energy along with a prolonged euphoria.

method planned, organized technique, activity, or experience that instructors use to help sutdents achieve certain objectives.

methotrexate a drug approved for use only in the treatment of certain cancerous conditions, severe psoriasis, and adult rheumatoid arthritis, but also prescribed along with misoprostol as a two-drug abortion producing method.

mind expansion psychedelic state characterized by heightened awareness of sensory input, enhanced sense of clarity, diminished control over experiences, distortion of objective reality, and general alteration of the conscious state.

minipill type of oral contraceptive containing only progestin.

minor tranquilizer antianxiety agent that functions somewhat like a sedative-hypnotic, including meprobamate and benzodiazepine.

modeling adoption by one individual, often a child, of another's (usually a parent) practice or attitude.

moonshining illegal production of distilled spirits.

morning after contraception use of higher dosage oral contraceptive pills for the prevention of conception, if taken within seventy-two hours of sexual intercourse.

morphine naturally occurring narcotic drug, derived from opium and used medically as a sedative and analgesic.

MPTP a chemical sometimes found in the designer drug meperidine whose use damages nerves and has resulted in permanent symptoms of Parkinson's disease.

multifactorial theories explanations based on two or more interacting factors or causative influences.

multimodality therapeutic approach comprehensive treatment and rehabilitation program for narcotic-dependent individuals, based upon several components providing various services to meet the physical, mental, social, and spiritual needs of patients.

mutagenic effect production of a sudden change from the parent that appears in an offspring due to a toxic or adverse force, such as a drug, on a gene or chromosome.

mutation change, alteration, or damage to genes within cells of an organism.

naltrexone drug used to treat alcoholism by helping reduce the craving for alcohol in many abstinent patients and stopping the reinforcing effects of ethanol.

naproxen sodium relatively new over-the-counter analgesic, originally available only as a prescription drug for the treatment of arthritis.

narcolepsy neurological disorder characterized by recurring attacks of sleep, often induced by emotional excitement.

narcotic drug that has a sleep-inducing and pain-relieving action; an opioid or opiate.

narcotic antagonist drug that tends to block and even reverse the effects of narcotics, thus making the antagonist useful in treating opioid dependence.

narcotics anonymous a self-help group patterned after Alcoholics Anonymous in which recovering drug addicts offer help to others seeking recovery from drug dependence.

National Drug Control Strategy the nationwide antidrug strategy aimed at preventing and reducing the use and abuse of illegal drugs through both supply reduction and demand reduction procedures (originally was called the "War on Drugs").

natural "high" feeling of elation or temporary euphoria sometimes associated with regular, vigorous exercise over a sustained time, and possibly related to the increased production of endorphins.

neuron nerve cell (the basic unit of the nervous system) capable of receiving stimuli and transmitting electrical messages.

neurotransmitter chemical substance manufactured in the axon; conducts a nerve impulse from one nerve cell to the dendrites of another nerve cell.

nicotiana tabacum the tobacco plant whose leaves are processed for smoking, chewing, or sniffing.

nicotine a major component of the particulate phase of tobacco cigarette smoke; colorless, oily compound in tobacco that has a central nervous system stimulant effect.

nonsalicylates nonaspirin over-the-counter analgesics, specifically acetaminophen and ibuprofen.

nonsmokers' liberation movement efforts of nonsmokers of tobacco products to prohibit cigarette advertising in the media and to restrict or segregate smokers in specific and public places, in order to promote a tobacco-free environment.

normative beliefs ATOD curriculum strategy that provides information to students about the actual rates of alcohol and other drug use, based on surveys, and thereby corrects the false belief that there is near-universal drinking, smoking, and other drug use among peers.

norplant surgically inserted subdermal implants of Silastic capsules containing slow-release progestin-only chemicals that exert a contraceptive effect for as long as five years.

nsaid abbreviation for a nonsteroidal anti-inflammatory drug, such as aspirin, ibuprofen, or naproxen sodium, that produces desirable effects by blocking the action of specific prostaglandin chemicals in the body.

on-the-job absenteeism frequent disappearances from the work station, lengthy breaks from assigned tasks, sleeping on-the-job, and accomplishing nothing of substance at work, all due to the effects of alcohol or drug abuse on work performance.

opioid narcotic drug so named because it is derived from the opium poppy plant or made synthetically to have the same drug actions of morphine, a major ingredient of opium.

opium naturally occurring narcotic drug derived from the opium poppy, *Papaver somniferum,* and considered as the "mother drug" or main source of nonsynthetic narcotics.

oral gratification satisfaction or need fulfillment obtained through the mouth, or by placing something in the mouth.

over-the-counter (OTC) drug drug substance sold as medicine without a physician's order or prescription.

oxidation process in which oxygen is combined with a chemical substance.

panic sudden overpowering terror marked by numerous fears, overexcitation, and uncontrollable behavior.

papaver somniferum the opium poppy plant from which opium is derived.

paraquat herbicide or plant killer that has been used to reduce the growth of cannabis plants; a marijuana contaminant associated with both temporary and permanent damage to specific body organs.

particulates extremely small solid particles found in tobacco smoke, primarily nicotine and tar.

passive smoking involuntary inhalation of secondary, unfiltered "sidestream smoke" from the burning tobacco products of others.

patient medication instructions (PMIs) printed information dealing with specific drugs and their effects, available to practicing physicians for distribution to their patients, to promote effectiveness of drug therapy and patient compliance with instructions for proper use.

peer-group influences any attitude, value, or practice of one's age-mates or companions that is perceived as significant, and which a person may eventually adopt.

peripheral nervous system major division of the nervous system consisting of all the nerves that branch from the central nervous system and connect it to other parts of the body, including the extremities. The two subdivisions of the peripheral nervous system are the somatic system and the autonomic system.

personal commitment ATOD curriculum strategy that encourages students to voluntarily make public or private pledges not to use or abuse alcohol, tobacco, or other psychoactive drugs.

peyote fleshy green cactus tips or mescal buttons of the peyote cactus, which, upon chewing, swallowing, or smoking, will cause stomach disorders, nausea, vomiting, and a variety of LSD-like effects.

pharmacology branch of science dealing with the effects of drugs or chemicals on living systems or organisms.

phencyclidine unique psychoactive drug having psychedelic, stimulant, depressant, hallucinogenic, psychotomimetic, analgesic, and anesthetic properties, used only in veterinary medical practice, because of its unpleasant side effects in humans; PCP.

physical dependence state of physical need for a drug; functional adaptation to a drug in which the presence of a foreign chemical becomes normal and necessary.

physician's desk reference annual publication compiled by representatives of pharmaceutical companies that provides detailed information on prescribed drugs.

placebo effect production of a specific drug action or effect resulting from use of an inert substance (placebo) that has no pharmacologic effect; fake medicine or nonmedicated item administered for psychological benefit.

polycyclic aromatic hydrocarbons cancer-producing chemicals found in tobacco tar.

polydrug use simultaneous use of two or more drugs (or medicines).

polypharmacy use of two or more drugs at the same time during the course of treatment for a particular illness.

potentiation drug interaction drug interaction in which one drug intensifies or increases the action of another that originally had no clinical effect or only a minor drug effect, resulting in an exaggerated effect on the central nervous system.

potentiation effect greatly exaggerated drug effect or response obtained when two drugs, taken together, produce a joint effect much greater than the sum of the effects of the two drugs when taken separately.

predisposing factors influences that make certain people susceptible in advance to use and abuse psychoactive drugs, for example, level of existing knowledge about drugs, personal beliefs and attitudes, and human biological and/or psychological characteristics.

prescription physician's order to a pharmacist to dispense a specific drug product to a patient.

prescription drug medicine that can be obtained only by the direction (oral or written prescription) of a physician.

primary prevention first level of intervention; prevention activities begun before an individual becomes diseased or impaired.

problem drinking use of alcohol that results in damage to the drinker, the drinker's family, or to the drinker's community.

prohibition forbidding of a certain act; period in American history (1920–33) during which time the manufacture, sale, transportation, and importation of intoxicating liquors was forbidden by national law.

pseudostimulation false or deceptive stimulation manifest as increased activity, animated feelings, and noisy behavior, caused by the disinhibition and depressant effects of alcohol.

psilocybin psychedelic drug derived originally from so-called sacred or magic mushrooms, having effects similar to but less intense than LSD.

psychedelics drugs that can affect one's perception, awareness, and emotions, which sometimes cause hallucinations and illusions.

psychoactive drug mind-altering drug that affects thinking, feeling, and behavior.

psychodynamic expeience psychedelic experience marked by a revelation in which subconscious material is brought to the surface of one's consciousness.

psychological dependence condition marked by a strong desire and intense craving to repeat the use of a drug for various emotional reasons, for example feeling of well-being and reduction of tension.

psychopathology one or more severe mental disorders, such as major depression, schizophrenia, organic brain syndrome, and bipolar manic-depression.

psychosis severe mental disorder characterized by loss of contact with reality.

psychotherapy purposeful conversation between two or more individuals through which trained therapists attempt to help clients achieve greater self-understanding, objectivity, and maturity.

psychotic experience psychedelic experience marked by panic, paranoid feelings, confusion, isolation, and/or mental depression; bad trip or bummer.

public health prevention model prevention model that focuses on three major intervention points or targets, within a conceptual framework of a host-agent-environment relationship.

pulmonary emphysema disease in which the lungs' ability to exchange gases is impaired due to the loss of alveolar elasticity and the stretching, rupture, and destruction of the lungs' tiny air sacs.

pure food and drug act 1906 law prohibiting interstate commerce in misbranded and adulterated drugs.

rapid eye movement (REM) characteristic movement of the eye during the sleep phase marked by dreaming.

rauwolfia serpentina Indian snakeroot shrub from which was derived reserpine, the first major tranquilizer used as an antipsychotic drug in treating mental illness.

receptor specific site on or within the brain or other body organ or cell to which drug molecules must attach to produce the characteristic effect of the drug.

referral process directing, convincing, and encouraging a drug abuser to contact a drug and alcohol treatment program for assistance in resolving drug-related problems.

reinforcing factors influences that usually encourage the continuation of drug-taking behavior once it has begun, for example, experience of pleasure or relief of pain.

reserpine one of the major tranquilizers used as an antipsychotic medication to relieve symptoms of schizophrenia and paranoia.

resistance skills general term describing refusal or avoidance behaviors that help an individual say no to drug use or prevent drug abuse by giving reasons for nonuse.

resources instructional media such as books, pamphlets, films, slides, projectors, videocassette tapes, and government and private agencies, community groups, and individuals that can support edcuational programs.

responsible drug use use of any drug in such a way so as to eliminate, reduce, lessen, or minimize the negative consequences often associated with such use.

revolving door routine process of arrest for public intoxication, followed by a brief incarceration in jail, release, and then rearrest upon the next episode of drunkenness.

Reye's syndrome a rare, acute, brain-damaging and sometimes fatal condition, characterized by vomiting and lethargy that may progress to delirium and coma; occurs in young people and teenagers recovering from certain viral infections, namely, chickenpox and flu.

risk factor condition or characteristic that increases the probability of some behavior or event.

rohypnol in the United States, an illegal benzodiazepine, flunitrazepam, that is a powerful sleeping pill also producing disinhibition and short-term memory loss. As such, this drug has become notorious for its use to incapacitate unsuspecting females, leaving them with no memory of sexual assault ("roofie rape") or robbery.

RU-486 antiprogesterone drug, mifepristone, used within the first forty-nine days of pregnancy to cause menstruation and thus prevents the implantation of a fertilized egg or causes pregnancy termination, that is, an abortion.

rush short-lived jolt and tingling sensation of intense well-being or euphoria experienced soon after injecting heroin directly into a vein.

rush reaction see *flash*.

salicylates a family of painkilling, fever-reducing, and anti-inflammatory drugs, such as aspirin, containing salicylic acid.

salicylism toxic condition resulting from excessive intake of acetysalicylic acid, marked by nausea, vomiting, ringing in the ear, deafness, and even severe headache.

secondary prevention second level of prevention; prevention activities applied during the early stages of a disease and aimed at restoring health to those who have become ill or impaired.

sedative drug that has a calming effect, relaxes muscles, and relieves feelings of tension, anxiety, and irritability.

sedative-hypnotic drug induces sleep and has a calming effect.

sedativism chemical dependency on sedative-type psychoactive drugs, particularly barbiturates, minor tranquilizers, and ethyl alcohol.

self-limiting condition disease condition, usually of a minor nature, that tends to run its course to recovery without treatment, such as the common cold.

self-medication practice of treating oneself with nonprescription medicine for relief of symptoms associated with relatively minor diseases or disorders.

sexual dysfunction difficulty in achieving sexual arousal and/or reaching orgasm.

side effect drug effect other than the intended or anticipated one.

sidestream smoke smoke inhaled from the burning tobacco products of others and originating from the lighted tip of a cigarette between puffs.

sinsemilla seedless variety of high-potency marijuana, prepared from unpollenated female cannabis plants.

skin-popping subcutaneous injection of a drug just beneath the skin's surface.

sleep aid over-the-counter drug for the promotion of mild sedation and sleep, usually containing an antihistamine that may produce drowsiness as a side effect.

smokeless tobacco tobacco products, such as chewing tobacco and snuff, that are not burned as they are used.

snorting drug-taking method in which a substance, such as cocaine, is inhaled or sniffed, with the finely chopped cocaine powder being absorbed through the mucous membrane lining of the nose.

snuff preparation of powdered tobacco introduced into the nostrils by inhalation.

snuff dipping insertion of powdered tobacco between the gum and cheek, where it is absorbed through the mucous membrane.

social drinking particular group's customary way of using beverage alcohol; drinking that promotes interpersonal relations and enhances feelings of camaraderie and solidarity.

social drug any chemical substance, especially alcohol and marijuana, used to help people better enjoy the company of others.

solubility the ability of a drug to dissolve in body tissue, in other words to spread from an area of high concentration to an area of low concentration.

speed methamphetamine.

speedball mixture of cocaine and heroin; combination of any central nervous system stimulant and depressant.

speed runs prolonged periods of heavy stimulant use in which an amphetamine solution is injected as often as every hour.

standard serving the quantity of an alcoholic beverage defined as one 5-ounce glass of table wine; one 12-ounce wine cooler; one 12-ounce can or bottle of regular beer; or one shot glass of "hard liquor" with 1.5 ounces of 80 proof whiskey or an equivalent distilled spirit.

stimulant chemical substance that tends to speed up central nervous system function, resulting in alertness and excitability.

stimulation increase in the rate of functional activity; speeding up of central nervous system function.

student assistance program (SAP) organized approach for intervening in and preventing alcohol, tobacco, and other drug (ATOD) problems among school-age youth; focuses on behavior and performance at school and uses a referral process that includes screening by teachers and other school personnel for ATOD involvement.

subdermal implants silastic capsules inserted beneath the surface of the skin where, for example, a slow-release, progestin-only chemical exerts a prolonged contraceptive effect.

subject matter topical content, such as facts, theories, controversies, projections, and ideas appropriate to the needs, interests, and developmental levels of the target audience.

supply reduction strategy for preventing drug abuse by lowering, restricting, or eliminating the availability of a drug.

surveillance secret and usually continuous watching of suspected individuals, objects, places, or vehicles in order to obtain information about criminal activities.

synapse junction or meeting place between two nerve cells.

synergistic drug interaction drug interaction in which there is a cooperative, facilitative, supra-additive effect between two or more drugs, resulting in an exaggerated drug effect or a prolonged drug action.

synergistic drug reaction drug reaction produced when one drug enhances or intensifies the action of another substance (with or without drug effect), and results in an exaggerated drug effect or in a prolonged drug action.

synesthesia drug-related effect in which there is a mingling of the senses, in which one sensation may be translated into another, for example, sounds may be seen and smells may be felt.

systematic planning process plan that considers both design and implementation of a curriculum, usually consists of a written document stating what the learning experiences are designed to accomplish, how the knowledge, attitudes, or skills will be taught, the resources needed for effective teaching, and the measures used to determine whether the plan achieved its objectives.

tar particulate matter in cigarette smoke containing various polycyclic aromatic hydrocarbons, phenols, cresols, radioactive compounds, agricultural chemicals, additives, and flavoring agents, all of which appear as a yellow-brown sticky mass when condensed.

temperance moderation or restraint in the practice of some behavior or use of some substance, such as an alcoholic beverage.

teratogen agent that causes defects in a developing embryo.

tertiary prevention third level of prevention; prevention activities initiated during the advanced stages of an illness or disease, aimed at stopping the reactivation of the disease process after recovery.

THC most active and principal psychoactive ingredient of marijuana; delta-9-tetrahydrocannabinol.

therapeutic agent drug substance used for treating and preventing disease or in preserving health.

therapeutic community treatment approach to chemically dependent individuals consisting of ex-addicts and other trained personnel who work with drug abusers through encounter group therapy, tutorial-learning sessions, remedial and formal education, and assignment of various housekeeping chores within a drug-free residential environment.

therapeutic index index for assessing the relative safety of drugs for use in large populations; ratio between the median lethal dose (LD_{50}) and the median effective dose (ED_{50}) of a particular drug used for a specific effect; more realistically calculated as the ratio between the effective dose in nearly all patients (ED_{99}) and the lethal dose in practically no patients (LD_1).

therapeutics use of drugs in treating and preventing disease and in preserving health status.

tobacco leaves of the tobacco plant, *Nicotiana tabacum,* prepared for smoking, chewing, or sniffing.

tobacco additives cellulose-based tobacco substitutes added to cigarettes during manufacture to enhance flavor or facilitate processing.

tolerance reduction in the pharmacological response to a particular drug in which continued intake of the same dose has diminishing effects; reduced sensitivity resulting in the need for increased dosage to achieve the desired drug effect.

toxic reaction disturbance of function in one or more body systems caused by a drug overdose; poisonous condition, such as intoxication.

toxic syndrome undesirable physical and mental experiences ranging from tremors and agitation to hostility and panic, resulting from chronic use of high dose levels of central nervous system stimulants.

trafficking unauthorized manufacture, distribution, or possession with intent to distribute any controlled drug substance.

transcendental (mystical) experience a psychedelic response known as the "peak" or mystical experience and characterized by development of a sense of unity, lack of time and space limits, deeply felt moods, feelings of awsomeness and reverence, and meaningfulness of philosophic insight.

tricyclic compounds potent drugs used as antidepressants to elevate mood and relieve certain types of mental depression.

trip variety of mind-altering effects induced by a psychedelic drug and subjectively interpreted.

valium a frequently prescribed brand name of diazepam that functions as an antianxiety drug or minor tranquilizer; a benzodiazepine derivative.

values classification use of teaching methods that foster decision making based upon the recognition of values; instructional techniques that promote choosing freely from alternatives, prizing, and acting on one's beliefs and choices consistently and regularly.

war on drugs the nationwide antidrug strategy aimed at preventing and reducing the use and abuse of illegal drugs through both supply reduction and demand reduction procedures (more currently called "The National Drug Control Strategy").

wine alcoholic beverage containing 10–14 percent alcohol by volume and made from fermented juice of grapes or other fruits.

withdrawal symptoms withdrawal sickness or abstinence syndrome consisting of drastic changes in physical functioning and behavior (insomnia, tremors, nausea vomiting, cramps, elevation of heart rate and blood pressure, convulsions, anxiety, psychological depression) due to overactivity of the nervous system, observed or experienced after use of a drug by a physically dependent person has been stopped.

withdrawal syndrome drastic alterations in physical function and behavior, experienced after drug use is terminated.

xanax an intermediate-acting benzodiazepine frequently prescribed as an antianxiety drug.

youth rebellion rejection of parental values and conflict between parents and children over independence and self-identity, as symbolized by the sudden increase in the use of illegal psychoactive drugs.

zero tolerance limits lowered blood alcohol concentration limits of 0.02 percent or less for young drivers under the age of twenty-one years.

credits

Photographs

Chapter 1
p. 1: © Dave Schafer/Uniphoto Picture Agency; p. 10 © Larry Mulvehill/ The Image Works

Chapter 2
p. 25: © G. Savage/Vantstadt/Photo Researchers, Inc.; p. 28 © Michael Newman/Photo Edit

Chapter 3
p. 44: © Tony Freeman/Photo Edit; p. 48: © James L. Shaffer; p. 57: © Bob Daemmrich/The Image Works

Chapter 4
p. 63: © Bob Daemmrich/The Image Works; p. 69: © The Bettmann Archive; p. 73: © James L. Shaffer; p. 82: © Video Surgery/Photo Researchers; p. 82: © Biophoto Associates/Science Source

Chapter 5
p. 93: © Peter Menzel/Stock Boston; p. 96: © Stacy Pick/Stock Boston; p. 103: © James L. Shaffer; © p. 108: © U.S. Department of Health and Human Services

Chapter 6
p. 124: © Kurt Weidmann/Photo Researchers; p. 131: © Bettmann Archive; p. 135: © J. Griffin/The Image Works

Chapter 7
p. 141: © Tony Freeman/Photo Edit; p. 148: © Courtesy of the Drug Enforcement Agency; p. 150: © Ann Marie Rousseau/The Image Works

Chapter 8
p. 159: © Charles Gupton/Uniphoto Picture Agency; p. 163: © Lee Snider/The Image Works; p. 173: © Stephen M. Brady/ The Picture Cube; p. 176: © American Cancer Society; p. 179: © M. Edrington/The Image Works; p. 184: © National Cancer Institute, U.S. Department of Health and Human Services

Chapter 9
p. 191: © Jonathan Nourok/Photo Edit; p. 194: © Drug Enforcement Agency; p. 195: © Jeffrey L. Rotman/Peter Arnold, Inc.; p. 201: © Liewellyn/Uniphoto Picture Agency; p. 204: © James L. Shaffer

Chapter 10
p. 211: © Chromosohm Media/The Image Works; p. 215: © Lisa Lau/The Image Works; p. 219: © Drug Enforcement Agency; p. 223: © Drug Enforcement Agency; p. 223: © Drug Enforcement Agency

Chapter 11
p. 233: © Drug Enforcement Agency; p. 235: © James L. Shaffer; p. 237: © Drug Enforcement Agency; p. 241: © Mark H. Walker/The Picture Cube

Chapter 12
p. 251: © Dion Ogust/The Image Works; p. 255: © Dion Ogust/The Image Works; p. 257: © Didier Ermakoff/The Image Works; © James L. Shaffer; p.265: © James L. Shaffer; p. 268: © Felicia Martinez/Photo Edit

Chapter 13
p. 275: © Jeff Greenberg/Photo Edit; p. 279: © U.S. Food and Drug Administration; p. 284: © James L. Shaffer; p. 286: © Courtesy Wyeth-Ayers Laboratories

Chapter 14
p. 295: © Bob Daemmrich/The Image Works; p. 299: © Bob Daemmrich/The Image Works; p. 302: © R. Sidney/The Image Works; p. 305: Mark Richards/PhotoEdit; p. 310: © Photo Uniphoto Picture Agency

Chapter 15
p. 323: © Toni Michael/The Image Works; p. 329: © Bob Daemmrich/The Image Works; p. 342: © Office of the Attorney General. State of California and the U.S. Drug Enforcement Administration

Chapter 16
p. 355: © Rick Berkowitz/The Picture Cube; p. 360: © l995 Len Berger/Picture Perfect; p. 364: © Jeff Greenberg/The Picture Cube

index